BIRTH *of a* SPECIALTY

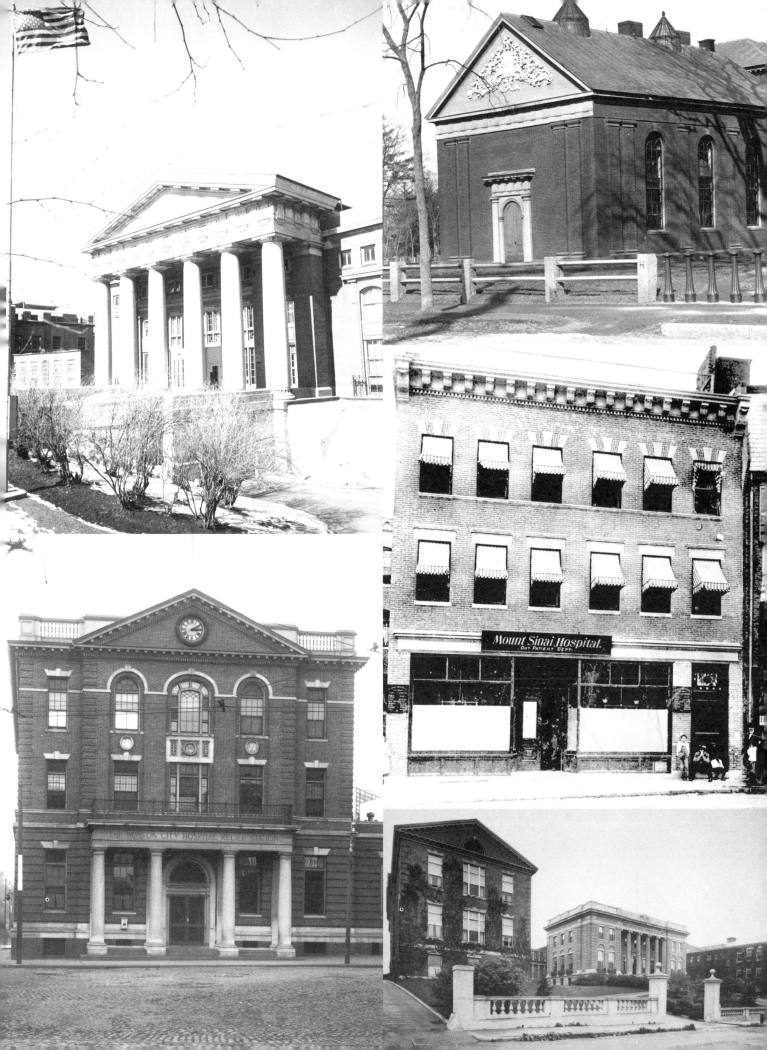

BIRTH
of a
SPECIALTY

A History of Orthopaedics at Harvard
and Its Teaching Hospitals

VOLUME 4

by
James H. Herndon, MD, MBA

Peter E. Randall Publisher
Portsmouth, New Hampshire
2021

© 2021 James H. Herndon
All rights reserved.

ISBN: 978-1-942155-36-2
Library of Congress Control Number: 2021916147

Published by
Peter E. Randall Publisher LLC
Portsmouth, NH 03801
www.perpublisher.com

Volume 1: Harvard Medical School
Volume 2: Boston Children's Hospital
Volume 3: Massachusetts General Hospital
Volume 4: Brigham and Women's Hospital, Beth Israel Deaconess Medical Center, Boston City Hospital, World War I, and World War II
Volume 5: Bibliography (available only in PDF form, visit www.birthofaspecialty.com)

Cover images:
Front:
   Volume 1: Boston Medical Library collection, Center for the History of Medicine in the Francis A. Countway Library.
   Volume 2: *Images of America. Children's Hospital Boston.* Charleston, SC: Arcadia Publishing, 2005. Boston Children's Hospital Archives, Boston, Massachusetts.
   Volume 3: Massachusetts General Hospital, Archives and Special Collections.
   Volume 4: Brigham and Women's Hospital Archives.

Back:
   Volumes 1–4: Warren Anatomical Museum collection, Center for the History of Medicine in the Francis A. Countway Library.

Endpaper images:
Front: **Top:** (l) Exterior view of the Old Harvard Medical School, Boston, Mass, ca. 1880. Photograph by Baldwin Coolidge. Courtesy of Historic New England; (cl) Boston Children's Hospital Archives, Boston, Massachusetts; (cr) Brigham and Women's Hospital Archives; (r) Theodore Roosevelt Collection in the Houghton Library, Harvard University.
   Center: (l) The Ruth and David Freiman Archives at Beth Israel Deaconess Medical Center; (c) Boston Children's Hospital Archives, Boston, Massachusetts; (r) The Ruth and David Freiman Archives at Beth Israel Deaconess Medical Center.
   Bottom: (l) Massachusetts General Hospital, Archives and Special Collections; (c) Boston City Archives; (r) Brigham and Women's Hospital Archives.
Back: All: Kael E. Randall/Kael Randall Images

All reasonable efforts have been made to obtain necessary copyright permissions. Grateful acknowledgment for these permissions is made at point of use (for images) and in Volume 5 (for text). Any omissions or errors are unintentional and will, if brought to the attention of the author, be resolved.

Book design by Tim Holtz

Printed in the United States of America

Contents

Section 6	**Brigham and Women's Hospital**	
Chapter 44	Peter Bent Brigham Hospital and Robert Breck Brigham Hospital: The Beginning	1
Chapter 45	Robert Breck Brigham Hospital and Peter Bent Brigham Hospital: Orthopaedic Service Chiefs	43
	Robert Breck Brigham Hospital	44
	Peter Bent Brigham Hospital	72
Chapter 46	RBBH and PBBH: Other Surgeon Scholars, 1900–1970	79
	Robert Breck Brigham Hospital	80
	Peter Bent Brigham Hospital	104
Chapter 47	Origins of BWH and Organizing Orthopaedics as a Department	113
Chapter 48	Clement B. Sledge: Clinician Scientist	125
Chapter 49	BWH: Other Surgeon Scholars: 1970–2000	143
Chapter 50	BWH's Modernization and Preparation for the Twenty-First Century	191
Section 7	**Beth Israel Deaconess Medical Center**	
Chapter 51	Beth Israel Hospital: The Beginning	199
Chapter 52	Albert Ehrenfried: Surgeon Leader at Mount Sinai and Beth Israel Hospital	215
Chapter 53	Beth Israel Hospital: Orthopaedic Division Chiefs	223
Chapter 54	Augustus A. White III: First Orthopaedic Surgeon-in-Chief at Beth Israel Hospital	257
Chapter 55	Stephen J. Lipson: Chief of Orthopaedics at Beth Israel Hospital and Beth Israel Deaconess Medical Center	267
Chapter 56	Beth Israel Deaconess Medical Center: A History of New England Deaconess Hospital and Its Merger with Beth Israel Hospital	273
Chapter 57	BIDMC: Modernization and Preparation for the Twenty-First Century	283
Section 8	**Boston City Hospital**	
Chapter 58	Boston City Hospital (Harvard Service): The Beginning	293
Chapter 59	Frederic J. Cotton: Orthopaedic Renaissance Man	309

Chapter 60	The Bone and Joint Service at Boston City Hospital: Other Surgeons-in-Chief	333
Chapter 61	Boston City Hospital: Other Surgeon Scholars	357
Chapter 62	Pedagogical Changes: Harvard Leaves Boston City Hospital	377

Section 9 Harvard Orthopaedists in the World Wars

Chapter 63	World War I: Trench Warfare	385
Chapter 64	World War II: Mobile Warfare	463
	Index	495

Volume 1 Contents

Acknowledgements		xiii
Foreword		xv
Preface		xvii
Introduction		xix
About the Author		xxv

Section 1 — The First Family of Surgery in the United States

Chapter 1	Joseph Warren: Physician Before the Revolution	3
Chapter 2	John Warren: Father of Harvard Medical School	21
Chapter 3	John Collins Warren: Co-Founder of the Massachusetts General Hospital	31
Chapter 4	Warren Family: Tradition of Medical Leaders Continues into the Twentieth Century	71

Section 2 — Orthopaedics Emerges as a Focus of Clinical Care

Chapter 5	John Ball Brown: The First American Orthopaedic Surgeon	95
Chapter 6	Buckminster Brown: Founder of the John Ball & Buckminster Brown Chair	105
Chapter 7	The Boston Orthopedic Institution: America's First Orthopaedic Hospital	113
Chapter 8	House of the Good Samaritan: America's First Orthopaedic Ward	123

Section 3 — Harvard Medical School

Chapter 9	Orthopaedic Curriculum	133
Chapter 10	The Evolution of the Organization and Department of Orthopaedic Surgery	171
Chapter 11	The Harvard Combined Orthopaedic Residency Program	183
Chapter 12	Harvard Sports Medicine	245
Chapter 13	Murder at Harvard	291

Volume 2 Contents

Section 4	**Boston Children's Hospital**	
Chapter 14	Boston Children's Hospital: The Beginning	3
Chapter 15	Edward H. Bradford: Boston's Foremost Pioneer Orthopaedic Surgeon	19
Chapter 16	Robert W. Lovett: The First John Ball and Buckminster Brown Professor of Orthopaedic Surgery	45
Chapter 17	James W. Sever: Medical Director of the Industrial School for Crippled and Deformed Children	83
Chapter 18	Arthur T. Legg: Dedicated to Disabled Children	101
Chapter 19	Robert B. Osgood: Advocate for Orthopaedics as a Profession of Physicians and Surgeons Who Restore Function	113
Chapter 20	Frank R. Ober: Caring Clinician and Skilled Educator	143
Chapter 21	William T. Green: Master in Pediatric Orthopaedics	167
Chapter 22	David S. Grice: Advocate for Polio Treatment	207
Chapter 23	BCH: Other Surgeon-Scholars (1900–1970)	217
Chapter 24	Melvin J. Glimcher: Father of the Bone Field	319
Chapter 25	John E. Hall: Mentor to Many and Master Surgeon	333
Chapter 26	Paul P. Griffin: Southern Gentleman and Disciple of Dr. William T. Green	349
Chapter 27	BCH Other Surgeon Scholars (1970–2000)	357
Chapter 28	Boston Children's Hospital: Modernization and Preparation for the Twenty-First Century	427

Volume 3 Contents

Section 5   **Massachusetts General Hospital**

Chapter 29	Massachusetts General Hospital: The Beginning	3
Chapter 30	Henry J. Bigelow: The First Orthopaedic Surgeon at MGH	23
Chapter 31	Charles L. Scudder: Strong Advocate for Accurate Open Reduction and Internal Fixation of Fractures	53
Chapter 32	Orthopaedics Becomes a Department at MGH: Ward I	67
Chapter 33	Joel E. Goldthwait: First Chief of the Department of Orthopaedic Surgery at MGH	77
Chapter 34	Ernest A. Codman: Father of the "End-Result Idea" Movement	93
Chapter 35	Elliott G. Brackett: His Character Was a Jewel with Many Facets	147
Chapter 36	Nathaniel Allison: A Focus on Research and Education	163
Chapter 37	Marius N. Smith-Petersen: Prolific Inventor in Orthopaedics	179
Chapter 38	Joseph S. Barr: A "Gentle Scholar" and a Great Teacher	201
Chapter 39	William H. Harris: Innovator in Hip Replacement Surgery	215
Chapter 40	MGH: Other Surgeon Scholars (1900–1970)	227
Chapter 41	Henry J. Mankin: Prolific Researcher and Dedicated Educator	381
Chapter 42	MGH: Other Surgeon Scholars (1970–2000)	395
Chapter 43	MGH: Modernization and Preparation for the Twenty-First Century	453

Volume 5 Contents

Bibliography

Copyright Acknowledgments

"Military Orthopedic Surgery," World War I by R. W. Lovett

Harvard Faculty Who Served as Presidents of Major Professional Organizations

James H. Herndon, MD, MBA Curriculum Vitae

Volume 5 is available as an electronic version only and is included with purchase. It is available for download at www.birthofaspecialty.com.

To access link directly, go to https://pathway-book-service-cart.mypinnaclecart.com//peter-e-randall/birth-of-a-specialty-bibliography-only/

Section 6

Brigham and Women's Hospital

"At the entrance of the Robert Breck Brigham Hospital there are two bronze tablets. On one of them are the names of the benefactors, Robert Breck Brigham and his sister, Elizabeth Fay Brigham. On the other are excerpts from the will stating that the hospital was for the study and treatment of those people who were suffering from chronic disease. The interesting part of this excerpt is that the hospital was for the study and treatment of people, and not primarily for the study of their diseases."

—**Dr. Lloyd T. Brown**. Correspondence, 1954. "History of the Robert Breck Brigham Hospital for Incurables" by Matthew H. Liang, MD, 2013, pg. 17.

"I have seen today what I have always wished would come here in Boston, what I have always thought would come; I have seen a new and perfectly striking departure in hospital growth. You are part of a great organization, you are taking a very important step in medical education, and this is a great thing for the city and for the country in the future development of medicine."

—**Sir William Osler**. Statement given by Osler upon his visit to the PBBH, April 30, 1913, *Nicholas L. Tilney. A Perfectly Striking Departure*, 2006, pg. 17.

CHAPTER 44

Peter Bent Brigham Hospital and Robert Breck Brigham Hospital

The Beginning

Orthopaedics evolved as a specialty within two distinctive hospitals, each with their own rich history: the Peter Bent Brigham Hospital (PBBH) and the Robert Breck Brigham Hospital (RBBH). This chapter details the origins of these hospitals and the development of orthopaedics as a specialty ahead of their later merger to form Brigham and Women's Hospital. Both were established in the early 1900s, opening to admit their first patients near or during the beginning of World War I.

PETER BENT BRIGHAM HOSPITAL (PBBH)

The Peter Bent Brigham Hospital (PBBH) opened its doors in 1913 in affiliation with Harvard Medical School (HMS). Like Johns Hopkins, Peter Bent Brigham's fortune was willed into a trust to form the hospital. Brigham, whose family "had lived in New England for six generations," was born on February 4, 1807, in Bakersfield, Vermont, more than 100 years before the hospital opened (**Box 44.1**).

Brigham was a successful businessman, investing in restaurants, real estate, and local railroads as well as acting as a founding director of the Fitchburg Railroad (**Box 44.2**). Throughout his life, he was known as a man of integrity in all his affairs and someone who had "great compassion for the poor" and who "stood strongly against slavery" (McCord 1963). He never married nor had

Box 44.1. History of the Brigham Family

"John Bent Brigham, who made the Atlantic crossing, arrived in 1638, just two years after the founding of Harvard College. His descendants took a prominent part in the affairs of Sudbury and Marlboro in Massachusetts. Uriah Brigham (1757-1820), [with] wife… Elizabeth Fay, migrated to Vermont about 1796…in the decade of 1790–1800…Vermont's population almost doubled…Uriah Brigham's death in 1820 left a widow and nine children, of whom Peter was the seventh. He was then thirteen; but not long after he made his way to Boston…In Boston master Peter prospered from the first, and when he died on 24 May 1877 in his Boston house at the corner of Bulfinch and Allston Streets, he was considerably more than a millionaire"

(McCord 1963).

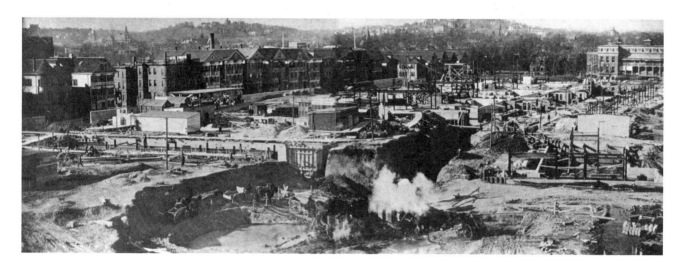

Aerial view: PBBH under reconstruction, 1911. Brigham and Women's Hospital Archives.

children; he died on May 24, 1877, and was buried in Mount Auburn Cemetery. His will (including assets of $1.3 million at the time) transformed him into one of Boston's greatest philanthropists; it stated:

> at the expiration of twenty-five years from his decease the executors of his estate should dispose of the residue of his property and of all the interest and accommodations that should have accrued thereon for the purpose of founding a hospital in Boston for the care of sick persons in indigent circumstances residing in the County of Suffolk. (quoted in McCord 1963)

The Founding of the PBBH Corporation and a Partnership with Harvard

Around 1899, twenty-two years after Brigham's death, HMS realized that it would need to expand beyond its building on Boylston Street, which it had occupied since 1883. Charles S. Minot, a professor there, began lobbying HMS President Charles Eliot to consider bringing together teaching and laboratory facilities in one place. Minot suggested building on a piece of land in the Roxbury neighborhood. Although initially inclined against this idea of consolidation and location, HMS faculty eventually realized that this might lure the new Peter Brigham Bent

Box 44.2. Peter Bent Brigham: From Shucking Oysters to Captain of Industry

> "Young Peter started his career by selling fish and oysters from a wheelbarrow, advanced through the restaurant business (cutting pies into six pieces, says the legend...) and made his investments shrewdly in real estate and local railroads. For many years he owned and operated the restaurant in Concert Hall which stood in the corner of Scollay Square and Hanover Street...Above Peter's restaurant, Concert Hall offered a large auditorium for receptions, soirées, and the playing of secular music. The restaurant...remained one of the favorite dining spots for State Street merchants, bankers, and lawyers. Peter Brigham retired from the restaurant business when Hanover Street was widened in 1869. During the last eight years of his life, he gave full attention to real estate investments and to the celebrated Fitchburg Railroad of which he was long a director. Most of [his] holdings in real estate were concentrated within a half-mile radius of Scollay Square..."
>
> (McCord 1963).

Hospital Corporation to build its hospital nearby, easily allowing faculty to connect their work at both HMS and the hospital. That same year, HMS began soliciting the hospital corporation—even before the corporation had received the money from the trust.

One main difference between the trust willed for the hospital, for the PBBH, and Johns Hopkins, however, is that Johns Hopkins specified use of the funds for a medical school, whereas Brigham's cited only the Hospital Corporation. Thus, Harvard had to be sensitive and cautious in making this link between hospital and medical school—at the time, most people did not recognize the need for training in medicine in order to improve the quality of care and may not have realized the need for enhanced medical education for physicians-in-training.

In early 1900, the HMS faculty agreed with Minot's suggested location of the Francis estate in Roxbury—it was large enough for both the school and the hospital, and it was in Suffolk County, where Peter Bent Brigham's will dictated the hospital be built. Twenty benefactors from the city funded the cost of the land, but J. Collins (Coll) Warren (see chapter 4) and Henry Bowditch began focusing on fundraising to construct the school's new buildings. The two used the promising potential connection of HMS to the new PBBH—along with their dream of "an extraordinary school…controlling appointments in a great new hospital…[and] a national institution reaching beyond Boston for a distinguished staff" (Vogel 1980)—to entice donors.

In 1902, twenty-five years after Brigham's death and when the assets were ready to be released to the new hospital corporation, the value of the estate had almost quadrupled to $4.3 million. The Peter Bent Brigham Hospital Corporation was established on May 8 of that year, and the corporation "received from the trustees of the Brigham estate assets the extent of which would have pleased, and possibly surprised, the benefactor" on May 24. Afterward, HMS leaders approached the PBBH board to persuade them to officially connect the PBBH with HMS. As incentive, HMS offered the hospital a section of land on the lot it had purchased in Roxbury. Between Warren and Bowditch's convincing reasoning for an association and the land—located within "the most desirable section of the city" to which "neither the City Hospital nor the Massachusetts General Hospital [MGH] are near enough to this section [of Boston] to give it adequate service" (quoted in Vogel 1980)—the hospital's first eight-member board of trustees informally agreed to the affiliation and recommended that the hospital purchase the land Harvard offered it.

The hospital's board of trustees agreed that it would be mutually beneficial for HMS to use the new PBBH for both teaching and research, but it bristled against Harvard's wish to select hospital staff members. On this, the two institutions were at odds: Dr. George Rowe, then affiliated with Boston City Hospital, pushed for the PBBH to be fully independent from HMS, whereas Warren and Bowditch, along with HMS Dean William Richardson, advocated for affiliating with PBBH only if it would be designated as a university hospital. Coll Warren in particular was cognizant of the drawbacks of a lesser connection: he knew of the issues his grandfather, John Collins Warren, had dealt with when MGH had asserted its autonomy after initially being established as a Harvard-affiliated teaching hospital, and he noted in his memoirs that "They [had] made the mistake of placing this hospital [MGH] in the hands of an independent board of trustees, instead of uniting it intimately with the medical school" (quoted in Vogel 1980). But rather than contract such an agreement, Harvard simply stated its expectation and the PBBH board agreed to give it due consideration.

However, with an estate with such high stakes, a legal battle quickly ensued, initiated by the Brigham heirs. According to McCord (1963):

> The case was tried in the Federal Courts in Boston in October 1902…The Federal Court

ruled that the will had been executed properly. The Brigham heirs appealed; but in 1904 the U.S. Circuit Court of Appeals upheld the decision of the lower court...The Corporation, apparently sure of its ground, wisely took no steps to settle out of court. By 1906 the book value of the Corporation's assets had reached $5 million; by 1910 it was $5.3 million. In 1911 the Hospital took title from the Harvard Medical School to land "already conditionally purchased."

Appointment of Hospital Leadership

Construction of the hospital was delayed for almost a decade because of contestations in court, but HMS faculty were already thinking about who they would appoint as hospital staff. Eliot, however, worried in particular about the leadership roles of chief of medicine and chief of surgery—the men chosen for these positions would guide the hospital either toward the school's grand vision or toward becoming too insular and homogenous an endeavor.

William T. Councilman, then a pathologist at Boston City Hospital, held the same concerns as Eliot. He nominated Harvey Cushing as surgeon-in-chief and Henry A. Christian as physician-in-chief. In 1910, the hospital's board of trustees formally approved both Cushing and Christian to those respective positions; they named Councilman himself as pathologist-in-chief two years later. In May of that year, Eliot wrote to Dr. Christian:

> Now that you and Dr. Cushing have been put at the head respectively of the two Departments of Brigham Hospital, I feel as if the Medical School were entering on a happier future. Ever since I have been a member of the Medical Faculty I have seen clearly what a handicap on the School it was that the University had no hold on hospital appointments. Hereafter the school will be able to search all over the country for the very best men to fill vacancies. I hope you will see your way by and by to change the tenure of heads of departments of the Medical School. The heads are generally senior officers of the department, and they serve indefinitely...for many years. The method used at Cambridge of changing the head of a department every three, four or five years, but irregularly is, I am sure, a great deal more effective [though] not applicable in all departments of the Medical School...
> (quoted in McCord 1963)

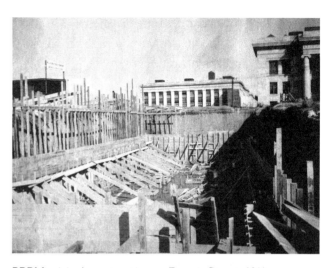

PBBH original construction on Francis Street, 1911.
The Teaching Hospital: Brigham and Women's Hospital and the Evolution of Academic Medicine by Peter V. Tishler, Christine Wenc, and Joseph Loscalzo. McGraw-Hill Education, 2014. Brigham and Women's Hospital Archives.

Opening Its Doors: A Twentieth-Century Hospital

About six months before the new PBBH opened, Drs. Cushing and Christian set about to fulfil their directives. At the time, "under a temporary arrangement entered into with Harvard University, the present surgeon-in-chief and the present physician-in-chief of the hospital occupy respectfully the chairs of surgery and medicine in the Harvard Medical School" ("Report of the President" 1914). The new hospital admitted its first patients on January 27, 1913. More than 35 years had passed since Peter Bent Brigham died and his

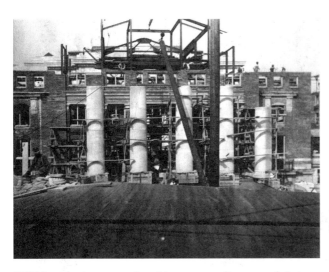

PBBH original construction. Limestone columns on Administration Building, September 16, 1912. Brigham and Women's Hospital Archives.

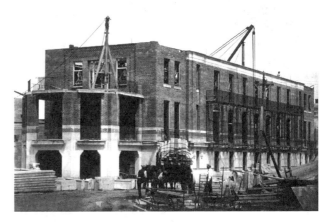

PBBH original construction. Ward A, August 2, 1912. Brigham and Women's Hospital Archives.

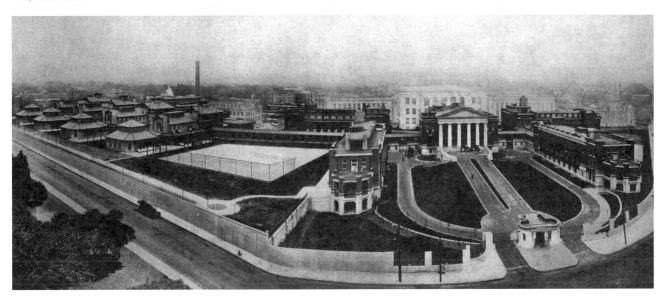

PBBH campus, ca. 1914. The Administration Building (right, with columns) was connected to Ward A (center building) and the wards (pavilions on the left) with a walkway, called the "pike" (center). Originally located on the ground floor, the pike was open. Later, after the pike was retained and enclosed (1940s), it was moved to the second floor and the pavilions were replaced by the BWH towers (1980s). Brigham and Women's Hospital Archives.

will had allocated funds toward a new hospital. In that time, the form that hospital would take had evolved significantly—from Brigham's notion of a hospital as providing a home and care to the poor, to a twentieth-century view of a hospital as an institution meant to advance the field of medicine.

During its first year, the surgical department of the PBBH consisted of three surgeons: Dr. Cushing as surgeon-in-chief and two other surgeons, Dr. David Cheever and Dr. John Homans. The department had 15 beds in the first completed ward (10 beds for a house officer service) and a temporary operating room. The resident staff included one resident surgeon and three assistant resident surgeons.

The new hospital kept statistics on all outpatient visits and inpatient admissions; as well as outcomes data. Patients discharged were listed in

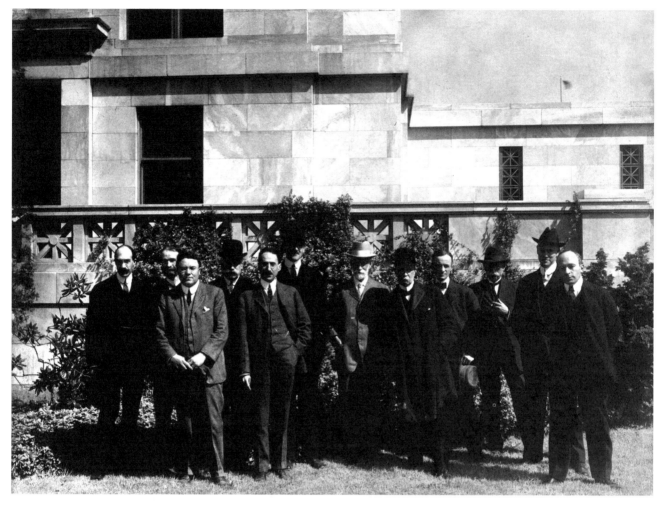

Opening of the new hospital (PBBH). Left to right: John L. Bremer, Theobold Smith, Walter B. Cannon, Harold C. Ernst, Milton J. Rosenau, David L. Edsall, Charles S. Minot, Sir William Osler, Harvey Cushing, W. T. Councilman, Henry A. Christian, S. Burt Wolbach. *A Perfectly Striking Departure: Surgeons and Surgery at the Peter Bent Brigham Hospital 1912–1980* by Nicholas L. Tilney. Science History Publications, 2006. Brigham and Women's Hospital Archives.

annual reports in the following categories: well, improved, unimproved, untreated, and died. From the beginning, surgical admissions were always larger than medical admissions. "An Out-Door Department [outpatient clinic] had been conducted for some two years by the Harvard Medical School through the generosity of one of the citizens of Boston," however, "it was transferred to [the PBBH] Out-Door Building" after the hospital officially opened ("Report of the Superintendent" 1914). Thereafter, "the doors were kept open for a continuous clinic from six in the morning until eight in the evening" ("Report of the Superintendent" 1914).

Each annual report of the hospital included reports of the president, the treasurer, the superintendent, the pathologist, the surgeon-in-chief, the physician-in-chief, and reports from nursing and social services, as well as a register of former members of the staff and officers of the institution. In the first annual report (1913–1914), Dr. Harvey Cushing wrote his first Report of the Surgeon-in-Chief. He included detailed statistics of the surgical diagnosis of each patient on the service in broad categories. Musculoskeletal or orthopaedic diagnoses were not listed separately but were included in each of the following categories: congenital abnormalities and

Peter Bent Brigham Hospital and Robert Breck Brigham Hospital

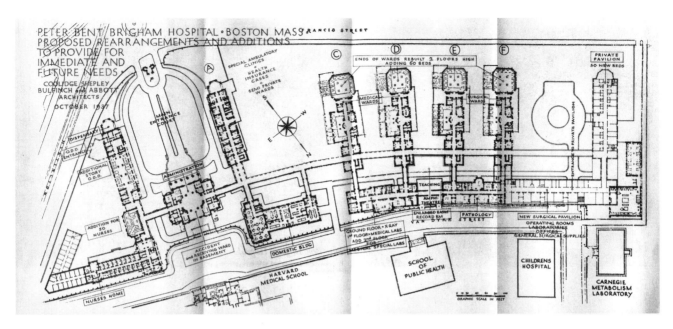

PBBH plans, ca. 1914. Brigham and Women's Hospital Archives.

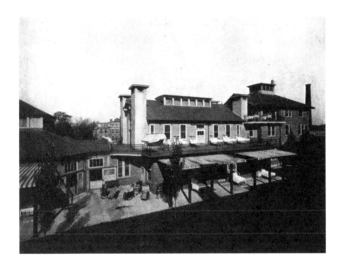

PBBH: Pavilion F.

The Teaching Hospital: Brigham and Women's Hospital and the Evolution of Academic Medicine by Peter V. Tishler, Christine Wenc, and Joseph Loscalzo. McGraw-Hill Education, 2014. Brigham and Women's Hospital Archives.

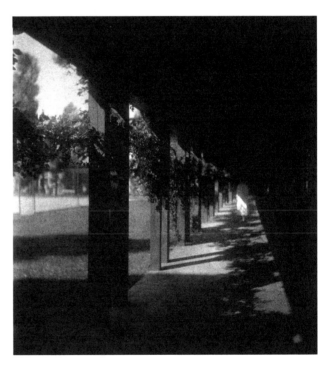

PBBH: Open air pike, 1930s.

The Teaching Hospital: Brigham and Women's Hospital and the Evolution of Academic Medicine by Peter V. Tishler, Christine Wenc, and Joseph Loscalzo. McGraw-Hill Education, 2014. Harvard Medical Library in the Countway Library of Medicine.

malformations; bones and cartilages; infective diseases; joints; miscellaneous diseases and conditions; muscles, fasciae, tendons and tendon sheaths; nervous system; tumors; injuries (bone contusions and dislocation, traumatic synovitis; and wounds (gunshots and stabs) and lacerated wounds (punctures). Surgical specialties were not accepted in the broad field of surgery at the time, but some interest was beginning to surface in the fields of neurosurgery, ophthalmology, urology, and orthopaedic surgery.

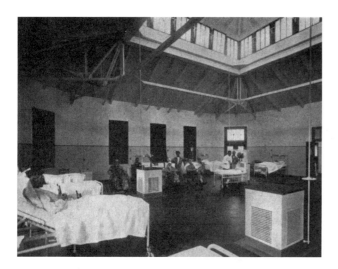

PBBH: Pavilion C (Ward I, 14 beds), ca. 1914.
A Perfectly Striking Departure: Surgeons and Surgery at the Peter Bent Brigham Hospital 1912-1980 by Nicholas L. Tilney. Science History Publications, 2006. Brigham and Women's Hospital Archives.

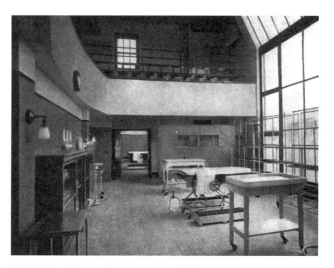

PBBH: large operating room, ca. 1914.
A Perfectly Striking Departure: Surgeons and Surgery at the Peter Bent Brigham Hospital 1912-1980 by Nicholas L. Tilney. Science History Publications, 2006. Brigham and Women's Hospital Archives.

> No one can be a good physician who has no idea of surgical operations, and a surgeon is nothing if ignorant of medicine.
> —Harvey Cushing, MD (*The Fabrick of Man: Fifty Years of the Peter Bent Brigham Hospital*. David McCord, 1963, pg. 125.)

Although musculoskeletal conditions did not have a unique listing, they "were treated at the Brigham from the day it opened in 1913. The first patient treated for a musculoskeletal problem was a nine-year-old with spasticity. Her adductors were released by Harvey Cushing who postoperatively noted that both of her hips were dislocated" (Banks 1983). Some of the orthopaedic surgical cases admitted to the hospital during its first two years included spina bifida (3), syndactyly (1), osteomyelitis (12), bursitis (4), tuberculosis of bone or joints (7), ankylosis (2), acute arthritis (4), chronic arthritis (8), hallux valgus (3), tendon contracture (8), Dupuytren's contracture (50), acute myositis (1), hand tenosynovitis (1), benign bone tumors (3), neuroma (1), pelvis cancer (1), leg sarcoma (1), fractures (69), semilunar cartilage fracture (2), knee synovitis (2), hand wound (1), thigh wound (1), brachial plexus stab wound (1).

Except for an occasional subspecialty such as eye, ears, nose, and throat or urology, the PBBH maintained a general surgical service without major subspecialty development during Dr. Cushing's (1910–1932) and Dr. Elliot Cutler's (1932–1948) tenures as surgeon-in-chief. It was not until Dr. Francis Moore's tenure as surgeon-in-chief (1948–1976) that surgical subspecialty departments emerged, including orthopaedic surgery. Dr. Cushing wrote:

> At the Peter Bent Brigham Hospital we are in the interesting and somewhat enviable position of being able to begin our service without specialization, so that the entire field of surgery is more or less completely covered for it would appear that so-called general surgery in many institutions is somewhat emasculated by the withdrawal from it of the surgical disorders of the eye, ear, nose and throat, of the pelvic disorders of women, of genito-urinary, neurological, orthopaedic, proctological, vascular, thoracic diseases, and so on, so that "general surgery" has come to mean the surgery of the extremities and the alimentary canal. In consequence, the majority of so-called general surgeons, perhaps unconsciously have become more or less

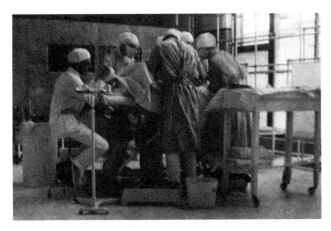

PBBH: Surgery under ether in large operating room, ca. 1918.
Brigham and Women's Hospital Archives.

specialized workers. My personal conviction… is that general surgery should cover all these fields and that groups of patients should be temporarily withdrawn from a general service to be under the direction of one who may be trained a specialist, only in the event of some individual arising in the clinic who shows a special interest in and a particular aptitude for a certain kind of special work…[would] such a special surgical service [be] justifiable. When such an offshoot…ceases to make progress, it would be wise to reabsorb it again within the general service. ("Report of the Surgeon-in-Chief" 1914)

At the end of the first year, following the careful and conservative guidance of Cushing and Christian, the hospital was treating 119 inpatients, whereas:

the highest number up to that date at any one time had been one hundred and seventy-three patients…This is one of the earliest hospitals to introduce what has become known as "fulltime" work, which means continuous service in the Hospital by members of the Staff instead of having changes several times a year. ("Report of the President" 1914)

Following that first year, the department of surgery began a yearly, but slow continuous growth in staff, residents, inpatients, outpatients and operations performed. McCord (1963) noted:

The original "chiefs" of the two services, Cushing and Christian, when faced with the pressure to enlarge the Hospital, wisely decided to keep it small, preferring a small number of patients, carefully selected and very thoroughly studied, to a larger more heterogenous hospital population without the integration in and between services and departments which would be lost by doubling or tripling bed capacity.

In 1915, the Brigham Department of Surgery established a new salaried staff position: resident surgeon. The resident surgeon was one of four house officers who ensured the smooth operations of the surgical service. Those in senior positions also supervised the Out-Door Department. The number and roles of the residents at PBBH was modeled after that in place at Johns Hopkins hospital, which had gained widespread recognition as a productive and competent scheme. The position of resident surgeon:

is one for which, particularly in surgery, a long preliminary training is necessary and hence is rarely attained until several years after graduation, but once attained it gives an intensive operative experience to the incumbent which should put him in his familiarity with the problems of general surgery years ahead of his contemporaries and will repay him for his long apprenticeship. ("Report of the Surgeon-in-Chief" 1915)

The PBBH and World War I

As the US became entrenched in World War I, in 1915, "Cushing was called by the Army to serve with the American Ambulance…Dr. Homans also served in the Army for two years" ("Report of the Surgeon-in-Chief" 1915). Cheever joined

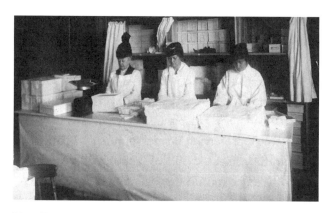

New England Dressings Committee (Red Cross Auxiliary), 1918. Six thousand women throughout New England (some seen here at PBBH) made and sterilized surgical dressings during WWI. Packed in sealed tins, the dressings were to be shipped with Harvard's Base Hospital No. 5 but were initially diverted to Halifax after the harbor explosion (see chapter 34). Brigham and Women's Hospital Archives.

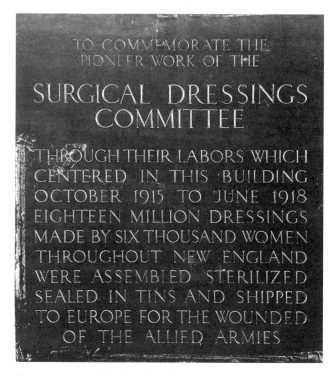

Memorial plaque for the New England Dressings Committee. During WWI, the committee made eighteen million sterilized dressings for the wounded Allied armies. Brigham and Women's Hospital Archives.

the British Expeditionary Forces. He and other Harvard physicians and surgeons joined a unit that served in Boulogne, France. After his tour of duty, he returned to Boston and took over the position of surgeon-in-chief, covering for Cushing while he was also serving in France. Cheever did the same again almost 30 years later, when he took the place of Elliott Cutler, who was in service overseas during World War II.

Dr. Robert Lovett and his associates at Boston Children's Hospital provided guidance on orthopaedic cases at the PBBH, as well as did specialists from other hospitals. The entire staff at both PBBH and Boston Children's Hospital also visited the other's wards every week. Two physicians from Boston City Hospital, Dr. Frederic Cotton and Dr. Edward Nichols, volunteered their time to teach at the PBBH surgical clinic.

The surgical service continued to grow during the war. In 1916, the average number of admissions had increased to 1,924 (from 1,142 in 1913), surgical beds had increased to 110, and the Out-Door Department growth had expanded to 26,134 visits (from 15,713 in 1914). Dr. Cheever, as acting surgeon-in-chief, wrote in 1917 that most of the junior staff had also enlisted in the military:

Of the Surgical Resident and House Staff at the outbreak of the war, thirteen in number, all but five have resigned during the year before completing their terms, in order to enter the army or navy and [after the US declared War] the surgical work has been conducted during the remainder of 1917 under considerable difficulties, and that it has gone forward without serious dislocation is due, in large part, at least, to the system and traditions…and to the unremitting devotion to its [hospital's] interests of the Chief Resident [Dr. Conrad Jackson]. ("Report of the Acting Surgeon in Chief" 1917)

In 1916, the first subspecialty of surgery was recognized in the department of general surgery: eye, ear, nose, and throat under Dr. C. B. Walker. In June 1916, "urology cases split off from surgery and [were] placed under charge of

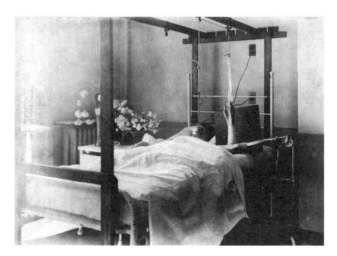

PBBH: Patient in traction in bed with a wooden Balkan frame, ca. 1917. Brigham and Women's Hospital Archives.

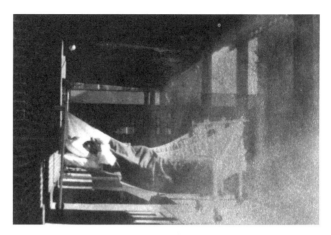

PBBH: Patient in a flu tent, 1918. Brigham and Women's Hospital Archives.

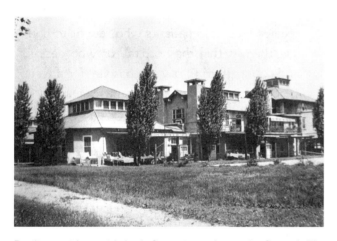

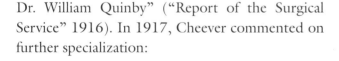

Pavilions with outside beds for patients during the Spanish Flu epidemic, 1918–1920. Brigham and Women's Hospital Archives.

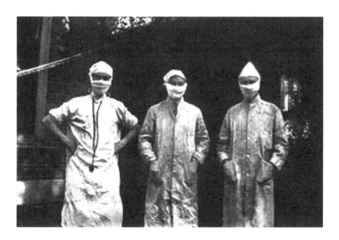

PBBH: Physicians in gauze masks during the Spanish Flu epidemic. Brigham and Women's Hospital Archives.

Dr. William Quinby" ("Report of the Surgical Service" 1916). In 1917, Cheever commented on further specialization:

> The opinion [Dr. Cushing's] was expressed that it was unwise to establish such specialties except when their need was clearly indicated and an individual was available capable of developing them beyond the point reached by the existing staff. No such new departments have been created during the year… Another group which might well be separated off into a specialty is orthopaedics (using the term in its stricter sense as the treatment of deformities, congenital and acquired). Such work requires as an indispensable adjunct a well-equipped mechanical appliance shop, — a project at present beyond our means. Such cases and others which we are not prepared to handle are referred to other clinics. It is pleasant to record the cordial coöperation between the medical and surgical services, and the many instances in which we have been helped with special knowledge by members of the staff of neighboring institutions, especially Dr. Lovett and his assistants at the Children's Hospital. ("Report of the Acting Surgeon in Chief" 1917)

That year, at the PBBH, orthopaedic operations numbered 76, including 38 fractures. One death occurred: a 69-year-old male with a fractured femur who underwent open reduction and plating under ether drop anesthesia and application of a hip spica cast. He died postoperatively from pneumonia.

Codman's End-Result System and Hospital Reorganization

Dr. Lovett was named consultant orthopaedist to the PBBH in 1919. In his report, Dr. Cushing also commented about surgical outcomes. He believed that Codman's end-result system (see chapter 34) was very important and that the hospital should support use of the annual questionnaire advocated by Codman. He thought "it was a colossal task that required a trained medical man" ("Report of the Surgeon-in-Chief" 1917), suggesting that an outgoing house officer be appointed as a registrar with a staff much like what he had seen in British hospitals.

In 1920, Dr. Cushing merged the Surgical Research Laboratory with the Laboratory of Surgical Pathology directed by Dr. E. H. Nichols. He was successful in establishing an end-result system. That year, he had also begun to modify his opinion about specialization:

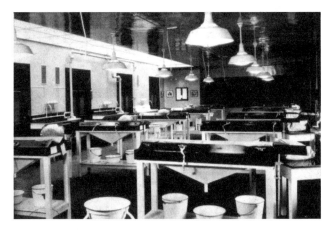

PBBH/HMS surgical research laboratory, ca. 1920.
A Perfectly Striking Departure: Surgeons and Surgery at the Peter Bent Brigham Hospital 1912–1980 by Nicholas L. Tilney. Science History Publications, 2006. Brigham and Women's Hospital Archives.

> We have a general surgical service with the same group of attendants on duty the year round; that within this general service specialization is encouraged, but the so-called surgical specialties are not segregated…In one respect, however, we have diverged from the custom… of the Johns Hopkins clinic…This concerns what has come to be known as the "full-time" clinical positions…for the first time in any general hospital, provision was made whereby the chiefs-of-service could give their individual time to the institution and their duties in the medical school with which it was closely affiliated… They were at the same time privileged to receive fees from patients who saw fit to consult them within the hospital, or who desired and could afford to pay the hospital for private accommodations. Within the past year a corresponding arrangement for officers in the hospital, for assistant physicians and surgeons in attendance, has been made so that…the entire staff…at work throughout the day somewhere in the institution and all on the same basis… receive a nominal academic salary [and] are at liberty to augment as their consciences permit, by charging fees to those persons [if] they are able to pay. ("Report of the Surgeon-in-Chief" 1920)

The following year, Cushing wrote in his yearly annual report that: "The chief advantage we of the Brigham Hospital hold over our sister institutions in Boston, lies in the fact of our immediate proximity to Harvard Medical School, and it is incumbent upon us to make the most of this fortunate circumstance" ("Report of the Surgeon-in-Chief" 1921). In an attempt to differentiate the PBBH from the MGH and the Boston City Hospital, he stated:

> A friendly rivalry between local institutions is something to be encouraged; and competition for house officers, associates and even staff

Table 44.1. First Report of Bone Diseases and "Organs of Locomotion" in 1924

	Medical		Surgical		Outdoor Department
	Discharged	Died	Discharged	Died	
Bones (no tuberculosis)	35	–	41	1	39
Joints (rheumatism, no TBC)	49	–	21	–	360
Amputation	2	–	–	–	–
Other diseases	19	–	24	–	659

From "Report of the Superintendent" in the 1924 PBBH Annual Report, PBBH Records, 1830-[inclusive] 1911–1980 [bulk] BWH c 3, Box 1, Folder 2-29.

officers, we shall always have to face [with increased staff], we must strive against that habit of in-breeding which fosters conservatism and sees no good in other schools and hospitals…Every hospital has a distinct character of its own, which is nothing more than the composite of the characters of those who came in contact with its patients…It is this—the local color or spirit of a hospital—which no possible effort or desire for standardization, beneficent as the moment may be, can alter or should be permitted to alter…Our proximity to the Medical School has from the outset obliged us to accept the unqualified rôle of a university hospital…In the Brigham Hospital all of its chiefs of service are appointed by mutual agreement with the school in which they hold professional posts. ("Report of the Surgeon-in-Chief" 1922)

During this period, he had also begun to preserve protected time for residents from their clinical and teaching obligations so that they could research and write. The surgical labs remained in the medical school, while the department of medicine's laboratories were in the hospital. By 1923, Dr. Cushing recalled that the hospital, for the past decade, had supported a geographic fulltime system where the academic staff received a small salary which they could supplement with fees collected from private patients. A special private ward had been established. This contrasted with the Johns Hopkins system in which all full-time faculty were on a fixed salary.

> The balance sheets of surgery should periodically be audited by those not actively engaged in its practice.
> —Harvey Cushing, MD (*The Fabrick of Man: Fifty Years of the Peter Bent Brigham Hospital*. David McCord, 1963, pg. 125.)

In the 1924 Report of the Superintendent, diseases of bones and the organs of locomotion were first reported in one category (**Table 44.1**). In this same annual report, Cushing raised his concerns about the organization of surgery at the medical school and its teaching hospitals:

The relation of the Brigham Hospital to the Harvard Medical School is a peculiar one. In accordance with an unwritten agreement between the corporation of the University and the original Hospital Board of Trustees, it was understood that the Physician-in-Chief and the Surgeon-in-Chief should hold chairs of Medicine and Surgery in the Medical School…respectively the Hersey Professorship of the Theory and Practice of Physic and the Moseley Professorship of Surgery…It would appear, therefore, that the Brigham Hospital, more truly than in the case with any of the other general hospitals affiliated with the School, plays the rôle of a university hospital so far as that it is possible when boards of control are not interlocking and when the principle is not clearly and frankly acknowledged by both parties. [An alliance not in the founder's mind but] was accepted at the outset by the chiefs-of-service [at the PBBH]. ("Report of the Surgeon-in-Chief" 1924)

His additional concern was his prediction that there would be full-time teaching services in surgery at both the PBBH and the MGH, a concept he supported that:

> when fully attained, will necessitate some definite alteration in the present organization of the Departments of Medicine and Surgery...a question deserving careful consideration...one involving the principle of administrative centralization or decentralization of the clinical departments [the laboratory] for the past twelve years has been the only foothold the Department of Surgery has held in the buildings of the Medical School [for teaching medical students and research]...there are three general hospitals which are healthy rivals for school favor so far as clinical teaching in surgery is concerned... well-organized teaching units as a modified full-time basis...each of them a teacher of professional rank has been appointed...[the PBBH surgical laboratory at HMS] is the only common meeting ground...largely utilized by the Brigham Hospital group...different from other high-grade university medical schools, but at Harvard it is a stated principle that there are no acknowledged heads of departments...while authority is becoming more and more centralized in chiefs-of-service within the several hospitals, it at the same time is becoming decentralized so far as the school departments of medicine and surgery are concerned...the affairs of a department...of...surgery...must inevitably suffer... particularly...when its activities are so scattered as they are at Harvard between many hospitals. A committee may serve an equal purpose up to a certain point, even though its actions are usually influenced by its most active and interested members...The inevitable consequence [is] splitting of the existing department into three independent units.

("Report of the Surgeon-in-Chief" 1924)

Because of this trend, Dr. Cushing argued that HMS should distribute the resources, including students and teaching positions equally amongst the surgical services at the teaching hospitals. Cushing continued to prefer a surgical staff consisting of general surgeons, although he did accept an EENT and a urology service in the department. For other cases requiring a specialist's treatment, he preferred to send them to other hospitals rather than increase his surgical staff with subspecialists. By 1927, the Zander Room (see chapters 29 and 40), in the outpatient department, was designated "for installation of apparatus for mechanical therapy [which] has never been used for that purpose" ("Report of the Superintendent" 1927).

Beginning of a New Era

In 1931, regulations at the PBBH "specified... that all officers should retire at a given age and sixty-three was hit upon as a reasonable jumping-off place" ("Report of the Surgeon-in-Chief" 1931). The board of incorporators extended the time by three years, but Dr. Harvey Cushing declined stating it was an "unwise precedent" ("Report of the Surgeon-in-Chief" 1931). He retired in 1931 after 23 years as surgeon-in-chief at the PBBH.

Cushing demonstrated his strong support of orthopaedics and the strong relationship of the two hospitals by inviting Professor Vittorio Putti from Bologna as his last visiting surgeon-in-chief pro tempore (May 30–June 6, 1932). At the time of his retirement, Cushing also commented on the PBBH's relationship with Boston Children's Hospital:

> From the early days we have enjoyed the closest cooperation with the orthopoedic [sic] and surgical departments of the neighboring hospital for children. With the late Robert W. Lovett, the plan of having a weekly exchange visit with the combined staffs of the two hospitals was put into effect. The primary idea on his part was that it would broaden the experience

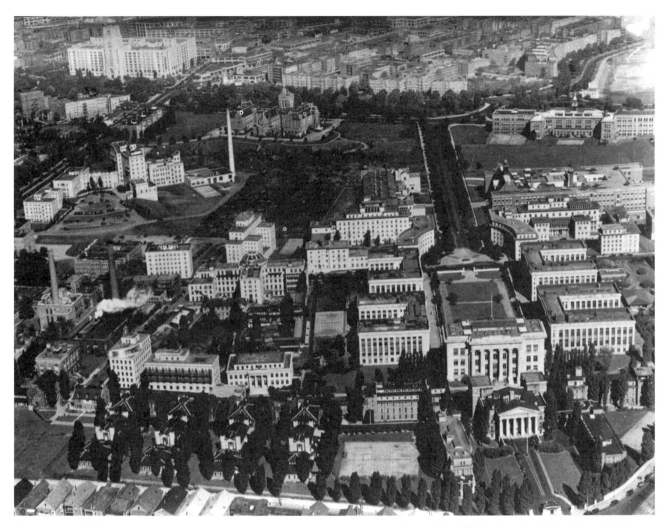

Aerial view of PBBH. The Administration Building is lower right; pavilions are lower left. HMS is directly behind the Administration Building, and Boston Children's Hospital is behind the pavilions. Brigham and Women's Hospital Archives.

of his group could they thus keep in touch with the problems of general surgery…his successors…Osgood and…Ober have kept on with the program and the attendance at these early Tuesday morning ward visits and demonstrations, alternating between the two hospitals, bears witness to the continued enjoyment and profit gained from them. ("Report of the Surgeon-in-Chief" 1931)

A change occurred in the philosophy of the department regarding specialty care in 1932 with the appointment of the new surgeon-in-chief, Dr. Elliott Cutler. Although Cutler also favored generalist care in surgery, he wanted all patients admitted to PBBH "to obtain the most modern and expert form of therapy" ("Report of the Surgeon-in-Chief" 1932). In September 1932, Dr. Frank Ober was made a consulting orthopedic surgeon at the RBBH. Cutler wrote:

In a further attempt to strengthen orthopedic teaching and so as to make it unnecessary for us to send some of our O.D.D. [Out Door Department] bone and joint cases to MGH for therapy, Dr. William T. Green has been added as Junior Associate in Orthopedic Surgery as of April 1933. The position filled by Dr. Green bespeaks, perhaps my ideas as to a further direction in which the hospital might be enlarged. We already run a splendid orthopedic clinic two mornings a week in our O.D.D., at which times the third-year students have experience in this important surgical specialty...many cases...have [recently] been admitted to the house and treated here, sometimes by the regular surgical staff and sometimes by our orthopedic consultants... [providing] considerable educational value to both the house staff and the students, as well as making the whole experience simpler and, I think, better for the patient. ("Report of the Surgeon-in-Chief" 1932)

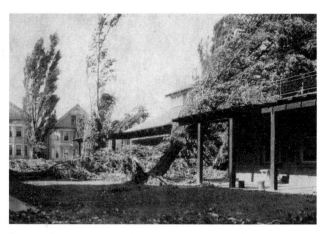

PBBH: Damage to the pavilions during the hurricane in 1938. Brigham and Women's Hospital Archives.

By 1933, Dr. Cutler had started new specialty clinics in orthopaedics, gynecology, vascular, tumor, and gastroenterology (where the surgeon attended the medical clinics). Dr. William T. Green and Dr. A. H. Brewster were attendings in the orthopaedic clinic, along with both interns at the PBBH and third-year students.

The hospital's annual reports during the depression were brief. Limited statistics were provided for bone and joint cases in the 1935 report (**Table 44.2**). In 1936, Cutler noted that there were 28 teachers of general surgery at the MGH and 10 at the PBBH. Dr. Paul Hugenberger was added to the staff as voluntary graduate assistant in orthopedic surgery.

In his 1937 report, Cutler expressed his desire for medical students to have closer contact with inpatients and to assist in surgery; a concept he originally proposed as a resident at MGH in 1915 to Dr. Washburn, the superintendent of the hospital. He also expressed his gratitude to Drs. Cushing and Christian for their original plan of a full-time service: "The full time service set up by our original chiefs-of-service has proven so valuable that it has found wide applications elsewhere...That our Chiefs-of-Service resisted the more strict 'free-time' service for clinicians as proposed by Mr. Flexner we should be very grateful" ("Report of the Surgeon-in-Chief" 1937).

The PBBH had continued to treat fractures and dislocations within the confines of general surgery throughout Cushing's tenure and the beginning of Cutler's tenure, but by 1938, Dr. Carl Walter "was asked to organize a fracture service," which still fell within "a division of general surgery" (McCord 1963). One specialty area was assumed by Dr. Cutler: "The assignment of septic hands to the Surgeon-in-Chief represents a sense of responsibility to our patients...no field for surgical endeavor [is] more difficult [where] the surgeon is confronted with a complicated anatomy" ("Report of the Surgeon-in-Chief" 1940). In 1940, Dr. Cutler demonstrated his continued but limited support of orthopaedic surgery as a specialty:

> In an attempt to continue the Brigham Hospital in the tradition of a single surgical service, with the surgical specialties as integral parts and not

Table 44.2. Statistics for Bone and Joint Cases, 1932–35

	1932	1933	1934	1935
Fractures	25	10	33	35
Other diseases	103	76	54	53
Plasters	–	66	91	85

From "Report of the Surgeon-in-Chief" in the 1935 PBBH Annual Report, PBBH Records, 1830-[inclusive] 1911-1980 [bulk] BWH c 3, Box 1, Folder 2-29.

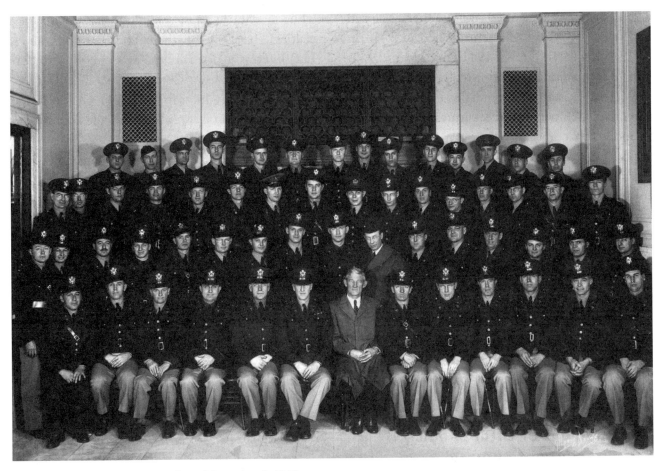

5th Harvard Hospital Unit in uniform, November 7, 1942.
The Teaching Hospital: Brigham and Women's Hospital and the Evolution of Academic Medicine by Peter V. Tishler, Christine Wenc, and Joseph Loscalzo. McGraw-Hill Education, 2014. Brigham and Women's Hospital Archives.

separate divisions – a method best suited to the education of our house staff and the students – and at the same time to permit a few to dig deep in special fields, a system of topical assignments has been set up. Assignments are as follows: Orthopedic Surgery, Dr. Brewster and Associates…Fractures, Drs. Walter and Quigley…The creation of special assignments has already proved particularly fruitful in the field of fractures. Here Dr. Walter and Dr. Quigley have revolutionized our care of patients through the utilization of modern apparatus, by which accurate reduction of fractures may be assured. I know of no single step in this Hospital in the last ten years which has brought greater benefit to our patients. ("Report of the Surgeon-in-Chief" 1940)

The PBBH and World War II

During World War II, the Harvard University Unit (5th General Hospital) was re-established. The unit that originally left Boston on May 7, 1917, during World War I, now included Drs. Cutler and Quigley (see chapter 64) and 17 others from the PBBH. It also included Drs. Edwin Cave, Augustus Thorndike Jr., and Carter Rowe. With Dr. Cutler recalled by the army on July 18, 1942, and sent to Europe, Harvard University successfully applied pressure to the surgeon general to allow Dr. Cheever to remain at the PBBH as acting surgeon-in-chief (for the second time). Dr. Brewster also continued to care for orthopaedic cases at the PBBH during the War.

Although short staffed, the number of closed and open reduction of fractures increased: 53 in 1939, 84 in 1940, 165 in 1941, and 213 in 1942. In 1942, the annual report listed the names of the physicians on staff in specific departments. There were 39 members of the surgical department, including six orthopaedic surgeons and two general surgeons that treated fractures (Dr. Carl Walter and Dr. Thomas Quigley). The orthopaedic surgeons included: Frank R. Ober (orthopaedic surgeon), Albert H. Brewster (senior associate in orthopaedic surgery), William T. Green (associate in orthopaedic surgery), and Meier G. Karp (associate in orthopaedic surgery) in absentia while on active duty, and two junior associates in orthopaedic surgery: William A. Elliston (also in absentia) and Paul E. Hugenberger. With the orthopaedic staff severely depleted by the war, Dr. Brewster oversaw the orthopaedic service as senior associate.

Development of Orthopaedics as a Specialty of Surgery

Dr. Cutler resumed his duties as surgeon-in-chief after the war ended. In his 1945 report (the first one after the war and three years of active duty), he wrote that for those who stayed behind:

> medical school and hospital obligations more than doubled…with service crippled and the staff overtaxed, the students themselves could not be so receptive. They in turn graduated and were pushed into hospitals inadequately trained to carry out the best care for sick people…their lack of training necessitated unusual efforts on the part of the staff to properly safeguard records and care. ("Report of the Surgeon-in-Chief" 1945)

The specialty services he named included orthopaedic surgery (Drs. Green, Brewster, and associates) and fractures (Drs. Walter and Quigley), and septic hands (Drs. Cutler and Quigley).

Thus individuals (and others in different subspecialties) "have one of [their] major responsibilities [an] interest in a small field of surgery" ("Report of the Surgeon-in-Chief" 1946). Dr. Ober remained a consultant in orthopaedic surgery and a new junior associate in orthopaedic surgery was added to the staff, Dr. David Grice.

The fracture clinic and the orthopaedic clinic were "spread over two mornings a week and on different days so that the new Resident in Bone and Joint Surgery [1946] can assist in the proper running of these very important clinics" ("Report of the Surgeon-in-Chief" 1946). Each service had eight inpatient beds; private patients were included with the public wards. Dr. Elliston was no longer listed on the staff, and Dr. Charles L. Sturdevant was added as a junior associate in orthopaedic surgery.

In 1948, Dr. Francis D. Moore was named surgeon-in-chief, replacing Dr. Cutler who had died on August 8, 1947. Moore had different opinions regarding specialization compared to his two predecessors. He wrote: "on the score of specialization, we must realize that in modern surgery no one man can be expert in all fields…The Brigham of the future cannot be a 'one man show.' It must be a collaborative enterprise on the part of several expert specialists in various branches of surgery… to satisfy our obligation to students and patients, we must cover the major fields of surgery with men who provide the highest quality of care" ("Report of the Surgeon-in-Chief" 1948).

Most medical educators, when gathered together in solemn conclave, bewail the growth of specialization. Generalization is far the superior. Yet the same educator, when seized with a primary carcinoma of the bronchus, will inevitably seek out the person who in his opinion has had the most extensive and effective special experience in this field. "No one wants specialization except the patient."

—Frances D. Moore, MD, *Peter Bent Brigham Hospital Annual Report, 1961* (McCord 1963: 106)

Dr. Hugenberger and Dr. Karp were now senior associates; the junior associates included Drs. Grice, Sturdevant, and Frank H. Stelling. Dr. Moore also had strong feelings about the role of residents in surgery: "The teaching of young surgeons requires that the Resident be given the final operating room responsibility of performing operations himself. This responsibility is the sacred trust of the staff...since it must be granted only when it can be granted without jeopardizing the individual safety of the patient" ("Report of the Surgeon-in-Chief" 1948).

In his 1951 annual report, Moore added a new section: Surgical Divisions and Enterprises. Both neurosurgery and bone and joint surgery were included as surgical divisions. Dr. Albert B. Ferguson Jr. joined the staff as a junior associate in orthopaedic surgery. At the time, Dr. Moore stated that Dr. Ferguson would "add strength to our clinical studies of the many problems encountered in corrective orthopaedics and the surgery of skeletal trauma. In addition Dr. Ferguson is embarking on a study of histo-chemistry and muscle dynamics of prolonged immobilization... Under the leadership of Dr. Green, Dr. Quigley, and Dr. Walter, the Brigham deals effectively with a large volume of orthopaedic problems and fractures from the neighboring communities" ("Report of the Surgeon-in-Chief" 1951).

The following year, Ferguson was given an office in the Brigham (the first office in the hospital provided for an orthopaedic surgeon). Dr. Arthur Trott from Boston Children's Hospital was also added to the staff. Ferguson remained on the staff for two years, resigning in June 1953 to accept the position of professor of orthopaedic surgery at the University of Pittsburgh. Dr. Henry Banks replaced him in October 1953. With clinical responsibilities for orthopaedics given first to Dr. Ferguson and then to Dr. Banks; Dr. Green, the head of the orthopaedic department at Boston Children's was designated, "Chief of our Orthopaedic Division," at the PBBH by Dr. Moore.

Between 1950 and 1955, the yearly volume of orthopaedic inpatients increased from 400 to 600; ward cases 140 to 240. The average types of cases operated on by the residents included 80 fracture reductions and internal fixations and 50 reconstructive orthopaedic cases. The private staff increased, and a total of 575 fracture cases were treated in the previous year and 870 industrial accident cases were treated in the emergency department. A need for an industrial clinic was identified.

Fractures remained the responsibility of Walter and Quigley, although after Banks arrived, he began a long-term study on hip fractures. Both orthopaedics and the fracture service were very busy in 1955, treating 500 patients and about 3,000 outpatients. They were the most active clinics in the department of surgery. Orthopaedics and the fracture service met regularly for conferences and teaching rounds under Green's leadership and met monthly to review research projects and discuss administrative issues. The two services decided not to treat polio cases at the PBBH, referring all cases to the Boston Children's Hospital. Dr. Banks was given an office in the hospital that year in order "to strengthen our geographic full-time staff in orthopedic surgery" ("Report of the Surgeon-in-Chief" 1958). Three orthopedic residents from Boston Children's rotated through the PBBH as well.

The hospital began to treat large numbers of industrial accident cases (969 in 1955), and, in January 1956, the Boston police began bringing patients to the PBBH from the area west of Ruggles Street. That year the orthopaedic service "care[d] for approximately one-sixth of the total patients on the surgical service" ("Report of the Surgeon-in-Chief" 1956). A total of 585 patients with fractures were treated by the service. Seventy-eight (mostly hip fractures) underwent open reduction and internal fixation. In the previous year, 240 fracture patients and 400 general orthopaedic cases were admitted. In the busy clinic, the "resident staff...sees more patients than all the other surgical specialty clinics put together" ("Report of the Surgeon-in-Chief" 1956). At the same time, the entire hospital was feeling a financial and space-related pinch:

> Eighty-five % of the hospital beds were in semi-private and public wards, with only 15% private. There was an immediate, desperate need for: a) increased endowment; b) a new pavilion; c) additional and improved radiology facilities; d) a new blood bank and pathology laboratory...[After] long years of deficit operations, the added problems of change of business methods and procedures [led to leadership changes and] a long-term need of $7 million to be raised [for endowment and administrative needs]. (McCord 1963)

Before, during, and immediately after World War II, "in what Robert Cutler calls the 'doldrum years' certain individuals close to the Hospital contributed to offset the relatively small annual deficits" (McCord 1963). A plaster room was built in 1958, and an amputee clinic was started under the leadership of Dr. Richard Warren (vascular surgeon) and Dr. Banks. Banks continued to expand both clinical and basic research in orthopaedics (see chapter 45). In addition to surgeons Drs. Green, Quigley and Walter, the staff consisted of Dr. Albert Brewster (senior associate in surgery), Drs. Banks, Hugenberger, and Karp (associates in surgery), Drs. Sturdevant and Trott (junior associates in surgery) and Drs. Bates and Elliston (assistants in surgery).

As the hospital continued to grow, the trustees pursued legal recourse with the state supreme court "in order not to violate the terms of the Founder's will respecting the care of sick persons in indigent circumstances residing in Suffolk County" (McCord 1963). On June 30, 1958, the court decreed:

> limiting that portion of the Hospital's remaining unrestricted funds to be used for the "indigent sick of Suffolk County," but broadening the charter powers to care for patients regardless of their place of residence, and to provide specifically broad powers to operate all...facilities necessary to a modern hospital functioning today. (McCord 1963)

The next year, Dr. Albert Brewster, "a valued member for 26 years," reached retirement age ("Report of the Surgeon-in-Chief" 1959). The orthopaedic service now included chief residents. The number of cases treated the previous year was about 10,000. In May 1959, some designated space for orthopaedic research was provided for the first time in the pathology department (Dr. Dammin's laboratory). By 1960, discussions had begun regarding a possible consolidation of five different hospitals (see chapter 47). Only minimal changes occurred on the orthopaedic clinical service. A combined hand clinic (surgery and orthopaedic surgery) was started. Each outpatient clinic was staffed by an orthopaedic surgeon for consultations and to teach residents and third-year students. A junior assistant surgical resident no longer rotated on the orthopaedic service. Drs. Griffin and Tachjian were added to the staff as junior associates. Drs. Bates and Elliston were assistants in surgery.

In the hospital's annual report 1960–1961, the chairman of the board of trustees and the president jointly reported that the consolidation project continued to progress: the "Affiliated Hospitals Center, Incorporated was established" ("Joint Report" 1962). The Brigham property on the corner of Shattuck and Huntington Streets, which was the location of the Carrie M. Hall Nurses Residence, was sold. The area is now occupied by the Francis A. Countway Medical Library.

At the hospital's 50th anniversary, in 1963, the chairman of the board of trustees and the president of the Hospital quoted David McCord, a poet and fundraiser, in their annual report: "In fifty years [this] astonishing small teaching hospital, with eighty percent public wards and twenty

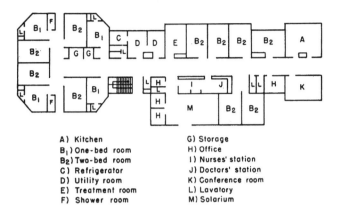

PBBH: Clinical Research Center floor plan, 1960.
The Teaching Hospital: Brigham and Women's Hospital and the Evolution of Academic Medicine by Peter V. Tishler, Christine Wenc, and Joseph Loscalzo. McGraw-Hill Education, 2014. Brigham and Women's Hospital Archives.

Box 44.3. Dr. Francis Moore's Report at the 50th Anniversary of the PBBH

> "The fragmentation of surgery is a well-known phenomenon dictated by the technical applicability of its methods and by the fact that intensive activity in one area yields the greatest skill and effectiveness in relieving suffering. From a teaching point of view, such specialization seems undesirable, but 'Everyone is against specialization except the patient'…
>
> "One of the largest areas of surgical responsibility is that designated as orthopedic surgery. Orthopedic surgeons care for a remarkably large fraction of those total patients designated as 'surgical' because their diseases are amenable to treatment by surgeons and by the operative sterile anesthetized dissection known as an operation. Orthopedic surgery is a low mortality area in surgery. It is an area that has to do with disease of the bones and joints, and injuries. The orthopedic surgeon sees but rarely the patient with acute life-endangering injury, and the threats to life…Possibly because of his concern for very long-term illness with low threat to life but high threat to socio-economic effectiveness, Orthopedics seems to have gone the farthest along the way of separation from the rest of surgery…of all the fields discussed during the 'Career Day,' this was the one that showed the widest difference of opinion as to what constituted a proper and well-balanced university service…"
>
> ("Report of the Chairman" 1963).

percent private, contending often with inadequate facilities, has greatly and honorably achieved for itself an enviable position both here and abroad" ("Report of the Chairman" 1963). The celebration continued for two days, including a scientific program. Dr. Joseph Barr presented a lecture on "Orthopaedic Surgery as a Career," followed by discussion with Dr. T. B. Quigley, Dr. R. A. Milch (Baltimore) and Dr. A. B. Ferguson Jr. (Pittsburgh). Dr. Green closed with comments summarizing the presentations and addressing future needs in orthopaedic surgery.

Dr. Moore's report (**Box 44.3**) was long and thoughtful, summarizing his thoughts about specialization, the field of orthopaedic surgery, and the importance of research. Regarding research in surgery, he stated: "The essence of this revolution [relationship between biological research and clinical surgery] is to resolve the conflict between the clinic and the laboratory without a fight, realizing that the two must be united in the career of an individual surgeon so as to produce any significant new advance" ("Report of the Chairman" 1963).

Further organization of the staff at the PBBH occurred in the fall of 1963 with the formation of the Peter Bent Brigham Hospital Surgical Associates, which was the hospital's second venture into the form of a faculty group practice. The first was the Industrial Accident Clinic. The Surgical Associates, after two years of preliminary study, determined their "purpose [was] to make it possible to collect and return for educational use, any fees arising from the care of public ward patients who have made third party premium payments…It has been our conviction that such fees should not be retained for the personal use of the surgeons concerned" ("Report of the Surgeon-in-Chief" 1964).

Both outpatient visits and fractures treated increased; supported in part by an agreement in 1961 between the PBBH, the Beth Israel Hospital, and the town of Brookline "whereby [each hospital] would care for approximately half the patients that the police bring to the hospital as emergency cases" (McCord 1963). According to the 1964 Report of the Surgeon-in-Chief, "Orthopedics continued to grow...the Brigham is approaching twice the number of orthopedic admissions and questions recorded ten years ago." Dr. Banks remained as medical director of the division of orthopaedic surgery and senior associate in orthopaedic surgery under Dr. Green as visiting orthopaedic surgeon. Dr. Richard Eaton was added as a junior associate and Drs. Oh and Pappas as assistants.

Dr. John B. McGinty returned from military service in 1965 and joined the staff at Boston Children's Hospital and the PBBH as well as the West Roxbury VAMC where he was responsible for the orthopaedic service. By 1967, the surgical staff had grown significantly: 32 in 1940, 60 in 1950, and 117 in 1967. Dr. Moore raised the issue about whether the HMS faculty should establish a faculty group practice plan similar to those at the following clinics: Mayo, Cleveland, and Lahey. He took a six-month sabbatical to study academic faculty practice plans in the United States. At the time, there were three faculty group practices at the PBBH: the Surgical Associates, the Industrial Accident Clinic, and the Brigham Anesthesia Associates. Dr. Moore stated further that the purpose of the Surgical Associates was "to provide a mechanism for the receipt of medical insurance payments for patients cared for on the Residents' Service...obligated to distribute this income for teaching, research and academic enterprise" ("Report of the Surgeon-in-Chief" 1967).

On June 30, 1968, Dr. Green reached retirement age after about 40 years of service. Banks succeeded Green as chief of the orthopaedic division at the PBBH. He had "under the leadership of Dr. Green, carried a large share of the responsibilities for Brigham Orthopedics for many years" ("Report of the Surgeon-in-Chief" 1968). In addition to Dr. Banks as visiting surgeon, the staff consisted of Drs. Griffin, Hugenberger, Pappas, and Trott (associates); Drs. Bates, Manson, and McGinty (junior associates); and Drs. Michael A. Ashworth and Panos G. Panagakos (as assistants). That year, a podiatry service was started as well, including both inpatient and outpatient.

Orthopaedic admissions in 1969 increased to 781 from 693, fractures to 734 from 620, and 671 surgical procedures were performed. Improvements, initially under Banks' direction, included new office space, conference rooms, increased laboratory space, and additional staff. New assistants in surgery included Drs. Bierbaum, Bland, and Thomas. Robert Keller was a new junior associate. Grand rounds were changed to include a weekly fracture service and guest speakers were invited. In 1970, Banks resigned from the PBBH, accepting the position of professor and chairman of orthopaedics at Tufts University School of Medicine.

ROBERT BRECK BRIGHAM HOSPITAL

The Robert Breck Brigham Hospital (RBBH) opened its doors on April 1, 1914, a little more than a year after the PBBH admitted its first patients and just a few months before World War I erupted across Europe. It was initially named the Robert Breck Brigham Hospital for Incurables. Its origin story dates back to Robert Breck Brigham (1826–1900), who was born in Bakersfield, Vermont. At age 16, he shucked oysters in Peter Bent Brigham's (his uncle's) restaurant. He became a highly successful and innovative businessman in his own right and went on to found a restaurant and a hotel. When he died on January 2, 1900, he bequeathed a generous donation in his will toward the founding of the hospital (**Box 44.4**).

Box 44.4. Robert Breck Brigham's Life and Career

"Ten years [after he began work in his uncle's restaurant], Robert would establish a restaurant of his own [the] 'Brigham's Oyster Saloon' [and] start to build his future… 'The restaurant became famous for his lemon pies as well as its oysters. It was also the first restaurant (in Boston) to serve liquor with meals at the tables instead of at the bar. Brigham's competitors declared, and his friends admitted, that he had an eye for business – to the extent that he had discovered how to cut a pie into five quarters.'

"Robert Breck Brigham…lived simply. He spent his time in a small room over his restaurant…His social life was modest: he rarely traveled, was not interested in sports, and was not a member of any church or club…'His only foray into public life was to build the Hollis Street Theater, at which he maintained a private box'…[His] sister, Elizabeth Fay Brigham (1824–1909), who was to become an important benefactor of the hospital bearing her brother's name, came to live with him after he left an unhappy marriage with a young cousin.

"Robert Brigham's holdings expanded beyond the original restaurant. 'Brigham's Hotel' was added about 1882… Its location was a historical site. In 1636 [almost 250 years before the hotel was built] an elm tree [was planted and] in 1765…an effigy of a British Stamp Officer was hung from the elm, which came to be known as the Liberty Tree. The site is marked [today] in…Boston…on the corner of Washington and Essex Streets. When Robert Brigham was sixty-five, he sold the Brigham's Oyster Saloon, but he and his sister both continued to live over the restaurant and saved their money.

"While the foundation of his fortune was in the restaurant and hotel business, the bulk of Robert Brigham's fortune was in real estate—property valued at around three million dollars and all within a mile of his home…[Seeking] advice about disposing his estate after death [his lawyer's daughter and a] Associated Charities volunteer visitor, [suggested]… Having found it difficult to find proper places for the care of 'incurable' patients…that Mr. Brigham build them a hospital. Robert Breck Brigham died on January 2, 1900, at age 73. His will included bequests to relatives and friends and provisions…to numerous charitable institutions [and] directed that the balance…be set aside for the erection, equipment and maintenance of a hospital 'for the care and support and medical and surgical treatment of those citizens of Boston who are without necessary means of support, and incapable of obtaining a comfortable livelihood by reason of chronic or incurable diseases or prominent physical disability'…

"The Robert Breck Brigham Hospital for Incurables [RBBH] was formally chartered by the Commonwealth of Massachusetts on February 11, 1903, after the purchase of a ten acre site on top of Parker Hill…Parker Hill—once an enclave for prosperous settlers…was on the northern tip of the village of Roxbury…The neighborhood became known as Mission Hill in the 1920's…The Parker Hill population grew in the 1860s when German families settled at the base of the hill and built the first of many breweries there… Working-class Irish families soon moved into underdeveloped areas like Parker Hill…In the last years of the nineteenth century, a homogenous Irish Catholic community filled the…wood-frame tenements that were in the area… After 1910, the fields on the hill gradually disappeared in the wake of another building boom, during which new houses and more hospitals were constructed…A tuberculosis hospital was built adjacent to the reservoir on top of the hill in 1908…[Later] the reservoir was drained and the construction of the Robert Breck Brigham Hospital started"

(Liang 2013).

The first meeting of the hospital's board of trustees was held three years later on January 30, 1903. Bylaws or articles of the corporation were written, and election of officers was planned on February 7, 1903. Drs. Ernest W. Cushing, Robert B. Dixon, and J. Theodore Heard were elected to membership on the corporation, and, the following year, "Louis M. Spear was appointed the first physician-in-chief" (Liang 2013).

At the annual meeting of the corporation on January 14, 1907. Dr. Joel E. Goldthwait (see chapter 33) was elected a member. Also, a

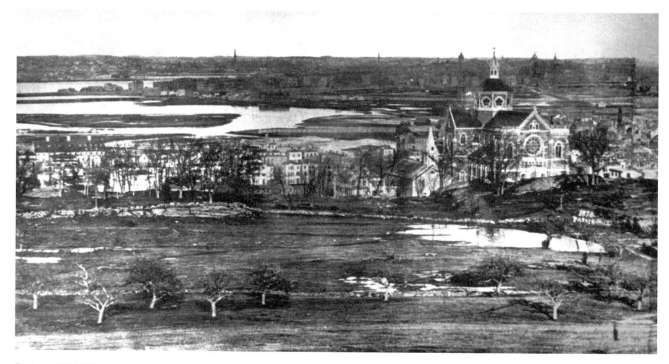

Parker Hill, 1878. *The Teaching Hospital: Brigham and Women's Hospital and the Evolution of Academic Medicine* by Peter V. Tishler, Christine Wenc, and Joseph Loscalzo. McGraw-Hill Education, 2014. Brigham and Women's Hospital Archives.

member of the hospital corporation was Robert Breck Brigham's sister, Elizabeth Fay Brigham who "until her death in 1909…'spent her last days devoting herself to the support of her brother's favorite charity.' Her will directed that $1.5 million of her estate be given to the Robert Breck Brigham Hospital" (Liang 2013).

In 1911, Dr. Goldthwait emphasized to the trustees at their annual meeting "the necessity of preceding at once with the construction of the buildings and of the pressing demand for such a hospital" ("Meetings of the Corporation" 1911). Typical of the early trustee's meetings, the agenda focused on planning, building the hospital and "consider[ing] the hospital organization including the medical staff, superintendent and head nurse; [and] general character of the cases to be admitted" ("Meetings of the Corporation" 1911). By 1912, there were 28 members of the board of trustees. Goldthwait was chairman of a committee of five (including four physicians) that reported to the board about the hospital's organization and the medical staff. He was also appointed to be on

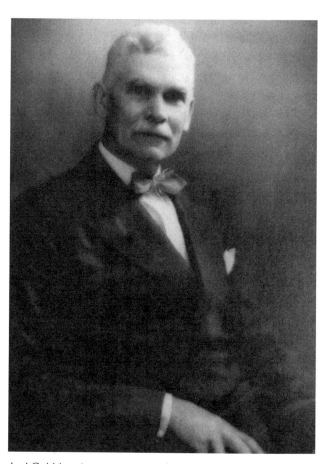

Joel Goldthwait. Brigham and Women's Hospital Archives.

Box 44.5. Dr. Joel E. Goldthwait's Influence on the RBBH's Philosophy of Care

"At the entrance to the Robert Breck Brigham Hospital there are two bronze tablets...On one...are the names of the [two] benefactors...On the other are excerpts from the will stating that the hospital was for the study and treatment of those people who were suffering from chronic disease...Charles Rosenberg (1987) noted that early twentieth-century hospital leaders were increasingly aware of the need to keep hospital care humane, partly due to growing criticism that such was not the case...At the Robert Breck Brigham Hospital, measures would be taken to prevent this [with] the impetus for these measures [coming] directly from the man largely responsible for the fledgling philosophy and goals of the institution—the orthopedic surgeon, Joel E. Goldthwait (1866–1961).

"...Physicians at the Robert Breck Brigham Hospital would espouse specialty care [at a time when most hospitals were general hospitals]. Not long after its founding, the hospital came to focus on [arthritis and] rheumatic disease.

"...At the turn of the century, no hospital in Boston had facilities for the care of the so-called 'crippled' and 'disabled' after the age of twelve. [Dr.] Goldthwait's concern for the continued care of these patients finally convinced leaders at the Carney Hospital in Dorchester to give him the use of a third-floor room where he started the first clinic for 'crippled' adults in America. Many of the patients seen in this clinic improved to the point where they returned to useful lives. When Goldthwait's work became known, the Massachusetts legislature voted $10,000 to support a clinic for the care of the adult 'cripple.' In 1899 Goldthwait organized and directed MGH's first orthopedic service...

"...Goldthwait became one of the original trustees of the Robert Breck Brigham Hospital Corporation—a group charged with the management of the hospital...formed before the construction...began...Goldthwait became president of the corporation in the early years of the hospital's existence"

(Liang 2013).

another subcommittee of the board to recommend individuals for the position of superintendent and head nurse. He would serve as a member of the board of trustees for about 53 years (1907–1961) and president of the board for 15 years (1916–1932) (**Box 44.5**).

The RBBH and World War I

By January 8, 1912, six physicians had been appointed to the staff of the soon-to-open RBBH. Of those early appointments, two were orthopaedic surgeons—Charles F. Painter and his assistant Lloyd T. Brown; "the primary emphasis of the hospital in its early years was orthopedic surgery, and orthopedists had primary responsibility for patient care" (Liang 2013). After the RBBH officially opened in 1914, Painter and Brown remained the only orthopaedic surgeons on the staff until 1918, when Robert Osgood (see chapter 19) was appointed to an advisory committee.

World War I began the same year that the RBBH admitted its first patient. While this external turmoil was unfolding, the hospital trustees were quickly realizing they did not have the funds to support the mission of the large hospital they had originally planned. Dr. Goldthwait noted that "this meant that the Robert Breck Brigham Hospital was forced to admit paying patients only a year after its opening" (Liang 2013). Goldthwait was elected president of the board of directors in 1916. During the war, even though he sometimes missed meetings while in Europe, he continued to be reelected. If in Washington, DC, he always returned to Boston for trustee meetings.

The financial troubles continued. By 1918, paying patients were assigned to the East Wing. Despite these difficulties, long-term patient "care from the physicians and orthopedists was set up in a coordinated fashion and each patient was under the purview of the entire staff and not divided among services...research also began at

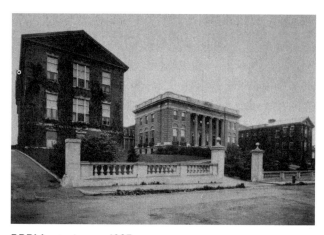

RBBH exterior, ca. 1927. Brigham and Women's Hospital Archives.

the hospital" (Liang 2013). During those first few years, Dr. Goldthwait also "pioneered a multidisciplinary treatment model at the Robert Breck Brigham Hospital to help patients become self-sufficient. The hospital had not only top surgeons and medical physicians, but also a social service department...and the first hospital-based 'industrial' or occupational therapy (OT) department in the country" (Liang 2013).

In the "summer of 1918 negotiations were entered with the Directors by Government officials looking to the taking over of the Hospital for the use of sick and wounded Soldiers to be returned from the front" ("Meetings of the Corporation" 1918) (see chapter 63). The directors signed a lease for $55,000 per year from October 1, 1918, until June 30, 1919. The hospital, however, had to move all their patients to other hospitals or "private houses" ("Meetings of the Corporation" 1918). For the next five years, the hospital:

> was leased by the government to care for the wounded and for those with diseases that resulted from the war...In many ways, the war was ultimately beneficial to the mission of the hospital. The war helped the hospital to survive financially...Goldthwait returned from the service eager...to put the Robert Breck Brigham Hospital on a more progressive course throughout the 1920s...In these years, the Robert Brigham was still primarily noted for orthopedics. Increasingly, the hospital received referrals from larger institutions like Boston City Hospital. (Liang 2013)

In 1919, the control of the hospital, which had been under the War Department during World War I, was transferred to the Treasury Department. Because of the large numbers of men injured in Europe and returning to the US for care, Goldthwait reported that "there is no definite idea of how long the Government may wish to hold the hospital [at $6,000 per month]" ("Meetings of the Corporation" 1920). That same year, to raise needed money, the board of directors sold some adjoining land: "the transfer of property to the New England Baptist has been carried through and $30,000 has been paid to us" ("Meetings of the Corporation" 1921). In his 1924 physician-in-chief's report, Dr. Spear stated:

> During the time that the government occupied the hospital, the work with the patients was more or less at a standstill except for the nursing care which they would be given. Since our return to the Robert Breck Brigham Hospital in June 1923, it has been possible to take up the active work of caring for and for studying the cases. ("Annual Reports" 1924)

Orthopaedics and Arthritis at the RBBH: 1913–1925

Treatment of the arthritic, damaged, or stiffened joint was difficult, almost impossible, in the early twentieth century. According to Liang (2013): "Even the more sophisticated practitioners in Boston did not know how to treat arthritis medically, and they often distained the 'quackery' associated with its treatment." In 1913, the year following Dr. Painter's appointment and before the hospital admitted its first patient, Dr. Osgood published a paper on the then state-of-the-art treatment of stiff joints (**Box 44.6**).

Box 44.6. Dr. Robert Osgood and "The End Results of Attempts to Mobilize Stiffened Joints"

"This report is made with some reluctance, because in the majority of cases the results of the attempts at the mobilization of stiffened joints which have been made by the writer have been far from satisfactory…no criticism is intended of the work of other men who have been more successful in their attempts…One of the maxims of surgery must be still, *Primum Non Nocere*. The report of failures which have resulted from at least considerate attempts may aid good judgment…

"In a recent [report in] the *Journal of the American Medical Association*…the writer…said 'in aggravated cases of post-rheumatic ankylosis in which there is osseous union it becomes necessary to resort to arthroplastic operations. When…correctly performed in a suitable case and the proper after-treatment is carried out, there is a reasonable assurance that the patient will have a freely movable joint, free from pain, and which will support weight and withstand traction'…There can be no doubt as to the impression given that arthroplasty is no longer in the experimental stage…such a report in our opinion may be productive of much harmful surgery. By personal observation and personal conversation…no such rosy prognosis is warranted… We urge as far as possible the concentration of these cases in the hands of a few men, preferably only one in a city, who will fit himself by study to be at least conversant with the most successful methods. The mobilization of stiffening joints peculiarly concerns orthopaedic surgeons, and the profession has a right to expect most careful consideration by them of a matter so important…

"The charts will outline quickly the scope of these operations. I have included two private patients of Dr. J.E. Goldthwaite's [sic] in which the unsuccessful operation was performed by the writer [Dr. Osgood] at his request; two cases of Dr. E.G. Brackett's, and one case of Dr. C.F. Painter's, operated on by them…We have used to prevent ankylosis recurring, either chromicized pig's bladder as recommended by Baer or pieces of free fascia removed from the fascia lata at the time of operation…in every case there has been a slight discharging sinus…In three cases the membrane itself, in whole or in part, has been extruded several weeks after the operation. In the cases where free fascial flaps have been used, the healing has been by first intention, and no sinuses have occurred…

"I confess the end results of some of the cases have given me pause. When we obtain a joint with useful motion persisting for six months and then gradually see this motion disappear, in spite of careful after-treatment, owing to joint sensitiveness and to soft part contractures, and when we may watch the overgrowth of bone about our seat of the operation continue for long periods, we owe it to our patients to explain these possible contingencies until we know how to surely prevent them…our prognosis should be most guarded as to painless or useful motion and as to function"

(Osgood 1913).

In 1917, Dr. Spear, the physician-in-chief, listed the types of cases admitted to the RBBH: spastic paralysis, muscular dystrophy, nephritis, pernicious anemia, and cardiac disease. By January 1918, he wrote: "The staff and the laboratory are still making one of their chief duties the study of arthritis" ("Annual Reports" 1918).

The change in the types of disease selected for admission and research at the RBBH was partially supported by a grant of $2,700 from the Goldthwait Research Fund. In 1915, Mrs. Ellen W. R. Goldthwait—along with two other beneficiaries—had donated $60,000 "to constitute a fund to be known as the "Joel and Ellen Goldthwait Research Fund…[and] the income therefrom to be used for research to increase the knowledge of chronic disease" ("Meetings of the BWH" 1915). The identity of Ellen Goldthwait is unclear in the historical records. She was not one of Dr. Joel Goldthwait's wives, a sister, or his mother. It's possible she was another relation. Her estate left the RBBH $50,000, and two other beneficiaries provided another $10,000. In addition to supporting

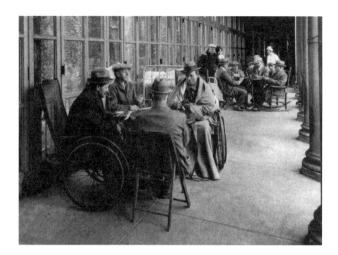

RBBH patients, ca. 1920s. Brigham and Women's Hospital Archives.

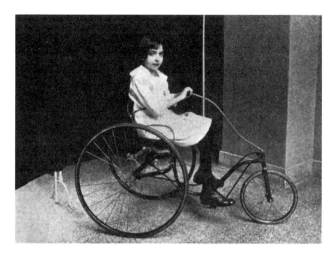

RBBH: Patient in physical therapy, ca. 1920s. Brigham and Women's Hospital Archives.

research, the fund was often used to help cover hospital deficits.

Dr. Goldthwait had also "realized the importance of allied health professionals in arthritis care" (Liang 2013). He understood the value even before serving during World War I, and after reentering:

> [in] civilian life, he was instrumental in establishing and nurturing these professionals, some of whom were studying in fledgling—now historic—schools such as the Boston School of Physical Education and the Boston School of Occupational Therapy…Goldthwait emphasized that treatment needed to go beyond surgery. He agreed with fellow Robert Breck Brigham Hospital surgeon Robert Osgood [who was on the courtesy staff in 1925], who noted: "Orthopedic surgery has a very large part to play in…conserving and restoring the function of the locomotive apparatus…providing the physical possibility…by which…cripples may become happy, productive, wage-earning citizens, instead of…idle derelicts." (Liang 2013)

By 1924, Dr. Loring T. Swaim was listed as orthopaedic surgeon, with Dr. Philip D. Wilson (see chapter 40) as consultant, and, by 1925, a courtesy staff was added. It numbered 27 members and included two orthopaedic surgeons, Drs. Charles Painter and Robert Osgood. A recently added new department of occupational therapy reported: "Many of our cases are arthritic and definite mechanical problems confront us" ("Annual Reports" 1924).

An Identity Crisis and Financial Difficulties

In 1924, the occupational therapy department treated an average of four new patients per month and an average of 52 patients per year. The 1925 physician-in-chief's report for the first time also included the types of cases admitted to the hospital with their outcomes (**Table 44.3**). Dr. Louis Spear, in his physician-in-chief's report also commented about a new trial:

> having a graduate physician [house officer] residing in the hospital…has demonstrated beyond doubt that we need a man who has had an all-round orthopedic training, who is particularly interested in chronic work and who can give at least half of his time to the hospital. This would relieve the staff of considerable routine work and enable them to use their time to somewhat better advantage. For some time now the practice has been in operation of having two fourth-year Harvard medical students living in the

Table 44.3. Conditions and Outcomes among Admitted Patients, 1925

	New patients (n)	Total patients (n)	Relieved (n)	Unrelieved (n)	Died (n)	Operations (n)
Arthritis						
Chronic infections	17	33	8	1	—	3 (1 capsulotomy; 1 femur osteotomy; 1 synovectomy)
Chronic atrophic arthritis	1	16	—	1	2	1 (1 elbow arthroplasty)
Hypertrophic arthritis	3	3	2	—	—	—
Marie-Strumpell disease	1	2	1	—	—	—
Still's disease	—	2	—	—	—	—
Tuberculosis						—
Ankle	1	1	—	—	1	1 (1 foot amputation)
Ilium	—	1	—	1	—	
Hip	1	2	—	—	—	2 (1 I&D; 1 hip arthrodesis)

Adapted from "Physician-in-Chief Report," 1925.

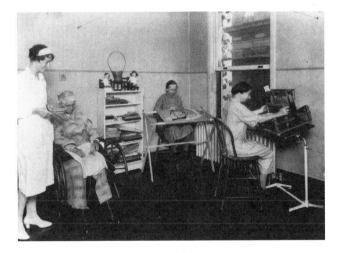

RBBH: Occupational therapy, 1923. Brigham and Women's Hospital Archives.

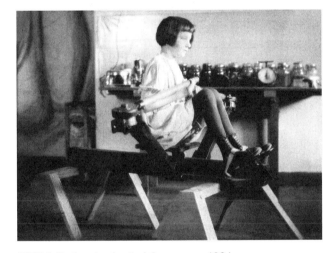

RBBH: Patient in physical therapy, ca. 1924.

The Teaching Hospital: Brigham and Women's Hospital and the Evolution of Academic Medicine by Peter V. Tishler, Christine Wenc, and Joseph Loscalzo. McGraw-Hill Education, 2014. Brigham and Women's Hospital Archives.

hospital and giving part of their time, who carry on the routine laboratory work, take histories, and do such other clinical work as the staff man may delegate to them. This has been very satisfactory both to the hospital and to the students.

("Physician-in-Chief Report" 1925)

By 1925, the RBBH faced a lawsuit (**Box 44.7**), and an "interpretation of Robert Breck Brigham's will" was contested in court (Liang 2013). The hospital leadership had already approved that a limited number of private patients could be admitted by the staff. However, the corporation, the board, and the staff had continued to clash over what the hospital's overarching mission should be and how best to serve the patients. The corporation's perspective included the belief:

that the Robert Breck Brigham Hospital should be a haven for humane custodial care.

Box 44.7. The Lawsuit: Determining the RBBH Could Treat Both Curable and Incurable Patients

"[T]he difference between the trustees and staff came to a head over whether or not the hospital could continue to admit curable and private patients. It had been charged that admission of these categories of individuals violated the will's terms. The Robert Breck Brigham Hospital staff predictably [argued] that the hospital was not a rest home, and that the sole admission of free [public] patients…would quickly bankrupt the hospital…Private patient admissions were also important to keep physicians on staff [needing] private practice for their financial survival…

"The court ruled that Robert Breck Brigham Hospital patients need not be destitute or 'incurable.' [The hospital's president] Hollis French…wrote about what the ruling meant for the institution: 'The decree…confirms us in our methods of managing the hospital…that applicants…need not be entirely destitute of all property…we might admit an applicant suffering from a chronic disease even if there were reasonable probability that…such person's condition might be alleviated. In other words, we are not obliged to confine our ministrations only to incurable cases'…

"After the court decision, the hospital came to be known as simply the Robert Breck Brigham Hospital, though the phrase 'for Incurables' was not legally dropped until 1954… The charity hospital that was started for 'incurable' would completely shift its ethos and basic character. From being a custodial, palliative warehouse for the infirmed, the Robert Brigham would fully embrace active treatment for rheumatic diseases, research into their root causes, and critical analysis of long-term results…

"Under the leadership of Dr. Joel E. Goldthwait, the hospital was changed from a chronic disease facility to a hospital actively involved in the care of patients with chronic bone and joint disease. This attracted patients with arthritic problems who had been neglected by the medical profession…"

(Liang 2013).

The alternative view [the staff's perspective] held that the hospital should embrace a more aggressive approach towards treating chronic illnesses, and toward actively restoring function and productivity even in patients for whom cure, or prevention of some disability was impossible. An additional discussion to the debate involved whether or not "private pay" patients should be admitted, or whether the hospital should be devoted exclusively to those who had no means to pay for their care. (Liang 2013)

The court determined the RBBH could treat both curable and incurable patients, or both private and public patients. The Robert Breck Brigham Hospital for Incurables did not officially remove "for Incurables" from its name until 1954.

After the lawsuit was resolved, the hospital's 1927 annual report provided more statistics for patients treated in the public and private wings (**Table 44.4**). The free ward beds remained fully occupied; 50% of requests were turned down because of lack of available beds. The RBBH had also become a major source for teaching Harvard medical students, residents at Boston Children's Hospital, and students from the Boston School of Physical Therapy and the Boston School of Occupational Therapy:

> The work of the Hospital is becoming better and better known throughout the city and the country in general…Also we are having visiting doctors from all parts of the country who…show a great deal of interest and enthusiasm…During these years of quiet working…the Hospital has convinced itself and any of those who know of its work that the problem of chronic disease is far from a hopeless one and that many of those conditions which have been thought hopeless are in fact hopeful. ("Report of the Superintendent" 1927)

Table 44.4. Outcomes among Treated Patients, 1926

Public wing	
Total patients	136
Total surgical procedures	18
Outcomes	
Discharged	
Relieved	50
Unrelieved	5
Died	6
Private wing	
Total patients	445
Total surgical procedures	228
Outcomes	
Discharged	—
Died	—

Data from the 1927 Report of the Superintendent.

Arthroplasties began to increase: 4 elbows, 2 knees, and 3 knee posterior capsulotomies. Dr. L. T. Brown had been elected to the board's executive committee; Dr. Swaim was the orthopaedic surgeon; Dr. Philip Wilson was orthopaedic consultant; and orthopaedic surgeons on the courtesy staff included: Drs. L. T. Brown, J. E. Goldthwait, R. B. Osgood, and C. Painter. In Dr. Spear's chief report (1927), he highlighted additional changes within orthopaedics:

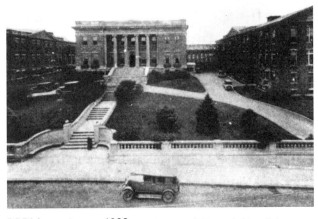

RBBH exterior, ca. 1928. Brigham and Women's Hospital Archives.

A special nurse has been engaged to take care of some of the detail Orthopedic work [to] relieve the Orthopedic physician of much of the routine work…A new departure in the hospital histories has been inaugurated. Routine photographs are now being taken of patients as they are admitted and at intervals during their stay…taken from the point of view of posture, pre-and-post-operative condition of special joints, and changes in condition resultant from Orthopedic means of correction of joint.

By December 1928, there was a total of 75 beds in the hospital for free patients. New orthopaedic additions to the courtesy staff included Dr. M. Smith-Petersen (see chapter 37) and Dr. William A. Rogers (see chapter 40). Dr. Sumner M. Roberts (see chapter 40) became assistant orthopaedic surgeon in 1929. The average length of stay was 7 months, 18 days. At the time, the average length of stay in an acute general hospital in Boston was 18 days. Outpatient clinics were held three days each week.

Despite growth, the hospital continued to have financial difficulties. It did not have enough funds from the endowment to cover the expenses of impoverished patients who required longer treatments. The president reported: "financially we had a very hard time…[the expected deficit was about $11,000] due entirely to the affairs of the Robert Brigham Estate" ("President's Report" 1929). The following year, Dr. John G. Kuhns joined Dr. Sumner M. Roberts as an assistant orthopaedic surgeon. Because of the continued deficit and lack of financial support from the Brigham estate, the president announced a new effort at fund raising.

Dr. Goldthwait was eventually succeeded as elected president of the corporation by Dr. Lloyd T. Brown, who had started a posture clinic with Goldthwait at the MGH (see chapter 46). Brown had previously been a member of the executive committee, chairman of the medical committee, and a member of the corporation (board of trustees) since 1927. In 1932, he helped steer the hospital through one of its most difficult periods while chairman of the medical committee. That year, during the stock market crash, "was undoubtedly the hardest one for any hospital during a very long period...It was during the past twelve months we learned from our new trustees that the Robert Brigham Estate was nearly insolvent and that we should certainly have to do without any income for several years...that loss of income might continue indefinitely" ("Corporation Records" 1934).

Finances continued to be problematic for the RBBH, as it had been and would continue to be for many years. Fundraising became a priority, starting with a campaign in 1934. Brown gave a speech at Copley Plaza about the Emergency Campaign of 1935, which was broadcast over the radio (**Box 44.8**). The Emergency Campaign failed to reach its goal that year, however. Only

Box 44.8. Dr. Lloyd T. Brown's Speech at Copley Plaza

> "We all know that Boston is well equipped with Hospitals to take care of the ordinary acute surgical and medical cases of the community. There are, however, very few hospitals which are properly equipped to take care of those suffering from chronic diseases. The Robert B. Brigham Hospital was founded for the care of cases of a chronic nature such as Arthritis, Heart Disease, Chorea, etc. In itw [sic] twenty years of experience it has shown that many sufferers from arthritis and other diseases considered incurable, not only can be cured but can also be made self-supporting. During 1934, out of 75 beds in the public wards it has been possible to keep full only 50 beds because of lack of funds…The work of the Robert B. Brigham Hospital…was helped to a great extent by the Emergency Campaign of 1934. If the campaign of 1935 is not a success the work of the hospital will have to be still further curtailed" ("Corporation Records" 1934).

$28,637.42 was raised. Importantly, in 1935, the hospital received no financial support from the Robert Breck Brigham estate; the income from the estate had stopped in 1931.

Orthopaedics and Arthritis at the RBBH: 1934–1939

In 1934, the RBBH had been receiving patients for 20 years. In that year, Dr. Robert Osgood published a book with Dr. Ralph Pemperton (professor of medicine at the University of Pennsylvania), *The Medical and Orthopaedic Management of Chronic Arthritis.* In the preface, the authors stated that orthopaedists shouldn't need to treat patients with arthritis because the condition is mainly a medical one. Because of the meager therapeutic options to treat arthritis and physicians' disinterest in and poor knowledge of the condition, orthopaedists had to step in after the disease has progressed. Surgery for the arthritic patient in 1934 included manipulation under anesthesia, aspiration, arthrotomies to remove loose bodies, synovectomy of the knee, posterior capsulotomy for knee contractures, osteotomies near joints (trans-and subtrochanteric for the hip), distal femur, distal radius or proximal row carpus, arthrodesis (especially for hip or ankle), arthroplasty (Jones pseudoarthrosis of the hip; use of fascia in the hip and elbow), and sympathectomy to improve local circulation.

By 1936, Dr. Louis Spear had resigned as physician-in-chief and was replaced by Dr. John G. Kuhns; Dr. Lloyd T. Brown remained president of the board of directors. In Kuhn's report of the medical committee in 1937, he noted there had been an increase in clinical services and teaching, not only including Harvard's students, but also students from Tufts Medical School. Students at the Boston School of Physical Education and the Boston School of Occupational Therapy trained at the RBBH.

Dr. William B. Elliston was appointed as assistant orthopaedic surgeon in 1939. Evening clinics were started that year and medical students from

Boston University now rotated at the RBBH. In his president's report, Dr. Brown stated, "for many years the President of the Board [Dr. Goldthwait], whose vision of more than twenty-five years ago was the incentive that started the present interest in the treatment of patients suffering from chronic disease…the most common disease and the one causing the greatest economic loss was chronic arthritis" ("Corporation Records" 1939).

> Since the disease affects all parts of the individual, to get the best results we must treat the whole individual, not only his body and mind but his soul…Evidence accumulates that physical health is closely related to spiritual health…Rheumatoid arthritis is no exception.
> —Loring T. Swaim, MD
> The President's Address, American Rheumatism Association, *Annals of Internal Medicine*, 1941; 19:118–121.

That same year, Dr. J. J. R. Duthie published on "The Sociological Aspects of the Treatment of Arthritis" in the US from a European perspective. Echoing Osgood's thoughts from five years earlier, Duthie noted that orthopaedists often treat patients with arthritis-induced deformities that could have been prevented or avoided. He described the process for treating such deformities at the RBBH, which incorporated collaboration between the orthopaedic surgeon and the treating physician along the entire continuum—from patient preparation before the surgery to in-home visits after discharge. For Duthie, this cooperation and continued involvement with the patient help explain the positive functional gains and outcomes patients treated at RBBH achieved.

Research was increasingly emphasized at the RBBH; both an intramural research committee and an extramural research council were formed in 1939 as well. Duthie lauded the "hospital's reputation as a leading institution for the care of those with rheumatic disease…in a report in the Annals of Rheumatic Diseases" He went on to describe: the collaborative approach to care that the hospital espoused, as well as, the innovative services arrived at supporting patients in the community [, and he] noted, "As a result of…close association of the physician and orthopaedic surgeon in the treatment of patients during and after their stay in the hospital, a surprisingly high proportion of cases of chronic arthritis return to active occupations and become wholly or partially self-supporting." (Liang 2013)

The RBBH and World War II

World War II began in 1939, but it wasn't until Pearl Harbor was bombed in 1941 that the US entered the conflict. That same year, Dr. Loring T. Swaim became chairman of the Medical Committee. Dr. Brown remained as president of the Board of Directors, but "the staff of the Robert Brigham was drained as younger staff…went into the armed services [at 5th General Hospital]. Senior physicians, including Louis Spear and Loring Swaim, stayed on to help run the hospital" (Liang 2013). Research efforts were stopped during this period in the hospital's history.

The orthopaedic cases were cared for by Dr. Swaim and Dr. Kuhns until Dr. Swaim eventually went to Europe. The volume of admissions continued to increase, even with the reduced staff, especially the nurses. In 1945, Dr. Brown wrote in his president's report: "[last year] has been the most difficult one in the history of the hospital" due to the lack of medical and nursing staff coupled with increasing demands of patients for admission and evaluations, which Brown felt was due to the increased knowledge and sophistication of patients. He went on to state: "In these days with the enormous number of wounded service men returning to this country (30,000 during the month of December) the problems of rehabilitation are staggering" ("Corporation Records" 1945). **Table 44.5** shows hospital statistics for 1945.

Table 44.5. RBBH Statistics, 1945

Admissions (n)	
Private	519
Public/ward	291
Mean length of stay (days)	
Private	21
Public/ward	101
Procedures (n)	
Operations	
Major	164
Minor	95
Plasters	764
Joint manipulations	115

Data from the 1946 Annual Meeting of the Corporation.

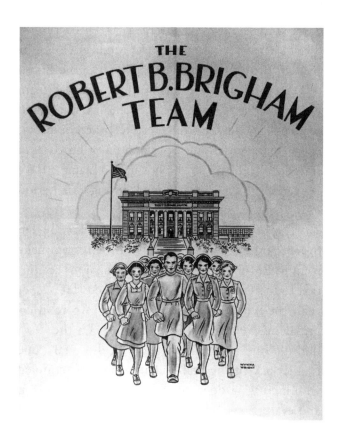

Drawing of the Robert B. Brigham Team of doctor, nurses and therapists.
Brigham and Women's Hospital Archives.

"The Robert B. Brigham Team"
When Jack and Jill come up to Parker Hill,
We greet them with a welcome and a will.
R.N.s, G.A.s, students on the beam!
Each doctor, supervisor, we're all a team!
We're out to put the nation on its feet,
And strengthen every pulse and every heart beat!
A wealth of new health is the gift we're out to bring;
So, if you're a patient, be patient, and we'll sing!
For we're the ROBERT B. BRIGHAM TEAM here together,
And there's no limit to all the things we can do.
Because, no matter how tough the job or the weather,
You can bet your sweet life we'll always come through!
So give a shout and a cheer for ROBERT B. BRIGHAM!
We've got a spirit here that's bound to see us through.
So, we'll work, and we'll fight!
We will work and fight as one!
For we're the ROBERT B. BRIGHAM Forever!
For we're THE WER!
—Words and Music by Richard H. Hadden.
Brigham and Women's Hospital Records, c 4,
Box 2, Folder 19 [1944]

The Post War Years and Continued Financial Difficulties

By 1946, some of the RBBH physicians were discharged from the military and returned to Boston and resumed their practices. For the next decade, President Brown would repeatedly report annually that costs usually exceeded revenues (**Box 44.9**), and in 1947—just two years after World War II ended—the hospital became affiliated with the Peter Bent Brigham Hospital (PBBH). The Hospital Council of Boston, in 1950, suggested that all patients (private or public) "should be charged the daily per capita cost of the hospital" ("Corporation Records" 1950).

Nevertheless, after affiliation with the PBBH, medical resident rotations were started at the

Peter Bent Brigham Hospital and Robert Breck Brigham Hospital

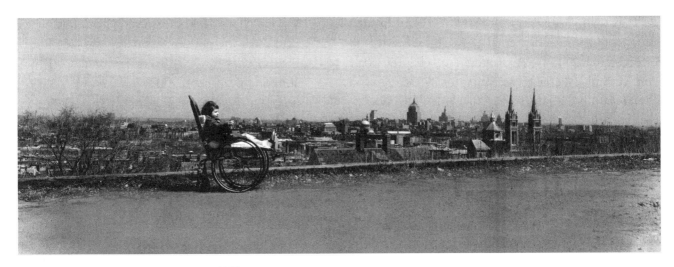

RBBH patient on top of Parker Hill, ca. 1950. Brigham and Women's Hospital Archives.

Box 44.9. Financial Difficulties: Hemmed in on All Sides

> "The financial problems of the hospital continued. In addition to operational shortfalls, the hospital faced costs associated with state-mandated improvements for the aging buildings [and] struggled to find sufficient numbers of trained personnel…In 1949…it had sold a strip of land [where] its residence housing for nurses stood, to the adjacent New England Baptist Hospital for the sum of $125,000…to build a new nurses' residence [but unable to] still accommodate the hospital's Training School for Attendant Nurses…the 1949 President [L.T. Brown]…noted…we have decided with deep regret, to give up our school when our present class graduates next Fall. By giving up the School, we will be able to build a much less expensive Nurses' Home'…In 1949 the RBBH which had received no income from the Brigham estate for eighteen years, was forced to pass on more of the operating costs to patients" (Liang 2013).

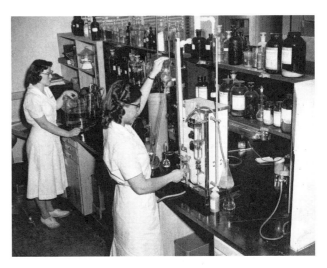

RBBH laboratory, ca. 1950. Brigham and Women's Hospital Archives.

RBBH which "proved very satisfactory" ("Corporation Records" 1948). Grand rounds were held every other Thursday morning, and "ward visits [were] conducted by an orthopedist and an internist, one each being assigned to each ward, for periods of three months…each week…they jointly consider[ed] patients who present[ed] combined problems" ("Corporation Records" 1949). Dr. Theodore A. Potter taught students from Boston University and Dr. John G. Kuhns taught Harvard medical students.

By 1951, Dr. L. T. Brown remained as president of the board, Potter was chairman of the medical staff, and Kuhns was chief of the orthopaedic service and visiting orthopedic surgeon. The orthopaedic visits increased to include Dr. William A. Elliston, Theodore A. Potter, Robert S. Hormell, and Joseph W. Copel. Dr. Loring Swaim was a senior staff member and John A. Reidy (see chapter 40) was a consultant orthopaedic surgeon. The orthopaedic courtesy staff consisted of Drs.

L. T. Brown, A.B. Ferguson Jr., J. E. Goldthwait, R. J. Joplin (see chapter 40), Robert H. Morris (see chapter 23), W. A. Rogers (see chapter 40), and M. Smith-Petersen (see chapter 37).

Dr. Brown retired as chairman of the board on January 15, 1952, after "twenty years of loyal and devoted service to the hospital" ("Annual Reports" 1952). He had been a member of the board for 35 years (1921–1956) and had served as president for twenty years (1932–1951). In April 1954, on the 40th anniversary of the opening of the hospital, newly inaugurated President Upton wrote:

> we continue to perform the functions of a specialized hospital and to play a major role in the treatment of rheumatoid arthritis and related chronic disease [but because of financial problems] the directors have recognized that to carry out literally the restricted purposes of the Robert B. Brigham will...is impracticable because of the failure of the financial provisions of Mr. Brigham's will [in addition to] the changes and advances in medical knowledge and practice particularly in the field in which the hospital has specialized. ("Meetings of the Corporation" 1954)

The directors filed a petition to the Massachusetts Supreme Judicial Court to approve a name change of the hospital (to officially drop the phrase "for Incurables" and to allow greater flexibility in choosing patients, i.e., to increase the number of private patients in the hospital. That year total expenses exceeded total revenue from operations by $37,401.61.

The term "for incurables" was legally dropped from the hospital name in 1954, and at the Board of Directors meeting it was approved:

> to adopt at the next meeting of the Corporation the change of purposes and change in name set forth in the decree of the Supreme Judicial Court entered October 22, 1953...to maintain and operate a hospital, with related out-patient services [for] patients suffering from any type of disease or physical disability...to admit to the hospital for treatment as many patients suffering from chronic disease, chronic disability or recurrent disease as may be treated on a wholly charitable basis with current funds available from all sources, with preference...to be given to citizens domiciled in the City of Boston and secondarily to citizens...served by United Community Service of Metropolitan Boston and...For all the foregoing purposes to hold, use and apply (i) all property of every nature now or hereafter owned by the Petitioner and received from the trusts under the wills of Robert B. Brigham and Elizabeth F. Brigham and all income received from paid property and said trusts, and (ii)...all income received...from any other source or from any other trust, now in existence or established in the future...That the name of the corporation be changed so as to be Robert B. Brigham Hospital. ("Meetings of the Corporation" 1954)

Leadership at the hospital continued to make changes to improve the bottom line. Later that fall, they started a private consultation clinic for patients with arthritis, staffed by internists and orthopaedic surgeons. They began to collaborate with the PBBH with the departments of radiology, pathology, and pharmacy. The chiefs of radiology and pathology were made consultants at the RBBH. Dr. Henry H. Banks was placed on the courtesy staff. They continued to draw from investment funds. The RBBH staff began to cover the wards of the West Roxbury Veterans Administration Hospital (WRVAH) with junior and senior assistant residents. Medical interns from the PBBH now rotated monthly at the RBBH to help care for patients and expand the patient volume. The medical interns were "mature enough [medically speaking] to run the wards without the direct supervision of a resident physician" ("Annual Reports" 1954). The professional fees were adjusted to the patients' ability to pay.

> I had enough wine but was not well enough to drink;
> My hand was stiff, I stopped playing my lute.
> Excerpt from an old Chinese poem which depicts the tragedy of "years without life." Cover, *1955 Annual Report*, Robert Breck Brigham Hospital

The consult clinic proved successful (fee for service), admissions from the specialty clinic increased, and Dr. Joel E. Goldthwait's Research Fund had a balance in 1954 of $123,724.10. Dr. Joel C. Goldthwait (Joel E. Goldthwait's grandson) applied for a large federal grant to support a new rehabilitation service. A clinical fellowship in medicine was started (one per year). The rehabilitation project was funded, and, in 1956, the hospital finally reported a gain from operations of $8,275 in 1955 (versus a deficit of $56,481 the previous year) and $15,882.22 in 1956. That year Dr. L. T. Brown resigned, Dr. J. E. Goldthwait remained on the board, and Dr. Thornton Brown (see chapter 40) was appointed as a member of the Corporation.

In 1957, Dr. J. Sidney Stillman, the chief of the medical staff, reminisced in his report about the following changes: in 1933 the average length of stay was 3 months, 8 days; now it was 21 days. In 1933, there was a fourth-year student house officer; now there were two student house officers, one resident physician and two graduate clinical fellows. In 1958, Dr. Potter became a member of the board of directors, and the annual meeting of the corporation included for the first time a report from the chief of medicine. He reported that the current staff consisted of ten visiting physicians and five visiting orthopaedists. In 1959, 13 interns from the PBBH rotated for four weeks at the RBBH. That year admissions had increased 12% and outpatient visits increased 14%. The consultation clinics had grown by 35% over the last five years. Yet the hospital was still in the red from operations by $15,591 because of increased operating costs. There was strong resistance against increasing patient charges:

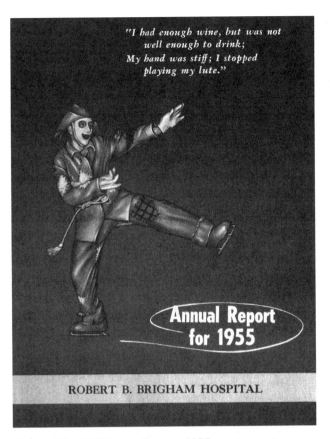

Cover of the RBBH annual report, 1955. Brigham and Women's Hospital Archives.

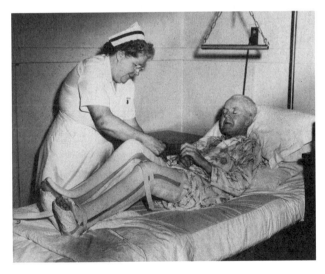

RBBH patient in bilateral, long-leg bivalved casts, 1960s. Brigham and Women's Hospital Archives.

"Already at a high level" ("Meetings of the Corporation" 1960).

That same year, Dr. Joel E. Goldthwait "made an unrestricted gift of $100,000 to the Hospital. [He had been president from 1916 to 1923] and

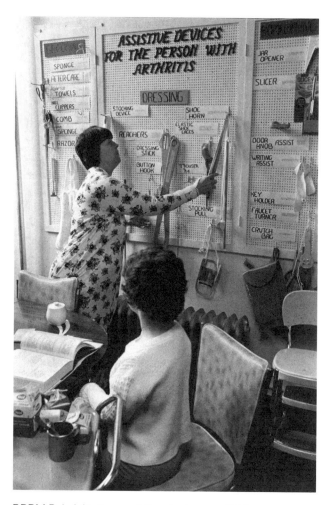

RBBH Rehabilitation: assistive devices, ca. 1960s. Brigham and Women's Hospital Archives.

the first time: "Drs. Theodore A. Potter and John G. Kuhns continue a constant review—and critical approval of the important part that orthopedic surgery plays in the rehabilitation of our patients" ("Meetings of the Corporation" 1960). At the time of Goldthwait's death in 1961, the average occupancy of the hospital was 60 patients.

Dr. Potter remained chairman of the medical committee. Dr. Edward Nalebuff joined the staff as a junior visiting surgeon. Other orthopaedic staff included Drs. Elliston and Hormell, as visits, and consultant, Dr. Reidy. Dr. Kuhns had submitted his resignation as chief of the orthopaedic service (held since 1939). The hospital was "barely in the black" ("Meetings of the Corporation" 1960); the first ever formal audit of the hospital's finances was ordered by the trustees. A major milestone for the hospital occurred that year; it was designated a "Clinical Research Center" by the National Institutes of Health (NIH), funded by a grant of $1,175,000.00. The research program was divided into five sections ("Director of Research Report" 1961):

1. Plasma proteins (studying abnormal proteins in R.A.)
2. Pathology and experimental pathology (inflammatory lesions in R.A.)
3. Cartilage and bone metabolism (biochemistry of cartilage protein polysaccharides)
4. Pharmacology and endocrinology (utilization of aspirin in R.A.)
5. Clinical facilities (orthopedic research on surgical approaches to repair and prevent damaged joints in arthritis

remained active in many capacities associated with the Hospital and its development" ("Corporation Records" 1959). The president's report of 1960 paid a tribute to Goldthwait: "The hospital in particular in its early years is in debt to Dr. Goldthwait for his inspiring leadership. Thereafter, his continued association with the affairs of the hospital and his great loyalty and conviction during its difficult periods have done much towards enabling us to reach our present status" ("Meetings of the Corporation" 1960). He died on January 15, 1961, and the corporation passed a resolution in his honor (**Box 44.10**).

In the previous year, Dr. Joseph Copel had resigned from the staff, and orthopaedic research had been mentioned in the president's report for

The orthopaedic research program was under the direction of Potter and included studying various prostheses, interposition membranes, and the use of plastics and metals in joint reconstruction. The clinical research ward could admit eight to ten patients. Goldthwait's grandson, Dr. J. C. Goldthwait, an internist, was largely responsible for obtaining the federal grant for rehabilitation, which began on July 1, 1961. The hospital

Box 44.10. Resolution Passed in Honor of Dr. Joel E. Goldthwait

Resolution relating to death of Dr. Joel E. Goldthwait

The following resolution was read by Mr. Wallace L. Pierce, Vice President:

"WHEREAS, the member of the corporation, the Medical Staff and the personnel of the Robert B. Brigham Hospital were saddened when on January 15, 1961 Dr. Joel E. Goldthwait died in our, or rather as some of us like to think, his hospital. We might find words to express our gratitude for the many financial and material things he gave to the hospital, but there are no words that could express what he did for the hospital by his ideals and vision.

"His long experience in the care of patients suffering from all kinds of chronic disease made him realize how little was being done for these badly neglected people. So when the opportunity came, he gave everything he had to improve their condition.

"About 1910 the Trustees of the Funds left by the wills of Robert B. Brigham and his sister Elizabeth F. Brigham felt that sufficient funds had accumulated so that they could proceed to carry out the provisions of the wills. In the lobby of the hospital there is a tablet showing in part what were their desires. When the Trustees had the plans for the hospital they looked around for a staff. Knowing that Dr. Goldthwait had been instrumental in starting the first adult Orthopaedic Clinic in Boston at the old Carney Hospital in South Boston, and that this had filled such a need in the city that the Massachusetts General Hospital asked him to start a similar clinic at their hospital, which he did with equal success, the Trustees asked him to help them select a staff for their proposed hospital. When he left the Carney, he selected Dr. Charles F. Painter, one of his associates, to take over the clinic. Dr. Painter later became the Chief of the Orthopaedic Department at the Robert B. Brigham Hospital.

"In Boston at this time the medical profession as a whole was not interested in chronic disease except as they had to take care of these patients, and since there was no place where proper care and study of their conditions could be found, Dr. Goldthwait persuaded the Trustees that they had a golden opportunity to provide such a place. There were very few medical men in Boston who had the temperament or the training to care for such patients, so the difficulty of finding such a doctor to become the Chief of the Medical Department was hard indeed to meet. However, they were fortunate in finding such a man in Dr. Louis Spear. With this as a beginning, it is not necessary to continue the story of the hospital. We know it survived two World Wars and that at the present time it is in a stronger position in the Medical World than ever before. It is recognized all over the world for its care, treatment, and research in the causes of chronic disease.

"WHEREAS, we have the satisfaction of knowing that the work of Dr. Goldthwait and his hospital was the forerunner of the interest that is not being taken by the medical profession in the care of the aged and all kinds of chronic disease, and

"WHEREAS, we as Corporators of this hospital are fortunate to have had so many years of advice and association with such a man as Dr. Joel E. Goldthwait,

"BE IT THEREFORE RESOLVED, that this expression of gratitude and appreciation by recorded in the minutes of this meeting and that copies of this resolution be tendered to the members of his family as an expression of the Hospital's great sense of loss and of it sympathy in their bereavement.

"Upon motion duly made and seconded, it was unanimously

"VOTED: That this resolution be adopted."

("Meetings of the Corporation" 1961)

(with 90 beds) now had two graduate fellowships, one sponsored by the NIH and the other by the Arthritis and Rheumatism Foundation. Junior medical residents from the PBBH continued to rotate at the RBBH as well as second year students from HMS and third year students from Boston University.

Dr. Lloyd T. Brown died in 1961; it was noted that "he was one of Dr. Goldthwait's group, came on the Board in 1921, was President of the Board from 1932 through 1951, and meant much in these halls and to our people" ("Meetings of the Corporation" 1961). A resolution for Brown was passed by the Board in December 1961.

Orthopaedic Advancements

In the chief of medicine's report in 1962, "the total number of patients treated in the clinic and wards more than tripled" ("Chief of Medicine's Report" 1962). Potter was elected to replace Kuhns as chief of the orthopaedic service that year; and he wrote the first report of the Chief of the Orthopedic Service (**Box 44.11**), which was included in both the hospital's Annual Reports and the Corporation Records.

In 1964, Dr. Thornton Brown (son of Dr. Lloyd T. Brown) remained a member of the board of trustees, but Dr. L. T. Swaim died early in the year: "He did much to guide our Robert Breck Hospital in its early years. We are grateful to his memory" ("Corporation Records" 1965). In his president's report, Howard Gambrill Jr. wrote: "We can point with pride to the orthopedic residency program conducted by Dr. Potter [3rd year orthopedic residents began rotating at the RBBH in 1963] in connection with the Children's Hospital and at the same time to the [now] Juvenile Arthritis Program [first patients admitted September 1963] under Drs. Stillman and [J. C.] Goldthwait" ("President's Report" 1964).

The orthopaedic residents rotated quarterly. The orthopaedic service benefitted from the addition of a fulltime anesthesiologist (Dr. James Krisher) from the PBBH, beginning September 1, 1965. In his chief's report, Dr. Potter stated: "the bulk of our work has been in the reconstructive procedures on the chronic arthritis individual" ("Report of the Chief of Orthopaedics" 1964).

There had been a two-fold increase in the volume of work since 1950. In 1964, there had been 302 orthopedic operations, 239 joint injections, 2,419 casts applied, and 29 joint manipulations. Orthopaedic involvement in the Clinical

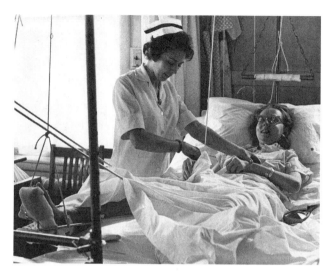

RBBH patient in balanced suspension, 1965. Brigham and Women's Hospital Archives.

Research Center included Potter's clinical series on the use of tibial plateau metal prostheses and with Nalebuff a study on prophylactic synovectomy in the hand; results of synovectomy of the knee by Dr. Weinfeld; Hormell's study of hallux valgus; and Dr. Elliston's early efforts at standardization of follow-up of hip arthroplasty cases. The next major orthopaedic advance at the RBBH in the treatment of arthritic patients was the metal spacer, which was an implant called the McKeever prothesis designed by Dr. Duncan McKeever. Used for knee arthroplasty by Potter in the 1960s, it was followed by metal and polyethylene total hip and total knee replacement and other joint replacements by Dr. Clement Sledge (see chapter 48) and colleagues in the 1970s.

Harvard medical students in their second year attended orthopaedic seminars at the RBBH; third-year Boston University students (three or four students) rotated on orthopaedics every two to four weeks and were offered a one-month orthopaedic elective at the RBBH in their fourth year. Dr. William T. Green had been added to the staff as a consultant in 1965, and, in 1967, Dr. William Thomas was named to the orthopaedic outpatient service. Two orthopaedic consultants were listed: Drs. Henry Banks and Kenneth Christophe.

Box 44.11. The First Report of the Chief of the Orthopedic Service

Report of the Orthopedic Service

Theodore A. Potter, M.D., Chief

"In April 1962, upon the retirement of Dr. John Kuhns as Chief of the orthopedic Service, I was asked to take up this post. At that time in the reorganization of the department, it was felt that new members should be added to the Service. Accordingly, three recently trained, qualified surgeons have been added to the staff. These are Drs. Edward Nalebuff, Ralph Bender and Marvin Weinfeld.

"These three physicians, with former members of our staff, Drs. Robert Hormell, William Elliston and myself, constitute the active orthopedic group in our hospital.

"In addition, we were very happy to offer an orthopedic fellowship for the year July 1962 through June 1963 and this has been ably filled by Dr. Rosario Tomaselli who came to us from the Rhode Island Hospital, having had five years of orthopedic training. While in our hospital, Dr. Tomaselli has performed a yeoman's service to the institution.

"Upon the retirement of Dr. Franklin Balach. Dr. Stewart Armstrong assumed the position as Chief consultant in General Surgery and he has been very active in this particular area.

"A year ago we were very distressed to learn that our anaesthesia coverage from the Boston Lying-in-Hospital suddenly terminated as of August 1962. However, we have been most fortunate in obtaining several free-lance anaesthetists, two of whom have been very faithful to our hospital. These are Drs. Frances Evans and Charles Hauck. It is hoped, however, in the near future that anaesthesia coverage from the Peter Bent Brigham Hospital anaesthesia department will service our hospital.

"Our Orthopedic Service has been very active in reconstructive work on the arthritic patients and patients with other musculo-skeletal diseases. There have been 232 major operations, 252 minor procedures. 190 joint injections, and 75 blood transfusions and numerous corrective plaster casts have been applied.

"This Orthopedic Service has been very active in orthopedic research problems during the past year. The major ones have been the anatomy of the rheumatoid deformities of the hand and that of the knee joint reconstructive procedures, using metal replacements. Improvement in surgical techniques in all phases of corrective surgery has gone on concomitant with other work.

"Papers in print are by Kuhns and Potter on "the Surgical Treatment of the Knee Joint of Chronic Arthritis." Scientific exhibits have been carried out across the breadth of the land and an exhibit on 'The Rheumatoid Foot" was presented in Nevada to the American Academy of General Practice. A cooperative exhibit with the Buffalo and New York groups was presented to the American Medical Association in June.

"At the annual meeting of the American Rheumatism Association members of our staff participated in a panel discussion on 'The Treatment of the Arthritic Knee.' This theme was carried out later in 1962 at the New Jersey Rheumatism Society and also at a postgraduate course at the New York University School of Medicine.

"As already mentioned, most members of our group were particularly active in the course that was presented at the Robert B. Brigham Hospital and which, incidentally, was very well received by the American College of Physicians participants.

"In the area of teaching most of our time has been consumed with the third-year medical students from Boston University School of Medicine. Eight students come to the hospital one day a week each month for orthopedic and surgical seminars. There is also a course offered to the class which is divided into two parts for a two-hour session. This is very similar to the course offered to the second-year Harvard students in pathology. Additional teaching has been carried out throughout the year for the residents, fellows, house officers and nurses.

"We have been asked to participate in a new elective course for the Boston University fourth-year students which will take place in the fall and winter of 1963-1964. This course will be attended by two or three students for an entire month and it is felt that this will be most instructive and stimulating, not only for the students but for the group who will be participating in this concerted effort.

"Our plans for the future are for expansion of services, particularly in the operating room. Preliminary discussions are being carried out at this moment relative to establishment of a recovery room and intensive postoperative care, relocation of the plaster room, acquisition of special instruments and safety devices in the operating room"

("Director of Research Report" 1962).

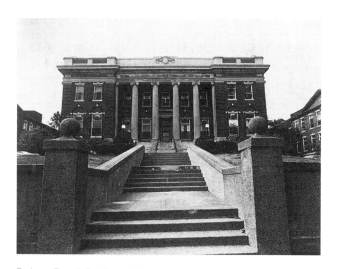

Robert Breck Brigham Hospital.
History of the Robert Breck Brigham Hospital for Incurables by Matthew H. Liang. The Brigham and Women's Hospital, Inc., 2013. Brigham and Women's Hospital Archives.

That year, Dr. Frank F. Austen, from the MGH, was named physician-in-chief. He brought his research team with him and the basic and clinical research program greatly expanded over the next few years. New laboratories were built. There were no more orthopaedic service chiefs' reports in the hospital's annual reports until orthopaedics became a department, only physician-in-chiefs' reports by Dr. Austen. In 1968, after spending a year on sabbatical studying rheumatoid hand surgery in Europe, Dr. Nalebuff returned to the RBBH and started the hospital's first-hand clinic.

In his 1968 physician-in-chief's report, Dr. Austen described the newly structured teaching service on two teaching units, Brigham East and Brigham West, each with 20 beds. Both units had service and private patients that were cared for by an assistant resident in medicine with visit coverage. The orthopaedic residents, from Boston Children's Hospital, or the post-doctoral fellow saw all other patients. Every patient was a teaching patient; private patients' care was supervised by the private physician, and service patients were supervised by the visiting physician/surgeon on service. The president in his 1969 report to the corporation noted the increase in full time faculty. "The growth of the hospital's pre-eminence in the field of rheumatic diseases has now reached a point where there is little doubt throughout the country as to our unique character" ("Corporation Records" 1969).

As a means to address its ubiquitous financial difficulties, the RBBH had previously begun discussions to merge with the PBBH and the Boston Hospital for Women. They had established the Affiliated Hospitals Center, Inc.—a charitable corporation—in 1961. By 1967, the hospitals had officially agreed to merge; but the negotiation process was exceedingly complex, and the hospitals would not officially complete the merger until 1980. (See chapter 47 for details on the merger and the ensuing organization of the new orthopaedic department. See chapter 50 for discussion of new growth and development in orthopaedics as a result of that merger).

CHAPTER 45

Robert Breck Brigham Hospital and Peter Bent Brigham Hospital

Orthopaedic Service Chiefs

The distinguished orthopaedic surgeons described in this chapter include those orthopaedic service chiefs who served at the Robert Breck Brigham Hospital (RBBH) 1912–1970 and the Peter Bent Brigham Hospital (PBBH) ca.1951–1970, before these two hospitals merged with the Boston Hospital for Women to form Brigham and Women's Hospital. The history of the RBBH is a history of the many challenges in treating severe chronic arthritis and, specifically, for the orthopaedic surgeon, it is the history of the many challenges in treating severe painful joint deformities, often damaged beyond repair, and stiff joints. The following orthopaedic chiefs, along with their medical colleagues, were largely responsible for a cooperative management program and its numerous successes during the rapidly changing field of arthroplasty over the 65 years of the RBBH's existence. Dr. Henry H. Banks, as the orthopaedic chief at the PBBH, advanced the understanding of the pathophysiology and treatment of hip fractures and other intra-articular fractures as well as pathologic fractures.

Dr. Clement Sledge served as the first full-time professor of orthopaedic surgery at the RBBH and PBBH; he was also surgeon-in-chief at the RBBH and orthopaedic surgeon-in-chief at the PBBH from 1970–1980 (see chapter 48). Orthopaedic surgery became a department at Brigham and Women's Hospital in 1980 (see chapter 47). The orthopaedic service chiefs covered in this chapter include:

Charles F. Painter	44
Loring T. Swaim	51
John G. Kuhns	59
Theodore A. Potter	67
Henry H. Banks	72

ROBERT BRECK BRIGHAM HOSPITAL

CHARLES F. PAINTER

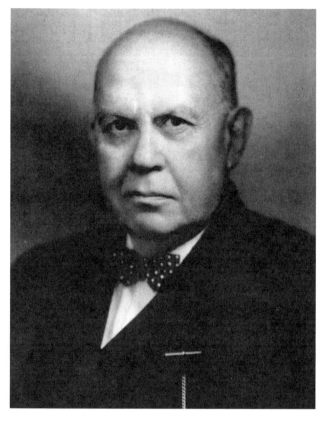

Charles F. Painter. "Charles Fairbank Painter 1869-1947," *Journal of Bone and Joint Surgery, 1947*; 29: 541.

Physician Snapshot

Charles F. Painter

BORN: 1869

DIED: 1947

SIGNIFICANT CONTRIBUTIONS: First chief orthopaedic surgeon at the Robert Breck Brigham Hospital (ca. 1912–1917); chief of the service at Carney Hospital 1902–1913; coauthor with Drs. Joel Goldthwait and Robert Osgood on the book *Diseases of the Bones and Joints: Clinical Studies* (1909); served as orthopaedic surgeon to the Chelsea Naval Hospital during World War I; president of the American Orthopaedic Association (1916); dean at Tufts Medical School (1913–1922); acting editor the *Journal of Bone and Joint Surgery* (*JBJS*) (1943)

Charles Fairbank Painter was born in Grand Haven, Michigan, in 1869. He was "descended from an old Virginia family [and was] the son of a clergyman. He went to school in Great Barrington, Massachusetts" ("Obituary. Charles Fairbank Painter" 1947). He attended Williams College for a year before continuing his undergraduate education at Johns Hopkins and receiving an AB degree in 1891. He graduated from Harvard Medical School (HMS) four years later in 1895 "with such men as…Amory Codman and Harvey Cushing" ("Obituary. Charles Fairbank Painter" 1947).

After graduation, he was a surgical house officer at Massachusetts General Hospital (MGH) for one year (1895–1896). After spending two years in general practice, he began to specialize in orthopaedic surgery and was mentored by Dr. Joel E. Goldthwait (see chapter 33). At the end of 1896, "he received the appointment as surgeon at the House of the Good Samaritan and two years later…was acting as Assistant Orthopedic surgeon at the Carney Hospital" ("Dr. Painter Named Dean of Tufts Medical School" 1913). Painter was appointed the first instructor in the Division of Orthopedic Surgery at Tufts in 1897; he taught simultaneously at HMS. He published his first paper shortly thereafter in 1898—titled "Inflammation of the Post-calcaneal Bursa Associated With Exostosis." This paper:

> reflect[ed] the thinking of the time…Perhaps owing to the radiographic appearance of exostosis, Painter, directed his attention to that feature…[x-rays were discovered the year he graduated from medical school]…there was great confusion at the time, so it is not surprising Painter focused on the obvious: the calcaneal exostoses that result from longstanding inflammation of the Achilles tendon. (Brand 2008)

Dr. Painter eventually became a professor and chairman of the division at Tufts, when he became chief of the service at Carney Hospital in 1902 following Dr. Goldthwait's retirement. Medical students at Tufts received their clinical instruction there, and the Carney Hospital had:

> the oldest mixed [orthopaedic] clinic of its kind in Boston; it was established by Dr. J.E. Goldthwait and was until recently under the charge of Dr. C.F. Painter. Dr. MacAusland is now surgeon-in-chief. [MacAusland] has interested himself particularly in the operative treatment of fractures, using bone plates as his means of fixation. He believes in the deliberate removal of the plate in most cases after a few months. I [Sir Henry Platt] was privileged to see a good deal of the work of Goldthwait and Painter in their private clinics. The former has now relinquished his hospital appointments and the latter will shortly take over the orthopedic service of a new hospital for the treatment of chronic diseases only [RBBH] which has been built on a hill on the outskirts of Boston.
> (Platt 1914)

Painter would go on to publish about 70 articles throughout his career; he also edited one book and, in 1909, was coauthor with Drs. Goldthwait and Osgood on another, *Diseases of the Bones and Joints: Clinical Studies.* In a paper he published the same year, "Myositis Ossificans," he described the condition, and he stated, "it is likely to be a long time before the medical profession will be in a position to offer the sufferer from myositis ossificans any material aid" (Brand 2008).

At the annual meeting of the board of directors of the newly organizing Robert Breck Brigham Hospital (RBBH) on January 8, 1912, Dr. Goldthwait was elected chairman of a committee of five to evaluate hiring potential hospital staff. On March 5, 1912, he presented his committee's report to the trustees, recommending six physicians be appointed to the staff, including Dr. Charles F. Painter as orthopaedic surgeon (eventually appointed the chief of the service that same year) and Dr. Lloyd T. Brown (Dr. Painter's request) as assistant orthopaedic surgeon. Dr. Louis M. Spear was appointed physician-in-chief with a salary of $3,000 and Dr. Painter was given a salary of $500. Six house officers were also approved by the trustees. At this time, there was no surgeon-in-chief or orthopaedic surgeon-in-chief appointment.

The following year, 11 years after his promotion to chief at Carney Hospital, Painter left Carney to join MGH in addition to RBBH. He retained his affiliation with Tufts and was named dean of the medical school that same year. A pivotal year, he also published "The Development of Orthopedic Teaching in America" in 1913. In this article, he wrote about the basic foundation for the development of the specialty of orthopaedic surgery:

> A desire to solve some of the problems presented by chronic disease has been the fundamental incentive…the establishment of courses of instruction in a few of our medical schools has been instrumental in bringing about the present results…those who have been engaged at the outset of this…propaganda to further the cause the most, particularly those who were instrumental in gaining…specialty recognition on the medical facilities. The best evidence… of the value of [these] courses…is the fact that only one or two subjects in which electives are offered in the Harvard Medical School are more popular than the elective in orthopaedics.
>
> The prime reason for the advance of specialization…was not to shirk the responsibilities of general practice or to amass a fortune speedily through the charging of the larger fees… but the earnest hope that something might be added to the sum of knowledge in a particular subject…Another fact significant of the growth of interest…of the specialty is that between the years 1825 and 1860 there were only 172 titles in medical literature on orthopedic subjects. In the years 1889-1900 there was compiled a list of 583 titles on orthopaedic subjects and this was without doubt incomplete [but it wasn't]

until…the International Congress of Physician and Surgeons in 1900 formally acknowledged the existence of such a specialty that the schools generally offered systematic courses… From that time on…schools of this country, one after another, created [teaching] positions… for the instruction of students. An influence… was the fact that several institutions have been founded for the treatment of cripples…

The stigmen [sic] of "harness makers" and other similar terms indicated that at first the surgical management of the diseases… being treated was not to be undertaken by those practicing orthopedic surgery and even by those practicing the specialty there have been differences of opinion on this score and at times the practice has been predominantly mechanical and at other times predominately operative…[one] must be competent technically as a surgeon and also must possess, for the greatest success, the temperament for handling chronic diseases and considerable appreciation of mechanical problems…It is our duty in inculcate in our students the necessity of never abandoning a fight against chronic difficulties until the last gun has been fired…

Together with many others it was my privilege to be initiated into the study of orthopedic surgery at the time that the specialty was getting on its feet and systematic instruction was just beginning in most of our larger schools… One could not work with those early engaged in developing orthopedics as a specialty without being fired by their inspiration and it is the pleasure as well as the privilege of all who had the advantage of such personal contact to pay what tribute they may to the sources from which they received their incentive. (Painter 1913)

There is almost no information about Dr. Painter's activities as chief of the orthopaedic service at the RBBH. His salary was increased by $125.00 in 1916. The hospital had "opened for indigents with chronic incurable diseases or permanent disabilities" ("Robert Beck Brigham Hospital as a Regional Resource" 1914)—more than 50% of whom had arthritis or rheumatic disease. While chief of the orthopaedic service at the RBBH, Dr. Painter was also a member of the editorial committee of the American Orthopaedic Association (1908–1914), and he "gave freely of his time and interest to *The Journal*, the publication of which was then the function of that Committee" ("Obituary. Charles Fairbank Painter" 1947).

In 1916, he became president of the American Orthopaedic Association. In his presidential address (**Box 45.1**), he argued for major changes in the organization:

[T]hose who possessed mechanical ingenuity in devising and adjusting apparatus, and patience and resourcefulness in managing chronic patients became known as Orthopedic Surgeons…therefore qualified to handle chronic bone and joint diseases better than the general surgeons [but] through the thirty years of existence of this Association the pendulum has been swinging back and forth between these two extremes [mechanotherapist versus operative surgeon]…Latterly certain conditions have been added to the realm of orthopedics which have been purloined from the field of the internist, viz: non-tuberculous arthritis, largely because it is so essentially chronic that its best management is secured through the medium of men accustomed to deal with chronic processes…the time has come…when the good resulting from the development of specialization must be winnowed from the bad effects which follow in its wake…the occasion has arisen for this Association to take cognizance of this fact and make its organization effective toward the adjustment of specialization to the new demands which are bound…to be made upon it…We should go further [and] must institute and foster more collective investigations [and] standardize the teaching of orthopedic surgery in our various schools…

I am convinced that as an Association we have striven too long to promote the individual interests of the Association members...an object [that] has ceased to be a vitalizing influence in this organization. It is time to change our policy, it seems to me. We must have a little different organization to make any new policies decided upon effective...Instead of electing your president to serve for one year and act merely as a presiding officer at the [annual] meeting...I believe...the following [plan] would work well. As it is now, every member is slated to become your president, if he lives long enough. There is no incentive to shape any policy...on the part of either the President or the Executive Committee...I believe that dignity of the office could be enhanced and the purposes as above outline could be brought to fruition, if there were a president-elected chosen the year before he is to serve, and if the executive committee were not made up entirely of ex-presidents, but was, partly at least, composed of future presidential timber. With such an organization, some consistent policy might be originated and carried out through a series of years and not be at most a "flash in the pan" at the end of one administration. (Painter 1916)

During World War I, Painter served as orthopaedic surgeon to the Chelsea Naval Hospital. By 1918, after the war, the RBBH was devoting its entire effort toward treating rheumatic diseases. Clinical growth continued to increase with the ambulatory center seeing more than 10,000 patients per year. Specialty clinics were started in juvenile rheumatoid arthritis, immunological diseases, systemic lupus erythematosus, and hand surgery. Eventually there were 15 rheumatologists on the staff and six orthopaedic surgeons. Clinical research was growing. In addition to 24 medical residents from the PBBH, 16 surgical residents and 8 fellows were trained each year. Admissions to the hospital numbered greater than 1,900 per year. Staff were consultants at the PBBH, Beth Israel Hospital (BIH), New England Baptist Hospital (NEBH), Boston City Hospital, Cambridge City Hospital, and the West Roxbury Veterans

Box 45.1. The Orthopaedic Surgeon Versus the Orthopaedic Physician

> For most of the twentieth century, leaders in orthopaedic surgery have discussed and debated the role of an orthopaedic surgeon versus that of an orthopaedic physician. Dr. Charles Painter was no stranger to this debate.
>
> In 1916, "[he] observed [in his AOA presidential address] that orthopaedists had become 'infected with the virus of operative furor.' In 1931, Willis C. Campbell declared, 'Many of the problems are often more medical than surgical. Operative technique is of less consequence, as this can always be acquired by experience!' In 1933, Arthur Steindler declared that the term orthopaedic surgeon was inadequate and that we should be called orthopaedic physicians. Joel E. Goldthwait...in the Robert Jones lecture of 1933 stated: 'In our special line of work, with the great interest in the operative side of the work, with its general indifference to the non-operative...one can but wonder if the basic ideals which justify our work have not been lost sight of. If we are to see only the operation...we cease to be true orthopaedic surgeons, but just surgeons doing bone and joint work...if we choose operative work only, which is the easier, instead of the harder and more general, some other specialty or school will take this over.' In 1948, R. I. Harris predicted: 'The future of orthopaedic surgery will be intimately concerned with the broadening of the structure and function [through basic sciences] of the tissues with which we deal...We shall not retain mastery of our field if we limit ourselves to operative therapy and depend upon others for the fundamental knowledge upon which rational therapy can be based'...In 1954, president [AOA] Alfred R. Shands, Jr. declared, 'We should ask ourselves seriously whether we are not giving too much attention in our training and teaching to the surgical procedures of our specialty and thereby risking a problematical existence in the future'" (Lipscomb 1975).

Administration Hospital. It is unclear whether Painter had continued as chief during this period; the date he resigned as chief of staff of the orthopaedic service at the RBBH is not known. Dr. Loring T. Swaim may have been appointed the second chief of orthopaedics in 1917, but Swaim was listed as chief orthopaedic surgeon in the hospital's annual report in 1924 so Painter may have continued as chief past 1917.

Dr. Painter continued to publish, and the cases he reported were seen in the orthopaedic clinic of the Boston Dispensary, Carney Hospital, and other hospitals. At the Boston Dispensary, he had previously reported cases in a paper on inflammation of the calcaneal bursa and exostosis. **Case 45.1** is an example of one of his case reports from 1919, documented while serving at the Chelsea Naval Hospital during World War I. He served as the fourth dean of Tufts Medical School for eight years until 1922, and he maintained his academic appointment until 1924. He remained in private practice with staff privileges at the Beth Israel Hospital, the House of the Good Samaritan, the Massachusetts Women's Hospital, and Brockton Hospital.

Case 45.1. Internal Derangement of Knee-Joints

"S.P.G. U.S.M.C. 27 years. Christmas Day, December 25, 1916. In practicing high jumping he fell on the left knee, striking on the side, with the leg in a position of flexion. Had to be picked up and carried to quarters. Leg could not be completely extended for three months. There was much swelling and pain with tenderness over the inner aspect of the left knee.

"He remained in bed with knee bandaged for four days, and was then returned to duty on December 30, 1916, with diagnosis of sprain. On January 6, 1917, reported again to 'sick bay' because of synovitis and pain in knee. Then was transferred to hospital where the diagnosis of synovitis was continued. He was kept in bed ten days where he was given exercises and massage. On January 17, 1917, there was limitation in motion in flexion of the knee. On the 28th there was still some swelling and disability. On March 9, 1917, it is recorded that he was 'exercising freely without marked discomfort.' He was discharged to duty on this date.

"From that time to November 18, 1918, no mention in his health record of any further trouble with the knee-joint, though the patient says that after March, 1917, when the hospital discharged him to duty with a diagnosis of sprain of the knee, that there had been about a dozen occasions when there had been a slip in the joint accompanied by pain, swelling, and limitation in motion. In the above mentioned interval he had had the diagnosis of mumps, urethritis, influenza, and chronic articular rheumatism.

"On the third of March, 1919, he had a displacement of something in the left knee-joint, which was accompanied by effusion and pain. At that time he stated that from time to time this had occurred during the previous three or four months, with comparatively little provocation. He could do no bayonet drill without causing a slipping of the cartilage.

"On the 12th of March I had opportunity to examine this man's knee. He stated that there had been recently three or four slips of the same sort that he had been having before. There was a moderate effusion: tenderness over the inner meniscus of the left semilunar and a palpable mass to be felt filling up the sulcus between the tibia and the femur. Forced extension and flexion are slightly painful. Calf and thigh show slight atrophy.

"In view of the history and physical signs, it seems certain that this man's semilunar cartilage had been displaced on Christmas Day, 1916, but the diagnosis has been carried as 'synovitis' or a 'sprain,' so far as the knee-joint lesion was concerned, ever since…

"The operative removal of this is the only method of treatment that gives permanent relief. The bursa should be dissected out and tied off from the knee-joint. Care should be used in the dissection because the external popliteal nerve is close to the head of the fibula and the biceps tendon; it has been injured in this operation with a troublesome peroneal paralysis."

(Painter 1919)

Dr. Painter gave the annual discourse before the Massachusetts Medical Society in 1926, 16 years after Flexner published his report. Painter spoke about medical education, "Educational Requirements for Twentieth Century Practice: Who Should Determine Them, and How May They Best be Achieved" (**Box 45.2**). He stated:

> We have recently been righteously indignant because certain institutions, licensed to grant degrees in medicine have been guilty of exercising this right without reference to the

Title of Painter's Annual Discourse of the Massachusetts Medical Society in which he discussed educational requirements for physicians in the twentieth century.
Boston Medical and Surgical Journal 1926; 194: 1057.

Box 45.2. Excerpt from "Educational Requirements for Twentieth Century Practice: Who Should Determine Them, and How May They Best be Achieved"

Painter emphasized:

"[T]he importance of research in the medical curriculum. No one deny....that discipline in the methods of the scientific approach to the solution of medical problems is 'desirable for all medical students...The man with the right balance between art and science...consists of two things, point of view and time to think...We are turning out...a body of graduates with perhaps a greater store of information then was possessed by graduates of twenty years ago but with no greater ability to make use of this knowledge, if as much, and with scarcely any incentive to culture in its broad sense...From the day he enters the medical school until he leaves, the time is fully occupied...I am confident [that time could be saved by] restoration of much of the subject matter taken away from medicine and surgery and allotted to special departments [as well as] material reduction in the time allotted to undergraduate teaching in throat, nose, ear, eye, orthopaedic surgery and other subjects...[to] provide time for...clinical work, preferably in dispensaries...and also for free time to read and think... The pedagogic value of research as an undergraduate education method...in teaching medical students, has not as yet been demonstrated, whatever its graduate educational importance may be...

"Before passing on to a consideration of who shall determine the requirements of medical training, it may be well to refer to one of the chief reasons that the medical profession should interest itself in this subject. The growing popularity of cultists is not based on the successes of their particular procedures...but rather the blind faith that a very considerable portion of humanity are constitutionally disposed to place in anyone who makes the more extravagant claims of what he is able to do. The high cost of being sick in this day when the doctor calls for all sorts of special examinations and consultations which have to be paid for outside his personal fee...have driven many a heretofore perfectly satisfied patient into the hands of the cultist [who] has no need for such examinations and tests...For such an individual it is easy to promise far more than the conscience of an intelligent and well trained physician will permit him to promise...The patient reasons that, economically, the cultist is his best buy for relatively the difference in the results may be very slight. Whoever, therefore, is responsible for introducing into practice the cost-raising features which lead to the division of patients to quacks and cultists, without contributing a commensurate practical advantage to the sufferer in a percentage of cases whose such service is necessary (10–20%), can be credited with being the cause for the present situation in the practice of medicine...that the weight of the evidence lays this at the doors of the medical schools and those regulative bodies to whose advice the school authorities have listened."

(Painter 1926)

qualifications of the applicant...this has been done in the case of one or more such institutions...for a fee amounting to...the annual tuition in many of our medical schools without regard to the previous general education of the candidate, his moral character or his professional attainments...In our own state...we are...one of only three or four commonwealths where it is legally possible for practitioners of this class to settle...[Adam] Smith said no harm would come to the state from the irregular practitioners and opposed an investigation of the methods of the schools. Flexner, very properly pointing out defects in the system, set in motion correction machinery which has been so drastic in its effect that it is difficult to keep in control. (Painter 1926)

Painter referred to Dr. Frederick C. Waite's publications on fraudulent medical diplomas and licensing of graduates of inadequate medical schools. Two were in Massachusetts: the College of Physicians and Surgeons, in Boston, and the Middlesex College of Medicine and Surgery, in Cambridge. Neither was recognized by most state licensing boards and eventually closed. Dr. Painter argued for improved standards of medical education; increasing the number of properly educated physicians to meet community needs, especially general practitioners and supply more physicians for rural areas; the need to increase clinical skills and minimize the use of special tests, especially regarding therapeutics. He noted, "The graduated student in these days has his bag packed full of tricks; his mind is like the pocket of a boy's pants—so full of things, he can't find the bit of string he wants" (Painter 1926).

Painter continued to contribute to the literature, and he wrote "many articles of a scientific nature, including 'The Uses and Limitations of Vaccine Therapy in the Management of Arthritis[,]' 'Prognosis in Chronic Arthritis'[and,] 'Surgery Treatment of Arthritis of Infectious Origin.'"

("Dr. Painter Named Dean of Tufts Medical School" 1913). From 1937 to 1944, he was a member of the Board of Associate Editors; and for seven months, following the death of Dr. Murray S. Danforth in June 1943, he served as acting editor of the *Journal of Bone and Joint Surgery*. During all these years, he contributed richly to the growth and development of the journal, both in the editorial work and later as administration and councilor:

> Besides all these activities, he became Librarian of the Boston Medical Library, a position he held for eight years. In 1940 he assumed the editorship of the Year Book of Industrial and Orthopedic Surgery, which became valuable as a critical review of each year's important literature on these subjects. His choice of subjects for review, cleverness of expression, fair and judicial comments on the new controversial reports were of great value, coming as they did from one who had had so many years of contemplative and surgical experience. ("Obituary. Charles Fairbank Painter" 1947)

Box 45.3. Charles Painter's Professional Memberships

Member

- American Orthopaedic Association
- American Medical Association
- Massachusetts Medical Society
- American Academy of Orthopaedic Surgeons
- General Committee of the Nutritional Clinics for Delicate Children
- Boston Orthopedic Club
- Other
- President, American Orthopaedic Association, 1916
- Fellow, American College of Surgeons
- President, Boston Orthopedic Club (1929)

Robert Breck Brigham Hospital and Peter Bent Brigham Hospital

For many years, Dr. Charles Painter was a member of the Medical Committee of the Industrial School for Crippled and Deformed Children. He was also an active member of various clubs and associations (**Box 45.3**). He died on January 6, 1947, at around age 78. Upon his death, the *Journal of Bone and Joint Surgery* honored him in its April 1947 issue: "As a person he was delightful, —modest, with a strong ease of humor, one who was a good companion and full of common sense…Orthopaedic Surgery has lost a great scholar.'"

LORING T. SWAIM

> **Physician Snapshot**
>
> Loring T. Swaim
> BORN: 1882
> DIED: 1964
> SIGNIFICANT CONTRIBUTIONS: Chief orthopaedic surgeon at the Robert Breck Brigham Hospital (ca. 1917–1938); cofounder of the American Rheumatism Association and president in 1942; published *Arthritis, Medicine and the Spiritual Laws* (1962)

Loring Tiffany Swaim, the son of Joseph Skinner Swaim and Caroline Tiffany (Dyer) Swaim, was born on December 11, 1882, in Claremont, New

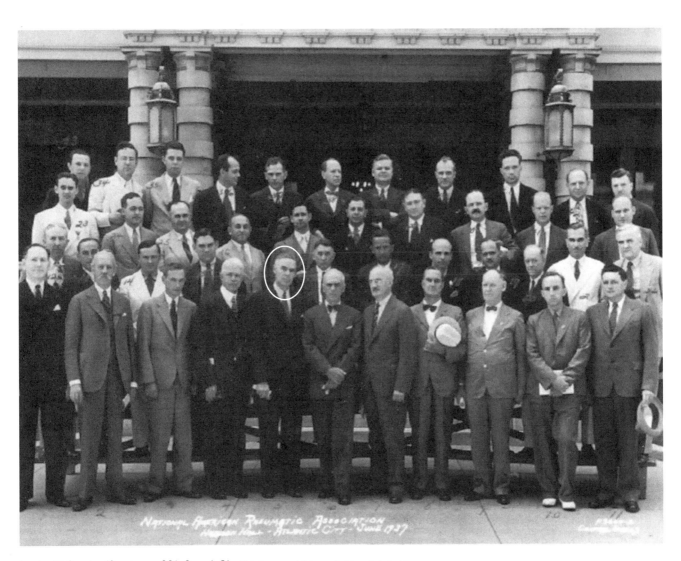

Loring T. Swaim (front row, fifth from left). Brigham and Women's Hospital Archives.

Hampshire. His early education was at the Volkman School, where he graduated in 1901 at age 19. The Volkman School, on Dartmouth Street in Trinity Court (Back Bay), was an all-boys school that prepared students for college or polytechnic school. It was a small school with only eight teachers. A few decades later, after World War I, the school eventually merged with Noble and Greenough in Dedham because it "had faced a drastically declining student population due to the headmaster's German origins" ("Noble and Greenough School" 2020).

Swaim entered Harvard College where his father had graduated in 1873. In his ninth report of the secretary for the class of 1873, his father commented that his three sons had all crewed in college: "My second son Loring Tiffany Swain was bow-oar on freshman crew and bow-oar on the varsity crew one year" ("J.S. Swaim" 1913). After receiving an AB degree in 1905, Swaim entered Harvard Medical School, graduating in 1909. He was an excellent student, having been elected into Phi Beta Kappa and graduating cum laude from medical school. He was also elected into Alpha Omega Alpha. In medical school, he had been a member of Sigma Xi. For the next two years, Dr. Swaim was a surgical house officer at the Massachusetts General Hospital (MGH) on the West Surgical Service.

After completing his internship, Swaim briefly travelled to the West Indies and to South America. He sought to specialize in orthopaedics immediately thereafter; he noted, "Dr. Joel E. Goldthwait [see chapter 33] asked me to join him for a while to see whether I liked orthopaedic practice. Those three months were priceless. Dr. Goldthwait was a stimulating teacher and ahead of his time in his vision and concept of the causes of chronic disease" (Swaim 1962). During the summer of 1912—about three years after graduating from medical school—he remembered that:

Dr. James Mumford [a surgeon at MGH] took charge of Clifton Springs Sanatorium in New York State. He asked me to organize an orthopaedic department there [beginning that fall]. The following three years at Clifton Springs were rewarding. The patients were mostly chronic cases not often treated in the big city hospitals. At that time there were so many gaps in our knowledge of chronic medicine that the staff discussions under Dr. Mumford's expert leadership were exciting and stimulating. (Swaim 1962)

Drs. Swaim, Goldthwait, L. T. Brown, and Robert Osgood each had a strong interest early in their careers in chronic disease and the effects of posture on health. In 1913, Swaim published an article in the Clifton Medical Bulletin, "The Orthopedic Surgeon's Relation to Chronic Disease." In it, he stated:

Orthopedic surgery as practiced in a Sanatorium Hospital of the Clifton Springs type, is frequently a study and treatment of such visceroptosis [a flat chest, round shoulders, angel-wing scapulae, a very acute sterno-costal angle and a prominent abdomen] cases; resulting in long continued deformities and handicaps of the body. A man's inability to carry on continuously his work without nervous breakdown or excessive fatigue can in most cases, I believe, be traced to some mechanical disorder in the human machine. This mechanical handicap interfering with the proper functioning of the body.--produces what is usually called the chronic case, —so-called because of its apparent hopelessness or its progressive nature. The arthritis cases, the chronic stomach, intestinal, and back cases…yearly have returned to a Sanitorium Hospital for a rest or baths, going away slightly relieved, only to come back again the next year. From a study of these chronic invalids I am convinced there is among them much work for the orthopedic surgeon…

The cry of the so-called chronic care patient is constantly "All we want, is to have further progress of this disease stopped; to get no worse," and the physician must in accordance with his professional duties do his best so to arrange the machine and life of such unfortunates as to make them run more smoothly and efficiently. The great cry of the age is economy and efficiency, and to this end in chronic disease the orthopedic surgeon is a necessity. ("The Orthopedic Surgeon's Relation to Chronic Disease" 1913)

In an article in the same journal edition, Dr. Goldthwait also discussed posture. He emphasized:

The way in which the human body is used many times determines the question of its health or disease. When it is used rightly, upright, extended, there is no undue strain on any of the structures...the parts may be used in perfect balance [allowing] full space available in the different cavities of the body for all the important viscera. The functions of the organs thus properly housed are carried on with the greatest possible ease...When the body droops all of its parts suffer. The spine is strained; the shoulders...strained; the neck becomes painful because of the undue curve...the pelvic joints become painful because of an unnatural use of the muscles and the severe strain upon the ligaments; the knees are necessarily sprung, with...symptoms...the feet who are necessarily sprung, with resulting painful symptoms... the natural support of the viscera is taken away, and the pelvic organs are exposed to the downward thrust of the abdominal viscera...with the unnatural strain on the spinal muscles and the unnatural curves of the spine, there follows interference with the vessels having to do with the spinal circulation...Accidently observed symptoms usually determine just what parts of the body or what functions are disordered, whether joints, muscles, viscera...the whole or any part of the being may suffer from these states of faulty poise. (Goldthwait 1913)

Dr. Swaim was the only orthopaedic surgeon on the staff of the Clifton Springs Sanitorium from 1912 to 1915. In 1913, there was an orthopaedic intern on his service, Dr. Fergus A. Butler. Afterward, he rejoined Drs. Goldthwait, Robert Osgood, and L. T. Brown at 372 Marlborough Street in Boston in private practice.

Over his career, Swaim published about 40 articles (most on arthritis) and two books, one of which he coauthored with Drs. Joel Goldthwait, Lloyd T. Brown, and John Kuhns: *Body Mechanics in Health and Disease*, 1934. While at Clifton Springs, he published six papers, four on arthritis. In one, "The Mechanically Unfit. A Study of Type Forms in Chronic Invalids," he stated:

Faulty posture is one of the most common defects met in practice...the figures have been gathered entirely from the sanitarium [Clifford Springs] class of patients...From recent observations and study, it would seem that the large majority of chronic invalids of a sanitarium are of the hyper-onto-morph type of [Dr. Robert B.] Bean, the carnivorous type of Treves and the congenital viseroptosis type described by Goldthwait. The proof of this statement—that the chronic invalid of the sanitariums is of the visceroptoses' type—is found in the radiograms of the viscera. Of 397 sets examined, but 53 showed normally placed stomachs and properly supported intestines...of 64 cases of polyarthritis, 23 had visceroptosis...[In] Discussion of Dr. Swaim's paper. Dr. Freiberg [asked] – I should like to know from what number of patients Dr. Swaim deducts his conclusions. How many normal individuals has he examined? Dr. Swaim. – I think in the last three years we have seen in all something like 3000 patients. I do not believe I have seen more than ten normal individuals...Dr. Freiberg. – I rise to discuss this paper simply because I feel that it is necessary to call a halt to our process of reasoning on this type of question. I believe we need to go back to the Baconian method of reasoning. We lay down one theory unproved and upon that we build another unproved, and so we go on...Dr. Painter. – I think I am getting more and more in Dr. Freiberg's position of wishing to investigate the normal quite as thoroughly as the apparently abnormal. In the hospital [possibly RBBH] with which I am now connected, we are commencing to study as many normal individuals as can be examined with the x-ray...we have found about as many normal individuals who show x-ray evidence of viseroptosis as we have those who have had symptoms. (Swaim 1915)

Dr. Swaim's early papers on arthritis demonstrated his comprehensive thinking regarding treatment of the whole patient with chronic arthritis. In his second publication (1915) on chronic arthritis, "Postural Treatment of Chronic Arthritis," Swaim proposed the following "steps in the diagnoses and treatment...(1) to locate and eliminate all sources of infection; (2) to study and improve metabolism; (3) locally to treat the joints and muscles; (4) and lastly, so to remodel the body by the postural treatment that permanent improvement may be maintained."

During World War I, Dr. Swaim "taught three times a week at the Massachusetts General Hospital Outpatient Clinic of Medical Officers, who were sent to the hospital for instruction in orthopaedic surgery. This was organized at the declaration of war and was carried on steadily for a year" ("Loring Tiffany Swaim" 1920). For many years, he worked in the outpatient clinic there every other day. With the onset of World War I, Swain wrote:

There was a shortage of doctors at the Massachusetts General Hospital, and I was assigned to the staff for the duration of the war. When the old staff came back, I asked to be permitted to start a clinic for arthritic patients. There were two reasons for this clinic. First, these arthritics were wandering from one hospital to the other, patiently seeking help. Secondly, they seemed to face real problems of fears, resentments, and hopelessness, which I felt some were in some way connected with their arthritis...

The plan for the clinic developed as it went along. The people who came were, of course, treated for their physical ailments, but the primary aim was to find out about their inner lives – what conflicts they had, what strains they were under; in short, what made them tick!... As the clinic grew, it became increasingly evident that, for the purpose I had in mind, an appointment a week for each patient was not sufficient. So, after five years, the project was moved to the Robert Brigham Hospital where there were endowed beds for the care of chronic cases. Here patients could be seen daily when necessary. Many of these men and women spent six months or more in the hospital and became more than patients – they grew to be my friends...At this time psychoanalysis was beginning to be popular. I hoped it might be the solution for my patients. I felt I ought to try it for myself before recommending it... So I was psychoanalyzed...My wife had been helping me in the clinic and wanted to go along with me in this experiment, so she also was analyzed. We had hoped that psychoanalysis would show us how to deal successfully with... family conflicts...But...The fact remained that we did not know how to change ourselves or anyone else...I had prayed for an answer to the emotional problems of my patients. (Swaim 1962)

For Dr. Swaim, the answer lay in his very strong religious beliefs and his eventual commitment to be honest in his relationships with his family and his patients (**Box 45.4**). He humbly wrote, "This time I decided to be honest about myself—first, which meant climbing down from my self-erected pedestal" (Swaim 1962). He immediately observed that his relationship with his patients and family improved, and "thus, began a new phase in living, a new adventure in the practice of medicine" (Swaim 1962).

He continued to publish about arthritis (**Case 45.2** provides an example of a later case on chronic arthritis). In 1922, he described chronic arthritis as having "been divided into three groups by Goldthwait, Painter, and Osgood: the infectious, the atrophic and the hypertrophic; by Nichols and Richardson into two: the proliferative and the degenerative; and by the English into rheumatoid and osteo arthritis" (Swaim 1922).

After describing infectious arthritis, atrophic or proliferative arthritis, hypertrophic or degenerative arthritis he commented on treatment, that "involves two parts, the medical and the orthopaedic [which] are so closely interwoven that they cannot be separated...medical deals with the arresting of the disease...orthopaedic deals with the prevention and correction of deformity, leaving the patient in as nearly normal functional capacity as is possible" (Swaim 1922). In the same article, he went on to say:

> Body mechanics, as shown by Brown, Goldthwait, and others, is a tremendous factor in the functional derangement of the viscera and nutrition...The orthopaedic care of the joints presents many problems, because of the tendency after cartilage destruction to bony ankylosis. The more motion a patient can keep during the active stage...the greater the advantage...Very little can be done operatively in the reconstruction of these joints. The hands, however, offer a huge field for more reconstructive surgery, as the hands usually are badly deformed and cause much incapacity. (Swaim 1922)

One of his insightful observations/conclusions was that: "Clinical data seem valueless unless these types are studied as separate pathological entities" (Swaim 1922).

It is unclear from the historical record when Dr. Swaim became chief of the orthopaedic service at the Robert Breck Brigham Hospital (RBBH). One source stated that he became chief in 1917, but in the annual reports, his name first appears as the orthopaedic surgeon in 1924. In 1924, Dr. Philip D. Wilson joined him as a consultant in orthopedic surgery. A courtesy staff was appointed for the first time the following year. It

Box 45.4. Dr. Loring Swaim's Outlook on Patient Care

> "During the early years of practice, I cared for my patients to the best of my ability, using all the approved methods of medical and orthopaedic treatment when in use (ACTH and cortisone were unknown at that time). But I was not satisfied – some important factor was missing. My patients did not improve as much as I felt they should, and recurrences of arthritis happened too frequently. Then, midway in my forty years of active practice...[this] profound change took place in my life...I still continued the same medical care but added the spiritual laws of 'change' as an answer to my patients' 'emotional' problems. I believe that this was the missing factor... [He followed his patients carefully for] twenty-five years before drawing conclusions...it was found that the first attack was almost always preceded by unhappy events and by periods of sustained emotional strain...[and] any further emotional conflict caused a recurrence. The feelings and emotions most frequently found were bitterness and resentment...It was chronic resentment that was so devastating...The root of these emotions is the hurt feelings of unsatisfied selfish demand, and selfishness can only be cured by obeying spiritual laws...[which] meant a willingness to give up first the demand...It cannot be done lightly... The decision must be intelligent...[and] the whole mind that acts...Once having given up the ill-will, the guidance usually was for the person to sincerely apologize for his or her part in a strained or unhappy relationship... the necessary price we must pay for the wrong that resentment does to others...an essential part of permanent change and peace...Now...of what happened to the rheumatoid arthritis. It definitely improved in those who went the whole way. The active disease actually subsided and remained quiescent for unusually long periods of time."
>
> (Swaim 1962)

Case 45.2. Growth Disturbances in Children with Chronic Arthritis

> "A Hebrew girl, was 8 years of age on her admission to the hospital and at the time of this report is 16 ½ years. The onset of the disease occurred at the age of 3 years, without any immediately preceding illness or injury. Swelling and stiffness developed in the wrists, fingers and right knee. There was gradual spreading of the disease, with development of deformities of the ankles, knees, spine, shoulders and elbows. The patient had been treated elsewhere with autogenous vaccine and baking and massage of the joints, which brought no improvement. The past history was unimportant except for frequent attacks of sore throat prior to tonsillectomy and adenoidectomy at the age of 4 years. The father died of multiple sclerosis at the age of 32. The family history was otherwise irrelevant. The general physical examination gave negative results, except for decayed teeth, a slight rachitic rosary, enlargement of the liver (two finger-breadths below the costal margin) and slight enlargement of the spleen. Examination of the extremities showed fusiform swelling in the finger joints of both hands; the shoulders and knees were limited in motion, and the elbows, wrists and ankles were almost completely ankylosed. X-ray films showed marked atrophy of all bones, periarticular thickening and irregular growth of the epiphyses. The results of all laboratory tests were normal, including the Wasserman and tuberculin reactions...photograph show[ed] the infantile proportions in the hands and the short forearms of this patient; ulnar deviation of the hand, due to disproportion in radial and ulnar growth.
>
> "The patient remained in the hospital for four years. Progress was delayed by acute nephritis. This partially disappeared, and the general condition improved. Treatment consisted of general hygienic measures, rest, physical therapy and calipers to straighten the knees. Eight years after the patient's first admission an arthroplasty was performed on the left elbow, and both wrists were manipulated.
>
> "At the time of this report the child walks with crutches and calipers and is able to feed and dress herself. X-ray films show: marked atrophy of all bones; marked narrowing of the articular spaces at the hip joints; fusion of the articular facets in the cervical region, and ankyloses at the right elbow, wrists and carpal and tarsal joints. Laboratory tests are all negative except that her urine shows a trace of globulin...Roentgenograms taken in 1929...the right knee...the right foot and the hands showing obliteration of the articular spaces; marked bone atrophy and premature union of the epiphyses, and early ossification of the ulnar epiphysis with disproportionate growth.
>
> "The measurements of the patient are as follows: height, 50 ¾ inches, weight, 79 ½ pounds (36.1 Kg); occipitofrontal circumference, 23 ¼ inches.
>
> | | Right (inches) | Left (inches) |
> | --- | --- | --- |
> | Femora | 13 | 13 |
> | Tibiae | 12 ⅝ | 13 ¼ |
> | Feet | 6 | 6 |
> | Humeri | 10 | 10 |
> | Ulnae | 6 ⅞ | 6 ¾ |
> | Hands | 4 ⅝ | 4 ⅝ |
>
> "The dwarfism of this child, with lack of growth in many bones, was due to early union of the epiphyses. The arthritis was extensive and severe, affecting general nutrition as well as particular epiphyses."
>
> (Kuhns and Swaim 1932)

included two orthopaedic surgeons, Dr. Painter and Dr. R. B. Osgood. At the RBBH, Dr. Swaim:

> Guided...the orthopaedic care of the patients and the formation of many of its pioneer policies. He will long be remembered by the patients for his unfailing kindness and his personal interest in all of their problems. For many years...he was a popular teacher on the study and treatment of clinical arthritis to medical students and to many visiting physicians. He sought to find the total treatment of his arthritis patients. This included the emotional and the spiritual. (Kuhns 1964)

Dr. Swaim gave frequent talks on a variety of topics covering arthritis at regional and national meetings, and locally at the RBBH and at Harvard

Medical School (HMS). By 1924, he had an appointment as assistant in Orthopaedic Surgery at HMS; from 1926 to 1946, he was an instructor in orthopaedic surgery.

In 1926, Swaim published additional orthopaedic recommendations for joint deformities. He commented that he had tried to induce arthritis in rabbits with strains of streptococci but failed. He wrote:

> Deformity must be prevented. Positions, protection, and rest do this. Joints at this time should never be manipulated or strained... Painless active motion is encouraged. After the acute stage has passed, however, the second great principle dominates. The joint function must be restored if possible. Our best results have been secured through very gradual use of the joints in exercise and occupational work. Manipulation is used less and less...If later, operative procedures are necessary to get joint motion, the muscles...are ready to do their share in securing motion much sooner after operation and the chance of adhesions becomes less...Discussion...Dr. Melvin Henderson, Rochester, Minnesota [stated that at] the Mayo Clinic...in the last few years we have operated on some of these [severe] cases and by multiple arthoplasties on the same individual we have succeeded in placing them in such condition that they can at least feed and care for themselves and probably get about a bit by the aid of crutches. (Swaim 1926)

A decade later, Dr. Swaim included more details about recent surgical procedures (after manipulation, wedge plaster splints and calipers) that were being used at the RBBH. He advised:

> The joints which are most successfully operated on are the elbows and knees...Operations on the shoulder, fingers, and hips have not been as successful. Although some hands have been reconstructed by doing arthroplasties on the finger joints, really satisfactory hands have not resulted. Arthroplasties on the hip have been successful in but a very small percentage of the cases. The tendency to ankylosis is very great. Arthoplasties on the elbow give satisfactory results in practically all cases. Arthroplasties on the knees are successful in most cases, but there is the possibility of limited motion. In knees, which are flexed and have motion, with the patellae free, the posterior capsuloplasty as developed by [Dr. Philip D.] Wilson, has given the best results...Another operation which has been successful in certain selected cases is synovectomy [knee]...Arthrodesis is an operation which in certain cases gives a stable knee or hip, making painless use possible. The aim of orthopaedic surgery, however, should be to secure motion whenever possible...Operations should never be performed during the active stage of the disease. (Swaim 1936)

Dr. Swaim was active in the Moral Re-Armament program, also known as the Oxford Group and the nondenominational movement referred to as Buchmanism, beginning in 1938. He sometimes traveled with its founder, Frank N. D. Buchman. The group aimed to encourage people to become involved or maintain their involvement in their current churches and enhance their spiritual growth. At the Moral Re-Armament Assembly in Michigan (headquartered on Mackinac Island) in 1939, Swaim and others called for leaders in every discipline worldwide to push for and lead people toward a new "age of faith" (quoted in "M.R.A. Issues Call to World Leaders" 1939).

In December 1941, Swaim began his tenure on the American Rheumatism Association's editorial committee. A year later, he became the association's president. Previously, in the late 1920s, Swaim had been part of a group of men interested in forming an organization devoted to arthritis and rheumatic disease. Osgood was heavily involved with this group, and they eventually formed the American Rheumatism Association (now called the American College of

Rheumatology). Osgood pushed for arthritis and rheumatic disease to be considered the domain of internal medicine because only that field could initiate the wide-reaching approach their treatment required. Swaim had been "one of the founders in 1933 [and] its first Secretary" (Kuhns 1964).

In his presidential address in 1942, given as the US became more deeply enmeshed in World War II, Swaim described the role medicine would play after the war, connecting it not only to healing wounded bodies but also helping people grow spiritually and finding the ability to forgive and love after the horrors of war. He cited evidence that connects both physical and spiritual health, and suggested that physicians should treat the entire individual, both their physical body and their soul. He discussed rheumatoid arthritis as an example, describing patients with the condition as experiencing resentment, anxiety, and problematic relationships with others. Swaim pointed toward his belief of the need for purposeful work by the patient toward an "unselfish character"—recognizing their mistakes, caring for others, and being honest—which would help them achieve not only physical but also spiritual healing.

After his retirement in 1944, he published his observations, opinions, and experiences treating large numbers of patients over 25 years with chronic arthritis. Using his memory, his clinical records and many letters from patients, in 1962 he published his book, *Arthritis, Medicine and the Spiritual Laws*. He traced his own history of understanding the many complexities in patients with arthritis with detailed case analyses. Dr. George Cheever Shattuck (1962) wrote in the book's foreword: "I feel that this book is an important contribution to psychosomatic medicine which deserves careful study by practicing physicians and by the clergy as well."

Swaim was a member of the American Medical Association, a diplomate of the American Board of Orthopaedic Surgery; and a member of the American Electro Therapeutic Society, Aesculapian Club, Harvard Club of New York, Boston Orthopaedic Society and the Union Board Club. In addition to being on the staff of MGH and the RBBH, he was "orthopaedic surgeon to the New England Baptist Hospital, consulting orthopaedic surgeon to Devereaux Mansion [rehabilitation], Marblehead, and New England Tubercular Sanitorium, Rutland" ("Loring Tiffany Swaim" 1964). Dr. John Kuhns (1964) noted that Dr. Swaim's:

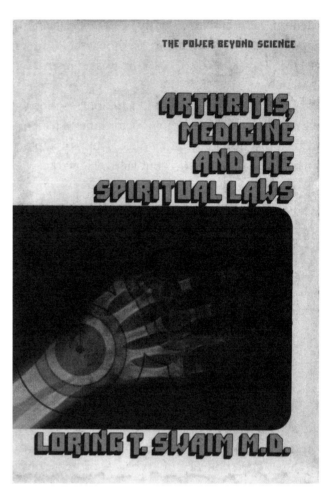

Cover of Swaim's book, *Arthritis, Medicine and the Spiritual Laws*. Philadelphia, Chilton Book Company, 1962.

> counsel was widely sought in the organization and development of arthritic societies in Europe and South America. He was the first secretary of the Pan-American League against Rheumatism. Besides membership in the American Orthopaedic Association and the American Academy of Orthopaedic Surgeons, he held honorary membership in the Royal Society of

Medicine of England, membership in the Ligue Internationale contre le Rheumatisme, the English, Brazilian, Argentine and Danish Rheumatism Associations.

Dr. Loring Swaim died at 82 on March 4, 1964. He lived at 8 Coolidge Hill Road in Cambridge; his office was 372 Marlborough Street, Boston. He was survived by his wife (Madeline K. Gill) and three children.

JOHN G. KUHNS

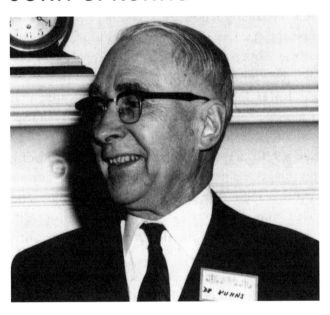

John G. Kuhns. Brigham and Women's Hospital Archives.

Physician Snapshot

John G. Kuhns
BORN: 1898
DIED: 1969
SIGNIFICANT CONTRIBUTIONS: Chief orthopaedic surgeon at the Robert Breck Brigham Hospital (RBBH) 1939–1962; chief of the staff at the RBBH 1936–1966; head of the Scoliosis Clinic at Boston Children's Hospital; expert in the treatment of arthritis; co-leader with T.A. Potter in research on nylon arthroplasty of the knee; early advocate for the use of roentgenotherapy for chronic arthritis; coauthored *Body Mechanics in Health and Disease* (1934) with Drs. Joel Goldthwait, Lloyd T. Brown, and Loring T. Swaim

John Groves Kuhns was born in 1898 in Pennsylvania Dutch country in Mount Joy, a small borough in Lancaster County. In 1900, the population in Mount Joy was only 1,900. He graduated from Elizabethtown College, a small college six miles from his home, in 1920. The college had been founded by the Church of the Brethren in 1899 and formally accredited in 1921, the year after Kuhns had graduated. Its mission was to educate students for service and leadership by fusing teaching in the classroom and experience through courses that build in students a groundwork of critical thinking, honesty and principles, and social responsibility. He then graduated from Johns Hopkins Medical School in 1924.

Following medical school, he was an orthopaedic intern at Boston Children's Hospital. Joseph A. Freiberg was an orthopaedic intern with Dr. Kuhns for eight months that year. Freiberg's research focused on chronic arthritis. Boston Children's Hospital had started a program "to give House Officers time to search for new knowledge as to the causes of disease as well as to learn the practice of an art" ("Report of the Orthopaedic Department" 1927). Kuhns was "engaged in another piece of research concerning the lymphatic supply of joints, which [had] already been fruitful" ("Report of the Orthopaedic Department" 1927). He was appointed a resident teaching fellow of orthopaedic surgery at Boston Children's Hospital (BCH) and Harvard Medical School (HMS) on September 1, 1926. Instructors at the time included Drs. H. J. Fitzsimmons, R. K. Ghormley, A. T. Legg, F. R. Ober, J. W. Sever, M. N. Smith-Petersen, R. Soutter, and L. T. Swaim.

After one year at Boston Children's Hospital, Kuhns passed his National Board Examination and was registered in Massachusetts. He was also listed at the HMS as a resident teaching fellow at Boston Children's Hospital and admitted into the Massachusetts Medical Society. His address at the time was 300 Longwood Avenue.

He presented his work on the lymphatic supply of joints in 1928 at a meeting of the Boston

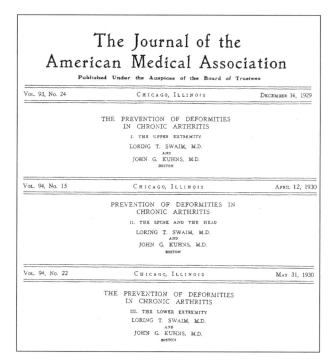

Titles of three articles on prevention of deformities in chronic arthritis by Swaim and Kuhns.
Journal of the American Medical Association 1929; 93: 1853; *Journal of the American Medical Association* 1930; 94: 1123; *Journal of the American Medical Association* 1930; 94: 1743.

Orthopedic Club in Sprague Hall of the Boston Medical Library: "He reviewed the literature on lymphatics of the lower extremities and reported some experiments in which he injected India ink and other substances into the knee and ankle joints of rabbits. He found that drainage of the knee joint takes place into the iliac lymph glands and of the ankle joint into the popliteal and inguinal glands" ("News Notes" 1929). However, I was unable to find any publication of this research. That same year, Kuhns published his first paper, along with coauthor, Philip D. Wilson. It was a review of 420 major amputations. They reported that:

> drainage is rarely indicated…if infection exists the wound should be left open and sutured secondarily. The Gritti-Stokes results were better than amputations higher in the thigh. Early temporary apparatus for walking is important. Some amputations gave good results…of thirty-four cases of amputations of the upper extremity only six used apparatus. (Ghormley et al. 1929)

In the orthopaedic department's report at Boston Children's Hospital in 1928–1929, Dr. Kuhns, along with Dr. Albert Brewster and Miss Janet Merrill (director of the physiotherapy department) oversaw "the special clinic for lateral curvature of the spine and faulty posture" ("Report of the Orthopaedic Department" 1929). HMS listed Kuhns as an assistant in orthopaedic surgery in 1930, along with Drs. E. F. Cave, R. H. Morris, and W. A. Rogers. Instructors in orthopaedic surgery that year included Drs. A. H. Brewster, L. T. Brown, H. J. Fitzsimmons, A. T. Legg, R. Soutter, and L. T. Swaim. Dr. Frederic C. Bost was a teaching fellow. At this time, his name also first appeared as an assistant in orthopedic surgery at the Robert Breck Brigham Hospital (RBBH), along with S. M. Roberts.

It was during these early years of his career that Kuhns began to publish papers on a variety of topics, but he showed an interest in arthritis. In 1929 and 1930, he published three papers with Loring Swaim on the prevention of deformities in chronic arthritis and in the upper extremity, the spine, and head, and the lower extremity. They did not differentiate between the different types of arthritis in these papers.

Swaim and Kuhns emphasized the importance of prevention in each of their papers; Kuhns did as well in his paper on foot care in arthritis. In order to prevent contractures in the upper extremity, Swaim and Kuhns suggested that nighttime wear of a cock-up splint and beginning occupational therapy as soon as possible can help prevent finger deformity. They mentioned traction in a banjo splint or a plaster of Paris splint could help correct deformities—as well as surgical procedures in severe cases—but they emphasized that prevention is always a better choice than correction. To do so, only a few things are necessary: proper positioning, rest, and mild use during everyday activities. They noted that bed rest over weeks while maintaining appropriate positioning is the most effective method for preventing deformity in the spine. In cases where a deformity already exists, a fully reclined position (into hyperextension for brief periods) and heat will help in correction, though months of such treatment might be necessary. Once a patient is able to get up and move around, a back brace or a jacket may be needed to continue to enforce the correction.

They reviewed their principles of prevention at each joint in the lower extremity: the hip, the knee, and the foot. At the hip, they noted that:

- Flexion contracture, then adduction and potentially internal rotation all indicate deformity. Dislocation and ankylosis can also occur.
- Prone positioning and traction are necessary, as is a plaster cast when the deformity is painful and resists correction through other methods.
- Such a cast should be able to be removed to allow therapeutic exercises, and excessive force should be avoided so that fractures and exacerbation of the arthritis do not occur.
- Surgical procedures are a last resort, and usually only after at least two years following an arthritis flare.

In the knee-joint, incomplete extension at the knee and backward tibial subluxation indicate deformity. A plaster case worn at night can help prevent a flexion deformity, and they recommended:

- Physical therapy to enhance thigh strength
- Bed rest for patients with pain and edema in the knee
- Gentle periodic traction to help correct contracture (capsuloplasty will help achieve this in a fixed deformity)
- Arthroplasty or osteotomy to treat any ankylosis

Finally, in the foot, arthritis most often causes rigid valgus, equinis, a flat anterior arch with cocked-up toes. Kuhns also found that hallux valgus and contracted toe deformity can also occur. Swaim and Kuhns recommend fixing a sagging arch through the use of support plates and well-fitted shoes. Exercises for the foot can be beneficial for patients with inverted feet and toe flexion. Patients with edema and pain in the feet should avoid all weight bearing. Existing deformities can be treated with plasters worn overnight; surgical procedures should be held for only severe deformity.

Dr. Kuhns remained an assistant in orthopaedic surgery at HMS in the year 1931 to 1932. In addition to Drs. E. F. Cave, R. H. Morris, and W. A. Rogers, the following assistants were appointed that year: Drs. J. S. Barr, W. T. Green, and S. M. Roberts. The same group was reappointed in 1932 for another year. His office address was 371 Marlborough Street in Boston.

Kuhns was also the lead author on two of the major Progress in Orthopaedic Surgery publications in the *Archives of Surgery*, the 48th report in 1932, and the 71st report in 1940. But the majority of his publications throughout his career focused on arthritis, a total of 32 of his 48 publications. Following his papers co-authored with Swaim, he published throughout the 1930s on disturbance of growth in children with arthritis, hypertrophic arthritis of the hip and spine, convalescent care of patients with chronic arthritis, and chronic arthritis of the shoulder.

During this period, he retained his same position at Harvard, and in 1934 he was appointed an assistant orthopedic surgeon at Boston Children's Hospital and the RBBH. Later his office was

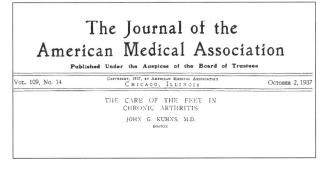

Title of Kuhns's article on the treatment of chronic arthritis in the feet. *Journal of the American Medical Association* 1937; 109: 1108.

located at 416 Marlborough Street in the Back Bay, where he practiced with Dr. Joel Goldthwait. Under the influence of Dr. Goldthwait's interest in posture and mechanics, Kuhns, along with Lloyd T. Brown and Loring T. Swaim, published a book in 1934 with Goldthwait, *Body Mechanics in Health and Disease*. It was republished in five additional editions over the next 18 years. A later review of the third edition stated: "The main theme of this work is the effect of poor body mechanics on the various systems of the body [including] the secondary effects on digestion, circulation and respiration...The book deals largely with end results and, by emphasizing the evils, points the way to prophylactic care in early life, when habits are formed" ("Book Reviews" 1942).

His publications were especially prolific during the early 1930s, and in 1934 he also reviewed 77 patients with congenital scoliosis. He wrote three papers from his experience at the scoliosis and posture clinic at Boston Children's Hospital, one on funnel chest deformity and two on congenital scoliosis. In his first paper, he concluded:

> 1. Congenital scoliosis is not an uncommon spinal deformity. It comprises 11 percent of the cases of structural scoliosis seen at the Boston Children's Hospital. 2. The vertebral deformities occur in early fetal life. We do not know as yet how to prevent their occurrence. 3. Early diagnosis is made too rarely. The deformity is usually the only physical sign. 4. Multiple deformities scattered throughout the spine were found in all except three children. 5. Treatment must begin early if good functional anatomic correction is to be obtained. 6. Supervision must be continued until full growth has occurred. (Kuhns 1934)

In 1935, Kuhns was secretary of the staff of the RBBH; he was appointed chief of staff the following year, a position he held until 1966. In 1937—following the publication of his three papers with Swaim on deformities seen in chronic

Table 45.1. Surgical Procedure to Correct Fixed Deformities in the Foot

Severe hallux valgus	Excision of the proximal part of the first phalanx of the great toe	Best functional result
Ankylosis of the phalanges	Excision of the entire proximal phalanx	Resolves pain
External deformity	Amputation of all toes and excision of the heads of the metatarsal bones	Unsatisfactory results
Hallux rigidus	Excise dorsal bone overgrowth of the 1st metatarsal head; sometimes must excise the proximal one-third of the proximal phalanx of the great toe	Relieves symptoms
Ankylosis of the tarsal-metatarsal joints	Excise ½ in. from the metatarsal bone Osteotomy proximal to the head of the metatarsal bone (if not enough motion at the distal end can be achieved) Remove metatarsal head in severe deformities	Relatively good function
Ankylosis of the tarsal joints	Wedge osteotomy through the subtalar joint or through the dorsal foot	Some improvement

Data from Kuhns 1937.

arthritis—Kuhns published a paper on the care of feet in chronic arthritis. He published on the experience of treating 1,200 patients with chronic arthritis (atrophic and hypertrophic) of the feet at the RBBH. Just as he had written with Swaim, he emphasized prevention, but he reported in more detail about deformities of the foot, especially the mid and forefoot and the toes. On the basis of serial roetgenography, Kuhns recognized that such abnormalities seem to progress in about 75% of patients with chronic arthritis. He outlined surgical procedures that provided positive results (**Table 45.1**), though he noted that the

> **The New England Journal of Medicine**
> Copyright, 1942, by the Massachusetts Medical Society
>
> VOLUME 227   DECEMBER 24, 1942   NUMBER 26
>
> TREATMENT OF ARTHRITIC CONTRACTURES OF THE KNEE
> JOHN G. KUHNS, M.D.*
> BOSTON

Title of Kuhns's article on the treatment of knee contractures secondary to arthritis. *New England Journal of Medicine* 1942; 227: 975.

best outcomes are often obtained with simple procedures that preclude trauma to the anatomy and obtain proper positioning.

Surgical treatment for arthritis continued to develop during this period. The following year, in his paper on the diagnosis and treatment of chronic arthritis of the shoulder, he made the following statement about surgical treatment at the time:

> Where no motion is possible at the shoulder joint as a result of fibrous or bony ankylosis... little abduction is possible it may be necessary to perform an osteotomy through the humeral neck. Attempts to produce a new joint at the shoulder have so far resulted in very unstable shoulder joints which have been quite inefficient for function. Arthrodesis...is rarely necessary...it is justifiable only in rare cases of subluxation with marked disintegration of the joint. (Kuhns 1938)

The year before, Roberts and Joplin had reported on arthroplasty of the elbow (23 cases) in which they acknowledged Dr. Kuhns: "We are indebted to Dr. John Kuhns of Boston for permission to include a case of his on which arthroplasty of both elbows was performed" (Roberts et al. 1937). The authors credited Dr. Philip Wilson for developing the surgical technique using fascia lata to cover the remodeled ends of the humerus and ulna; all patients had rheumatoid arthritis and were treated at the RBBH.

Dr. Kuhns was appointed chief of the orthopedic service at the RBBH in 1939, a position he held until 1962. Kuhns' associate from the early 1940s (following Dr. Swaim) was Dr. Theodore A. Potter, who later became chief of orthopaedics. During World War II, both Kuhns and Swaim were the only orthopaedic surgeons remaining on the hospital's staff at RBBH, and they cared for all the ward patients.

From his early experience at Boston Children's Hospital, Kuhns published a paper on congenital flatfoot in 1942. He concluded that it was fairly common among young children (~0.5%), and it is characterized by excessively relaxed ligaments and calcaneovalgus. Kuhns suggested appropriate shoes and arch and heel support to alleviate mild or moderate symptoms, but he noted that surgical procedures may be necessary for severe impairments. In his final remarks after the discussion of this paper, which he presented at the annual meeting of the American Medical Association that same year, Kuhns stated his preference for overtreating patients with congenital flatfoot, rather than risk not providing enough remedy.

In 1942, Kuhns also presented a paper, "The Treatment of Arthritic Contractures of the Knee," at the annual meeting of the American Rheumatism Association. Both he and Swaim made some interesting comments in the discussion: Swaim believed that prevention should allow orthopaedists to avoid the need for correction with most of the procedures Kuhns suggested; Kuhns acknowledge his different opinion, particularly as it applied to flexion contractures, and wondered, on the basis of his previous experience with manipulation at RBBH, whether that method should be avoided. He also mentioned his ongoing work with patients with flexion contracture in the knee, noting that although he hasn't been able to fix the contracture, those patients aren't completely incapacitated.

Three years later, Kuhns reported poor results of 12 arthroplasties performed at RBBH on patients with rheumatoid arthritis and bony ankylosis. Arthroplasty using interpositional tissues had begun in Europe and followed in the United States by Murphy in the early twentieth century. Murphy used both fat and fascia. MacAusland, in Boston, reported the results in four cases of knee arthroplasty utilizing fascia lata. He pushed for arthroplasty to be recognized as a standard procedure for knee joints with ankylosis. Kuhns and Potter became interested in arthroplasty of the knee, observing that work was still needed because, despite the many relatively successful procedures, many failed. They also recalled Osgood's 1913 study reporting only a very small increase (just a few degrees) in range of motion in the knee after fascial arthroplasty.

In Kuhns' paper in 1945, he described his efforts to identify a material that could be used as a membrane between articular surfaces of the knee in such patients; the material had to not cause irritation and last over time. One plastics manufacturer provided thin sheets made of six materials—polytheme, butacite, pliofilm, ethocel, and two nylon membranes. Although most caused only slight irritation in white rats, the nylon sheet produced none. He found similar results (normal movement and no adverse reaction to the nylon) in rabbits at autopsy. Eventually, he began to use the nylon membrane in patients with stiff knees resulting from chronic arthritis. They reported results on 25 cases, followed for as long as five years.

Kuhns told the *New York Times* that even unexceptional surgeons could achieve similar results in just one hour. The knees had severe fibrous or bony ankylosis and were painful, and many of the patients had rheumatoid arthritis. All experienced no pain postoperatively and could achieve 90° range of motion; most needed no support 12 months after the procedure. Radiographs taken over time and follow-up arthrotomy in three patients showed results similar to those of fascial arthroplasty, but Kuhns suggested that these results probably occur more quickly with nylon arthroplasty.

Throughout his surgical career as chief orthopaedic surgeon at the RBBH, Dr. Kuhns continued to present and publish papers on all aspects of the management and rehabilitation of patients with chronic arthritis, including the spine and upper and lower extremities. In 1946, he and Sidney L. Morrison reported their 12-year experience in using roentgenotherapy for chronic arthritis, 30 years before Sledge treated patients with radiation synovectomy using dysprosium-165 ferric hydroxide macroaggregate (see chapter 48). In addition to advances in arthroplasty and the use of synovectomy, on which Kuhns had presented papers, this type of synovectomy had been reported as early as 1906 in the United States. They treated 370 patients (252 with rheumatoid arthritis, 118 with osteoarthritis). Kuhns and Morrison (1946) wrote: "The dosage depended on the stage of the disease and the general condition of the patient… As a rule 200 r was given twice a week over two to four target areas [different joints] for six treatments, 1,200 r in six treatments during a period of three weeks comprised a course of treatment."

They observed objective changes and measured the joint circumference and the range of active painless motion. It was not known what the effects of irradiation would be on the joints and soft tissues. They reported:

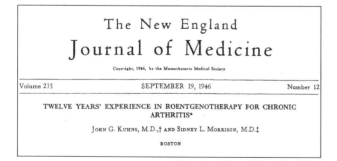

Title of Kuhns and Morrison's article on the use of roentgenotherapy for arthritis. *New England Journal of Medicine* 1946; 235: 399.

> NYLON ARTHROPLASTY IN RHEUMATOID
> AND OSTEO-ARTHRITIS*
> BY
> JOHN G. KUHNS and THEODORE A. POTTER
> Boston, Mass., U.S.A.
>
> Annals of the Rheumatic Diseases
> March 1951
> Volume 10, Issue 1

Title of Kuhns and Potter's article on nylon arthroplasty in arthritic knees. *Annals of the Rheumatic Diseases* 1951; 10: 22.

a diminution in swelling, frequently rapid subsidence of articular exudate, extensive local analgesia and a decrease in muscle spasm followed by an increased range of active, painless motion. In x-rays films taken two months to ten years after roentgenotherapy, no significant changes were observed in the bones... the improvement occurred in 78.4%, was mild in 24.1%, moderate in 37.2% and marked in 17.1%...The greatest improvement (84.5%) was seen in rheumatoid arthritis of the spine... The decrease in subjective symptoms almost paralleled the objective changes...In 80 patients who showed no response to roentgenotherapy the principal reasons for failure were severe deformity or mechanical derangement of the joint...Roentgenotherapy should be regarded as a local treatment only – a helpful adjunct to the medical and orthopedic measures that are usually prescribed. (Kuhns and Morrison 1946)

Kuhns also published two smaller books or pamphlets—one on low back pain and another with Dr. Robert Osgood on famous American orthopaedists—and translated a book on skeletal tuberculosis from Spanish into English. He translated papers into English from German and French as well. During the last 19 years of his practice, he wrote frequent book reviews, a total of 24 for the *New England Journal of Medicine* and the *Journal of the American Medical Association*. He was also consulting orthopaedic surgeon at Sturdy Memorial Hospital in Attleboro, the MGH and the Boston Home for Incurables. In a meeting of the Massachusetts Medical Society in 1948, Kuhns spoke about the surgical management of arthritis. At that meeting, he was still listed as chief of the orthopaedic service at the RBBH. In the 1950s, Dr. Kuhns was responsible for teaching the Harvard medical students and Dr. Potter taught the students from Boston University.

In 1952, eighteen years after his first paper on congenital scoliosis, he published a second one. He maintained that he had worked in the scoliosis clinic for 25 years. Kuhns and his co-author Robert S. Hormell described two types of congenital scoliosis: one (in only five patients) caused by muscular and ligamentous contractures, easily corrected by stretching exercises and corrective casts; and another more common type that occurred secondary to bony deformation of the spine and ribs. In this second group, Kuhns and Hormell grouped the patients at Boston Children's Hospital into five categories as described by Putti. They observed that in most of those patients, the curve of the spine does not change (increase) or does so only minutely. In the almost 50% of patients in whom the curvature does progress, appropriate support and physical therapy can help reduce the increase. Patients with severe scoliosis (a curve >30°) required spinal fusion after partial correction.

Kuhns also continued to publish on nylon arthroplasty of the knee; he published two additional papers with Potter and was sole author on another over a 14-year period (1950–1964). He published a description of his operation method using the material in 1951 (**Box 45.5**). In 1964 Kuhns reported that:

> nylon has proved to be less durable than was originally supposed. In all of the knees later subjected to arthrotomy three years or more after operation, the nylon membrane was found to be worn through over the weight-bearing portion of the femoral condyles. Despite this, function was usually satisfactory...We now

Box 45.5. Nylon Arthroplasty: Technique of Procedure in Patients with Arthritis

> "Our method of formatting new knee joints is a simple one modified from that of Hass (1930). All the earlier students of this problem soon learned that intricate reconstruction of articular surfaces was a waste of time since the bone ends were greatly changed in shape by weight-bearing and by use. The knee joint is exposed by a long medial parapatellar incision. The patella is chiseled free from the femur, which, with the attached quadriceps tendon, is retracted laterally. The bony ankylosis between femur and tibia is chiseled away. The knee is then flexed. The lower end of the femur is fashioned into a rounded wedge transversely. A shallow groove is formed in the tibial plateau to fit the lower end of the femur. About one inch of the joint is resected in most instances, to permit unobstructed motion. The intercondylar notch is deepened for the patella. The patella is made thin and coin-like. All roughened areas are made smooth with a rasp. A single layer of nylon is sewed to the periosteum and bone of the femur covering all articular surfaces and the supra-patellar pouch. Pleats in the nylon are burned down smoothly with the electrocautery.
>
> "In the postoperative care the leg is usually kept elevated upon pillows for 48 hours. Transfusion of one to two pints of blood are usually given as well as penicillin as prophylactic measures. The dressing is not changed for four or five days. Muscle-setting exercises are begun before the end of the first week after operation. Active exercises are begun after one week. Movement against gravity is begun as soon as the wound is healed. Weight-bearing with crutches and a plaster cylinder are begun in three weeks unless there is much bony atrophy. Resistance exercises (DeLorme and Watkins, 1948) are given to regain normal strength in the extensor muscles. Six months are usually required to regain normal strength and good function" (Kuhns 1951).

can report on 104 arthroplasties using nylon membrane in eighty-five patients…fifty-three had 60 degrees or more of painless stable motion five years after operation, but with the passage of time, there has been a gradual decrease in the range of active motion…The two most common causes of poor function… were: exacerbation of the rheumatoid arthritis producing further crippling and instability [and] with deformity from weight-bearing on cystic or osteoporotic bone. Usually function did not change very much after two years…Through the years, our ideas regarding arthroplasty have changed somewhat…Our chief indication for arthroplasty of the knee is ankylosis or severe restriction of motion in both knee joints.

Dr. John Kuhns retired from the orthopaedic service at the Robert Breck Brigham Hospital in 1966, two years following this last publication on arthritis. Two years prior, in April 1962, he had retired as chief of the orthopaedic service there; Dr. Theodore Potter was named his successor by the Trustees. Dr. William T. Green, in his 1963 annual report of the department at Boston Children's Hospital, said that "Dr. John Kuhns reached the age of retirement in June 1963. Dr. Kuhns has not been active at the Children's Hospital in recent years but was for a long time head of the Scoliosis Clinic here and was Chief of Orthopedics at the Robert Breck Brigham Hospital" ("Annual Report of the Department of Orthopaedic Surgery" 1963). Previously, in 1955, Kuhns had donated his books and journals to the Boston Medical Library. In 1956, at the second meeting of the Boston Orthopedic Club in the Boston Medical Library, Kuhns presented a memorial in honor of the late Dr. Robert Osgood.

In addition to the Boston Orthopedic Club, he had been a member of the American Medical Association, the American Academy of Orthopaedic Surgeons, the American Orthopaedic Association, the American College of Surgeons, and the Orthopedic Guild. He was also active in Newton's Highland Glee Club and the First Baptist Church in Newton. He died three years after he retired at the age of 71 in 1969. A long resident of Newton, he was survived by his wife Jane (Roper), two daughters, a brother, and a sister.

THEODORE A. POTTER

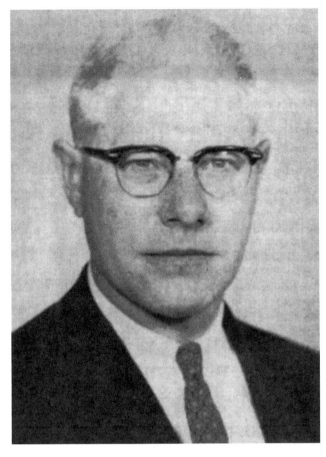

Theodore A. Potter. *BUSM Alumni News*, February 1963; 7: 1. Boston University Alumni Medical Library Archives.

Physician Snapshot

Theodore A. Potter
BORN: 1912
DIED: 1995
SIGNIFICANT CONTRIBUTIONS: Chief orthopaedic surgeon at the Robert Breck Brigham Hospital 1962–1969; coauthored an original article with Dr. John Kuhns on the nylon arthroplasty of the knee; early advocate of metal hemiarthroplasty of the knee in arthritis; section editor for Hollander's *Arthritis and Allied Conditions: A Textbook of Rheumatology*; president of the New England Rheumatism Association; president of the Boston University School of Medicine Alumni Association

Theodore Alexander Potter of West Newton graduated from Boston University and Boston University School of Medicine in 1938. He was a surgical intern at Boston University Hospital and completed his orthopaedic residency at the New York Orthopaedic Hospital in New York City in 1942. After his training, he went back to Boston to begin work in Dr. Joel Goldthwait's private practice at 372 Marlboro Street. He also began an affiliation with the Robert Breck Brigham Hospital (RBBH), where he mainly treated patients with arthritis.

Dr. John Kuhns was chief of the orthopaedic service when Dr. Potter joined the staff of the RBBH. Potter was first mentioned in the minutes of the meeting of the corporation in 1947; he was responsible for teaching students from both Harvard Medical School (HMS) and Boston University School of Medicine. In 1950, he divided the teaching with Dr. Kuhns, with Kuhns taking the Harvard students and Potter the Boston University students.

That same year, Potter published his first three of about 25 articles, including the original article he coauthored with Kuhns on the nylon arthroplasty of the knee. More than 60% of his publications were about arthritis or the surgical management of arthritis, especially involving the knees. He became a recognized expert in the surgical management of arthritis and was a section editor for Hollander's *Arthritis and Allied Conditions: A Textbook of Rheumatology*.

In 1955, Potter was an instructor of orthopaedics and fracture surgery at Boston University's School of Medicine and a lecturer in orthopaedic surgery at Tufts University School of Medicine. Three years later, he was named a member of the corporation at the RBBH. In 1962, after Dr. Kuhns resigned, Dr. Potter was named chief of the orthopaedic service. He wrote the first orthopedic chief's report to be included in the hospital's annual report (along with the chief of medicine's report), which represented a significant change at the RBBH. The orthopaedic chief's report was included beginning in 1962 and every year thereafter until 1967 (see chapter 44).

> **Surg Clin North Am. 1969 Aug;49(4):903-15**
>
> **Arthroplasty of the knee with tibial metallic implants of the McKeever and MacIntosh design**
>
> T A Potter

Title of Potter's article reviewing 10 years of experience using McKeever and MacIntosh tibial prostheses at RBBH.
Surgical Clinics of North America 1969; 49: 903.

During Dr. Potter's tenure as chief of the orthopedic service at the RBBH, the service continued to expand. This expansion process had begun initially with Dr. Kuhns. A decade before Dr. Potter's appointment, the visiting orthopaedic surgeons included Drs. Kuhns (chief), William Elliston, Robert Hormell, and Potter in 1951, adding Dr. Joseph Copel as well in 1952. Dr. Edward Nalebuff (see chapter 46) joined the staff in 1961, the same year Dr. Potter was appointed chief. Medical student teaching increased with second-year students from HMS and third-year students from Boston University. Plans were in place for a new elective course for fourth-year students from Boston University in the winter of 1963–1964. Drs. Marvin S. Weinfeld and Ralph H. Bender joined the staff in 1962 as junior visiting orthopaedic surgeons. By 1964, the orthopaedic service admitted 1,383 patients (1,223 in 1963) and treated 6,171 outpatients (5,550 in 1963). The average length of stay was reduced to 18.8 days from 19.8 days in 1963. Eighty-six patients remained on the waiting list for admission despite the hospital's addition of nine beds.

Dr. Potter and Dr. William T. Green began an affiliation with the RBBH and the MGH/CH combined residency program in 1963. In his report the following year, the president of the RBBH stated: "We can point with pride to the orthopedic residency program conducted by Dr. Potter in connection with the Children's Hospital" ("Report of the President" 1964). Potter and Green "instituted a rotation program under the direction of Dr. William Green. Selected residents came to our service for a period of three months…Residency teaching has also been carried out with the Peter Brigham Hospital medical residents in which some of members of the staff [RBBH] and the orthopedic residents participate on ward rounds, examinations, observations in the operating room and other advanced postgraduate forms of education" ("Annual Report" 1964).

The orthopaedic service was so busy that Potter stated in his 1964 chief's report his hope "that in the near future the volume of surgical cases will increase and that we will be able to run multiple major operative procedures simultaneously" ("Report of the Chief of Orthopaedics" 1964). He also summarized his frustration in that "We have come to the crossroads in which the demand far exceeds the supply…I cannot foresee any reversal of this ratio" ("Report of the Chief of Orthopaedics" 1964). The first full-time anesthesiologist was hired in 1965 as a member of Dr. Leroy Vandam's department at the PBBH.

Dr. William Thomas was added to the staff in 1967, initially on the outpatient service. After 1967, Dr. Potter no longer wrote a chief's report from the orthopaedic service. The newly appointed physician-in-chief, Dr. R. Frank Austen, included all issues regarding the physician staff, clinical care, and research in his annual physician-in-chief report, beginning in 1966. He included the following about orthopaedics: one orthopaedic surgical resident from Boston Children's Hospital rotated at the RBBH; Dr. Potter continued with his important clinical work on knee arthroplasty (140 tibial implants) and in the spring, would complete his ten-year follow up study; and

Dr. Nalebuff was on a one-year sabbatical visiting well known orthopaedic hand surgeons in major centers in Europe. By 1967, Harvard medical students were taught by the RBBH staff in the second, third and fourth years, including lectures and demonstrations for the second-year class, an introduction to the clinics for third-year students, and assignments to inpatients including involvement with ward rounds and consultations for the fourth-year students. The next year, Austen highlighted the ongoing reconstructive surgery research on the orthopaedic service, stating, "Dr. Potter and associates are pioneers in the reconstructive surgery of the knee…currently reviewing the results of tibial plateau metallic implants in patients with rheumatoid arthritis and osteoarthritis of the knee" ("Report of the Physician-in-Chief" 1968).

By 1969, Potter was also assistant clinical professor of orthopaedic surgery at HMS. The date of his initial clinical appointment at Harvard is unknown. One of his first publications dealt with a topic he enjoyed his entire professional life: arthroplasty of the knee. He described his experience with John Kuhns in performing more than 100 knee arthroplasties using a nylon membrane during an almost 15-year period (1944–58), noting that the rate of recurrence and deterioration of the nylon precluded them from continuing use of the procedure. This was the same experience with fascial arthroplasties reported earlier by Osgood and others. In 1969, Potter reported a series of cases (>170 arthroplasties) treated with either McKeever or MacIntosh tibial metallic implants at the RBBH over the years 1958–67. He summarized his experience, noting successful results in >55% of patients with rheumatoid arthritis and good or excellent outcomes in 90% of patients with osteoarthritis.

Potter had served as chief of the orthopaedic service at the RBBH for seven years, 1962–1969. After the RBBH, the Peter Bent Brigham Hospital, and the Boston Hospital for Women merged, he moved his practice to the New England Baptist Hospital. Not long thereafter, he was promoted in 1972 to clinical professor of orthopaedic surgery at Tufts, where he was active in educating residents. That year, Dr. Potter, with coauthors Drs. Weinfeld and Thomas, reported their long-term follow-up (one to nine years) of 142 arthroplasties using McKeever and MacIntosh implants in 119 patients (**Box 45.6**). They wrote:

> Using the described method of evaluation, fifty-six of the ninety-nine rheumatoid knees and seventeen of the nineteen osteoarthritic knees which could be evaluated, had good or excellent results…it is concluded that knee arthroplasty of the type described when performed in properly selected patients is an effective method to relieve pain and restore function. (Potter, Weinfeld, and Thomas 1972)

Dr. Theodore Potter was a member of the Massachusetts Medical Society (since 1942), the American Medical Association, a fellow of the American College of Surgeons and a member of the New England Rheumatism Association, of which he was president. He also served as president of the Boston University School of Medicine Alumni Association. He enjoyed ice skating and was a member of, and at one time served as vice president and a member of the board of, the Skating Club of Boston. He also held membership in and was secretary of the Miramichi Renous Club ("Dr. Theodore Potter" 1995), a salmon fishing club in New Brunswick, Canada, where Ted Williams had a summer home for over 30 years. Dr. Potter retired at age 81 in Kearsarge, New Hampshire, and died two years later in the Maine Medical Center in Portland, Maine, at the age of 83 in 1995. He was survived by his wife of 60 years, Constance, and two daughters.

Box 45.6. Knee Arthroplasty in Patients with Osteoarthritis or Rheumatoid Arthritis

"The operation is usually performed using a tourniquet and a long medial parapatellar incision. The vastus medialis with a narrow strip of its tendinous attachment is reflected medially to expose the capsule. After opening the joint, it is thoroughly examined to evaluate the extent of destruction of the articular surfaces of the tibia, femur, and patella. In every case, the operative findings showed more extensive destruction than had been anticipated from either the appearance of the joint on the roentgenograms or the clinical findings during the preoperative examination.

"Initially a synovectomy is performed, starting in the suprapatellar region and removing all viable synovium including that in the posterior part of the joint. In cases of osteoarthritis, a synovectomy is performed only when there is marked hypertrophy or proliferation of the synovium. The menisci are also excised, since they are generally involved by the arthritis process. The anterior cruciate ligament is often absent or attenuated. If it is markedly involved by the synovitis, it may be removed since loss of the anterior cruciate ligament in these patients does not noticeably interfere with joint function.

"Large marginal spurs along the femoral condyle are excised, but since the resulting raw bone surfaces provide potential sites for adhesions, smaller spurs and those which do not interfere with motion are left intact. There is usually a transverse ridge along the anterior aspect of both femoral condyles which appears to be the result of repeated impingement of the anterior margin of the tibia against the femoral condyles. This bone ridge is excised in order to improve knee extension. A bone rasp is used to smooth each femoral condyle and provide it with a rounded contour. Multiple parallel straight cuts three millimeters apart are made with a thin straight osteotome in the areas of exposed eburnated bone on the femoral condyles. Then, by directing additional parallel cuts at right angles to the first set of cuts, a crosshatched appearance is produced. We believe that cutting through the eburnated cortical bone facilitates vascularization and the formation of fibrocartilage on the femoral condyles."

McKeever Prosthesis

"A slotted template is used to determine the appropriate site of insertion of the McKeever prostheses. Each component should be placed so that it forms a posteriorly opening angle of about 10 degrees with the mid-sagittal plane to conform to the angulation of the femoral condyles. The curved outer margins of each prosthesis should not protrude beyond the outer margin of the corresponding tibial plateau or impinge on the collateral ligaments. The inner margins of the medial and lateral prostheses when properly placed should outline on the tibia a wedge-shaped area which encompasses the tibial spines and is pointed anteriorly. An osteotome is used to mark the tibial surface along the straight side of the template which is placed in one side of the joint. A vertical cut is then made along this mark to form a buttress against which the straight side of the prosthesis will impinge. A horizontal anteroposterior cut is then made with a slightly curved 12.7 millimeter osteotome so that it joins the vertical cut. This cut surface should be slightly concave paralleling the surface of the tibial plateau and conforming to the shape of the under-surface of the prosthesis. In making the horizontal cut an effort should be made to preserve the subchondral bone. After the fragment formed by the osteotomies is removed a similar fragment is removed from the opposite joint compartment using the same technique. The template is then reinserted to determine the sites of the slots for the fins of the medical and lateral prosthesis. The longitudinal (sagittal) slots are six millimeters from the corresponding inner vertical buttress near the base of the tibial spines while the transverse (frontal) slots are twelve millimeters behind the anterior margin of the tibial plateaus. A small reciprocating saw is useful to cut these T-shaped slots to prevent fracture of the tibial plateaus; however, a thin osteotome can be used if a saw is not available. The cuts should extend through the subchondral cortex into cancellous bone.

"With the knee in maximum flexion the longitudinal fin of the McKeever prosthesis is inserted into the appropriate longitudinal slot in the tibia. The prosthesis is then tamped in a posterior direction using a nylon hammer. Then the transverse fin overlies its tibial slot, the knee is gently extended to seat the prosthesis firmly in place. A similar procedure is carried out in the other compartment. To correct a valgus deformity, the medial prosthesis should be inserted first. The lateral prosthesis, which should be sufficiently thick to correct the deformity yet still permit full knee motion, is then inserted in the same manner. If there is difficulty inserting the implant due to a narrow joint space, a few millimeters of bone may be removed from the posterior non-weight-bearing portion of the corresponding femoral condyle. Similarly, if the anterior tibial spine impinges against the femur in in the intercondylar notch, full extension of the knee is prevented. Under these circumstances a rectangular block of bone should be removed from the femoral intercondylar area to create a sufficient space to accommodate the tibial spines when the knee is in full extension.

"Once inserted the prosthesis should be stable and not move in the knee if flexed and extended through an arc of a least 90 degrees. The anterior edge of the implant may project just beyond the edge of the tibial plateau. If this edge of the implants is too far posteriorly, it will abut against the femoral condyle and block full extension. The prosthesis must be inserted correctly the first time. A new set of slots should not be made because the prosthesis may then be unstable."

MacIntosh Prosthesis

"For insertion of the MacIntosh prosthesis, the buttresses along the tibial spines are cut initially in the same manner as for the McKeever device. Bone is then removed from each tibial plateau to provide flat surfaces. These cuts should not be made so deeply that they extend entirely into cancellous bone. It is important to remove the posterior lip of each tibial plateau so that the prosthesis can be seated far enough posteriorly to prevent anterior displacement of the implant during knee flexion.

"A patelloplasty is performed when there is loss of patellar articular cartilage and extensive marginal osteophytes. To do this the soft issues are dissected subperiosteally away from the periphery of the patella, and using a reciprocating saw, the posterior two-thirds of the patella is removed, leaving a slight central ridge, corresponding to the femoral intercondylar groove. The cancellous surface of the patella is usually covered with fascia lata. However, the infrapatellar fat pad or articularis genu muscle has also been used. The layers of the wound are then closed with interrupted silk sutures, and the extremity is immobilized in a long plaster cast with the knee in maximum extension. The cast is bivalved on the day of surgery."

(Potter, Weinfeld, and Thomas 1972)

PETER BENT BRIGHAM HOSPITAL

HENRY H. BANKS

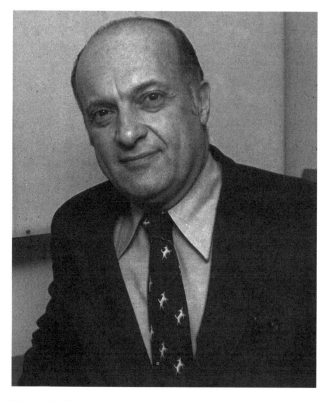

Henry H. Banks. Digital Collections and Archives, Tufts University.

Physician Snapshot

Henry H. Banks

BORN: 1921

DIED: —

SIGNIFICANT CONTRIBUTIONS: Chief orthopaedic surgeon at the Peter Bent Brigham Hospital (PBBH) 1968–1970; chairman of the Committee on Evaluation of Treatment in Cerebral Palsy for the American Academy for Cerebral Palsy; President of the American Academy for Cerebral Palsy (1971); served as both secretary and president (1979), then executive director (1979–1986) of the American Board of Orthopaedic Surgery; chairman of orthopaedics at Tufts University School of Medicine (1970–1972); associate dean for hospital affairs at Tufts (1972–1982); dean of the school of medicine at Tufts (1983–1990); published *Orthopaedic Surgery at Tufts University. The School of Medicine 1893-1998* (1999)

Henry H. Banks came of age during World War II, and the war allowed him to graduate early both from Harvard College, where he was an undergraduate in the class of 1943 but graduated in 1942, and from Tufts Medical School, from which he graduated in 1945. He spent nine months in a surgical internship at the Beth Israel Hospital before joining the US Army Medical Corps. He spent his period of active duty in the United States and Italy. In 1947, after about 18 months of service, Banks went back to Beth Israel Hospital for further surgical training.

Two years later, he turned toward orthopaedics, completing another nine months studying bone and joint pathology with Dr. Sidney Farber. His later career was heavily shaped by this early training. He published his first paper from his experience in Dr. Farber's laboratory: "The Effect of Hyaluronidase on the Absorption of Parenterally Administered Radioactive Plasma Proteins in the Dog."

After one year as a resident at Boston Children's Hospital with Dr. William T. Green (see chapter 21), followed by one year at Massachusetts General Hospital (MGH), Dr. Banks was chief resident at the Peter Bent Brigham Hospital (PBBH) from April 1, 1952, until October 1, 1952 (**Box 45.7**), and then chief resident at Boston Children's Hospital from October 1952 until October 1953. Dr. Francis Moore, the surgeon-in-chief at the PBBH commented about Banks in his 1952 annual report. It was the first time that Moore had stated anything about the residents on the bone and joint service: "Dr. Banks's period as a resident was marked by superb care of his patients and a very active teaching program which will give all other orthopedic residents a very high standard to equal" ("Report of the Surgeon-in-Chief" 1952).

It was during this period that Banks published his second paper—his first with Dr. William Green—titled "Osteochondritis Dissecans in Children." Dr. Banks wrote about his experience:

> While I was a resident at Children's, I wrote a paper with Dr. Green about Osteochondritis

Box 45.7. Banks Remembers His Chief Residency at the PBBH

Dr. Banks described his experiences as a resident at the Brigham in his memoirs:

"On April, 1, 1952, I arrived at the Peter Bent Hospital as Chief Resident in Orthopedic Surgery. It was a small, remarkable teaching hospital across the street from Harvard Medical School and connected by an enclosed bridge to Children's. Smaller than the other teaching hospitals in Boston, it…was modeled on the two-story cottage system in vogue at the time. It was distinguished by the presence and contributions of many famous faculty members…In keeping with the Hopkins tradition where Dr. Cushing came from, all surgical specialties were a part of the Department of Surgery. I, therefore, had two masters at the Brigham… Dr. Moore and Dr. Green who was Chief of Orthopaedics at both Children's and the Brigham. Orthopaedics was a Division of the Department of Surgery. General surgeons Thomas Quigley and Carl Walter were my supervisors in the management of fractures. A separate visit from Orthopaedics was responsible for supervising my care of strictly orthopaedic patients. It was an awkward arrangement but Drs. Quigley and Walter had something special to add to the residency. Dr. Quigley was a charismatic teacher, who…was very knowledgeable about sports injuries. Due to his wartime experience in England, he also managed fractures well. Dr. Walter was an acerbic, highly talented writer and engineer…He too was knowledgeable about the management of fractures and taught me how to us external fixators in the management of Colles fractures of the radius…Neither of these two men were card carrying orthopaedic surgeons. I, therefore, had to walk a tightrope between Surgery and Orthopaedics and the personalities in both areas. I was able to become a friend of both…

"The academic environment of the small hospital was outstanding. All residents, including those on Orthopaedics were expected to attend hospital Grand Rounds and Complications meeting each week unless patient care demanded otherwise…while the staff was relatively small, it was closely knit. Both it and the House Staff ate lunch together in a private dining room equipped with cloth tablecloths and napkins. A Surgical Senior Assistant Resident and an intern were assigned to me as the Chief Resident…We made rounds on all patients, ward and private, each morning and evening. Three outpatient clinics were managed by us and a Visit with students in attendance. Otherwise we were often in the operating room leaving one member of the team to cover the hospitalized patients and the Emergency Ward. We functioned as the hospital for the large neighborhood and the town of Brookline. It was a busy service. Orthopaedic Grand Rounds were held weekly on Thursdays at noon. Dr. Green was in charge…

"As there was no designated floor, private patients were scattered throughout the private and semiprivate areas. There were separate open wards of the old style for male and female patients…visiting fracture and orthopaedic surgeons made infrequent rounds during the week mainly to see problem cases. The Chief Resident, who often made decisions in their absence, was really in charge of the service. He had his choice of surgical cases and assisted the SAR [senior assistant resident] or Intern on less complicated cases. In the Hopkins tradition, the Chief Resident was expected to be able to perform in the Operating Room without supervision unless he asked for assistance from a Visit, especially in potentially difficult cases. Dr. Green usually had a few private patients in the Brigham where he operated from time to time. Not only did he expect the Chief Resident to assist him in the OR, but also to see his private patients with him. He usually made his rounds at about 7 PM after he had finished seeing his office patients at Children's…always a learning experience, but meant for a long day…I usually did not get home weekdays before 9 PM…The Korean War [which] began on June 24, 1950, was still raging when I was at the Brigham. Several young surgeons, who were in the reserves, were recalled to active duty…

"In the Spring of 1953, Dr. Green asked me if I would like to replace Dr. Albert Ferguson, who on July 1, 1953 would be leaving the Brigham to become the…Chairman of Orthopaedic Surgery at the University of Pittsburgh School of Medicine…[I] moved into the office [of Dr. Ferguson as the only orthopaedic surgeon at the PBBH] on A-Ground. It included small quarters: a secretary-reception room, small office and an examining room…fully furnished and equipped…He also left the records of his patients and had sent out a letter referring them to me… On September 30, 1953, I met with Dr. Green for final

> advice…I asked him what I should charge private patients for office visits…'Son,' he said, 'you charge the same as I do. $10 for the first visit and $5 for return visits.' I followed his advice for many years.
>
> "On October 1, 1953…I was the liaison between the hierarchy at the Brigham and Dr. Green. Dr. Moore expected me to attend as many surgical grand rounds and complication meetings as possible. To him I was the orthopaedic-surgeon-in-charge at the Brigham and, as a 'surgeon,' responsible to him. Orthopaedic Surgery from the time of Harvey Cushing was a Division of Surgery. To Dr. Green, I was his man 'in Havana.' He expected me not only to organize and run the service…but also to keep him informed of all events and problems. On many an occasion, I had to tread a fine line between Drs. Moore and Green. It was not easy. I was responsible for the schedules and assignments for the teaching of Harvard Medical Students, the schedules of staff coverage of the ward service and clinics as well as the organization of Orthopaedic Grand Rounds…
>
> "At this point, it is important to note that for the privilege of working at the Brigham, one received inadequate office space and a telephone free of charge. No salary was provided. All office expenses including secretarial services, repairs, furnishings, space improvements, and supplies were the responsibility of the staff member. In fact, one had to earn his own support. Fringes such as health care, life insurance and retirement benefits were not available. With about half my time being occupied with teaching students, supervising residents at the Brigham and Children's, and research, I had to work long hours including Saturday mornings to earn a living. I was 'on service' at the Brigham officially six months of the year, but actually all year long except for vacation in the month of June. At Children's I was initially 'on service' two months of the year, but in later years one month. This meant walk rounds with the residents every week day at 5 PM for about two hours and Grand Rounds every Tuesday morning for two hours. When not 'on service,' attendance at weekly Grand Rounds was expected. I also inherited the Cerebral Palsy Clinic at Children's from my predecessor, Dr. Ferguson. I had other assignments: consulting monthly for orthopaedic problems at the Middlesex Tuberculosis Sanitarium in Waltham…and covering a monthly Handicapped Children's Clinic with Dr. Green in Haverhill. In 1956, the Massachusetts Department of Health assigned the Hyannis Clinic to me and I discontinued my trips with Dr. Green…
>
> "There was no shortage of private patients to see, only available time. At the beginning pediatricians from the community and Children's referred about 60% of my patients. The other 40% were adults…referred by community practitioners and the Brigham staff. A decade later, the split was about 50/50. By 1970, about 60% of my patients were adults and 40% were children…While many ward patients at the Brigham were covered by BC/BS or later by Medicare, I never billed for them, because their procedures were all performed by residents. My care and supervision were free. [In addition to working at the Brigham and Children's Dr. Banks was] also at the Beth Israel Hospital…primarily to cover a weekly clinic [and later] a consultant [seeing only] an occasional patient in consultation… and rarely admitting one…My practice grew by leaps and bounds, and I needed help and more space. Sometime in 1968 I was able to convince the hospital president, Bill Hassan, about my need for more space. He agreed to having a trailer attached to my office in the parking space adjoining A Ground…A hole in the wall had to be made to connect the office to the trailer. For once I had enough office and examining room space."
>
> (Bank, n.d.)

Dissecans…in children. Dr. Barr, who that year was President of the American Academy of Orthopaedic Surgeons, invited me to attend so I could hear Dr. Green present the paper at the meeting in the Palmer House…It was an awesome experience.

Banks was intellectually curious throughout his life, and in 1957 he was a founding member of an academic orthopaedic traveling club, the Little Orthopaedic Club. In addition to his interest in cerebral palsy, Banks also developed an early interest in hip fractures. That same year he received a grant from the US Public Health Service to "study factors contributing to the final result in the treatment of fractures of the neck of the femur" ("Report of the Surgeon-in-Chief" 1958). Moore was very supportive of Banks and the orthopaedic service, but he did not provide research space for Banks until 1959. In his 1958 annual report, Dr. Moore stated, "The orthopedic service…represents [a] well-balanced community service, large in volume, varied in character, and from which is derived maximum teaching impetus. Research areas in this field have not been obvious or prominent in the past 25 years" ("Report of the Surgeon-in-Chief" 1952). In May 1959, lab space was provided to Dr. Banks in Dr. Dammin's pathology laboratory (**Box 45.8**). Here he began studies on the blood supply to the femoral head in dogs and in human cadavers. He also began collaborative studies with the Massachusetts Institute of Technology (MIT) on forces about the hip resulting in hip fractures. Each year in his annual report, Moore provided a brief status report on Banks' studies on femoral neck fractures.

Banks published his first paper on femoral neck fractures in 1962—a 20-year review of 301 intracapsular fractures of the femoral neck in 296 patients (1939–59). In a minimum of one-year follow-up, he personally examined 120 of the patients. The average follow-up was four years. He noted:

> Inadequate reduction, technical errors in fixation and premature weight-bearing appear to

---

Box 45.8. Banks Remembers Developing a Research Program at PBBH

Dr. Henry Banks was appointed the only fulltime orthopaedic surgeon at the PBBH after completing his residency. Here Banks recalls a conversation with Dr. David Grice, a senior faculty member of the BWH staff and one of Banks' teachers. Grice informed Banks that if he wanted to survive at the PBBH he would need to develop a research program:

"One day in the spring of 1953…Dr. Grice asked me [Dr. Banks] how I planned to succeed in staying at the Brigham. Surprised by the question, I asked what he meant. He said that unless I could develop a research program, my tenure there would be limited…Remembering my chief residency there [PBBH], it was clear that the most common problem seen on the service was…fracture of the hip in the elderly. At the time, it was considered to be the 'unsolved fracture' because of the high incidence of…complications…It was clear that the etiology, treatment and care of patients on the wards with this injury were problems that needed study. My plan [was to keep] a record and x-ray review of all patients treated for the problem at the Brigham during the previous decade…It [also] seemed reasonable to assume that a microscopic study of…removed femoral head[s] might yield more important information… For this purpose I would need a laboratory…some special equipment [and] a technician…I received grant support from the National Institutes of Health…Space became available across from my office on A Ground when Gabriel, the barber, moved out. A laboratory was constructed with funds from Dr. Moore and some patients of mine…Dr. Gustave Dammin, the Brigham Chief of Pathology, was very helpful in providing me with a lab bench in his department…The review of patient records and x-rays yielded important information…experiments in dogs showed that if the femoral head was devascularized, the fracture could heal only if the fragments were perfectly aligned and soundly immobilized by internal fixation. A motion picture was made of [the reduction and fixation] shown to illustrate the problem at the Forum of the American College of Surgeons, courses for the American Academy of Orthopaedic Surgeons, and a consensus meeting on avascular necrosis…of the hip at the National Institutes of Health… Dr. Moore strongly encouraged all surgical specialties to be involved in the many research projects in his laboratory…I participated in various radioisotope studies…pathological fractures in…metastatic disease from breast cancer, and the use of fluoride in multiple myeloma."

(Banks, n.d.)

be the main factors leading to non-union. Aseptic necrosis occurred in one-third of displaced fractures with more than a two-year follow-up and is the most serious remaining factor affecting the result...The incidence of non-union can be decreased and many aspects of the unsolved factors can be resolved by: (1) accurate reduction, (2) accurately placed, adequate internal fixation, and (3) carefully supervised postoperative care. (Banks 1962)

Dr. Banks also presented his findings in his thesis presentation to the American Orthopaedic Association in 1963. Two years later, he authored another paper, "The Healing of Intra-articular Fractures." On the basis of a 10-year review (1954–64), he concluded that:

intra-articular fractures, i.e., femoral neck, radial head, patella, humeral head, do not possess the ability to respond to injury with periosteal callus. Their mode of healing depends entirely on a medullary callus which appears to arise from the marrow-supporting structure... shows no temporary cartilaginous callus, begins early and can occur even with fragment separation. The importance of accurate apposition and rigid immobilization in the healing of these fractures is obvious. (Banks 1965)

He published a third paper in 1968; this one concerning the tissue response at the fracture site of femoral neck fractures. He studied:

100 specimens of the femoral head and neck obtained from 98 patients with intracapsular fractures of the hip [94-from PBBH; 6 from RBBH]...All the femoral heads were removed and replaced by a prosthesis as a primary procedure...There were 92 microscopically viable and 8 non-viable femoral-head specimens. The viability of the femoral head after an intracapsular femoral neck fracture is much more likely to be preserved if the ligamentum teres and the inferior retinaculum are intact...The femoral neck fracture heals, not by periosteal callus, but by callus arising from the marrow tissue. If the femoral head is not viable, repair from the neck side is theoretically still possible provided reduction and fixation are adequate, rigid, and without distraction. (Banks 1968)

That same year, Moore chose Banks to succeed the retiring Green as chief of the orthopaedic division at the PBBH, which "[had] under the leadership of Dr. Green, carried a large share of the responsibility for Brigham Orthopedics for many years" ("Report of the Surgeon-in-Chief" 1968). At that time Banks, was very active in professional organizations, including the Medical Advisory Committee of the American Physical Therapy Association, the New England Regional Committee, the AAOS Committee on Scientific Exhibits, the Massachusetts Blue Shield Fee Committee, the Program Committee of the American Academy for Cerebral Palsy, the Rehabilitation Committee of the American Hospital Corporation, the Research Committee of the AOA. He was also an examiner for the American Board of Orthopaedic Surgery (ABOS). Dr. Banks also started a podiatry clinic in 1968 at the PBBH, which was supervised by Donald Holmes.

Dr. Banks stepped down as chief and resigned from the PBBH and HMS in 1970, accepting a position as a professor and the chairman of orthopaedics at Tufts University School of Medicine. He had previously served as chairman of the committee on evaluation of treatment in cerebral palsy for the American Academy for Cerebral Palsy, and, in 1971, he was elected president of the organization. He quoted Dr. George Deaver (who did not deliver his own presidential address in 1949), reiterating Deaver's idea that the academy should do all it can to help people with cerebral palsy find work and become productive members of society. He also referred to Green, who in 1958 noted research had failed to examine the full effectiveness of the many methods that existed for treating cerebral palsy. Although such a study had been started, it ended prematurely because of a lack of funding. After reviewing the academy's accomplishments and problems, Banks recommended that the academy form a committee to address such concerns and help the academy to become a forerunner in the field.

In 1972, Dr. Banks moved into the role of associate dean for hospital affairs at Tufts. That year he was also appointed as an AOA representative to the American Board of Orthopaedic Surgery (ABOS) and became a member of the orthopaedic residency review committee. Banks served as both secretary and president of the ABOS, completing his term in 1976. The directors of the ABOS then asked him to accept the position of executive director which he did; remaining as executive director until 1986. In his memoir, he states, "When I was President, I was very proud of the Board's decision to require periodic recertification of orthopaedic surgeons. It wanted to encourage orthopaedic surgeons to maintain competence throughout their career."

Dr. Henry Banks became dean of the school of medicine at Tufts in the 1980s and then, in 1990, he was named professor emeritus of orthopedic surgery and dean emeritus of the medical school. In 1999, he published the book, *Orthopaedic Surgery at Tufts University. The School of Medicine 1893–1998*. He published over 40 articles and three books in his career; 12 on children's problems (7 on cerebral palsy), 11 on femoral neck fractures and basic science, and the remainder on a variety of orthopaedic topics. In pediatric orthopaedics, his major contributions included cerebral palsy (flexor carpi ulnaris transfer, adductor hip release and treatment of equinus deformities) with Dr. Green. Almost half of his publications dealt with fractures, especially intraarticular and pathologic fractures. **Case 45.3** includes an example of one of his many fracture cases.

Case 45.3. Fracture Resulting from Metastatic Malignant Melanoma

"[The patient], a 75-year-old white female, was admitted to Boston City Hospital June 20, 1970, with the chief complaint of excruciating left hip pain of 2 days duration. She gave a history of pain in the left hip associated with weight-bearing for the past 20 years, and periodic X-rays during this interval had shown findings compatible with degenerative joint disease confined to the left hip. Her symptoms during that interval had been readily controlled with analgesics and occasional periods of protected weight-bearing. In May 1970, some 4 to 6 weeks prior to her present admission, she first noted a distinct change in her symptoms. Her left hip pain began to occur at rest and was severe enough to awaken her from sleep. Two days prior to admission she suddenly noted excruciating left hip pain preventing any motion. No trauma preceded this further distinct change in her symptoms.

"Significant past history included hypertension of many years duration and a cerebral vascular accident with resultant left spastic hemiparesis in 1966. The hemiparesis had forced her confinement to a nursing home, where she had led a bed-to-chair existence for the 10 months preceding this admission.

"Of particular interest was the discovery during the 1966 admission to Boston City Hospital for hypertension, of a hairy pigmented nevus on the anterior left thigh 8 cm distal to the inguinal ligament, present for many years but which then seemed to be enlarging. A punch biopsy at Boston City Hospital on August 15, 1966 was interpreted as a 'compound nevus in which the junctional area has undergone early malignant transformation.' A wide excision of the primary site was recommended, but this was not performed because the patient was lost to follow-up. By 1969 the nevus had recurred. At the time a 5 by 3 cm area of multiple pigmented hair-bearing nodules, including 1 cm nodule at the margin of the lesion, was noted at the site of the previous biopsy. No inguinal adenopathy was palpable. A metastatic survey of the skeleton on August 7, 1969, was negative, and liver function studies were likewise within normal limits. On August 15, 1969, a 10 by 8 cm ellipse, including a 2 cm margin of skin around the nevus, was excised down to the deep fascia; the inguinal nodes were not excised. The pathologic interpretation of the specimen was 'malignant melanoma from an intradermal nevus, with the tissue margins tumor free.'

"Her condition remained stable from then until the onset of her present illness. Examination at the time of admission on June 20, 1970, revealed an alert, mildly obese white female with the left lower extremity externally rotated. With the exception of a blood pressure of 180/110 mm Hg and a mild left spastic hemiplegia without joint contractures, positive findings were confined to the left lower extremity. This extremity was held in 40° external rotation; there was 1 inch shortening of the extremity. Excruciating pain was elicited on any attempted passive motion of the hip; active hip motion was not possible. There was a healed stellate scar on the anterior aspect of the proximal thigh from the prior melanoma excision; no recurrent nevus was noted. Inguinal adenopathy was not present.

"Roentgenograms at this time revealed a pathologic fracture of the base of the neck of the left femur, with lytic lesions noted at the base of the neck, in the greater trochanter, and the posterior proximal shaft. A metastatic survey of the skeleton at this time revealed lytic defects in the anterior aspect of the proximal right femoral shaft and in the left fifth rib. The chest film showed no evidence of parenchymal involvement, although a left pleural effusion was suspected. Liver function studies were within normal limits. A liver scan, using ^{99}Technetium Sulfur colloid, revealed a minimally enlarged spleen and a 3 cm focal 'cold' area in the left lobe of the liver.

"On June 26, 1970, the patient underwent a Moore prosthetic replacement of the left femoral head. A greenish-brown, highly vascular tissue had penetrated the hip joint capsule and was dissecting between the planes of the external rotator muscles. Likewise, the medullary cavity of the femoral neck and proximal shaft was largely replaced with the same material; the cortex of the proximal femoral shaft was thin, fragile, and frequently invaded by the vascular tumor. Histologic examination of the tissue showed clumps of tumor cells and extensive areas of necrosis, 'the tumor containing cells with large nuclei and scant cytoplasm, 3 or 4 mitoses per high power field, and scattered intracellular clumps of golden brown pigment which stain black with the Fontana-Masson Technic.' Eburnated bone had replaced the articular cartilage of the femoral head. The patient's postoperative course was uneventful and her wound healed *per primum*. Ambulation was not attempted because of her left hemiparesis. At the advice of the oncologists and radiotherapists, local irradiation was administered to both proximal femora (1,000 rads to the left hip in one dose and 2,000 rads daily for 10 days to the right proximal femur).

"She was transferred to a chronic care facility on August 18, 1970. Roentgenograms of her chest on August 28, 1970, showed small patchy densities throughout both lung fields, distinctly increased since a previous study a week earlier and not present on her admission films of June 20, 1970. In addition, further destruction of the left fifth rib had occurred, markedly increased from June 20, 1970. Her general condition deteriorated, and she expired on September 9, 1970. Permission for an autopsy was denied."

(Paul, Craig, and Banks 1973)

CHAPTER 46

RBBH and PBBH
Other Surgeon Scholars, 1900–1970

The Robert Breck Brigham Hospital (RBBH) and the Peter Bent Brigham Hospital (PBBH) were established in the early 1900s. They opened to admit their first patients at a time of great turmoil after World War I had begun. Although musculoskeletal conditions were treated at the PBBH from the outset, orthopaedics was treated as a specialty at the RBBH first. Drs. Charles F. Painter and Lloyd T. Brown were the first two orthopaedic surgeons at the RBBH, appointed in 1912. The RBBH later became affiliated with the PBBH around 1947. It was not until four years later that Dr. Albert Ferguson was appointed the first full-time orthopaedic surgeon at the PBBH.

The visionaries and leaders who helped guide and weather the storms of the period included RBBH trustees Dr. Joel Goldthwait (RBBH president, beginning 1916) and Dr. Lloyd T. Brown (RBBH president, 1932–1952); RBBH physician-in-chiefs Dr. Louis M. Spear (1904–1939) and Dr. J. Sidney Stillman (1939–1960s); PBBH surgeon-in-chiefs Dr. Harvey Cushing (1910–1931), Dr. Elliott Cutler (1932–1947), and Dr. Francis Moore (1948–1976); PBBH physician-in-chiefs Dr. Henry A. Christian (1912–1938), Soma Weiss (1939–1942), and George W. Thorn (1942–1972); RBBH orthopaedic chiefs Dr. Charles Painter (ca. 1912–1917), Dr. Loring Swaim (ca. 1917–1938), Dr. John G. Kuhns (1939–1961), and Theodore A. Potter (1962–1969); Dr. Carl Walter, who organized and led the PBBH fracture service between 1938–1946; and Dr. William T. Green, who organized the first orthopaedic division at the PBBH in 1946.

The surgeon scholars—Harvard's name for these clinicians—covered in this chapter upheld the ideals of the RBBH and the PBBH in their commitment to the work between 1900 and 1970. They include:

Robert Breck Brigham Hospital	80
Ralph H. Bender	80
Lloyd T. Brown	81
Joseph W. Copel	88
William A. Elliston	90
Robert S. Hormell	92
Edward A. Nalebuff	94
Marvin S. Weinfeld	101
Peter Bent Brigham Hospital	104
Carl W. Walter	104
Albert B. Ferguson Jr.	109

ROBERT BRECK BRIGHAM HOSPITAL

RALPH H. BENDER

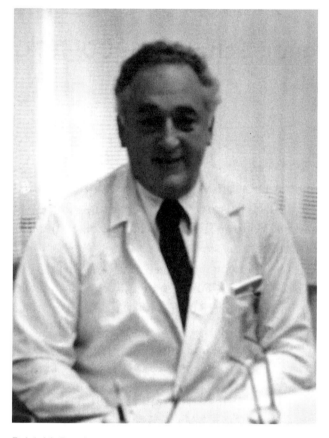

Ralph H. Bender. Courtesy of Walter Bender.

Physician Snapshot

RALPH H. BENDER
BORN: 1930
DIED: 1999
SIGNIFICANT CONTRIBUTIONS: Member of the Massachusetts Board of Bar Overseers

Ralph Herbert Bender was born in 1930 in the town of Peabody, Massachusetts. He played football on his high school team; they were state champions numerous times and undefeated in the 1946 season, when Ralph was a senior. Ralph excelled as a tight end, offensive tackle, and fullback. He stayed with the sport into his college years, playing on Harvard University's team as a lineman, defensive tackle, and offensive guard. After graduating from Harvard in 1951 and completing an additional year of premedical studies, Bender entered Tufts University Medical School, graduating in 1955. (I could not find any information about the location and type of Bender's internship.)

After medical school, Dr. Bender entered the US Air Force and served as a medical officer at the SAC base in South Dakota, after which he went to St. Louis to further his orthopaedic training. In 1962, he moved back to the East Coast, setting up a private practice in Newton, about ten miles southeast of Boston. He connected himself with three area hospitals: Beth Israel Hospital, the New England Medical Center, and the Faulkner Hospital. That same year, he was also appointed as junior visiting surgeon on the orthopaedic service at the Robert Breck Brigham Hospital, along with Dr. Marvin Weinfeld. He remained on the staff at the RBBH at least through 1965, but I was unable to determine if he worked at the RBBH after 1965 or if he had any faculty appointments.

I was also unable to locate any publications by Bender except for a foreword that he wrote for *Maggie's Back Book* in 1976, written by Maggie Lattvin, who taught at both MIT and Lesley College in Cambridge. Bender noted the glut of volumes available describing backache and the various, sometimes peculiar, ways they suggested to alleviate it. For Bender, physicians must focus not only on achieving an appropriate diagnosis and controlling pain, but also explaining to the patient the goals of rehabilitation and what the patient could do to help attain the best possible outcome. He recommended finding a single method for restoring function despite the cause of the condition—something that he argued Lattvin's book did through explanations of exercise and clear diagrams. Lattvin put forth an easy and straightforward method for rehabilitation that, if adhered to, would help people achieve more normal function—something Bender emphasized was much needed.

From 1985 until 1990, Bender was a member of the Massachusetts Board of Bar Overseers. The Massachusetts Supreme Judicial Court had created that 12-member board in 1974 with the goal of examining accusations and grievances against attorneys.

Dr. Ralph Bender died on August 31, 1999, from complications of cancer. He was 69 and left behind his wife Anita and their three sons and a daughter. In "Some Remembrances of Ralph," his friends and family recalled the type of man Bender had been. His son recalled the joy his father took in his chosen profession, through which he was able to "know and serve" many patients who deeply appreciated the care he gave. He described his father as an adept surgeon with sound judgment who cared for all his patients, and someone who knew his limits and lived by the motto "Do no harm." A friend remembered Bender as a loving, wise man who listened well and took pride in his work; he quoted a line from a poem written by the medieval Jewish poet Moses Ibn Ezra to characterize Bender: "the first virtue of wisdom is silence; the second is hearing; the third memory; and the fourth action."

LLOYD T. BROWN

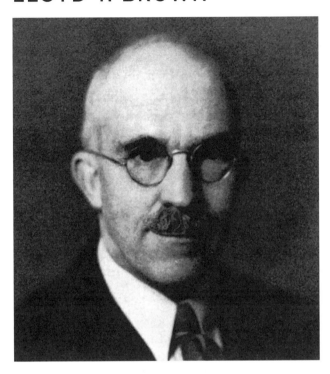

Lloyd T. Brown. L.T.S., "Lloyd Thornton Brown," *Journal of Bone and Joint Surgery* 1962; 44: 1252.

Physician Snapshot

Lloyd T. Brown
BORN: 1880
DIED: 1961
SIGNIFICANT CONTRIBUTIONS: Established with Goldthwait a popular posture clinic movement in the US and abroad; developed a posture chart with examples of good and bad posture; skilled executive: president RBBH board of trustees, chairman Milton Board of Health, trustee of the Massachusetts Medical Benevolent Society, and director of the Children's Island Sanatorium

Lloyd Thornton Brown was born on August 20, 1880, to Edwin and Marianna Mifflin Brown. He was raised with three brothers in Worcester, Massachusetts. "Despite his club foot," he participated in football and baseball while in secondary school at Milton Academy (L.T.S. 1962). He remembered that "his foot had been treated in the usual way for that time by manipulation, tenotomies, and later by osteotomy and removal of deformed bone, thereby giving him an unusual opportunity to see the end results of such treatment in later life." I was unable, however, to find any printed comments that he made about his condition and he made no mention of it in the three articles he published on the foot, including one on club feet. Before attending Harvard College, "he had another operation on his foot. This was done by Dr. Joel E. Goldthwait and thus began a lifelong friendship" (L.T.S. 1962). Brown graduated from Harvard in 1903.

Four years later—after graduating from Harvard Medical School (HMS)—Dr. Brown began a one-year surgical internship on the south surgical service at Massachusetts General Hospital (MGH). He remembered:

> recalling that as a house officer, he assisted in the first transfusion of whole blood from one patient to another [see Marble, chapter 40; recorded date of the first transfusion: July, 24, 1912]. This was a real operation, as it was thought that the only way it could be done was to attach the artery of a healthy person to the vein of the patient. It was a tremendous thrill to see the change in the patient as the blood went through the little tube, especially as the patient recovered. (L.T.S. 1962)

The following year, he completed a surgical and orthopaedic internship at Boston Children's Hospital, and:

> as soon as he graduated, Dr. Goldthwait asked him to join the office group at 372 Marlboro Street, where he worked until he retired. The two men seemed made for each other. They trusted, admired, and stimulated one another in the search to know more about the mechanics of the body, its care, and correct use. This cooperation resulted in a book, *The Education of Body Mechanics*, which was a group effort and went through [five] editions. (L.T.S. 1962)

One of Goldthwait's earliest papers on mechanics was about his beliefs regarding the relation of posture on function of the viscera, published in 1909. The following year, Brown coauthored his first paper with Goldthwait on the importance of body mechanics as a possible cause of rheumatoid disease. The authors wrote:

> The fact that the exacerbations of the joint symptoms so often follow…digestive or gastrointestinal conditions…the fact that attacks of vomiting so often were followed by improvement in the joint symptoms, the fact that with the administration of ether there was often a marked improvement in the joint symptoms, even though the joints themselves were not touched, the fact that pregnancy…was associated with improvement or often entire relief to the joint symptoms so long as the pregnancy lasted, the fact that many patients became markedly worse after being simply put to bed… the fact that a large number of the rheumatoid cases die finally of gastritis, intestinal obstruction, or by the newer term of gastromesenteric ileus…made it seem measurably more certain to the writers that there was some explanation of all these features…previous investigations…have been largely negative as to any clear reason being shown why such conditions [arthritis] exist…As a last resort, and in connection with some work carried on in relation to the poise of the body, the anatomical features were studied, with results that are at least suggestive and are offered here for discussion. (Goldthwait and Brown 1910)

Goldthwait and Brown had the assistance of Professor Thomas Dwight (the head of Harvard's Anatomy Department) and Assistant Professor John Warren (anatomist and great-grandson of John Collins Warren [see chapter 4, John Warren]).

The authors speculated about the problems associated with gastroptosis or downward displacement of the stomach, gastroenteric ileus or acute dilation of the stomach, and enteroptosis or downward displacement of the small intestines. They wrote:

> Imperfect stomach digestion due to the general atony of the organ...imperfect digestion with the function of the pancreas; together with...general atony of the bowel would result in definite disturbance of the digestion...After that, because of the presence normally of the bacteria in the ileum and colon, the disturbances might be chemical or bacteriological [which] might naturally result in...abnormal absorption and cause systemic manifestations of varying types...when there is distinct visceral ptosis...the liver also sags downward...with the possible interference with the circulation and innervation of that organ, so that its function also may be impaired [and] bacteria may develop in such quantities...that...undesirable absorption takes place. It seems probably that many of the cases of infectious arthritis are to be explained in this way...it is apparently a matter of accident whether the systemic manifestation takes the form of arthritis...of the arthritic conditions, the type in which there is true peripheral inflammation, the infectious arthritis, and...the one of degeneration or atrophy, the atrophic arthritis...are probably both explained in this way...
>
> The question of treatment with a problem having so many phases...involves so much that all that can be attempted...is to suggest the principles which must represent the basis of the treatment...Naturally the first thing to be desired is to restore the organs to as nearly as possible their usual position...[since] posture...is a definite factor [it] is most favorable for normal health [to have] the trunk erect, as it would be if one were to stand as tall as possible without rising on the toes...In the x-ray study of [one] subject it has been clearly shown that by merely changing the position from the droop to the erect position, the position of the bottom of the stomach can be raised from one to two inches...

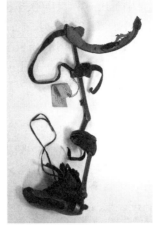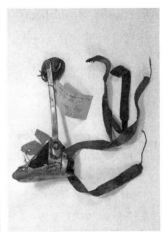

Examples of braces worn by Lloyd T. Brown as a child for a congenital club foot. He wore splints or braces from infancy. The braces were made for him between 1880 and 1898 by Edward Hickling Bradford. Warren Anatomical Museum in the Francis A. Countway Library of Medicine.

> If for any reason the organs cannot be brought back into place by the ordinary simple means [bed rest; braces; special exercises] and the general condition is such that radical steps seem indicated, operative measures for such purpose are indicated. Such occasion will probably not often arise, but in one case of the writers', because of a constantly recurring gastro-mesenteric ileus whenever the stomach was, by posture and support, brought up to the region of the duodenum, such an operation was performed with relief by Dr. F.C. Kidner...If for any reason the colon cannot be properly drained by cathartics or lavage...operations for the thorough drainage of this organ [colostomy] are to be considered. This will also not often be required, but [was] in two cases of the writers'... (Goldthwait and Brown 1910)

Brown held staff positions at various institutions, including MGH, Faulkner Hospital, the Boston House for Incurables, Children's Island Sanitarium, and the Robert Breck Brigham Hospital. The following year he married Marian Epes Wigglesworth on January 14, 1911. Brown continued with his interest in body mechanics and posture.

After his first publication on posture in 1910, he published approximately another 15 related articles over the next two decades. In addition to being a prolific writer, he was also innovative in his approach to technique:

> He developed his own technique for the treatment of club feet. During the first three weeks of a baby's life, he applied corrective plaster casts; changing them week by week until the deformity was corrected sufficiently to use rubber-band skin traction from the side of the leg to an outrigger on a tiny foot plate strapped to the infant's foot. The correction was thus completed in a dynamic fashion, reducing the number of visits required and preserving the flexibility of the foot. When Lloyd had perfected this method, he had the joy of successfully correcting the club-foot deformity of his youngest son. His skill with his hands was shown in those tiny plaster casts, in his surgery, and in his wood carving. He was a stickler for perfection, which won him many prizes on the squash court and in the tricky sailing-canoe races on the Charles River. (L.T.S. 1962)

During the interim of World War I, "he was assigned as a member of the staff at the Massachusetts General Hospital to teach orthopaedic surgery to medical officers" (L.T.S. 1962). It's unclear how long he held this position, but most likely he continued to teach medical officers throughout the war. He simultaneously continued to publish and probably his most notable was his study of Harvard freshmen and the development of a chart of normal and abnormal postures that were later used by Dr. Armin Klein in his reports published by the Children's Bureau, United States Department of Labor in 1926 (see chapter 53). Brown wrote:

> For the last three years at Harvard College, in October, a very thorough medical examination of the entering class has been made by Dr. Roger I. Lee [Department of Hygiene]

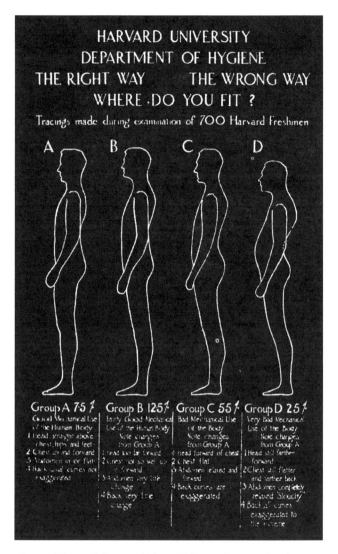

Chart of Roger I. Lee and Lloyd T. Brown's normal and abnormal postures they recorded in 700 Harvard freshmen. These posture groups became accepted as standards for evaluating posture in school-aged children and young adults in the US.

R. I. Lee and L. T. Brown, "A New Chart for the Standardization of Body Mechanics," *Journal of Bone and Joint Surgery* 1923; 5: 753.

> and his assistants. This year [1917] through the kindness of Dr. Lee, in addition to the regular work, an orthopedic examination, with special reference to posture, was also made of each man [by Dr. Brown] The method [used] was the schematograph [by the American Posture League]. This is not perfect, but it did allow records to be taken quickly [and] possible to get a fairly accurate record. It is a reducing camera, and the image of the object is focused by

means of a single adjustment of the lens and by a mirror upon a horizontal piece of tracing paper, which takes the place of the ground glass ordinarily used in cameras. The schematograph was placed on a table on one side of the room, and just in front of it was a reflector and a bright light projecting the rays upon a black screen on the opposite wall...after the medical men had finished their work...each man [without clothes] was made to stand...in a natural position...After the position was recorded, he was told to take his best standing position and another record was taken on the same piece of paper...The same method...was followed four years ago in an examination of 700 school children, and has been used with the nurses at the Massachusetts General Hospital for the last seven or eight years...The foot examination and the results of the medical examination, if anything out of the normal was found, were put on the same paper as the tracings. (Brown 1917)

It was difficult for Brown to choose a method of defining normal posture; there was a great difference of opinion amongst physicians. He noted:

The method used in this series included the vertical line test. In those tracings, which seemed to be up to standard, it was found that a line drawn upward from the external malleolus or the mediotarsal region, that it passed through the trochanter or the middle of the thigh, would also pass through the shoulders and the front of the ear [In the] 746 cases examined...only 20% of this selected group of educated men stood with their bodies in a normal or nearly normal position. (Brown 1917)

He also identified four types of posture in these young college students:

In the case of the bodily mechanics of the feet, the question of compensation and correction is somewhat different. It is decidedly more simple to compensate bad mechanics of the feet by the use of tight shoes or by plates then it is to correct their bad mechanics by sheer muscular power [as it is with posture]. We believe that it is because the results of bad use of the feet are relatively so promptly evident that...sounder opinions prevail in regard to correction versus compensation in the feet than in the back...Following correction we insist upon the fixation of correction by physical exercise in the corrected position and following...general, all-around physical exercise in order to fix more firmly the corrected habit. In other words, the stages are, 1, correction; 2, fixation of correction; 3, the habit of exercise in the corrected position; 4, form fixation of corrected habits. (Lee and Brown 1920)

In 1917 the *Boston Daily Globe* reported in an article about Dr. Brown's work. It stated:

After an exhaustive test of Harvard men... four out of five stood in a bad posture and that the college slump, instead of being a fad, is very much a reality...three out of five did not know how to take a correct posture when they tried to do so. In regard to...this slumped position [they] showed a greater variety and higher percentage of sickness [than the students with satisfactory posture] and that nearly two out of every 10 have feet which would prevent them from serving their country in time of war. ("Physical Faults of Harvard Students" 1917)

Dean Briggs—in his 1920 chairman's report of the Harvard Athletic Committee—wrote about these yearly examinations of incoming freshman students. He said:

The principle benefit of these physical examinations which are now held at Harvard is not in the detection of organic diseases among the men, but in the reassuring effect of the examination on many men. We find every year a number of students who fancy themselves to be afflicted with organic disease but are really perfectly sound and are glad to be reassured of the fact.

In summary, these studies were:

one of Brown's outstanding contributions to orthopaedics…his study of the relationship between health and posture. He [had] persuaded Norman Fradd, who was in charge of physical training at Harvard, to let him record photographically and classify the posture of all freshmen, correlating his findings with their records of achievement and health. This demonstrated that the men in the "A" posture group were out fewer days for sickness and were better athletes and students than those in the "D" class, who were sick more often and less efficient. Because of these findings, Harvard made the freshmen exercise program compulsory. National attention was drawn to the importance of correct posture in youth.
(L.T.S. 1962)

Beginning with an orthopaedic clinic at Carney Hospital that was started by Dr. Goldthwait and later moving to the MGH, Goldthwait and Brown, had established what would be the most well-respected posture clinic worldwide. MGH physicians traveled to clinics near and far, published articles, welcomed visiting physicians, and shared information with other providers and laypeople—all to spread the idea that posture could be adjusted and fixed by using exercise rather than pharmacology. They used spinal roentgenograms to illustrate and teach about various conditions and show how particular exercises would overcome the problems they caused. In 1920, Brown wrote in his 15th class reunion's report at Harvard:

Since 1913 I have been practicing orthopaedic surgery with Dr. Joel E. Goldthwait and Dr. Robert B. Osgood and more recently with Dr. Loring T. Swaim in Boston. I am now one of the orthopaedic surgeons to outpatients at the MGH. Also, assistant orthopaedic surgeon to the Robert B. Brigham Hospital. I have for the last two years been an assistant in the teaching of Orthopaedics [in the] Department of the Harvard Medical School. These positions keep me busy as I have any desire to be and are full of many interesting things.

At the time, he listed his home address on Highland Street in Milton, Massachusetts.

Brown was appointed a director of the board of trustees at the RBBH in 1923. RBBH had "opened for the care and study of patients with chronic disease" in 1914 (L.T.S. 1962). He would go on to assume the role of president over a 20-year span, from 1932 until 1951. Being very successful, he remained on the board of trustees for 35 years, until 1956 (see chapter 44). At one time, he also served as chairman of the Medical Committee at the RBBH. Brown also remained an Instructor in Orthopaedic Surgery at HMS until he retired. At HMS, he taught:

the Third-Year Class of the Harvard Medical School, demonstrating the principles of good body mechanics, so well demonstrated by his own posture, and the orthopaedic problems found in a hospital for patients with chronic disease. His students and his friends never found him too busy to drop whatever he was doing to lend a helping hand. People always came first in his thinking. As a conservative surgeon [he] never operated if he could find what he considered a less drastic way to solve the problem. He always tried to anticipate the long-range effect on the whole body of whatever he might decide to do. Despite his conservatism he investigated the still unsettled question of the suitability of heterogenous bone grafts. Beef bone, sawed into strips in his shop at home, was sterilized and used in spine fusions, with some success.
(L.T.S. 1962)

Brown retired from practice in 1951 at age 71 "because he felt it was only fair that the older men should make way for the younger ones. Besides this, the arthritic changes caused by years of strain from a club foot were increasingly painful" (L.T.S. 1962). He continued for another year on the staff of the Children's Island Sanitorium, a position he had held since 1917. He was "devoted to children" and "his weekly visits to Marblehead during the summer were a high point for the crippled children sent there from the Boston hospitals for sun and sea air" (L.T.S. 1962). His own children loved spending time there with him as well, and "one of the joys of their summer vacations was the occasional Tuesday afternoon sail along the coast from Manchester to Maine to Children's Island ["Cat Island"] to bring their father home, hopefully before the wind failed" (L.T.S. 1962). At the time of his retirement, "he had published about 37 articles and co-authored the books on body mechanics with Drs. Goldthwait, Swaim and Kuhns (5 editions)" (L.T.S. 1962). He hoped "to start a less strenuous life, with a chance to be outdoors on his daughter's Vitamilk Dairy Goat Farms [Harvard, Mass.]."

He was "remembered by many of Boston's former debutantes who served as volunteer nurses on [the Children's Island Sanitorium]. While they helped him put on plaster casts and carry out other treatment, he demonstrated the problems of chronic disease. To be a volunteer nurse on Children's Island was a much sought-after job in those days. He lived a robust and accomplished life and contributed to many professional organizations (see **Box 46.1**.) Others remembered him as demonstrating "real executive ability [as president of the board of directors at the Robert Breck Brigham Hospital for twenty years] and as chairman of the Milton Board of Health; as a director of the Children's Island Sanitorium, as chairman of the board of the Perkins School in Lancaster; as president of the Boston Orthopaedic Club; as a member of the Executive Committee of the Boston Tuberculosis Association; and as vice president of the American Orthopaedic Association [a Trustee of the Massachusetts Medical Benevolent Society; a member of the committee to study methods of re-education of disabled individuals for the Suffolk District Medical Society; and consulting surgeon to the Burrage Hospital on Bumpkin Island in Boston Harbor]" (L.T.S. 1962). He was also deeply admired by "the members of his beloved Eastern States Orthopaedic Club…Not only did he express sound opinions in the lively morning hospital discussions, where no holds were barred, but he was one of the top four golfers in the afternoon games. His enthusiasm carried over into the evening. He was the permanent secretary of the club" (L.T.S. 1962).

Box 46.1. Dr. Lloyd Brown's Professional Affiliations and Memberships

- Aesculapian Club
- American Academy of Orthopaedic Surgeons
- American Board of Orthopaedic Surgery
- American Orthopaedic Association
- American Medical Association
- Boston Orthopaedic Club
- Boylston Medical Society
- Eastern States Orthopaedic Club
- Fellow of the American College of Surgeons
- Massachusetts Medical Society

Dr. Lloyd Brown died suddenly at his home in Harvard, Massachusetts, on December 13, 1961 at 81 years old. He was survived by his wife, a daughter, and three sons (including Thornton, an orthopaedic surgeon and editor of the *Journal of Bone and Joint Surgery* [see chapter 40, Thornton Brown]). His friends and colleagues remembered him fondly as "full of fun," and they "also greatly respected [him] for his surgical judgment and/or his principles.

JOSEPH W. COPEL

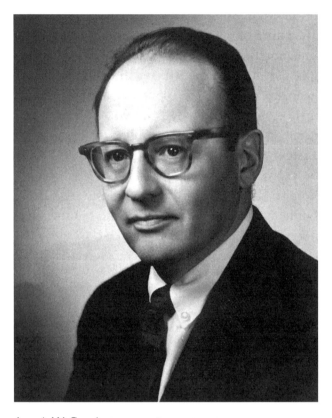

Joseph W. Copel. Courtesy of Dr. Joshua Copel.

Physician Snapshot

Joseph W. Copel
BORN: 1917
DIED: 1985
SIGNIFICANT CONTRIBUTIONS: Third chief of the Orthopedic Service at the Boston University Medical Center; chairman of the Department of Orthopedic and Fracture Surgery at the Boston University School of Medicine; studied the growth and senescent changes in vertebral bodies with Dr. Edgar Bick

Joseph William Copel was born in 1917 in Dorchester, Massachusetts, where he was a student at the Boston Latin School. After high school he attended Harvard, graduating in 1938 with a bachelor of arts degree with honors; his thesis was titled, "A Study of Lysine Deficiency in the Female Rat." After Harvard, Copel attended Tufts Medical School, graduating in 1942. He moved to New York City for a one-year internship at Mt. Sinai Hospital, but his training was interrupted by World War II.

Dr. Copel joined the US Army on August 13, 1943. He was stationed in Europe (shipped on October 22, 1944) and held the rank of captain. He served with the 564th Antiaircraft Artillery Battalion in France, Austria, and Germany. Upon returning to the U.S., he immediately married and entered the Mt. Sinai orthopaedic residency program. Mt. Sinai Hospital was organized as the 3rd General Hospital in World War II, officially activated in 1942. They trained at Camp Rucker in Ozark, Alabama, and eventually they were sent to Camp Shanks, Orangeburg, New York. Dr. Edgar M. Bick, an orthopaedic surgeon at Mt. Sinai, was the chief of the orthopaedic service of the 3rd General Hospital. The records are incomplete, but I believe that Captain Copel may have also served with the medical personnel of the 3rd General Hospital. They sailed for Europe with 300,000 troops on May 5, 1943. The 3rd General Hospital established hospitals in Tunisia and Algeria in North Africa; later moving to Italy and finally to southern France. They were officially deactivated on September 16, 1945.

While a resident at Mt. Sinai, he coauthored three papers with Dr. Edgar Bick on the development of human vertebrae. In the first, "Longitudinal Growth of the Human Vertebra," the authors studied 15 epiphyseal plates in:

> sagittally cut specimens taken from fresh autopsy material, ranging from one of an 8-centimeter foetus to one of a twenty-three-year-old adult...[their findings supported Dr. Schmorl's contention] that longitudinal growth of the vertebral body takes place by means of true epiphyseal-cartilage plates, as does longitudinal growth in the metaphyses of long bones...The vertebral ring, often observed in the roentgenograms of growing vertebrae, is an apophysis rather than on epiphysis, and takes no part in the longitudinal growth of the vertebral body. (Bick & Copel 1950)

In their second paper, they noted the vertebral ring apophysis does not contribute to longitudinal growth of the vertebral bodies (spine), and they went on to describe the changes in the vertebral bodies with aging: trabecular bone atrophies, peripheral osteophytes form, and small areas of necrosis that occur in the vertebral body. They concluded: "Histologically speaking it [ring apophysis] acts precisely as does an apophysis lying outside the line of longitudinal growth of its bone mass. In view of the attachment of the long vertebral ligament fibers, it may be classified as a traction apophysis. We, therefore, prefer to call it the vertebral-ring apophysis, or more simply, the vertebral ring…it adds nothing to the longitudinal growth of the vertebrae."

In their last paper on the senescent vertebra, they stated the following interesting observations:

> The process of senescence in the human vertebra…is characterized by three histological reactions…The fundamental characteristic is loss of trabecular substance due to the failure of formation of collagen while its normal, or possibly accelerated, absorption continues. A second manifestation…is that of osteophytosis about the periphery of the cephalic and caudal margins of the vertebral body…particularly permanent along the line of the anterior longitudinal ligament…a reaction of subchondral bone to the wear and tear of the articulating cartilaginous surface. The third histological characteristics is…one or more small areas of localized avascular necrosis or infarct spread through the spongiosa. (Bick and Copel 1951)

Copel then completed a fellowship at Tufts University's Lahey Clinic, and, in 1952, he opened an office at 483 Beacon Street for the private practice of orthopaedic surgery. He also became a fellow of the Massachusetts Medical Association. He lived at 33 Naples Road in Brookline during this period. That same year his name first appeared on the staff of the Robert Breck Brigham Hospital as a visiting orthopaedic surgeon. Dr. John Kuhns was chief and other orthopaedic visiting surgeons included Drs. W. A. Elliston, T. A. Potter and R. S. Hormell. Dr. John Reidy was listed as a consultant. After eight years, Dr. Copel resigned from Robert Breck Brigham Hospital in 1960. He had simultaneously been on the staff at Beth Israel Hospital; he continued in his position there, his affiliation spanning three decades. He also taught at the medical schools at both Harvard and Boston Universities. In 1966, Copel moved his private practice closer to home: he left Boston and opened an office in Brookline, where he practiced at 1180 Beacon Street with Dr. Ronald K. Kaplan.

In 1967, Copel stepped away from his private practice and his work at Beth Israel Hospital to succeed Dr. Kenneth Christophe as the third chief of the Orthopedic Service at the Boston University Medical Center and chairman of the Department of Orthopedic and Fracture Surgery at the Boston University School of Medicine. He was an active leader, and his involvement and direction engaged students and residents alike. Three years later Dr. Robert E. Leach took over, and he appreciated the work Copel had done to enhance the orthopaedic curriculum and expand the focus on the specialty. Later in his career, Dr. Joseph Copel was affiliated with Falmouth Hospital, where he died unexpectedly on December 30, 1985, at age 68. He left behind his wife (Marcia Kagno), two sons, and a daughter.

WILLIAM A. ELLISTON

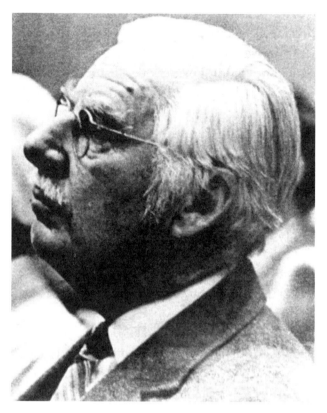

William A. Elliston. J.C., "William A. Elliston 1903–1984," *Journal of Bone and Joint Surgery* 1985; 67: 985.

Physician Snapshot

William A. Elliston
BORN: 1904
DIED: 1984
SIGNIFICANT CONTRIBUTIONS: Active on the staff of the Boston VA Hospital and the Robert B. Brigham Hospital; one of Weston's most influential residents; one of the founders of Weston's Forest and Trail Association; director of the Massachusetts Audubon Society

William "Bill" Arthur Elliston was born October 4, 1904. His family lived in Ipswich, England, where his father, William Rowley Elliston, was a barrister (the elder William eventually served as the town mayor). Bill attended Queen Elizabeth's Grammar School and Bradford College, where he received his secondary education. He went on to Christ Church College of Cambridge University and then St. Bartholomew's Hospital in London. In 1928, he received a bachelor's degree in both medicine and surgery and qualified to become a member of the Royal College of Surgeons and licentiate of the Royal College of Physicians of London. After further training at St. Bartholomew's, at Ancoats Hospital in Manchester, and at the Royal National Orthopaedic Hospital, he officially became a fellow of the Royal College of Surgeons in 1934. The following year, Elliston emigrated to the United States and joined the staff of the Massachusetts Memorial Hospital (now part of the UMass Memorial Health Care system). He married Harriet Hammond, daughter of Judge Franklin Hammond of Cambridge, in 1935. Harriet had a strong interest in anthropology, and she obtained her degree in it from Radcliffe College as the school's first female graduate in that field. Although officially women could not matriculate at Harvard until 1943, the university leadership had granted her dispensation to attend classes through Radcliffe College (A. Gomstyn 2002).

In 1937, Elliston became an instructor in orthopaedics at Harvard Medical School, a position he held for almost 30 years (until 1965), and joined the staff of Children's Hospital and the Robert B. Brigham Hospital (RBBH). He entered the US Army Medical Corps as a lieutenant colonel in 1941, and during World War II he was stationed at the US Army's 7th General Hospital back in England, at St. Alban's (1943–45). Upon returning to the US after the war, he continued teaching at Harvard, resumed his work at the Children's Hospital, and the RBBH. In 1946, he also began working at the Veterans Administration Hospital, where he held a role for ~25 years.

In 1953, he became certified by the American Board of Orthopaedic Surgeons.

Publications and Studies

Elliston cowrote orthopaedic progress reports for the *Archives of Surgery* in the late 1930s and

1940s. One of these reports, published in 1938, reviewed 123 papers selected from different medical publications between July and November 1937 in order to summarize the findings published throughout the literature.

In 1952, while at the VA Hospital, Elliston—in collaboration with Thomas DeLorme, Arthur Thibodeau, Dr. Joseph Hanelin (a radiologist), and Dr. Henry Musnick (research fellow)—completed a study of the outcomes of fractures of the scaphoid in military personnel. The study was supported by a Veterans Administration grant under the auspices of the National Research Council and published in the *Journal of Bone and Joint Surgery* in 1953.

In 1953, Elliston also cowrote a paper on nylon arthroplasty of the knee with Drs. John Kuhns, Theodore Potter, and Robert Hormell from the Robert Breck Brigham Hospital. They presented their results from 70 patients, reporting satisfactory outcomes in 58 of them, at the 20th meeting of the AAOS in Chicago. In that year, the *New York Times* reported that Elliston "originated" nylon arthroplasty.

In 1953, he became certified by the American Board of Orthopaedic Surgeons.

Life and Community Service in Weston

In 1937, the Ellistons moved to a historic farmhouse on South Avenue in Weston, Massachusetts, ~15 miles from Boston. A 1984 obituary for Elliston in the *Boston Globe* referred to him as one of Weston's "most influential residents," particularly in relation to developing and implementing the plan for the "open space" that defined Weston at the time.

In 1955, he was one of 12 founders of the Weston Forest and Trail Association, which maintains and protects the town's open spaces through conservation and stewardship of more than 200 acres of land and 100 miles of trails. The association's website (2015) characterizes Elliston as

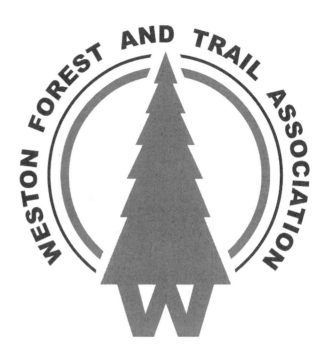

Logo, Weston Forest and Trail Association. Courtesy of the Weston Forest and Trail Association.

having long been "the heart of the organization," and a section of its conserved acreage is named "Elliston Woods" in the doctor's honor. In a 1979 town celebration recognizing Elliston's contributions to advancing and improving Weston, a fellow townsperson noted that only because of Elliston, who for years led monthly trail walks, are there "still paths and trails where we can walk and ride as we did when we were growing up" (*Boston Globe* 1984).

He was elected a member of the town planning board in 1958. He remained on the board for 22 years, serving as chairman for five terms.

The Ellistons shared their South Avenue farm with the community. Portions of the summer camps run by Roxbury-Weston Programs Inc., which brought together inner-city children with local kids from Weston, were held there. Not only were the Ellistons some of the founders of this program; he also acted as camp doctor and engaged in the camp's nature and storytelling programs. The farm sold raspberries from a farm stand along Massachusetts Route 30—the stand became a well-known fixture along the road—and all proceeds went to the camp.

The *Boston Globe* (1984) quoted Elliston's philosophy—"If you want to get things done, let someone else take the credit"—and the paper credited this perspective as being key to Elliston's successful efforts in advancing Weston.

Elliston also served as the director of the Massachusetts Audubon Society (1960–84) and president of the Massachusetts Federal Planning Board (1965–67). More locally he was a member of the executive committee of the Metropolitan Area Planning Council of Boston.

Harriet Elliston was a civil rights activist. Her involvement with Spain's postwar anti-Franco movement and her support of and aid to Spanish refugees resulted in both her and Dr. Elliston being questioned in 1947 by the House Un-American Activities Committee.

Elliston also enjoyed yachting. He often went out on the water with Maurice Griffiths, a friend he knew from Ipswich who designed boats and was the editor of the magazine *Yachting Monthly*.

Elliston died of heart failure at the Newton-Wellesley Hospital on November 26, 1984, leaving behind his wife, a son and a daughter, and four grandchildren.

ROBERT S. HORMELL

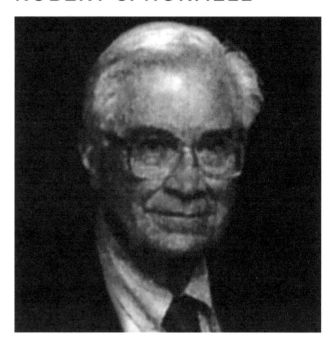

Robert S. Hormell. Courtesy of Bonnie Scalzi.

Physician Snapshot

Robert S. Hormell
BORN: 1917
DIED: 2006
SIGNIFICANT CONTRIBUTIONS: Interested in the history of rheumatism and gout; involved in the research and development of nylon arthroplasty of the knee

Robert Spaulding Hormell graduated from Harvard with an AB degree in 1935 and from Harvard Medical School in 1939. After receiving his MD degree, he was a surgical intern on the Fifth (Harvard) Surgical Service at Boston City Hospital. During his internship, he published two papers; the first described his modification of attaching a Wangensteen water suction siphonage to the hospital's vacuum system.

The second, "Notes on the History of Rheumatism and Gout," reflected his early interest in chronic arthritis. In that paper, Dr. Hormell traced the history of arthritis and its treatments, citing research that proved arthritis has long afflicted numerous creatures—as seen in 600-million-year-old fossils; in bones of 40-million-year-old cows and horses, 4-million-year-old camels; 1-million-year-old bear and saber-tooth tigers; and in 500,000-year-old human skeletons showing spondylitis deformans and rheumatoid arthritis in the fingers and spine. After providing a detailed history of the treatment of chronic arthritis, he referred to the experience of Dr. J. B. Bouillaud in 1832:

> It is strange that this man, who was so modern in his method of investigation [with use of the recently discovered stethoscope], should be the worst blood letter of whom we read. For the treatment of acute rheumatic fever, he recommended bleeding four or five bowls the first day, then three bowls each of the second and third days, followed by later bleeding by leeching, and venesection if the patient relapsed. He claimed to have treated 184 cases of acute rheumatic fever by the method, and said, "All of them have been cured except one." (Hormell 1940)

Dr. Hormell concluded stating: "The investigation is still going on, and our knowledge of specific causes is still incomplete. The nature, etiology and specific therapy of arthritis deformans remain among our most alluring medical problems, pre-eminent in medical, social and economic importance" (Hormell 1940).

World War II began the same year he graduated from medical school, but I do not know the details of Hormell's involvement. Hormell did, however, receive from Major General R. G. Breene a commendation for "outstanding conduct in the performance of duty" in 1945 while still in the army (though the site of his service is unknown). The commendation read: "[B]y denying himself sleep and rest did, during the month of April, save[d] the life of a colored soldier who was severely burned and injured in a gasoline explosion on 4 April 1943. For the first 48 hours following this accident, this officer remained constantly at the side of the injured soldier, and as a result of his personal knowledge and skill and through his perseverance when the rest of the staf[f] despaired of this solder's life, this soldier's life was saved" (quoted in "Decorations and Citations" 1945).

After the war, Dr. Hormell lived at 26 Poplar Street in Melrose and became a fellow of the Massachusetts Medical Society in 1947. That same year he was appointed assistant in surgery at HMS. In the 1951 annual report of the Robert Breck Brigham Hospital—the first report available after World War II—Hormell was listed as a visiting orthopedic surgeon along with Drs. Joseph Copel, William Elliston, and Theodore Potter. Dr. John Kuhns was the chief of the service. Dr. Loring Swaim was a member of the senior staff; Dr. John Reidy a consultant. The courtesy staff consisted of Drs. L. T. Brown, A. B. Ferguson Jr., R. Joplin, J. E. Goldthwait, R. H. Morris, W. A. Rogers and M. Smith-Petersen. Hormell also worked in the scoliosis clinic at Boston Children's Hospital, from which he coauthored a paper on congenital scoliosis in 1952 with Kuhns.

At the Robert Breck Brigham Hospital, Hormell coauthored two papers with Kuhns and others. In 1952, they published the paper "Replacement of the Femoral Head in Severe Osteoarthritis of the Hip." Hormell was listed as visiting orthopedic surgeon at the Robert Breck Brigham Hospital and instructor in the Department of Orthopedic and Fracture Surgery at Boston University School of Medicine. They reported 42 patients with severe osteoarthritis of the hip in whom they replaced the femoral head with a molded methyl methacrylate prosthesis fitted to a triflanged hip nail. All patients had improvement of function and decreased pain.

The following year the same group of orthopaedic surgeons described a new technique for treating arthritis of the knee, an arthroplasty that applied a nylon membrane to the joint surfaces (see chapter 45, John G. Kuhns). They had created stainless steel staples that would adhere the nylon "membrane" to the bone. Rehabilitation proceeded in stages:

- First, after the incision healed, the knee was put through range of motion exercises.
- Three weeks later, after applying a plaster cast, partial weight bearing was allowed.
- After six months, healing was usually complete, the leg muscles were stronger, and the nylon allowed the joint to move smoothly and painlessly.

Among 78 knees treated with this type of arthroplasty, 58 (74%) achieved "satisfactory functioning." This article, reviewed in *Newsweek* magazine, received national recognition.

Dr. Robert Hormell remained on the visiting staff at the RBBH, although little is recorded of his activities. In his chief's report for the year 1964, Potter mentioned that Hormell had started a research project on hallux valgus deformities; although I was unable to locate any publication of Hormell's on the subject. However, he did present a paper at the Boston City Hospital Centennial in 1964, "Arthroplasty of the M-P Joint of the Great Toe." He was last mentioned as on staff of the orthopaedic service in 1967. He retired to Meredith, New Hampshire, and died on October 26, 2006, at age 92. He left behind five children; his wife predeceased him on April 10, 2000.

EDWARD A. NALEBUFF

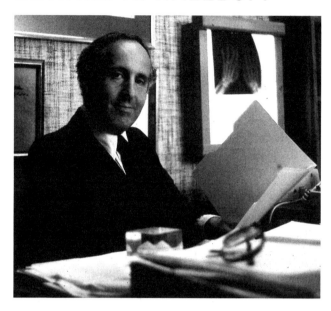

Edward A. Nalebuff. Digital Collections and Archives, Tufts University.

Physician Snapshot

Edward A. Nalebuff
BORN: 1928
DIED: 2018
SIGNIFICANT CONTRIBUTIONS: First orthopaedic hand surgeon at the RBBH and the MGH; started the first hand clinic at the RBBH; expert in arthritic deformities of the hand and wrist; established a classification system for thumb deformities in rheumatoid arthritis

Edward Alan Nalebuff was born on December 6, 1928, the firstborn of twins raised in New Jersey. Their dentist father wanted them to follow in his footsteps and become dentists, so he "sent [them] to Boston for college…so that they might both go to the Tufts Dental School. As fate would have it, Ed Nalebuff was left-handed at a time when there were no dental instruments made for southpaws. His brother, who was right handed [did go] to Tufts Dental School…[whereas] Edward took a [different] path, graduating from Tufts University and then attend[ing] its medical school, graduating in 1953" (Liang 2013). He graduated magna cum laude and was elected into Alpha Omega Alpha. He finished his surgical internship at Grace New Haven

Hospital the following year. In 1954, he joined the US Air Force as a general medical officer "and was stationed at Kessler Air Force Base in Biloxi, Mississippi, where he did obstetrics and gynecology for two years before returning to Boston to complete orthopedic training...During this period, polio and cerebral palsy were usually the [more common] hand problems that an orthopedic surgeon might encounter during training" (Liang 2013).

Early Orthopaedic Contributions

In 1956, after completing his military service, Dr. Nalebuff spent four years in various residencies: He enrolled in a three-year orthopaedic residency with the VA program, where he was supervised by Dr. Arthur Thibodeau and completed rotations at Boston City Hospital, the Boston VA, Lakeville Hospital, and MGH. After completing that program, he extended his orthopaedic training with an additional six months as a resident at Boston Children's Hospital. He then was named chief resident at the Peter Bent Brigham Hospital (PBBH), where he spent another six months. Nalebuff was a recipient of the:

> National Polio Foundation Award [from the National Foundation for Infantile Paralysis which eventually became the March of Dimes], which was given to outstanding candidates under 35 and supported 15 months of advanced orthopedic training wherever the awardee wished. Nalebuff, who wanted to eventually practice in Boston, chose the Peter Bent Brigham and Children's Hospital...led by William Green [while Nalebuff was chief resident at the Peter Bent Brigham Hospital] one of his interns was Joseph Barr, Jr., who introduced Nalebuff to his father...The senior Dr. Barr, impressed by young Nalebuff, gave him an opportunity to join the MGH staff. (Liang 2013)

Nalebuff published two papers from his residency experiences in 1960. The first was about delayed diagnosis of a congenital dislocation of the hip in children and treatment to provide a stable reduced hip. He published a series of 31 cases in 21 patients treated at Boston City Hospital with coauthor, Dr. Paul L. Norton. The VA Hospital had an affiliation with the Lakeville State Sanatorium where Norton was chief of orthopaedic surgery and a visiting orthopaedic surgeon at the MGH (see chapter 40). Later that same year Nalebuff published his second paper, coauthored with Dr. Alexander P. Aitken (see chapter 60) at the Boston City Hospital. The paper was a case report of a rare volar trans-scaphoid perilunate dislocation of the wrist.

After completing his residencies, Nalebuff began practicing orthopaedics at MGH and in 1961 became as a visiting orthopaedic surgeon at the Robert Breck Brigham Hospital. He had learned of the RBBH position from William Elliston. During that time, he chose hand surgery as his specialty. There were no orthopaedic hand specialists when Nalebuff joined as a staff surgeon:

> The senior medical clinicians did not refer patients to him for hand surgery for the first seven years after he came. Nalebuff recalls John Kuhns, who was nearing retirement, saying, "Son, you can make the hand look better but not work better!"...Theodore Potter, then 48, was more optimistic and encouraged Nalebuff's interest and focus on the hands...With access to almost unlimited patient material, Nalebuff compared the opportunity to being in a candy store. He set about to systematically and methodologically describe and classify the countless hand deformities in rheumatoid arthritis, including their presentations, course and patho-anatomy at surgery. (Liang 2013)

He took a two-year (1966 and 1967) sabbatical from the RBBH to study at the Derbyshire Royal Infirmary in Derby, England with Guy Pulvertaft, an Irish orthopaedic surgeon who specialized in surgery for hand injuries and disorders and who had helped found the British Society for Surgery of the Hand. During his fellowship

Nalebuff also visited other leading hand surgeons in Europe, including Claude Verdan in Lausanne, Switzerland, and Kauko Vainio "at the Rheumatism Foundation Hospital in Heinola, Finland—a 300 bed hospital for patients with rheumatoid arthritis" (Liang 2013). Nalebuff returned to Boston as a newly trained hand surgeon with a strong interest in arthritic deformities of the hand and wrist, and he started a hand clinic at the RBBH. The same year he returned, RBBH was:

> selected as one of nine centers [Nalebuff's hand clinic was part of the RBBH center] in the country to use the new Swanson silicone finger prosthesis...damaged MCP joints put the patient at risk for joint dislocation and deformity of the fingers. The early results were mixed and caused some controversy, as the view of the operation's usefulness differed between rheumatologists and surgeons. However, Nalebuff endured and the implant surgery gained popularity...It was not until some 40 years later that the Swanson arthroplasty's real role in management could be defined. For most patients, it improved hand deformities and some physical measures, but did not improve hand function when compared to medical management. (Liang 2013)

Later Orthopaedic Contributions

Over the course of his career, Nalebuff led new frontiers in the surgical treatment of patients with crippling deformities of the hands and wrists. He "was a colorful, enthusiastic, charismatic figure" (Liang 2013); these were important personality traits for an individual striving to correct severe deformities, relieve pain, and improve function in these patients, considering what Dr. Kuhns had told him early in his career. In 1968, Nalebuff began a more than 30-year period of publishing significant articles about rheumatoid arthritis of the hand and wrist as well as articles about other inflammatory diseases such as systemic lupus erythematosus, psoriatic arthritis, sarcoidosis, and systemic sclerosis.

Title of Nalebuff and Potter's article on surgical management of tenosynovitis of the hand & wrist in patients with rheumatoid arthritis. *Clinical Orthopaedics and Related Research* 1968; 59: 147.

He would eventually publish over 50 papers, two-thirds of which involved rheumatoid arthritis and other inflammatory conditions of the hand and wrist. His first paper from the RBBH, on rheumatoid tendonitis and tenosynovitis, was coauthored with Dr. Theodore Potter. Nalebuff was listed on the staff of both the RBBH and the MGH at the time, as well as on the clinical faculty at HMS.

In this initial paper on rheumatoid arthritis, the authors stated: "[We] have operated on over 500 patients with rheumatoid hand problems at the Robert B. Brigham and the Massachusetts General Hospitals during the past 7 years" (Nalebuff and Potter 1968). They reviewed the clinical patterns and their experiences with effective operations:

> The involvement of the tendon sheaths and the tendons themselves is not uncommon in rheumatoid arthritis...Dorsal tenosynovitis is common and easily recognized. Frequently, it is complicated by extensor rupture where the involved tendon passes adjacent to the distal ulna or Lister's tubercle. On the volar aspect of the hand and the wrist, tenosynovitis is often not recognized because of the overlying thick palmer fascia. This usually presents as a carpal-tunnel syndrome with median nerve compression. Flexor tendon ruptures occur, but are less common than extensor tendon ruptures. Direct involvement of the flexor tendons within the digital sheaths is also seen and can have a profound effect on finger function. (Nalebuff and Potter 1968)

> Bull Hosp Joint Dis. 1968 Oct;29(2):119-37.
>
> Diagnosis, classification and management of rheumatoid thumb deformities
>
> E A Nalebuff

Title of Nalebuff's article in which described his classification of thumb deformities in patients with rheumatoid arthritis.
Bulletin of the Hospital for Joint Diseases 1968; 29: 119.

They described their preferred treatments, which included early tenosynovectomy for dorsal tenosynovitis. For extensor tendon ruptures (commonly the EPL at Lister's tubercle), they preferred an extensor indicis proprius transfer; or in the case of other extensor tendons, a side-to-side juncture with an adjacent intact extensor tendon. They recommended a flexor tenosynovectomy with carpal tunnel release for flexor tenosynovitis; for tendon ruptures they preferred to use an adjacent sublimis tendon, transferring it to the involved digit's profundus tendon. They also classified trigger fingers in rheumatoid patients into four types, recommending surgical removal of the diseased tissue from the flexor tendons.

That same year Nalebuff published his classification of rheumatoid thumb deformities—a system still used today. Previous attempts at classification were based only on the condition of the joint as caused by the arthritis—for example, a weak, unstable joint or a rigid malformation, as described by Adrian Flatt. Since 1960, Nalebuff had performed surgical procedures on more than 600 hands with rheumatoid arthritis (in 100 of these, he had operated on the thumb in particular). His classification was based on his analysis of deformities as seen on radiographs, and on the joint that was most involved He elaborated on types I, II, and III. The type I deformity, the most common, encompassed MCP joint flexion with IP joint hyperextension (some refer to as a boutonnière deformity). Agreeing with Dr. Flatt that this deformity begins with extensive synovitis of the MCP joint, Nalebuff recommended an MCP joint arthrodesis and possibly an IP joint arthrodesis. Nalebuff had previously designed a new procedure—extensor pollicis rerouting—in 1965 for early intervention, a procedure he described as practical. The type II and type III deformities both begin with progressive synovitis and deformity at the CMC joint. In type II, the CMC joint subluxes or dislocates, the metacarpal is adducted, and the IP joint often hyperextends. Nalebuff recommended restoring the thumb metacarpal to an abducted position by CMC arthrodesis or resection arthroplasty and often an IP joint fusion as well. In type III, the thumb metacarpal is adducted with CMC subluxation or dislocation, the MCP joint is hyperextended, and the IP joint flexed (similar to a swan neck deformity). He believed this was the most difficult thumb deformity to treat, and he recommended a CMC joint fusion or resection arthroplasty or a metacarpal osteotomy followed by possible MCP joint arthrodesis. He emphasized the need for early treatment.

In a 1969 publication, Nalebuff recognized how even the smallest step toward treating rheumatoid arthritis (RA) can restore hope to patients who experience the condition—which in many severely affects their daily function to such an extent that they are in constant pain and believe they will never obtain relief. One of his patients, Mabel Hayes, had been so disabled from RA that she thought she would not ever leave her bed. After Nalebuff performed a metacarpophalangeal arthroplasty, she experienced such relief that she wrote a poem, "Dream Magic," to express her deep appreciation.

The same year as the 1969 publication, Nalebuff was appointed the chief of the hand service at the RBBH, assistant orthopaedic surgeon at the MGH, and instructor in orthopaedic surgery at HMS. Dr. Lewis H. Millender was Dr. Nalebuff's hand fellow, joining his practice afterward. At the RBBH, orthopaedic residents from the Chelsea Naval Hospital rotated on the hand service with Drs. Nalebuff and Millender. In 1973, Nalebuff

> Orthop Clin North Am. 1975 Jul;6(3):733-52.
>
> **Surgical treatment of the swan-neck deformity in rheumatoid arthritis**
>
> E A Nalebuff, L H Millender
>
> Orthop Clin North Am. 1975 Jul;6(3):753-63.
>
> **Surgical treatment of the boutonniere deformity in rheumatoid arthritis**
>
> E A Nalebuff, L H Millender

Titles of Nalebuff and Millender's articles reviewing the management of swan-neck and boutonniere deformities in patients with rheumatoid arthritis. *Orthopedic Clinics of North America* 1975; 6: 733, 753.

was promoted to assistant clinical professor of orthopaedic surgery at HMS, and he was chief of the hand service at the RBBH and on the staffs of the PBBH, the BIH, and the New England Baptist Hospital, as well as a consultant at the US Naval Hospital in Chelsea.

In the mid-1970s, Nalebuff wrote reviews of the surgical treatment of two major deformities that often occur in rheumatoid hands, the swan neck and boutonniere deformities. The swan neck deformity, one of the most common, is a result of reduced flexibility of the proximal interphalangeal joints and significant loss of flexion. He suggested three options for treating hands that retain finger motion: distal interphalangeal joint fusion, dermadesis, or flexor tendonesis. When finger motion is precluded, he advised initial manipulation and soft tissue releases to allow passive motion, and then a procedure to reinstate motion of the flexor tendons and, if necessary, fusion or arthroplasty. The boutonniere deformity often occurs initially at the proximal interphalangeal joint, resulting in its flexion, and expands to include the distal interphalangeal and metacarpophalangeal joints, which become hyperextended. Unlike the swan neck deformity, the boutonniere deformity affects function only when it advances to a severe state. Nalebuff suggested extensor tenotomy and dynamic splinting for patients with only a mild deformity. In those in whom the deformity is more extensive, he recommended repairing or restoring the extensor mechanism. For patients who have fixed boutonniere deformities, Nalebuff offered two options: arthroplasty or proximal interphalangeal joint fusion.

Nalebuff also made additional contributions regarding the surgical treatment of hand deformities in systemic lupus erythematosus (SLE), systemic sclerosis, and sarcoidosis. Until the 1980s, not much published research was available regarding the outcomes of procedures to rectify hand deformities resulting from SLE. In 1981, Nalebuff and his colleagues reported their experience with 51 reconstructive surgeries in 10 patients with such afflictions. They described positive results with distal ulnar excision for dorsal subluxation and suggested arthroplasty (over soft-tissue reconstruction) for intercarpal collapse. They pushed for early intervention when performing a metacarpophalangeal joint arthroplasty and suggested reconstruction of the volar ligament to retain a stable thumb carpometacarpal (CMC) joint and CMC arthrodesis or modified CMC arthroplasty to manage a fixed thumb CMC dislocation.

Fifteen years later, in a review of surgical reconstruction of the hand in patients with SLE, Nalebuff would write about the need for surgeons to grasp the role of soft tissues in the development of SLE-related hand deformities. Although he recognized metacarpophalangeal joint arthroplasty as a beneficial and widely used procedure, Nalebuff reiterated the importance of the gold-standard wrist, thumb, and finger fusions in treating such impairments.

Nalebuff's affiliation with Tufts University—which had started during his undergraduate years there and extended into the mid-1970s when he helped create a rotation on the hand service for residents and then a hand fellowship—solidified with his naming as a clinical professor in 1982. In a chapter on rheumatoid arthritis published that same year in Dr. David Green's book, *Operative Hand Surgery*, Nalebuff, Paul Feldon, and Lewis Millender summarized briefly the state of the art of reconstructive surgery in the hand. They referred to it as just one element in the scope of treatment of the condition, and one that can only do so much: it can relieve pain, fix or avoid deformity, and enhance the ability to use the hand, but it cannot completely restore function or strength. This indicates a definite improvement, but not a reversal of the observation made by Dr. Kuhns some 25 years earlier at the RBBH.

During this period in his career, Nalebuff had also brought attention to early treatment of the opera-glass hand deformity (*main en lorgnette*) seen in rheumatoid arthritis and psoriatic arthritis. With only about 40 published cases, he reported his experience in managing 13 patients, emphasizing prevention of shortening of the digits. Nalebuff enumerated three general elements that contribute to the deformity—namely, shortening of the fingers and thumb, unstable joints, and malalignment. He mainly used metacarpo- or interphalangeal fusion to preserve the ability to pinch, maintain length and reestablish stability in the digits. For him, however, preserving the length of the thumb and fingers was the main goal of such treatment, and early procedures to prevent such shortening were more effective than later procedures that are only attempts to recover or restore function. He made all attempts to preserve motion at the MCP joints and the thumb CMC joint.

In 1982, Nalebuff and his colleagues wrote about additional observations and their experiences with arthroplasty in the hands of patients with psoriatic arthritis. They found that such hands more often had spontaneously fused wrists that were functional, but the distal interphalangeal joints were often severely deformed with erosions and limited motion, and the involvement of the proximal interphalangeal joints more often resulted in severe flexion contractures than did hands with rheumatoid arthritis. Also, infection occurred more often after the procedure.

In his 1984 paper "Present Approach to the Severely Involved Rheumatoid Wrist," Nalebuff summarized his thoughts about handling the common involvement of the wrist (often the radiocarpal joint) in rheumatoid arthritis. Because the

> Orthop Clin North Am. 1984 Apr;15(2):369-80.
>
> **Present approach to the severely involved rheumatoid wrist**
>
> E A Nalebuff, K J Garrod

Title of article by Nalebuff and K. J. Garrod describing Nalebuff's surgical management of the rheumatoid wrist in the early 1980s. *Orthopedic Clinics of North America* 1984; 15: 369.

> **The Rheumatoid Hand**
> Reflections on Metacarpophalangeal Arthroplasty
>
> EDWARD A. NALEBUFF, M.D.*
>
> Clinical Orthopaedics & Related Research
> Volume 182   January/February 1984

Title of article reviewing Nalebuff's thoughts on the use of silicone flexible implant arthroplasty of the metacarpal phalangeal joints in rheumatoid patients.
Clinical Orthopaedics and Related Research 1984; 182: 150.

midcarpal joint is often not affected, Nalebuff and Garrod noted that they opt for partial wrist fusion at the radiocarpal level in almost a third of patients who necessitate a "salvage" procedure.

After leadership changes and reorganization of orthopaedics at the PBBH and the RBBH, Nalebuff moved his practice to the New England Baptist Hospital (NEBH). In 1984, he was chief of the hand service at the NEBH. With Dr. Len Ruby, Dr. Nalebuff established a Tufts hand fellowship program with rotations at the NEBH, the New England Medical Center and the Newton Wellesley Hospital. He had also been on the staffs of Milton Hospital, Carney Hospital, Braintree Rehabilitation Hospital, and St. Elizabeth's Medical Center.

In 1990, Nalebuff published a paper on the factors that influence results of implant surgery in the hand; it was one of at least eight articles he published on implant arthroplasty. He argued against the idea that poor outcomes occurred because of inadequate rehabilitation after surgery or a defective implant. He believed the latter had the least effect on results.

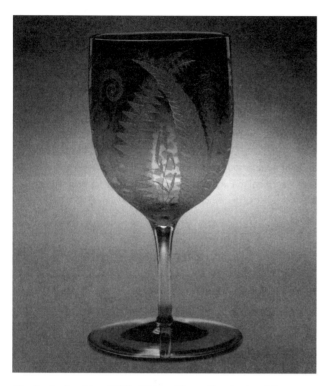

"Amberina" goblet, 1883. Object Place: Cambridge, Massachusetts. Made by: Joseph Locke, American, born in England, 1846–1936. Etched by: Joseph Locke, American, born in England, 1846–1936. Manufactured by: New England Glass Co., East Cambridge, Massachusetts, 1818–1888. Glass, blown and etched. Overall: 15.6 x 7.3 cm (6⅛ x 2⅞ in.). Museum of Fine Arts, Boston. Gift of Dr. and Mrs. Edward A. Nalebuff. 2011.223. Photograph © 2021 Museum of Fine Arts, Boston.

He preferred to use flexible Swanson implants, which he viewed as "spacers" and thus the least intrusive option. He rated the following important factors that contribute to the final outcome:

- four stars (most important): adjacent joints, controlling tendons, and stabilizing structures
- three stars: patient motivation, pain threshold, and tissue elasticity
- two stars: surgeon's judgement and technical skills as well as the occupational therapist's patient supervision and education (including supervising patients in their postoperative period with exercises, use of modalities to decrease pain and increase flexibility, and the proper use of splints and other apparatus to achieve the maximum benefit from the surgery)
- one star (least important): implant

Little had changed in his opinion. Six years previously, he had written about his thoughts on MCP implant arthroplasty: "The results of surgery depend more on the patient, the surgeon, and the therapist than on the prosthesis" (Nalebuff 1984).

Legacy

Nalebuff's last recorded membership on the staff of the RBBH was in 1994. The following year he was awarded the Marian Ropes Award "for his many contributions to the care of patients with arthritic hand deformities," which was presented by the Massachusetts Arthritis Foundation. In 2004, he retired from the editorial board of *Orthopedics* after serving as one of the original editors for 27 years. He retired from medical practice ten years later in 2014. Throughout his career, he had held memberships in the American Orthopaedic Association and the American Academy of Orthopaedic Surgeons as well as the hand societies of the United States (ASSH), United Kingdom, Canada, France, and Argentina.

Dr. Edward Nalebuff died on July 8, 2018. His accomplishments as a pioneer in hand surgery are widely renowned. Before his death, he also made many charitable contributions. His "parents collected 1880s New England Art Glass and they passed on their collection and this passion [to Nalebuff who] donated a large portion of his collection to various museums, including the Toledo Museum of Art" (Liang 2013). He also donated the Amberina goblet, blown and etched by Joseph Locke in 1883, to the Boston Museum of Fine Arts. At Tufts, he generously established the Edward A. Nalebuff Scholarship Fund over 30 years ago, the annual Thibodeau Visiting Professorship, and the Thibodeau room at the Medical School. He and his wife Marcia demonstrated their strong fondness for the New England Baptist Hospital by endowing a charitable remainder trust in their name.

MARVIN S. WEINFELD

Physician Snapshot

Marvin S. Weinfeld
BORN: 1930
DIED: 1986
SIGNIFICANT CONTRIBUTIONS: Developed an early classification system for patient outcomes after knee surgery

During my research I found almost no information about Marvin Sanford Weinfeld's early life. Details pick up once he begins his undergraduate education: he attended NYC's Columbia College, during which time he was elected into Phi Beta Kappa. He graduated in 1950 with a bachelor of arts degree. He then attended medical school at the State University of New York Downstate Medical Center and obtained an MD degree in 1954. Following an internship at Mt. Sinai Hospital in New York City (1954–1955), he was a surgical resident for one year at the Metropolitan General Hospital in Cleveland. He then spent two years as a captain in the US Army Medical Corps, then returned to Boston to complete an orthopaedic surgery residency at Boston Children's Hospital, MGH, Peter Bent Brigham Hospital, and at the West Roxbury VA Hospital. On April 1, 1960, he began as an assistant resident in orthopaedic surgery for one year at the MGH. He married Beverly D. Bunnin in January 1961.

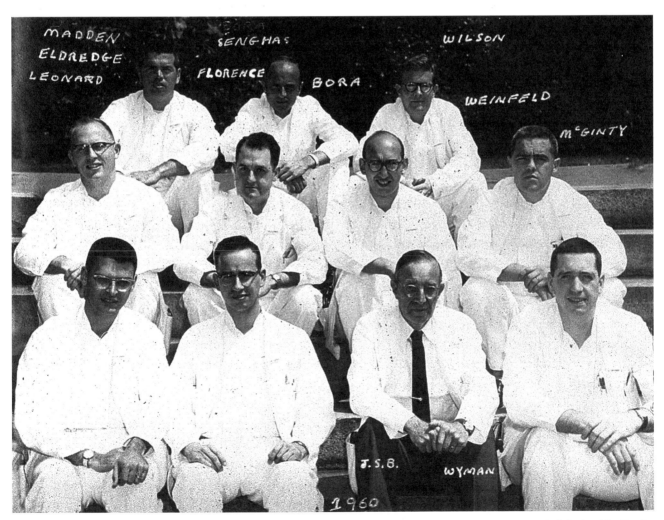

Group photo of orthopaedic residents with Dr. Barr at MGH. Marvin Weinfeld is in second row, third from the left (behind Dr. Barr).
MGH HCORP Archives.

Dr. Weinfeld entered private practice in Brookline after completing his residency. In 1962, he became a fellow of the Massachusetts Medical Society. That same year Dr. Theodore Potter, in his first report as chief of the orthopaedic service at the Robert Breck Brigham Hospital (RBBH), named three recently added orthopaedic surgeons to the staff: Dr. Marvin Weinfeld, Dr. Ralph Bender and Dr. Edward Nalebuff. Weinfeld remained on the staff of the RBBH throughout his career. He was also on the staff of the Peter Bent Brigham Hospital (PBBH) and the Beth Israel Hospital, and he was a volunteer assistant at Boston Children's Hospital. At Harvard Medical School (HMS), Weinfeld was also a teaching fellow in 1962.

Weinfeld published seven articles. His first was the product of his research with Dr. Jonathan Cohen at Boston Children's Hospital, "Experimental Excision of Muscles in the Weanling Rat." Expanding on previous studies by Dr. Albert B. Ferguson, Jr., who had moved from the PBBH to the University of Pittsburgh, Drs. Cohen and Weinfeld stated that:

> these experiments show that no substitutional hypertrophy occurred in any of the muscles in the myectomized extremity...only one muscle was heavier on the myomectomized side than on the intact side...the tibialis posterior...in the tibialis anterior excision group...hypertrophy of muscles which are substituted for those paralyzed is commonly seen in some patients...The discrepancy between the occurrence in those patients of substitutional hypertrophy and the lack of this change in these animal experiments invites speculation. The most attractive explanation is that the vastly higher level of integration of the nervous system of human beings compared with that of the rat prompts a substantial overuse of the appropriate muscles without conscious effort on the part of the patients...the data from these investigations serve to re-emphasize the marked discrepancies which may occur when experimental results in animals are compared with clinical situations.
> (Cohen and Weinfeld 1960)

In 1962, Weinfeld coauthored a paper on osteogenic sarcoma with Dr. H. Robert Dudley Jr., of the pathology department at MGH. They reviewed all the cases (164 patients) of osteogenic sarcoma between 1920–1960. Interestingly the authors referred to Dr. C. C. Simmons' review of bone sarcoma at the MGH in 1939—who found that several of the cases that had survived at least five years had tumors other than osteogenic sarcoma—and Drs. Ian Macdonald and J. W. Budd's review of 118 five-year cures in the American College of Surgeons Registry of Bone Sarcoma in 1943. However, they did not mention Dr. E. A. Codman (see chapter 34) from the MGH who was responsible for the founding of the Bone Sarcoma Registry of the American College of Surgeons.

Two years later, he moved his office from 475 Commonwealth Avenue to 454 Brookline Avenue in Boston, and in 1965 he was appointed an assistant in orthopaedic surgery at HMS, a position he held until at least 1969. Weinfeld's other five published articles were about arthritis. In 1969, he published two of these, one on the role of synovectomy of the knee in rheumatoid arthritis (see **Case 46.1**). He began by elaborating on the history of synovectomy of the knee to treat arthritis—mentioning the first procedure by M. Alfred Mignon in Paris in 1899, Joel Goldthwait's account of partial synovectomies in 1900, and the studies by Nathaniel Allison and Kenneth Coonse at MGH almost 30 years later—and highlighting the promising results they obtained. Weinfeld seemed to consider this procedure an initial treatment option to be performed early, with the goal of avoiding excessive damage from arthritis to the knee joint.

For Weinfeld, it was difficult to compare research results because of the different ways authors reported their findings, for example, as either only improved or not, or as simply good, fair, or poor results. In the second article he published that year. he proposed a rating system for use when evaluating knee arthroplasties. This system assigned various points to seven areas: pain, medial or lateral instability, knee motion, need for support while walking, flexion deformity, quadriceps power, and valgus or varus deformity. The points in each area are added together to achieve one of four outcomes: excellent (0–2 points), good (3–6 points), fair (7–10 points), or poor (≥ 11 points). He noted that only the pain category considers a subjective rating. Although Weinfeld initially created the system to indicate how well a knee arthroplasty succeeded, he indicated that it could also be applied in order to gauge the success of other knee procedures.

Dr. Marvin Weinfeld remained a junior visiting orthopaedic surgeon at the RBBH until the early 1970s when he was listed as a visiting orthopaedic surgeon. By 1976, he had been promoted to Clinical Instructor at HMS. He was board certified by the American Board of Orthopaedic Surgery and a member of the American Academy of Orthopaedic Surgeons (1967), the American College of Surgeons (1967), the American Medical Association, the American Rheumatism Association (American College of Rheumatology), the Massachusetts Medical Society, and the American Physicians Fellowship (APF, American Healthcare Professionals and Friends for Medicine in Israel). He died from a heart attack at Newton Wellesley Hospital on Sunday, September 28, 1986. He was 56 and was survived by his wife Beverly (Bunnin) and three sons.

Case 46.1. Knee Synovectomy in a Patient with Rheumatoid Arthritis

> "A 58-year-old woman had been experiencing moderate pain with weight-bearing and swelling involving both knees, more pronounced on the right side. X-rays did not show any joint space narrowing of the right knee, though there was slight narrowing of the joint space of the left knee. The lateral views showed moderate soft tissue thickening in the suprapatellar pouch area of both knees. Synovectomy of the right knee was performed and marked synovial thickening was observed with multiple white fibrin deposits covering the villi. The articular cartilage was intact except for a small area of erosion on the medial femoral condyle. She did well postoperatively but later developed increased pain in the left knee. X-rays taken 2 years later did not show any change in the joint space of the right knee, nor any recurrence of the soft tissue thickening. However, there had been further narrowing of the medial and lateral joint space of the left knee, and persistent soft tissue thickening. A synovectomy of the left knee was performed and the operative findings were marked synovial hypertrophy, with early articular cartilage destruction, though not sufficiently extensive for an arthroplasty procedure."
>
> (Marvin S. Weinfeld 1969)

PETER BENT BRIGHAM HOSPITAL

CARL W. WALTER

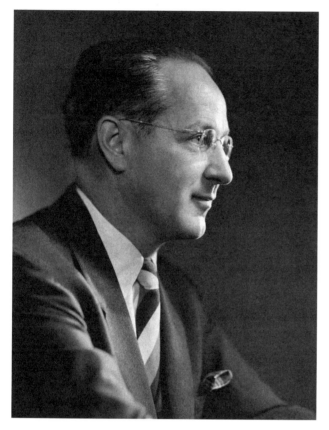

Carl W. Walter. Brigham and Women's Hospital Archives. Photo by Fabian Bachrach, courtesy of Louis F. Bachrach on behalf of Bachrach Studios.

Physician Snapshot

Carl W. Walter
BORN: 1905
DIED: 1992

SIGNIFICANT CONTRIBUTIONS: Advocate for surgical aseptic technique; published *The Aseptic Treatment of Wounds* (1948); director of the Surgical Research Laboratory at HMS; led the fracture service at the PBBH before the orthopaedic division was established; wrote a seminal paper about electrical effects on bone; pioneer in transfusion and storage of blood; founded the PBBH blood bank; a Harvard professorship is named for him (the Carl W. Walter Professor of Medicine and Medical Education)

Carl Waldemar Walter was born in Cleveland, Ohio, in 1905 to Carl Frederick and Leda Agatha Walter. He attended both primary and secondary school in Cleveland and was raised by parents who valued education. He excelled both scholastically and on the track. His mother was a teacher as well as a suffragist. His father worked as a stockbroker but had started as a minister before a career transition, having initially followed in the footsteps of his grandfather, who was also a minister. While in high school, Dr. Elliott C. Cutler, chairman of the Harvard Club, took Carl under his wing.

Walter graduated from Harvard College in 1928. He had continued to work while in school, having employment as a phone company lineman in high school and then completing odd jobs while in college. He graduated cum laude while balancing his studies with both work and running the quarter mile. He graduated from Harvard Medical School (HMS) in 1932 after Cutler, who had become a mentor, encouraged him to pursue medicine rather than chemistry.

The following year, Walter completed a surgical internship at the Peter Bent Brigham Hospital (PBBH). He later finished a residency there as well and began to pursue his lifelong passion for surgical asepsis. "He devised a method of properly sterilizing instruments using high pressure steam" as one of his earliest achievements (Brooks 1984). During his surgical residency under Dr. Elliot Cutler, the medical service under Dr. Henry Christian had a policy that:

> intravenous fluid therapy was not allowed because of the pyrogen reactions that resulted. Often patients would be transferred to the surgical service for fluid therapy and then returned to the medical service after correction of their fluid needs. Carl decided to try and eradicate the common problem of chills and fever that results from parenteral fluid therapy…he immediately went to work devising tubing, vents, flasks, and needle adapters…

Corning glass adapted his design for flasks that could be easily sterilized and centrifugalized. (Brooks 1984)

Advancing Aseptic Technique

After completing a Cabot Fellowship in 1936, Walter continued at the PBBH. Dr. Cutler, in his 1936 surgeon-in-chief's annual report, wrote:

> Of particular practical importance have been investigations of Carl Walter into the whole problem of antisepsis and asepsis, improvement of methods of sterilization, and the reverberations upon surgical technique. His studies have shown the many possible flaws in our present means of establishing asepsis and point to a more rigid setup if we are to protect our patients carefully. (quoted in "Carl Walter and the Evolution of the Surgical Research Laboratory" 1984)

Walter continued to pursue his interest in aseptic technique, and he was appointed director of the Surgical Research Laboratory at HMS in 1937, a position he held until 1949. He had an integral role teaching surgical technique using canine cadavers. Students would simulate surgical scenarios using the dogs (**Case 46.2**), following William Halsted's 1895 course as a model.

> The physicians, almoners, servants and all those who take care of the sick, before approaching them, and on quitting them, to wash their hands with chlorureted water.
> —Antoine Labarraque, Commissioner on Health of Marseilles, 1825

He used the course at HMS to teach aseptic technique to the second- and third-year students. He had some unusual but effective teaching methods:

Case 46.2. Dogs: a Medical Student's First Living Surgical Patient

> Dogs, Patients, and Physicians:
> "The emotional impact of a patient on the physician is a powerful determinant of each physician's concern and motivation. Sympathy, compassion, and identification complement the technical aspects of patient care and are reflected in a therapeutically positive patient response. The caring physician and the grateful patient are wed in a mutually beneficial alliance.
> "Similar emotional forces color learning and teaching situations. The choice of patient for teaching surgical technique has an enormous impact on the student's attitude and reaction to his responsibility for patients. Hence, teaching surgery using dogs as patients creates a poignant experience with many layers of perception, learning, and conditioning upon which is superimposed coaching of manual skill and surgical technique. The same degree of concern, often a paralyzing sense of responsibility, is not spontaneously evoked by a pig, or even a cat, simply because dogs have conditioned humans for eons in the proper posture and emotional response in a mutually gratifying relationship.
> "At the stage of emotional maturation when a student may faint while dissecting a cadaver or swoon at the sight of blood or be excused from helping a patient who is vomiting, the awesome responsibilities for a life that has related emotionally to him is often overwhelming. There is nothing like a wagging tail to put him in focus and to elicit the urge to care. The embryo physician's attitude toward future patient relationships crystallizes at that instant. If you doubt it, accompany me to any medical meeting and hear former students, some approaching retirement, recount the impact of dog surgery, a la Carl Walter, on their careers. The same emotion and identification that motivate antivivisectionists also create a physician who is dedicated to patient care because of the affection that glowed in the eyes of that dog – HIS first living patient!"
> —Carl W. Walter, unpublished, date unknown.
> (Reprinted from Barger 1984)

If the surgeon was bending too much over the operative field, he could expect a sharp blow in his back from the instructor, coupled with appropriate opprobrium. To learn scrubbing techniques, the students were blindfolded, and their hands covered with lamp black, and then they were challenged to get their hands clean. Finally, after scrubbing was completed, Carl would drop a quarter on the floor before the student. The victim's instinctive retrieval of the coin would be strongly commented on… surgeons to this day remember such training maneuvers with wry amusement and great appreciation. (Tilney "Carl Walter and the Evolution of the Surgical Research Laboratory" 1984)

In 1948, Walter published his classic book, *The Aseptic Treatment of Wounds* (**Box 46.2**). Later in his career, he established additional methods of infection control, including using "ethylene oxide for those substances that could not be placed in a fluid medium for sterilization" (Brooks 1984). Of his more than 150 publications, Dr. Walter published about 52 on hospital infections, the surgical environment, surgical gloves, scrubbing, and others. In his signature way, he stated "a mop reaches the wound more often than any surgical instrument." (quoted in Brooks 1984).

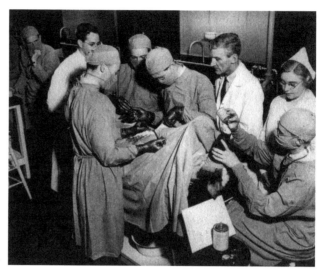

Surgical Research Laboratory during procedure under ether anesthesia. Dr. Walter is observing (second from left); Dr. Cutler is also observing (In the back, on the right, and without a mask).

A Perfectly Striking Departure: Surgeons and Surgery at the Peter Bent Brigham Hospital 1912-1980 by Nicholas L. Tilney. Science History Publications, 2006. Brigham and Women's Hospital Archives.

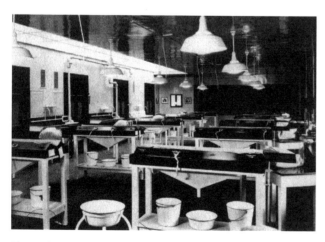

Surgical Research Laboratory, HMS, ca. 1920s.

A Perfectly Striking Departure: Surgeons and Surgery at the Peter Bent Brigham Hospital 1912-1980 by Nicholas L. Tilney. Science History Publications, 2006. Brigham and Women's Hospital Archives.

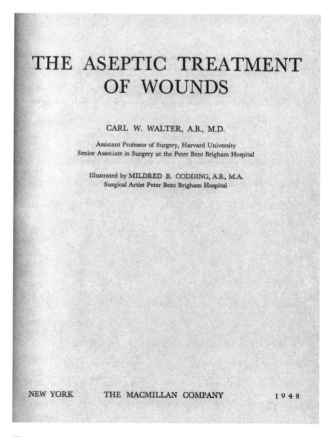

Title page of Walter's book, *The Aseptic Treatment of Wounds*. New York: The Macmillan Company, 1948.

Box 46.2. Publication of The Aseptic Treatment of Wounds

> In the preface, Dr. Carl W. Walter wrote:
>
> "The prompt, kindly healing of wounds, long a rarely attained goal of the most adept surgeon, has become so routine that modern surgeons habitually assume the miracle of the 1870s to be an attribute of their own skill rather than…chemotherapy. Indeed, a wave of chemotherapeutic hysteria has engulfed many surgeons, whose aseptic treatment is unknowingly so sketchy that wound complications plague their work…most surgeons think of asepsis only as the use of rubber gloves and a few sterile drapes… Carelessness, tradition, expediency, and habit dictate many techniques, whereas safety for the individual patient demands a basis of fact and a standardized technique…
>
> "The myriads of questions prompted in the minds of medical students, internes, and nurses by the inconsistencies and discrepancies in aseptic technique established the need for this book. Numerous adventures in hospitals where postoperative infections and sepsis presented problems broadened its scope. Even within one hundred miles of Boston, hospitals were visited where instruments were not sterilized routinely between cases; where the chamber of a steam sterilizer had never been connected to the steam supply; where waterproof duck was used as sterilizing wrappers; where the dry goods frequently burst into flames as they were withdrawn from the sterilizer; where the superintendent's hero was an orderly who 'sterilized' twice as much dry goods in half the time needed. In each instance, surgeons requested help to solve problems that basic knowledge would have avoided" (Walter 1948).
>
> Dr. Elliott Cutler wrote the forward:
>
> "The aseptic technique had its beginning in simple cleanliness…but it had to be established through the experience of antisepsis and its emergence was beclouded…Thus the notable book by Schimmelbusch published in 1893…*The Aseptic Treatment of Wounds*, fell in part on deaf ears… Every surgeon should know at least the principles which underly the working of an autoclave…he cannot escape full responsibility if the material supposedly sterile be not sterile…There can be little excuse now for sepsis following an operation of election, since the methods of avoiding it are presented here."
>
> (Cutler 1948)

Contributing to Blood Banks and Medical Devices

In 1937—the same year he was appointed to the Surgical Research Laboratory at HMS—he founded the PBBH blood bank, which he had initially started in the HMS basement. Walter contributed to red blood cell preservation and the invention of the plastic blood bags and other transfusion equipment:

> Walter is perhaps best known for inventing the plastic bags still universally used to collect and transport blood [and also establishing] one of the world's first blood banks, in 1934 in a basement room at Harvard – an obscure location chosen because some trustees thought storage and use of human blood was "immoral and unethical." He invented the blood bag 15 years

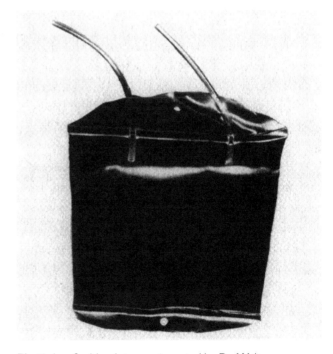

Plastic bag for blood storage invented by Dr. Walter.
C. W. Walter, "Invention and Development of the Blood Bag," *Vox Sanguinis* 1984; 47: 319.

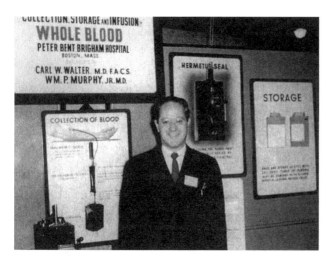

Photo of Dr. Walter with his (and Dr. W. P. Murphy Jr.s) exhibit on the collection, storage and transfusion of blood, 1950.

The Teaching Hospital: Brigham and Women's Hospital and the Evolution of Academic Medicine by Peter V. Tishler, Christine Wenc, and Joseph Loscalzo. McGraw-Hill Education, 2014. Brigham and Women's Hospital Archives.

later, making it possible to end a cumbersome and dangerous procedure by which doctors pumped blood directly from donor to patient via paraffin-coated glass tubes heated over alcohol lamps. ("Dr. Carl W. Walter; Inventor of Blood Bag" 1992)

He modified and improved the renal dialysis machine as well. In 1941, an article was published in the *Daily Boston Globe* about Walter's strong advocacy for the necessity of having blood banks in every community. The article quoted Dr. Walter:

> Transfusion is now a safe procedure for both donor and recipient…Careful study of the effect of blood loss on the donor has revealed no harmful results following donations of a pint of blood at intervals of four or five weeks… Records such as these should dispel the fear of giving blood which persists from the days when the ignorant were exploited by professional donor bureaus and bled so profusely that they suffered from severe anemia. Anyone in good health is suitable for service as a donor. ("Blood Banks Urged for Greater Boston" 1941)

Known as a pioneer in the medical device industry, he also contributed to industrial thermostats. He eventually became an industrial research entrepreneur.

Organizing the Fracture Service at the PBBH

One year after his appointment to the Surgical Research Laboratory at HMS, Dr. Walter was also asked to organize a fracture service at the PBBH. The service was to exist within the division of general surgery. He led the service for eight years. During this period, he:

> published a paper in 1941 [that] described the effect of electricity on bone. Two platinum bands were wrapped subperiosteally around the femur of an anesthetized rabbit…A 1½ volt battery was connected to the bands for…24 hours…He noted that there was bone produced about the positive electrode, but no change was noted about the negative electrode…one of the pioneer papers about electrical effects on bone. (Banks 1983)

He was creative and "fundamentally an engineer at heart" (Banks 1983). In his memoirs, Dr. Henry Banks wrote the following about Dr. Walter:

> He, too, was knowledgeable about the management of fractures and taught me how to use external fixators in the management of Colles fractures of the radius. It was a technique which was later copied and popularized by several orthopaedic surgeons. He was way ahead of his time in this regard and should have received more recognition but was outside of the "old boy" network in Orthopaedics. (Banks, n.d.)

He stepped down from leading the fracture service in 1946, when Dr. Cutler asked Dr. William Green to organize a new orthopaedic division. Although Walter continued on staff as a visiting surgeon, he eventually "withdrew from the Fracture Service and focused his attention on the control of infections on the wards and in the O.R." (Banks, n.d.).

Walter retired from the PBBH in 1973, after 40 years of service. He had spent most of his life living in Holliston, Massachusetts. Brooks (1984) described Walter as having "a strong dislike for inaccuracy and incompetence, which sometimes comes out explosively, and...a robust sense of humor. He sometimes riles his colleagues, but those who have known him through the years have tremendous admiration for his intellect, brilliance, innovative thoughts, and for his genuine devotion to his friends." Banks, a close friend of his, remembered that Walter "had a crusty, tough exterior, but we later became great friends. Indeed, his poodle, which was always present in his office, later fathered 'Blackie' which was given to the Banks' while I was recovering from neck (cervical disc) surgery in 1961" (Banks, n.d.).

Among his many achievements, Dr. Carl Walter was instrumental in supporting the Pound Bill in Massachusetts in 1957, which allowed researchers to obtain dogs and cats about to be put down by pounds; was chair of Harvard Medical School's committee on animal research; and was a major supporter and board member of the New England Regional Primate Research Center. He was a prolific writer "and won awards from the American Society of Mechanical Engineers and the Society of Manufacturing Engineers" (Lambert 1992). He died after a stroke at 86 years old on May 5, 1992, in the Stillman Infirmary in Cambridge, Massachusetts. He was survived by his wife, Margaret Davis Walter, four daughters (Martha, Alice, Linda, and Margaret), and two sons (Carl and David). A Harvard professorship (the Carl W. Walter Professor of Medicine and Medical Education) and amphitheater at HMS in the Tosteson Medical Education Center are named for him.

ALBERT B. FERGUSON JR.

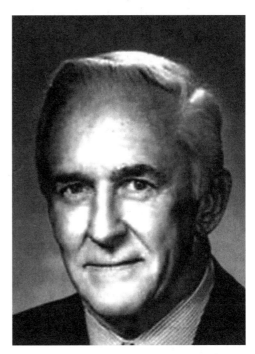

Albert B. Ferguson Jr. Courtesy of Dr. Freddie Fu and the Ferguson Laboratory for Orthopaedic and Spine Research.

Physician Snapshot

Albert B. Ferguson Jr.
BORN: 1919
DIED: 2014

SIGNIFICANT CONTRIBUTIONS: The first full time orthopaedic surgeon at the PBBH; established an orthopaedic surgery residency program at the University of Pittsburgh; served as president of the American Board of Orthopaedic Surgery and the American Orthopaedic Association

Dr. Albert Barnett Ferguson Jr. (who preferred to be called "Ferg") was born in New York City on June 10, 1919. He was the third physician in his family lineage; his grandfather, Dr. Jeremiah Ferguson, helped establish Cornell Medical School. His father, Albert B. Ferguson, performed pioneering work in radiography as one of the earliest x-ray specialists in the United States. His father also published the textbook *Roentgen Diagnosis of the Extremities and Spine* and led the department of roentgenology at New York Orthopaedic Hospital.

Ferg attended Dartmouth College, graduating in 1941. He completed two years of medical school at Dartmouth and graduated from Harvard Medical School (HMS) in 1943. Dr. Ferguson Jr. briefly deferred his medical training to serve in the US Marine Corps for three years, but he went on to complete a surgical internship and orthopaedic residency program at the Peter Bent Brigham Hospital (PBBH), the Massachusetts General Hospital (MGH), and Boston Children's Hospital (BCH). "While there, Elliot Cutler asked Dr. William T. Green to establish an orthopaedic division at the PBBH in 1946. Staff included "the orthopedic visiting staff from Children's as well as Doctors [Carl] Walter and [Bart] Quigley" ("Osgood Lecture," n.d.). Dr. Ferguson Jr. completed his internship training on June 30, 1947.

As a resident at the PBBH, Ferguson reviewed x-rays on 42 patients with solitary calcified medullary lesions in bone discovered on x-rays taken for other reasons, usually to visualize the adjacent joint in fractures. In one case, a fractured femur (see **Case 46.3**), he was able to obtain the lesion at the time of surgery by Dr. Walter and examine it histologically. He concluded the lesion was "an example of faulty development of bone from cartilage [and] classified as one of the many forms of chondrodysplasia" (Ferguson 1947).

To make his time spent teaching and completing research more efficient, Cutler arranged for Ferguson to have a small office on A-Main with a secretary-reception room and one examining room. In 1951 Ferguson was a junior associate in surgery at the PBBH. In addition to Dr. Green and senior associate in surgery, Dr. A. H. Brewster, the other orthopaedic surgeons on the clinical staff at the time included Drs. Paul Hugenberger and Meier Karp (associates in surgery) and Drs. David

Case 46.3. Spiral Fracture of the Middle and Distal Thirds of the Right Femur

"[The patient], a white male, sixty-eight years old, a stationary engineer, never engaged in construction work entered the Peter Bent Brigham Hospital with a spiral fracture of the middle and distal thirds of the right femur, following a fall on getting out of bed. A calcified developmental defect was found in the distal section of the fractured bone...

"At open reduction, this calcified area was removed, apparently intact and easily separated from the adjacent bone, leaving a round defect where it had been nesting. Postoperative roentgenograms revealed that the lesion had been removed except for two small flecks of calcification. The lesion consisted of reddish tissue, irregularly shaped into a rounded mass, approximately one centimeter in diameter and two centimeters in length, and containing hard yellow areas. It was found to be glassy hard and rang when dropped on a hard surface.

"Sections revealed a somewhat irregular area of calcified, non-viable cartilage, at the periphery of which a slow process of new-bone formation was taking place...a low-power photomicrograph taken at the periphery of this lesion...shows all features of the lesion, from calcified cartilaginous matrix on the left to bone spicules with small attached areas of viable cartilage on the right. A high-power photomicrograph of the cartilaginous matrix with an area of viable cartilage is shown."

(Ferguson 1947)

Grice, and junior associates Charles Sturdevant, and a man named Weston (first name unknown). According to the PBBH annual report (1951), Cutler stated that Ferguson would:

> add strength to our clinical studies of the many problems encountered in corrective orthopedics and the surgery of skeletal trauma. In addition, Dr. Ferguson is embarking on a study of the histo-chemistry and muscle dynamics of prolonged immobilization...Under the

leadership of Dr. Green, Dr. Quigley and Dr. Walter, the Brigham deals effectively with a large volume of orthopedic problems and fractures from the neighboring communities. (Banks, n.d.)

By October 1, 1951, Ferguson received an appointment at HMS. He also "became the first full-time orthopedic surgeon" at the PBBH ("Osgood Lecture," n.d.) because "it was clear that if the Brigham orthopedic service was to develop into something significant, it was going to require some full-time supervision" ("Osgood Lecture," n.d.). Ferguson remained at the PBBH for almost two years, resigning on July 1, 1953 to accept the position of chairman of orthopaedics at the University of Pittsburgh. While working at the PBBH, he had also been appointed to the courtesy staff of the Robert Breck Brigham Hospital (RBBH), along with Drs. Lloyd T. Brown, Joel E. Goldthwait, Robert Joplin, Robert H. Morris, William A. Rogers and Marius Smith-Petersen.

In 1953, Ferguson published a preliminary report demonstrating his early interest in muscle dynamics as Cutler had predicted. In the Laboratory for Surgical Research at the PBBH, he had studied the action of two opposing muscles, the tibialis anterior and the gastrocnemius. He concluded:

> the length-tension diagram of the tibialis anterior and gastrocnemius muscles of the rat reveals differences in the range of maximum… tension in relation to the resting tension…It is felt that the standard configuration noted by Blix in the gastrocnemius of the frog cannot be applied to all length-tension diagrams and…the point of maximum tension of a muscle will vary with structure and function. (Ferguson 1953)

After Ferguson left the PBBH and moved to the University of Pittsburgh, he continued his focus on muscles and the effects of immobilization by studying disuse atrophy of the tibialis anterior and gastrocnemius. After immobilizing 41 rabbits with 12 controls and measuring each muscle's weight, histologic changes, blood flow, and biochemistry changes, he concluded:

> 1. There is a fundamental difference in the reaction to immobilization of the tibialis anterior and the gastrocnemius in the rabbit. 2. There is an increased blood flow in both atrophy and hypertrophy of skeletal muscle in this animal. 3. Atrophy and hypertrophy appear to represent a change in intracellular constituents without change in the water content of the muscles studied. 4. Tension appears to protect against atrophy, in so far as the tibialis anterior is concurred in the rabbit. 5. Both atrophy and hypertrophy of skeletal muscles in the rabbit appear to represent a metabolic change. (Ferguson and Vaughan 1957)

He continued his basic applied research and clinical studies over the next 35 years at the University of Pittsburgh, publishing over 58 articles and several books. He started a residency program in orthopaedic surgery, which became highly sought after while developing a strong national and internationally known department of orthopaedic leaders. He also was elected president of several orthopaedic professional organizations, including the Hip Society, the American Board of Orthopaedic Surgery, and the American Orthopaedic Association.

Dr. Albert B. Ferguson Jr. died on August 20, 2014 at 95. He left behind a strong legacy of orthopaedic chairmen, residents, and staff who have great affection for him.

CHAPTER 47

Origins of BWH and Organizing Orthopaedics as a Department

Orthopaedics at Brigham and Women's Hospital (BWH) has a robust history. The hospital was initially established through a merger between the Robert Breck Brigham Hospital (RBBH), the Peter Bent Brigham Hospital (PBBH), and the Boston Hospital for Women. In 1958, an ad hoc committee at the Robert Breck Brigham Hospital was charged "with solving some of Peter Bent Brigham Hospital's financial problems by identifying ways to share costs of nursing education and laundry management among hospitals in the area. Informal discussions revealed an interest in cooperation in a broader basis to improve patient care among neighboring institutions" ("Historical Notes," n.d.). Harvard Medical School Dean George Packer Berry then "conceived, proposed, and initiated the combining of the six hospitals involved [PBBH, RBBH, Children's Hospital Medical Center, Boston Lying-in Hospital, Free Hospital for Women, and the Massachusetts Eye and Ear Infirmary] in one great medical complex" ("Annual Report, 1964–1965. Joint Report of the Chairman of the Board of Trustees and the President" 1965). By 1961, a charitable corporation known as the Affiliated Hospitals Center, Inc. (AHC) was established.

A PLAN FOR A MEDICAL CENTER

The 1964–1965 annual report of this newly established organization read that "this vital and tremendously complicated project may well appear to be far too slow for all concerned" ("Annual Report, 1964–1965. Joint Report of the Chairman of the Board of Trustees and the President" 1965). On July 1, 1963, Dr. Robert J. Glaser had become president of the Affiliated Hospitals Center, but he resigned in 1965 to become vice president and dean of Stanford's School of Medicine. On the day of Glaser's departure (June 30, 1965), Dean Berry also retired. There was a great deal of concern about the status of the mergers with the exit of these two leaders. However, Robert H. Ebert replaced Berry as dean. The annual report stated, "In one of his first pronouncements [Dean Ebert] indicated that bringing to fruition of Affiliated Hospitals Center, Inc. is to be one of his immediate and most important undertakings" ("Annual Report, 1964–1965. Joint Report of the Chairman of the Board of Trustees and the President" 1965). He remained in daily contact with the hospitals, administrators, and trustees involved in the project. Later that year, "Boston

Lying-in-Hospital [formed in 1832] and the Free Hospital for Women [formed in 1875] have...completed the details of consolidation into one women's hospital and the RBBH has strengthened its affiliations with Harvard Medical School" ("Annual Report, 1964–1965. Joint Report of the Chairman of the Board of Trustees and the President" 1965). The new hospital was named the Boston Hospital for Women.

Mr. F. Stanton Deland Jr., a prominent Boston attorney and member of the Lying-in-Hospital Board of Trustees, resigned from the board and was elected president of the Affiliated Hospitals Center, Inc. A governing body of the Affiliated Hospitals Center, Inc. was formed, and it included the presidents of the PBBH, RBBH, and the Boston Hospital for Women, as well as President Deland. The Children's Hospital Medical Center and the Massachusetts Eye and Ear Infirmary were no longer involved with the merger discussions. The joint venture was strengthened with the appointment of Dr. Frank Austen as Chief of Staff at the RBBH and associate professor at Harvard Medical School. February 14, 1967, was a momentous occasion. On that date:

> [A] working agreement called "A Plan for a Medical Center" was put together by the Robert B. Brigham, the Peter Bent Brigham, and the newly formed Boston Hospital for Women...the three hospitals formally resolved to support the plan for union without waiting for the other potential partners. This was followed by a centralization of power under a new Joint Venture Agreement giving the presidents of the participating hospitals and the Affiliated Hospitals Center president (F. Stanton Deland) authority to proceed with the creation of the new medical center "as quickly as possible."
> ("Historical Notes," n.d.)

The merger process for BWH would continue to unfold over the next 13 years, filled with many difficult negotiations, delays, and setbacks. Despite many challenges, the ultimate result would be successful: a new modern teaching hospital located across the street from Harvard Medical School (HMS).

ORTHOPAEDICS ORGANIZES AS A DEPARTMENT

In RBBH's 1969 annual report, the president wrote that the hospital had been sold to the Baptist (New England Baptist Hospital [NEBH]) for $4 million "to be paid over a period of years" ("Annual Report, 1969. Report of the President" 1969). The RBBH would continue to operate at its current site until it could move to a new facility in a joint venture near HMS. The president of RBBH also announced the "establishment of a full-time academic professorship in Orthopedic Surgery...to be shared with the PBBH...establishing a new Department of Orthopedic Medicine and Surgery equivalent to those of the Children's Hospital and Massachusetts General Hospital...The Board of this hospital and the Peter Bent Brigham have agreed to offer to appoint Dr. Clement Sledge to their hospital departments, upon his appointment to his academic post by Harvard College" ("Annual Report, 1969. Report of the President" 1969). Sledge (see chapter 48) was present at the hospital's corporation meeting.

Dr. Francis D. Moore, in his annual surgeon-in-chief's report (1969–1970) at the PBBH, wrote, "Sledge took over at the two Brighams [Peter Bent Brigham and Robert Breck Brigham] as the first Academic Full Time Professor of Orthopaedic Surgery at the Brigham...Dr. J. Drennan Lowell [PBBH 1954–1955] has been appointed Dr. Sledge's principal assistant in conducting orthopedic affairs at the Brigham. Coincident with this change, Orthopedic Surgery has been given department status at the Brigham" ("Annual Report, 1969-1970. Report of the

Origins of BWH and Organizing Orthopaedics as a Department

Surgeon-in-Chief" 1970). Dr. Sledge's appointment to the staff was dated March 1, 1970.

Three years after the three hospitals had officially resolved to merge, orthopaedic surgery became a department at the not-yet-named Brigham and Women's. The leadership had predetermined that there would be one department under one chairperson when the hospital merger was completed. It was initially organized as one department in two hospitals, RBBH and PBBH. Dr. Sledge was appointed surgeon-in-chief at the RBBH and orthopaedic surgeon-in-chief at the PBBH. It was an active time for change in orthopaedic surgery:

> [Dr. Clement] Sledge [see chapter 48] took over the two Brighams as the first Academic Full Time Professor of Orthopedic Surgery at the Brigham...Dr. J. Drennan Lowell (PBBH 1954–55) has been appointed as Dr. Sledge's principal assistant in conducting Orthopedic affairs at the Brigham. Coincident with this change, Orthopedic Surgery has been given department status at the Brigham. ("57th Annual Report, 1969–1970. Report of the Surgeon-in-Chief" 1970)

During the transition year of orthopaedic leadership at the Brigham hospitals, each orthopaedic service's statistics were: RBBH: 1,715 patients admitted, 88% occupancy, 17 days' average length of stay, and 7,416 outpatient visits; PBBH: 786 patients admitted, 728 operations performed, and more than 6,000 patients seen

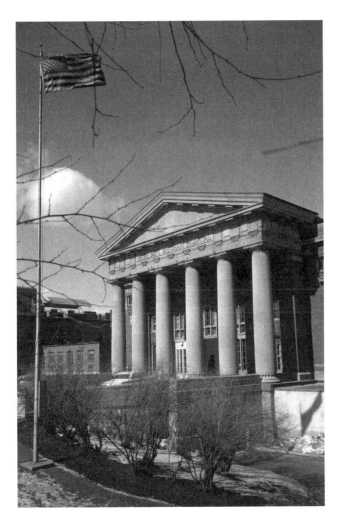

PBBH Administrative Building entrance, ca. 1960s. Brigham and Women's Hospital Archives.

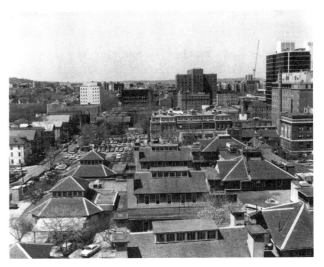

Pavilion wards at PBBH, ca. 1970s. Brigham and Women's Hospital Archives.

Box 47.1. Mandate to Unify Orthopaedics at the Brigham Hospitals

> In a 2009 interview with me, Dr. Clement Sledge discussed the mandate he received from hospital leadership, which: "was to unify two different groups of orthopedic surgeons. You can imagine some of the challenges. It wasn't bad though, because...Dr. Potter, who was chief at the Robert Brigham...a part time position...not salaried...gracefully moved over to the New England Baptist. And the only people on staff in orthopedics, other than Ted Potter, were Bill Thomas, Marv Weinberg and Ed Nalebuff. And so, I was happy to have them stay. Marv was never a contributor clinically or in terms of publications...But I was happy to have Bill, who also never wrote many papers, but was a wonderful teacher of residents and if you could afford to have someone to teach just bedside manner, you'd want to hire Bill. And Ed was Ed. Even then he was a pre-eminent hand surgeon and a very good teacher.
>
> "And at the Peter Bent Brigham the chief there [Henry Banks]—also a part time position, who left to go to Tufts—had hired a couple of former residents to be in the department...I was young and brash and knew no better [and] didn't think they really fit into our academic center that I was trying to build. I encouraged them to look elsewhere... Frank O'Connor and Larry Shields...so there was no one there because it had been a three-man department with Henry Banks...And so when Dren Lowell came...over time we would fall into the same trap. I guess most of us do. The devil you know—we would hire out of the residency program. These are people we'd observed for three to four years and knew they came from excellent backgrounds. In most instances we would send them away for further clinical or basic training. Steve Lipson was outstanding and spent time with the chemist named Helen Muir and he did some excellent work...I did set him up in the lab when he came back, but never to my final days discovered how you compensate a clinician for his time in the laboratory when he is losing clinical income and you have a reimbursement scheme that is based on the generation of clinical monies. So, though you can try and protect their time, you can't protect their money and so as he got busier and busier clinically, it became more and more difficult, even though I had a lab for him, paid his technician and so forth...so he drifted out of our lab. Barry [Simmons] went to France for his hand training and then came back. And that was sort of typical...we'd send people somewhere for special training, maybe based on my own experience with the Glimcher model...The Staff grew fairly slowly, but appropriate to the beds and the OR time we had."
>
> (Sledge, interview with the author, 2009)

in clinics. Orthopaedic growth at the PBBH was small (to 786 admissions from 781 in the previous year), but operations increased (to 728 from 671). Dr. Henry Banks, who had been at the PBBH since 1954, resigned on July 1, 1970. He had accepted an appointment as Professor and Chairman of Orthopaedics at Tufts University School of Medicine. In **Box 47.1**, Dr. Sledge discusses his mandate by the leadership of both Brigham hospitals.

Orthopedics was listed in the 58th annual report of the PBBH for the first time as the Department of Orthopedics (July 1, 1970, to June 30, 1971). Dr. Sledge was the orthopedic surgeon-in-chief (see chapter 48). Dr. Lowell was senior associate in orthopedic surgery. Associates in orthopedic surgery included Drs. Paul Hugenberger, Arthur Pappas, and Arthur Trott; junior associates in orthopaedic surgery included Drs. Frank Bates, Ben Bierbaum, Art Boland, Stuart Cope, Robert W. Hussey, Robert Keller, Jack McGinty, Larry Shields, and Bill Thomas. Dr. Panos G. Panagakos was an assistant in surgery. There were four orthopedic residents and four assistant orthopedic residents. Dr. Thomas Quigley remained in the department of surgery.

Dr. Sledge's additional staff included Bill Thomas, Fred Ewald, Ed Nalebuff, and Lew Millender—all from the RBBH—who joined Dren Lowell and Bill Head at the PBBH. In addition, staff from Boston Children's Hospital were a "devoted group of part-time visiting surgeons"

Origins of BWH and Organizing Orthopaedics as a Department

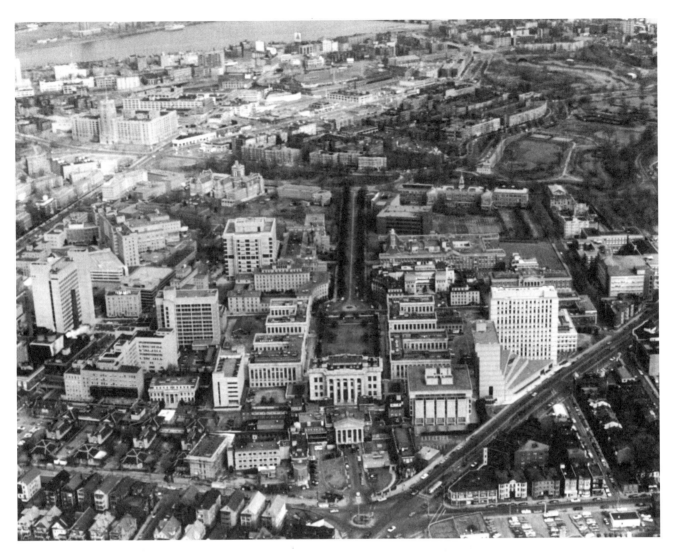

Aerial view of PBBH, 1973. Brigham and Women's Hospital Archives.

("58th Annual Report 1970–1971. Report of the Orthopedic Surgeon-in-Chief" 1971). In his first annual report of the orthopedic surgeon-in-chief, Dr. Sledge wrote: "[1970–1971] was a year of change for the Department of Orthopedic Surgery—changes in personnel, affiliations, residency training and even in the character of the patient population. A large amount of arthritic surgery at the RBBH compliments the trauma and reconstructive surgery at the PBBH and each gains from the other. The clinical research activities will be centered at the PBBH and laboratory research at the RBBH…" ("58th Annual Report 1970–1971. Report of the Orthopedic Surgeon-in-Chief" 1971).

Sledge recalled that most of the year was spent organizing a new department and coordinating the training program at both Brigham and the WRVA hospital. Orthopaedic statistics that year included: 800 admissions, 508 operations performed by residents and visiting staff, orthopaedic/fracture clinic visits: 4,441 patients, Industrial Accident Clinic visits: 5,390 patients, podiatry clinic: 1,305 patients, and 22,378 physical therapy treatments. Dr. Bruce Wood replaced Dr. Donald Holmes (who retired after five years) as chief of the podiatry clinic. Larry Shields went into private practice in Waltham. I asked Dr. Sledge if he had developed a practice plan separate and independent of the other departments. He replied:

Yes. As a matter of fact, because all salaries were [generated] from the practices...I don't think any had medical school money and only a couple had any hospital money. I wanted to give them a pension plan that they wouldn't otherwise have...I had to take it to the Trustees to be allowed to do that. But I did it so I could give them a pension/profit-sharing plan. It was a kind of insurance that I thought we wanted. It turns out that it became the model and the Department of Medicine later incorporated using the same lawyer I used...but as I said I never solved the problem of how do you get an appropriate compensation for people that doesn't penalize big earners when you need...to subsidize people whose skills you need, but they are in a section of orthopedics that insurance companies never thought should be remunerated very well [and subsidization] created great tensions. (Sledge, interview with the author, 2009)

Grand rounds were held on Thursday mornings at the RBBH (started by Dr. Sledge) and Friday mornings at the PBBH (with staff from Boston Children's Hospital), and the "three main teaching hospitals involved in the Combined Harvard Orthopaedic Teaching Program [included] the Brigham, the Massachusetts General and Children's" ("58th Annual Report 1970–1971. Report of the Orthopedic Surgeon-in-Chief" 1971). By 1978, Sledge had changed grand rounds to 5 PM on Wednesdays at the RBBH. During the transition into the new hospital, rheumatology continued to hold weekly grand rounds, but Orthopaedic Grand Rounds were briefly discontinued.

NEW FACILITIES FOR BWH AND ORTHOPAEDICS

The merger process was complex and there were many delays that affected the orthopaedic department. During this time of departmental transformation, the physical facilities simultaneously required extensive repair. Archival records indicate "the deterioration of [the] old hospital buildings has made new construction essential[, and in 1968] a capital funds campaign was organized to raise construction funds" ("Affiliated Hospitals Center," n.d.).

By 1971, their fundraising efforts had "surpassed its $15m goal...[and] the Massachusetts Department of Public Health granted the AHC, Inc. a Certificate of Need [in 1974] to enable construction of the new facility" ("Affiliated Hospitals Center," n.d.). Of the more than $15M raised, $0.5M was allocated to arthritic and joint disease:

> The Robert B. Brigham Hospital has achieved the reputation of being the outstanding center devoted to the study and treatment of arthritis...One of the more spectacular aspects of the program is the replacement of diseased joints with prosthetic devices. First hips, then fingers, and now knees and elbows are restored with plastic and metal appliances. Prosthetic replacements for shoulders are being developed. People who could no longer walk or even hold a cup of coffee can now emerge from the hospital with the ability to live a useful life. Because of its inclusion in the Seeley G. Mudd Research Building, a large portion of the research facilities needed by this program have been provided. ("Affiliated Hospitals Center," n.d.)

Other projects designated for funds included: $1.5M for primary and ambulatory care, $2M for obstetric and neonatal, $4M for cardiovascular devices, and $4M for transplant biology and immunology. The campaign was named "Campaign for Clinical and Academic Programs." Building plans included:

> a 16-story tower with 680 beds...Adjoining the hospital will be the Ambulatory Care Building... Each of the three divisions [PBBH, RBBH, and Boston Hospital for Women] will be assigned several floors. The Boston Hospital for Women

will occupy the lower levels, the Peter Bent Brigham the central section, and the Robert B. Brigham the upper floors. ("Affiliated Hospitals Center," n.d.)

They had originally planned to finish building the new hospital by 1974, but the work did not begin until the following year because "the escalation of building costs raised the project budget from the estimated 50 million dollars to 80 million. Political regimes changed and the expected amounts from government grants fell precipitously. Harvard University was no longer able to make land available for the construction." ("Historical Notes," n.d.). Although the initial certificate of need had not been granted, "Regulatory authorities were slow with the necessary approvals due to community protests [including Harvard students]" ("Historical Notes," n.d.). Community members feared losing their homes in the effort to secure enough space for the new hospital "and the potential environmental impact of Harvard's proposed power plant (Medical Area Total Energy Plant, or MATEP) designed to supply energy to the Affiliated Hospitals Center and nearby hospitals" ("Historical Notes," n.d.).

By January 1, 1975, the three hospitals had sealed their union "legally, finally, and irrevocably" as the Affiliated Hospitals Center, Inc., and "each hospital then operated as a division" of it (quoted in "Historical Notes," n.d.). Each had an executive committee (n=10) and a Board of Overseers (PBBH: 41 members; RBBH: 23 members). Dr. Sledge was on the executive committee with two other physicians and on the RBBH Board of Overseers (Class R) with the only other physician being Dr. Frank Austen. He was the surgeon-in-chief at the Robert Breck Brigham Hospital and orthopedic surgeon-in-chief at the Peter Bent Brigham Hospital.

By the end of that year, after receiving approval for a second certificate of need, "ground-breaking for the long-planned-for facility happened on December 20, 1975" ("Historical Notes" n.d.),

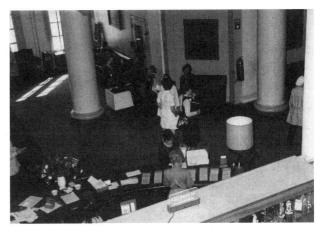

Francis Street lobby, PBBH, 1976. Brigham and Women's Hospital Archives.

and by "November 15, 1976 [after many meetings between the local community and AHC leadership] the City of Boston accepted the final plans" ("Affiliated Hospitals Center," n.d.). The three hospitals were expected to maintain operations with minimal disruption during the construction and merger process. Consolidation of functions and responsibilities were to evolve slowly and their initial efforts were focused on filling top-level administrative positions: VP for administration, VP for financial operations, VP for design and construction, and VP for external affairs.

Initially, Dr. Frank Austen was chair of the central planning committee; replaced by Dr. Eugene Braunwald in 1977. All department chiefs were members of the central planning committee. Decisions were made by consensus; no formal voting occurred. In 1977, Dean Ebert was replaced by Dr. Daniel Tosteson, who was very supportive of the merger. He stated, "I intend to support this happy alliance with all my vigor in the years ahead" ("Annual Corporation Meeting, February 9, 1977. Dean Tosteson's remarks" 1977). The Central Planning Committee reorganized their clinical strengths: reproductive biology, obstetrics, rheumatology, immunology, orthopaedics, renal diseases, and cardiovascular diseases. They also recognized a major need for more research space and often discussed one major problem: what to name the new hospital.

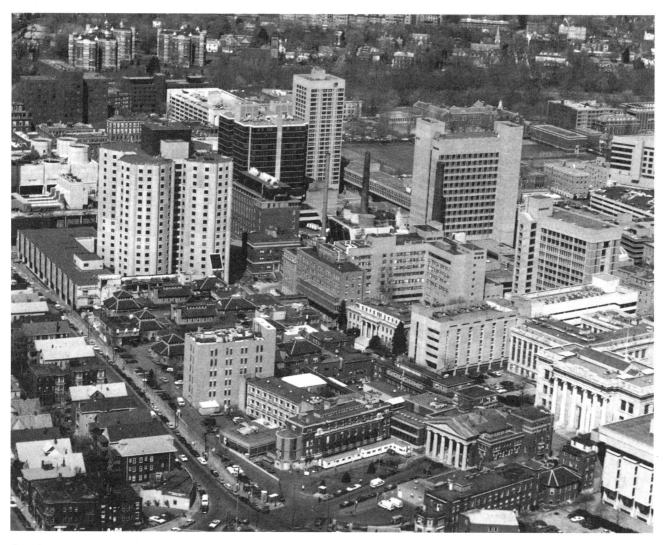
Aerial view BWH with towers. Notice the pavilions remain between the Administrative Building and the towers, ca. 1980s.
Brigham and Women's Hospital Archives.

OPENING ITS DOORS AS THE NEWLY NAMED BWH

The AHC, Inc. published annual reports which were divided into four sections: the AHC and three division reports (Boston Hospital for Women, PBBH and RBBH). The AHC report included status reports by the board of trustees, the president, financial and other reports. Lists of the boards of overseers, the administrative staff, and the medical staff were included in each division report. In addition, the PBBH included status reports provided by the director and the department chiefs of medicine, surgery, radiology, anesthesiology, pathology, and orthopaedics. The RBBH included status reports provided by the president and director, the physician-in-chief and the surgeon-in-chief.

Not surprisingly, physicians were concerned about adequate office space. President Deland stated: "There is too much of a 'we' and 'they' prevailing attitude, when in fact we are all in the same boat and striving for the same objectives. We must and will reach a compromise satisfactory to all concerned" ("Annual Report, 1977. President's Report" 1977). Professional staff (n=15) meetings were held frequently, and Dr. Sledge was an active participant. They completed the new staff by-laws early in 1979. By October 1, 1979, there were 14 orthopaedic beds and 15 rheumatology and orthopaedic beds in the new Tower Building. Orthopaedic staff were well represented on eight different major committees. That fiscal year was "the last full year that the hospital [RBBH] will spend on the heights at Parker Hill, as a move to the top three floors of the new AHC Tower is anticipated this summer" ("Robert Breck Brigham Hospital Division, 1978–1979" 1979).

After a 20-year negotiation process, the new BWH facility opened at 75 Francis Street in 1980. With the completed merger, the two divisions in orthopaedics—Robert Breck Brigham Hospital (RBBH) and Peter Bent Brigham Hospital (PBBH)—were discontinued and incorporated into a single department. Orthopaedic staff from both divisions became members of the new department. In his 1980 president's report, Dr. Robert G. Petersdorf (who replaced Mr. Deland) commented on the stresses and strains of the merger that were especially true for the staff of the RBBH: "who will be leaving their tight little islands for immigration into a large and perhaps unknown country [and] relations between the AHC and the community remain uneasy" ("Report of the President. May 29, 1980" 1980).

The RBBH buildings and land had been sold 11 years earlier to the New England Baptist Hospital (NEBH) in 1969. When the originally planned date for the merger did not happen, the BWH leadership had negotiated with the leadership at the NEBH to extend the sale until October 14, 1980. After that, the NEBH assumed ownership and occupancy of the RBBH buildings and land. At the RBBH, just prior to the opening of the new BWH hospital, "the volume of surgery…reached a plateau, dictated by the amount of available [operating room] time" (Annual Report 1977).

With the merger completed, the number of beds increased from about 500 to 680; the tower was 16-stories high and each floor had four circular pods. Lower level 1 contained 20 operating rooms. There were 14 orthopaedic beds and 15 rheumatology/orthopaedic beds in the upper floors. Each division comprised several floors, and the RBBH essentially became the Orthopedic and Arthritis Center in the BWH (upper floors). The PBBH was assigned the central area of the new building. At the professional staff executive committee meeting, Dr. Petersdorf presented a memorandum of understanding to the chiefs emphasizing the hospital's commitment to the public benefit:

> Memorandum of Understanding Harvard Medical School and other Institutions (patents and copyrights): Ideas, creative works…the public benefit should take precedence over profit-making by any Institution and its employees or appointees…Whatever any enterprise is made possible by the support of any institution, or wherever any Institution provides extra or special support, including but not limited to funding, facilities or equipment, for the development of ideas or the production of works, each Institution may reasonably expect to participate in the fruits of the enterprise…if such ideas or works are introduced commercially… The Inventor's share shall be 35% of the first $50K of the Net Royalty Income for the year… plus 25% of the Net Royalty Income for year between $50K and $100K, plus 15% of the Net Royalty Income for the year in excess of $100K; and such share shall be distributed equally between all joint Inventors…the remaining Net Royalty Income shall be distributed: a ___percent to Harvard University if the inventor shall hold a Harvard appointment. ("Professional Staff Executive Committee, February 29, 1980" 1980)

In April that year, tours were offered in the patient tower of the new AHC building. In July 1980, the certificate of need for a BWH Research Center, located between the new bed tower and the old PBBH, was approved. Four operating rooms at the PBBH were left open during the

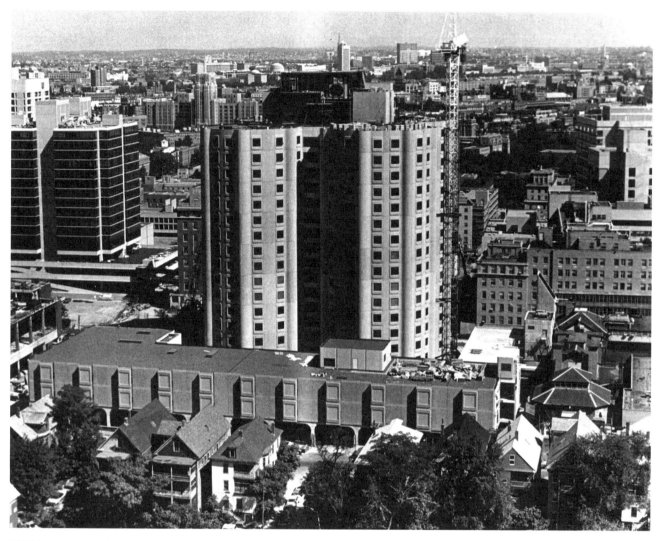
BWH towers and Amory Building, ca. 1980. Brigham and Women's Hospital Archives.

transition. The rest were closed on July 3. The majority were relocated on July 7 and 8 and the remaining four on July 9. Inpatients (n=250) from the PBBH were to be moved into the tower on July 9, 1980 (floors 7–12); inpatients from the RBBH were to follow on July 11 and 12. The new operating rooms opened on July 10, 1980. The RBBH continued to run two operating rooms through July 11 and were scheduled to completely relocate by August 1, 1980. Outpatients from the RBBH were moved to the new building on July 11 and 12; the others were to be moved on July 15.

Outpatients were seen in contiguous areas in the ambulatory building and each specialty (the Department of Orthopedic Surgery and the Division of Rheumatology in the Department of Medicine) had independent and expanding research laboratories. One of the hospital's most exceptional achievements was its research and work with prosthetic devices to treat diseased joints, and it was noted that the RBBH "has achieved the reputation of being the outstanding center devoted to the study and treatment of arthritis" (Campaign for Clinical and Academic Programs, 1977–1980). This is important because the RBBH was a specialty (arthritis) hospital and the PBBH was a general hospital.

With the merger, the leadership kept the specialty hospital (RBBH) within the general hospital

(BWH) in a separate unit, the Orthopaedic and Arthritis Center. According to the Campaign:

> One of the more spectacular aspects of the program is the replacement of diseased joints with prosthetic devices. First hips, then fingers, and now knees and elbows are restored with plastic and metal appliances. Prosthetic replacements for shoulders are being developed. People who could no longer walk or even hold a cup of coffee can now emerge from the hospital with the ability to live a useful life. Because of its inclusion in the Sealey G. Mudd Research Building, a large portion of the research facilities needed by this program have been provided. ("Affiliated Hospitals Center," n.d.)

That same year, Dr. Clement Sledge had established the Brigham Orthopedic Associates (BOA) while reorganizing the orthopaedic department. BOA was a for-profit organization for clinical practice formed the same year the merger was completed. The shareholders included Drs. Sledge, William Thomas, Frederick Ewald, and Robert Poss. All other staff were employees. Sledge also established the Brigham Orthopaedic Foundation (BOF), a nonprofit organization that managed the department's research program with contributions from the faculty (i.e., royalty's), grants, and donations.

After much discussion, the consensus on the name of the new hospital was the Brigham and Women's Hospital (BWH). The new facility was dedicated on November 14, 1980. All Harvard academic titles were changed to BWH from the PBBH, RBBH, and the Boston Hospital for Women. In BWH's 1977–1980 Campaign for

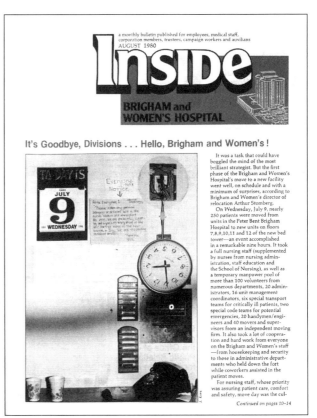

Cover of *Inside Brigham and Women's Hospital*, August 1980—announcing the opening of BWH and the successful transfer of patients from the PBBH and RBBH. Brigham and Women's Hospital Archives.

Clinical and Academic Programs, Dr. Robert H. Ebert (former HMS Dean) stated:

> Each unit gains the strength that comes from union and collaboration, while preserving the expertise that distinguishes each. We look forward now to the creation of a great new hospital complex which will contribute increased vigor to the search for knowledge, the enrichment of education and the improvement of health services. (Campaign for Clinical and Academic Programs, 1977–1980)

Growth in Patient Volume at the PBBH and BWH

	Year	Inpatients			Outpatient Visits	Emergency Department Visits
		Beds	Admissions	Mean Patients Per Day		
PBBH	1914	225	2,843	135+	30,434	—
	1915	—	3,417	165+	36,523	—
	1927	—	4,607	216	60,671	—
	1935	247	4,422	187	77,728	—
	1938	—	4,584	192+	84,365	—
	1950	—	5,169	208	48,360	—
	1963	311	7930	248	50,957	14,528
	1976	330	10,437	394	135,111	27,734
BWH	1982	698	28,201	—	131,830	28,583
	1988	720	35,136	640	179,596	44,510
	2009	777	46,432	713	396,000	59,323

Tishler, et al., "The Teaching Hospital," 2013. P. Tishler, J. Loscalzo, C. Wenc.

Clement B. Sledge

Clinician Scientist

Clement Blount Sledge, born on November 1, 1930, in Ada, Oklahoma, attended the University of the South in Sewanee, Tennessee, from 1948–1951. The university was known as "Sewanee" by students, faculty, and friends. Sewanee is "a private, residential coeducational liberal arts college… owned by 28 southern dioceses of the Episcopal Church, and its School of Theology is an official seminary of the church" ("Sewanee: The University of the South" 2018). Majoring in chemistry, during his junior year Sledge sought advice about a PhD in biochemistry. His advisor recommended that he get an MD degree first or "he wouldn't be allowed to touch humans" (Sledge, interview with the author, 2009). Concerned about keeping his deferment during the Korean War, he applied directly to medical school after his junior year at Sewanee. He had been elected to Phi Beta Kappa that year. Sledge was accepted at the Yale School of Medicine. By the time he was in his senior year at Yale, he had chosen a career in academic surgery. His first choice for a residency in surgery was the Massachusetts General Hospital (MGH), but his advisor recommended Washington University with Dr. Carl Moyer for academic surgery and MGH if he was interested in being trained as a community surgeon. He graduated from Yale School of Medicine in 1955.

EARLY CAREER AND TRAINING

After a surgical internship (1955–1956) at Barnes Hospital and enrollment in the Berry Plan (which deferred military service during the Vietnam War for some physicians until they completed residency training), he was activated in the US Navy, where he spent two years at sea as a ship surgeon. After discharge, he returned to Washington University to complete a second year of general surgery training (1958–1959). His naval experience had consisted mainly of orthopaedic problems, especially fractures. Approached by Dr. Fred Reynolds, the chief of orthopaedics at Washington University,

---

Physician Snapshot

Clement B. Sledge

BORN: 1930

DIED: —

SIGNIFICANT CONTRIBUTIONS: First full-time professor of orthopaedic surgery at RBBH and PBBH; surgeon-in-chief at RBBH; orthopaedic surgeon-in-chief at PBBH; chairman, department of orthopaedic surgery at BWH; recipient of the John Ball and Buckminster Brown Chair by Harvard Medical School; expert in cartilage growth and metabolism; advocate of radiation synovectomy; established an orthopaedic biomechanics laboratory at the BWH; president of the American Academy of Orthopaedic Surgeons (1985); founded a total joint registry at the BWH

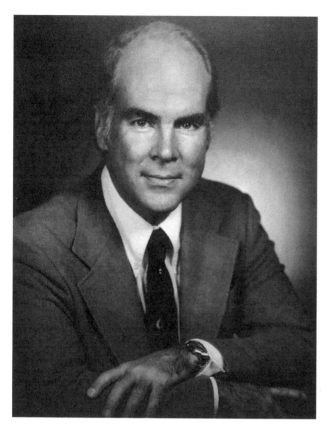

Clement B. Sledge. Courtesy of Francis Antupit.

about his interest in orthopaedic surgery as a career, he was initially not interested. However, after his naval experience, he switched his career choice from surgery to orthopaedic surgery.

Dr. Sledge selected the Combined Boston Children's Hospital/Massachusetts General Hospital residency program in orthopaedic surgery. He remembered, "I started in the middle of the year—so I spent the first six months after general surgery working in Jonathan Cohen's lab at Children's Hospital" (Sledge, interview with the author, 2009). His residency progressed between 1959 and 1962:

- assistant resident in orthopaedic surgery at Boston Children's Hospital, September 1959–December 1960
- assistant resident at MGH, January–December 1961
- resident at Boston Children's Hospital, January–June 1962
- senior fracture resident at MGH, July–September 1962
- senior resident at MGH, October–December 1962

He recalled that he received no salary in his first year at Boston Children's Hospital, but shortly thereafter small and slowly increasing salaries were provided to the residents. He noted:

At the urging of Mel Glimcher and Bill Harris… to stay on the staff, [I agreed to complete a fellowship]. Glimcher had instituted what turned out to be a short-lived requirement, that to come on the full-time staff in orthopaedics at Massachusetts General, you had to go away for a year of training somewhere else to keep from having a department that's too inbred and bring in new ideas. I was still interested in biochemistry and research and Bill Harris told me about the Strangeways Research Laboratory in Cambridge, England. And through the Massachusetts General, I got a fellowship…for three years. The idea would be that I would finally get my PhD in biochemistry. So, I enrolled as a graduate student at Cambridge University and I worked with the director, Honor B. Fell, who was one of the great pioneers in tissue culture. And I did my research there…doing mostly embryonic cartilage cells. (Sledge, interview with the author, 2009)

Upon completion of his residency, Sledge was appointed a research fellow in orthopaedic surgery by Dr. Joseph Barr. He spent six months studying pathology at the Armed Forces Institute of Pathology in Washington, DC. With a Medical Foundation Fellowship and a King Trust Fellowship, he spent the next two years in the Strangeways Laboratories in Cambridge, England, "studying tissue and organ culture with Drs. Honor B. Fell and Sylvia Fitton-Jackson" (Barr 1963).

Sledge never completed his dissertation for his PhD degree; instead, he had to return home for family reasons. Years later, however, he did receive an honorary ScD degree from his alma mater, the University of the South at Sewanee. He returned to the staff at MGH in 1965, joining Dr. Robert Boyd's practice. They shared an office and a secretary in the basement, next to the clinic.

His first publication, with J. Dingle, was in *Nature* that same year: "Oxygen-Induced Resorption of Cartilage in Organ Culture," which was part of a section of papers titled "Activation of Lysosomes by Oxygen." Their findings indicated that high oxygen concentrations had various compelling effects on the development of leg bones in chick embryos. Rudiments grew slowly longitudinally, remained soft and lost excessive amounts of metachromatic content, and the protease inhibitor epsilon-amino-*n*-caproic acid effectively reduced the creation of acid phosphatase and protease. On the basis of these two main findings, Sledge and Dingle believed that a high partial pressure of oxygen has physiological effects similar to those of vitamin A.

Sledge received an appointment at MGH as an assistant in orthopaedic surgery and as instructor in orthopaedic surgery at Harvard Medical School (HMS) on January 1, 1966. With this initial staff appointment, he was awarded the first Marion B. Gebbie Research Fellowship at MGH. Soon after his return to MGH and following his research fellowship at Strangeways, Sledge published his second article, "Some Morphologic and Experimental Aspects of Limb Development." By 1970, Sledge had published six articles, all dealing with embryonic cartilage, biochemical events at the epiphyseal plate, and limb bud development.

Toward the end of this short period (about 4–5 years) of Sledge's tenure on the staff, significant changes and movement of the faculty were developing at the MGH, with several surgeons departing from MGH. Approximately in late 1969 and early 1970, Dr. Ted Riseborough—a favorite teacher at MGH among students and residents as well as the only specialist in scoliosis surgery—moved from MGH to Boston Children's Hospital

> Nature. 1965 Jan 9;205:140-1
>
> **OXYGEN-INDUCED RESORPTION OF CARTILAGE IN ORGAN CULTURE**
>
> C B SLEDGE, J T DINGLE

Title of Sledge and Dingle's article on the effect of oxygen on embryonic cartilage. *Nature* 1965; 205: 140.

to join Dr. John Hall with his scoliosis practice (see chapter 27). About this time, Sledge recalled being asked by Dr. Glimcher to become the chief of a pediatric orthopaedic service at MGH, which Glimcher may have been considering establishing. However, Glimcher moved to Boston Children's Hospital as the chair of the department (see chapter 24) shortly thereafter, and Sledge became acting chief of orthopaedics at the MGH and associate professor of orthopaedic surgery at HMS. He was acting chief for less than one year.

MERGER AT RBBH AND PBBH: FIRST ACADEMIC FULL-TIME PROFESSOR OF ORTHOPAEDIC SURGERY

During this same period of unrest, the leadership of the Robert Breck Brigham Hospital (RBBH) and the Peter Bent Brigham Hospital (PBBH) was in the later stages of merger discussions (Affiliated Hospitals Center, Inc [AHC, Inc]) (see chapter 47 for complete discussion on the merger). Sledge recalled his reasons for leaving the MGH and becoming chairman of a new department at the Brigham: "If I stayed at the Mass. General…I won't know if I made a bit of difference. If I go to a place [without an established department of orthopaedic surgery], when I retire, I'll know if I had any impact or not, little knowing what my legacy would be. So, I went to the Brigham then at the end of 1969" (Sledge, interview with the

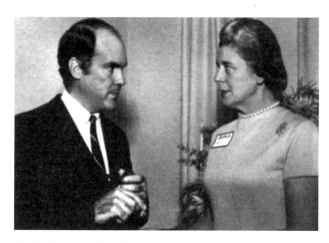

Dr. Sledge with Mrs. Steele, an active volunteer at the RBBH, 1970.

History of the Robert Breck Brigham Hospital for Incurables by Matthew H. Liang. The Brigham and Women's Hospital, Inc., 2013. Brigham and Women's Hospital Archives.

author, 2009). In 1970, Sledge was appointed surgeon-in-chief at the RBBH and orthopaedic surgeon-in-chief at the PBBH.

Dr. Frank Austen in his RBBH physician-in-chief's report, stated: "The bringing together of the Robert B. Brigham and Peter Bent Brigham Hospitals under the leadership of a single Harvard Professor heralds a particularly bright future for this aspect of our clinical endeavors" ("Annual Report, 1969, Report of the Physician-in-Chief" 1969, 2). During a 2009 interview with me, Sledge discussed the transition and the merger of the hospitals:

> I took Dren Lowell with me because I anticipated that it might be more than three years until we had one institution and knew I couldn't be at both places equally. My lab had been built at the Robert Brigham so I established myself at the Robert Brigham and asked Dren Lowell to be the clinical chief at the Peter Bent Brigham, succeeding Henry Banks. And that continued until the hospitals were physically combined in 1980. So, I think it was ten years before they were combined...at one time there were going to be four towers—the two Brigham's, Women's, and the V.A. was going to be rebuilt as the fourth tower, which makes a lot of sense [the medical and surgical staffs of the PBBH had traditionally covered the clinical cases, education and resident services at the WRVA]. I've always wondered why VAs are so remote from the academic center that supposedly controls them or governs or relates to them. But that didn't happen, obviously...too much expense. So, the three hospitals merged.

ORTHOPAEDIC SURGEON-IN-CHIEF AT THE PBBH

Dr. Banks had left the PBBH on July 1, 1970, after 16 years. In the staff booklet of the 58th annual report of the PBBH (1970–1971), the following staff were listed under the department of orthopedics: Orthopedic Surgeon-in-Chief Dr. Clement Sledge; Senior Associate in Orthopedic Surgery Dr. J. Drennan Lowell; Associates in Orthopedic Surgery Drs. Paul Hugenberger, Arthur Pappas, and Arthur Trott; Junior Associates in Orthopedic Surgery Drs. Frank Bates, Ben Bierbaum, Arthur Boland, Stuart Cope, Robert W. Hussey, Robert Keller, Jack McGinty, Larry Shields, and Bill Thomas; Assistant in Orthopedic Surgery Panos G. Panagakos. There were four residents and four assistant residents. In his 1971 PBBH annual report, Sledge wrote:

> 1971 was a year of change for the Department of Orthopedic Surgery...changes in personnel, affiliation, residency training and even in the character of the patient population...A large amount of arthritic surgery at the Robert Breck Brigham Hospital compliments the trauma and reconstructive surgery at the Peter Bent Brigham Hospital and each gains from the other. The clinical research activity will be centered at the Peter Bent Brigham Hospital and laboratory research at the Robert Breck Brigham Hospital. ("Annual Report, 1970-1971, Report of the Orthopedic Surgeon-in-Chief" 1971, 281)

Additional staff, including Bill Thomas, Fred Ewald, Ed Nalebuff, and Louis Millender (from the RBBH), joined Dren Lowell and William Head at the PBBH "to round out the full-time staff [plus staff at Boston Children's Hospital], a devoted group of part-time visiting surgeons. [Dr. Sledge spent] most of the year...organizing a new department and coordination of training at both Brighams and the West Roxbury V.A." ("Annual Report, 1970-1971, Report of the Orthopedic Surgeon-in-Chief" 1971, 281). There were 800 admissions at the PBBH that year, 508 operations performed by the residents and visiting staff, 4,441 patients seen in the orthopaedic and fracture clinic, 5,390 patients seen in the Industrial Accident Clinic, 1,305 patients seen in the podiatry clinic and 23,387 treatments given in physical therapy. Dr. Bruce Wood was named the new chief of the podiatry clinic, replacing Dr. Don Helems, who retired after five years. Grand rounds were started at the PBBH on Thursdays. Dr. Robert Hussey—who completed his MGH/CH residency and a spinal cord injury fellowship at Rancho Los Amigos in Downey, California—returned to the PBBH where his practice was centered at the West Roxbury VA Hospital.

SURGEON-IN-CHIEF AT THE RBBH

Meanwhile, in his first annual surgeon-in-chief's report at the RBBH (1970), Dr. Sledge reported that he and the RBBH were licensed by the FDA to use bone cement; 15 total hip replacements were done on average each month. Arthroscopy of the knee was also introduced at the RBBH that year and preliminary studies of total elbow replacement by Marvin Weinfeld and Bill Thomas were beginning. The orthopaedic department at the RBBH completed 700 operative cases. Two orthopaedic residents rotated to the RBBH; and Dr. Sledge began to increase the number of postdoctoral fellows, especially international fellows. He further stated:

A single orthopedic chair at the Robert Breck Brigham and the Peter Bent Brigham hospitals together with the West Roxbury V.A. Hospital comprise an equal partner with the Children's Hospital Medical Center and the Massachusetts General Hospital in a tripartite department at the medical school level...We have a common residency training program – the only such unified postgraduate training program within the Harvard Medical School...Because of the enlarged scope of my duties, greater responsibilities have fallen to Dr. William Thomas and Marvin Weinfeld here, and to Dr. J. Drennan Lowell at the Peter Bent Brigham Hospital...Dr. Nalebuff has assumed responsibility for the hand service...A milestone in surgery of the rheumatoid knee has been reached this year; Drs. Potter, Thomas and Weinfeld have completed their review of knee arthroplasties with metallic prostheses. This review will establish this procedure, now not widely appreciated, in its rightful place in the surgical armamentarium. ("Annual Report, 1970, Report of the Surgeon-in-Chief" 1970, 18)

KNEE ARTHROPLASTIES AND PROSTHESES AT THE RBBH

The year Dr. Sledge became surgeon-in-chief at the RBBH, the surgeons there had been performing knee arthroplasties with the tibial McKeever and MacIntosh prostheses. At the MGH the orthopaedic surgeons had focused their attention on the femoral side of arthritic joints with the use of the MGH femoral replacement prosthesis. In cases of failure of these hemiarthroplasties or in severe deformity, hinged implants (Guepar or Walldius) were used. Harris and Sledge (1970) noted:

The current era of knee arthroplasty began with the studies of Gunston in 1970 [who] created the first unlinked replacement knee, using polyethylene as one of the articulating surfaces and stainless steel as the other and fixing both to bone with methyl methacrylate cement. This prosthesis and the others that immediately followed were successful in relieving pain and providing about 90 degrees of flexion...To overcome the problems of inadequate motion and frequent loosening, Walker and Hajek pioneered the development of the more anatomical replacements [in an] attempt to duplicate the normal anatomy, motion, and stability of the knee and its ability to withstand the force of normal daily activities, which can easily reach five times body weight.

At the time, the McKeever prosthesis was more commonly used at the RBBH. In January of 1973, the surgeons began using the Marmor modular design prosthesis, followed shortly thereafter by the duo-condylar prosthesis (designed by Peter Walker, PhD, at the Hospital for Special Surgery). In 1974, two additional prostheses—the duopatellar and the total condylar prostheses—were developed by Drs. Peter Walker, Chit Ranawat, and John Insall. The two-piece, duopatellar prosthesis retained the cruciate ligaments, allowing better outcomes in patients with rheumatoid arthritis, and for this reason it was preferred at both Brigham hospitals. (In contrast, the total condylar prosthesis required excision of the cruciate ligaments.) Both prostheses contained a trochlear flange, which some surgeons at the Brigham altered to provide two versions, one for the left and one for the right, which allowed them to reduce medial overhang. The following year:

a comparison of 34 bicompartmental McKeever arthroplasties, 36 modular [Marmor] total knee replacements, and 143 duo-condylar total knee replacements were reported...The 34 McKeever arthroplasties represented failures from a large series...under consideration for conversation to total knee replacements...Sixteen had significant lateral subluxation of the

> Total Knee Arthroplasty
> Experience at the Robert Breck Brigham Hospital
>
> CLEMENT B. SLEDGE, M.D.,* AND FREDERICK C. EWALD, M.D.**
>
> Clinical Orthopaedics & Related Research
> Volume 145   November/December 1979

Title of Sledge and Ewald's article reviewing the RBBH results comparing the McKeever, Marmor, and duo-condylar prosthetic knee replacements.
Clinical Orthopaedics and Related Research 1979; 145: 78.

tibia on the femur...felt to be the major cause of pain...Of the 36 modular total knee replacements...7 of the 36...failed by this single mechanism. By contrast none of the 143 duocondylar total knee arthroplasties were radiographically subluxed. (Sledge and Ewald 1979)

Four years later, a one-piece plastic tibial component version of the duopatellar prosthesis was available, and, by 1979, two designs incorporating metal backing for the plastic component (Kinematic and Kinematic II) were the most used; this trend lasted into the mid-1980s. These prostheses allowed for good results at the Hospital for Special Surgery, but surgeons at RBBH expanded the use of the duopatellar approach, culminating in various versions of existing prostheses that saved the posterior cruciate ligament. Dr. Sledge and Ewald published the RBBH's 28-year (1950–1978) experience with total knee arthroplasty in 1979 (**Table 48.1**).

Sledge and his colleagues developed total knee systems that preserved the important posterior cruciate ligament—an essential feature in their opinion—for patients with rheumatoid arthritis. An additional essential feature is the preservation and proper balancing of the knee's soft tissues after the prosthesis is inserted. Early clinical outcomes and laboratory research appeared to support their premise. In summary, the authors stated:

Table 48.1. Total Knee Arthroplasties at RBBH, 1950–78

Prosthesis, by Years	Number
1950–57: Nylon interpositional membrane	104
1957–77: McKeever and MacIntosh	558
Feb 16, 1971–Dec 31, 1977	
Hinge joints	
Waldius	155
Guepar	39
Shiers	2
Metal-to-plastic	
Bicompartmental	
Duopatellar	983
Duocondylar	178
Marmor	23
Meniscocondlar	24
Total condylar	25
Total condylar II	7
Marmor-sled	8
Sled	4
Stabulocondylar	5
Cruciate condylar	5
Kinematic	13
Hemi-joint	
Unicondylar	184
Marmor	14
Sled	1
Total	2292

Reprinted with permission from Sledge and Ewald 1979.

Although the concepts are still evolving, and longer follow-up is necessary, recent experiences with nearly 1000 semi-constrained devices allowing cruciate retention strongly suggests that duopatellar and kinematic design concepts are correct. Soft tissue reconstruction is critical with these designs, since they rely heavily on soft tissue integrity and balance…The low incidence of radiolucency at the bone-cement interface…coupled with the results in vitro bench testing, suggest that the longevity of this generation of knee implants should be adequate. (Sledge and Ewald 1979)

SURGICAL CASELOADS AND ORTHOPAEDIC RESIDENTS AT THE RBBH

Two years after Dr. Sledge was appointed surgeon-in-chief (1972), the RBBH improved its single operating room, making it larger and installing ultraviolet lights to prevent infection in joint replacement procedures. By 1973, the number of surgical cases at the RBBH increased to 893, of which 762 were on rheumatoid patients. Surgical caseloads at the RBBH also increased overall (**Table 48.2**), as did the number of surgical procedures Nalebuff performed on patients with rheumatoid arthritis (**Table 48.3**). There were 1990 admissions in 1973.

That year, the orthopaedic residents rotated at the RBBH for three months (including hand) and three residents rotated there from Tufts. The staff consisted of Sledge, Nalebuff, Thomas, Weinfeld,

Table 48.2. Surgical Procedures Performed at RBBH, 1966–73

Year	No. of Procedures
1966	385
1967	420
1968	571
1969	624
1970	680
1971	695
1972	771
1973	890

Table 48.3. Surgical Procedures Performed by Edward Nalebuff, 1968–72

Year	No. of Procedures
1968	61
1969	37
1970	54
1971	107
1972	127

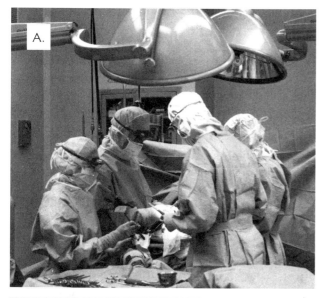

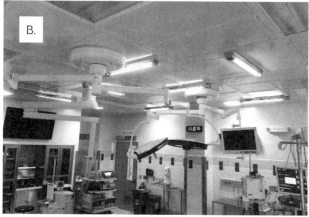

A. Surgical procedure at RBBH, ca. 1972. Brigham and Women's Hospital Archives.
B. Example of ultraviolet lights in an operating room ceiling. Courtesy of American Ultraviolet.

from the residency program, Drs. Robert Poss and Richard Scott. In the last annual report in the RBBH files, in 1976, Dr. Sledge reported that the number of surgical cases had more than doubled in six years: from 600 procedures in 1970 to 1251 in 1976. During this period, a second operating room had been added. Since 1969, when the first total hip replacement was performed at the RBBH, a total of 1,157 hip replacements, 1,013 knee replacements, and 61 elbow replacements were performed. In 1975, Nalebuff and Millender replaced 106 metacarpal phalangeal joints with silicone implants.

BRIGHAM AND WOMEN'S HOSPITAL: CHAIRMAN, DEPARTMENT OF ORTHOPAEDIC SURGERY

The Brigham Hospitals during the transition period consisted of two divisions: the PBBH (Class W) and the RBBH (Class R). Each had its own board of overseers. At the PBBH, only one physician (Dr. Warren E .C. Wacker) was a member of the 41-member board. At the RBBH, two physicians (Dr. K. F. Austen and Dr. Sledge) were the only physicians on the board (n=23). Dr. Sledge was listed as surgeon-in-chief at the RBBH and orthopedic surgeon-in-chief at the PBBH.

The professional staff of the three divisions (RBBH, PBBH, and Boston Hospital for Women) formed one professional staff committee in 1979 and completed the staff by-laws. The committee consisted of 15 members, mainly department chiefs and included Dr. Sledge. Sledge appointed many of the fulltime staff to subcommittees of the professional staff committee in 1980. That same year, he was given the John Ball and Buckminster Brown Chair by Harvard Medical School, which had been vacant since 1964. New titles were given to the clinical leaders as chairman of clinical departments. Dr. Sledge was named Chairman, Department of Orthopaedic Surgery, of the newly

Ewald, and Millender. Dr. William Elliston was now emeritus. Also, in 1973, the three divisions of the AHC, Inc. (RBBH, PBBH, Boston Hospital for Women) agreed to build a new research building (Mudd) with planned completion of approximately 1977. The RBBH research labs consisted of 24,000 square feet on the fifth and sixth floors of the new research facility. The clinical space for the RBBH was planned for the top three to five floors in the new tower, which was 16 floors.

By 1975, the total number of cases at the RBBH was 1,187. Sledge hired two new staff

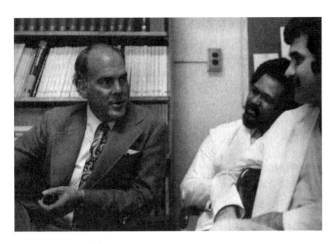

Sledge chatting with orthopaedic residents. *History of the Robert Breck Brigham Hospital for Incurables* by Matthew H. Liang. The Brigham and Women's Hospital, Inc., 2013. Brigham and Women's Hospital Archives.

named Brigham and Women's Hospital (BWH) from the now merged PBBH and RBBH.

LATER ORTHOPAEDIC RESEARCH CONTRIBUTIONS

During the merger transition period, Dr. Sledge was obviously busy as a leader in the frequent meetings and discussions; and he was equally busy in organizing a new two-hospital department structure and teaching program as well as in successfully moving his lab from MGH to the RBBH. Nevertheless, he continued his research on chondrocyte metabolism in cell culture. After a five-year delay in any publications, Dr. Sledge published eight articles over the next three years (1973–1975) on cartilage, synovium, and joint development.

Total Joint Replacement

While continuing his basic laboratory research on articular cartilage, synovium, and rheumatoid arthritis, Dr. Sledge published most of his clinical papers after 1976. Of his estimated more than 134 total publications, he published about 66 papers on joint replacement (including outcomes/complications): 21 on total hip replacement; 20 on total knee replacement; and about 25 on total joints in general, including four on the shoulder, three on the elbow, and one on the ankle. Earlier, in 1970, Sledge and the RBBH received one of the few licenses issued by the FDA in the United States to use methylmethacrylate, or bone cement, in total hip procedures.

Dr. Sledge, a clinician scholar, attempted to answer basic questions about joint physiology and arthritis in the laboratory with animal or cell culture studies, as well as outcomes regarding patient care and surgery with cohort studies. An early example of this latter effort regarded the question of whether or not to osteotomize the greater trochanter when doing a total hip replacement. In a paper published in 1976 (his first on total hip replacement), he and his coauthors reviewed the literature and stated: "According to Charnley and Lazansky, a trochanteric osteotomy must be performed; Müller and McKee and Watson-Farrar disagree. Harris contends that total hip replacement without trochanteric osteotomy has the advantage of decreased blood loss, shortened operating time, and earlier return to unsupported weight-bearing" (Parker et al. 1976).

In their study, Sledge and his coauthors compared 100 consecutive total hip operations with a trochanteric osteotomy to 100 consecutive

---

Comparison of Preoperative, Intraoperative and Early Postoperative Total Hip Replacements With and Without Trochanteric Osteotomy

HOWARD G. PARKER, M.D.,* HAROLD G. WIESMAN, M.D., FREDERICK C. EWALD, M.D., WILLIAM H. THOMAS, M.D. AND CLEMENT B. SLEDGE, M.D.

Clinical Orthopaedics & Related Research
Volume 121   November/December 1976

Article in which Sledge and coauthors reported that leaving the greater trochanter in place during total hip replacement had many advantages.
Clinical Orthopaedics and Related Research 1976; 121: 44.

procedures without the osteotomy. All patients were operated on at the RBBH. In their summary the authors concluded:

> Mean operating time was 3 hours for patients in the osteotomy group and 2 hours for those in the nonosteotomy group. Considerably more intraoperative and postoperative blood replacement was required in the patients having osteotomy. Patients sat, stood, walked and left the hospital sooner in the nonosteotomy group than in the osteotomy group. Trochanteric bursitis [was more common] in...patients having osteotomy...Hematomas developed in 15 patients in the osteotomy group and in 4 in the nonosteotomy group. Ectopic bone formation was observed in 12 of the osteotomy group, 8 with limitation of function, and in 5 of the nonosteotomy group; none had symptoms. Six osteotomized patients had troublesome abductor weakness secondary to wire breakage and proximal migration of the trochanter...When exposure was not difficult, leaving the trochanter intact had many advantages. (Parker et al. 1976)

Dr. Sledge was very interested in evaluating outcomes in patients with total joint replacements throughout his career. Another of his earlier papers reported complications of total hip replacement in patients with rheumatoid arthritis, which he wrote with Drs. Bob Poss, Fred Ewald, and Bill Thomas. They reviewed the results of hip replacement in 275 patients with rheumatoid arthritis and 382 patients with osteoarthritis over a five-year period. They reported: "It was our experience that there is an equal incidence of infection in the two groups" (Parker et al. 1976); this contrasted to other reports that found between 1.5 and 5 times the rate of infection in rheumatoid patients compared to osteoarthritis patients. However:

> Our finding of a thirteenfold difference (6/76 for revision versus 4/640 for a primary procedure) is worrisome...It is our contention that the patients with a revision operation who had a late infection probably were already infected... and that our diagnostic methods were not sufficiently sophisticated to identify the infection... We now obtain tissue for preoperative bacteriological diagnosis routinely and we perform the revision surgery without antibiotic coverage until biopsy specimens of the capsule are taken...Because of the increased risk that the revision operation entails [in rheumatoid patients: intraoperative fracture, malposition of the prosthesis and anesthesia difficulties], we now refrain from any "temporizing" operative procedures in young patients and recommend that definitive total hip replacement be performed even in younger adults...postoperative hematomas were associated with nerve palsy in three cases and with infection in one...we abandoned the use of coumadin (warfarin) prophylactically and began using aspirin for anticoagulation [with a significant decrease in wound hematomas]. (Parker et al. 1976)

Six years later, in 1982, Drs. Sledge and Poss from the RBBH, and Drs. Paul Pellicci, Phil Wilson Jr., Eduardo Salvati, and Chit Ranawat from the Hospital for Special Surgery reviewed 110 revision arthroplasties in 107 patients performed at both hospitals. They made some interesting observations on the status of the evolving art of total hip arthroplasty at that time:

> The majority of the primary total hip arthroplasties were performed without current knowledge and techniques, and would be judged suboptimal. Ninety-two per cent of the femoral components were in varus and/ or associated with poor cement technique. Sixty per cent of the acetabular failures were associated with subtotal osseous coverage, poor cement technique, or poor position. Of the fractured femoral components, 93% were inserted either with little proximal support, in varus position, or were too small (or of poor

design) for the heavy active patient. All of the revisions for dislocation caused by malposition and all those for protrusion acetabuli could possibly have been avoided with proper and modern, e.g., bone grafting, techniques. Thus 83% of the original failures would have been done differently on the basis of advances made in the last decade.

In this review, 110 hips in 107 patients underwent revision total hip arthroplasty [with a] minimum follow-up [of] two years (average 3.4 years). Failures of the original total hip arthroplasties were due to loosening of the femoral component (44 hips), loosening of both components (23 hips), loosening of the acetabular component (17 hips), fracture of the femoral component (14 hips), recurrent dislocation due to prosthetic malposition (7 hips), acetabular protrusion (3 hips), and fracture of the femoral shaft (2 hips). Sixty-six hips were categorized as good or excellent and 25 hips were rated as fair...Complications included infection (3.6%), trochanteric problems (13%), mechanical failure (14%) and progressive radiolucent zones (26%)...The extremely high incidence of progressive radiolucent zones at the bone-cement interface makes predictions for even longer-term results guarded. (Pellicci et al. 1982)

In a longer-term follow-up (8.1 years), of the above 110 total hip revisions, Pellicci et al. reported "twenty-nine [percent] of these arthroplasties have since failed...that there is an increased failure rate with longer follow-up... and that progressive radiolucency at an interface indicates a poor prognosis for the arthroplasty" (Pellicci et al. 1985). Over the next 15 years, Dr. Sledge and his colleagues published numerous articles on total hip arthroplasty results, complications and outcomes, including: infection affecting outcomes (1984), results in patients with rheumatoid arthritis (1984), prosthetic developments for the geriatric patient (1985), cost effectiveness of total hips (1986), modern cement technique and improvements in fixation, evaluation by the use of enhanced computed tomography (1989), clinical and radiographic analyses (1990), use of the AAOS outcome evaluation form (1991), validity of an outcome evaluation questionnaire (1995), a 10-year follow-up of patients under the age of 30 with juvenile rheumatoid arthritis (1997), and outcomes that were influenced by both timing (2002) and the preoperative functional status of the patient (1999).

In 1990, he coauthored a two-part article reviewing the current status of total hip and total knees replacement with Dr. William H. Harris in the *New England Journal of Medicine*. At the time, the authors favored low-dose warfarin over aspirin to prevent postoperative deep vein thrombosis and possibly fatal pulmonary embolism. Commenting on clinical outcomes, they mentioned:

> two major developments. The first has been the disquieting recognition that, over time, the failure of components to remain fixed to the skeleton [is due to] fragmentation of the methyl

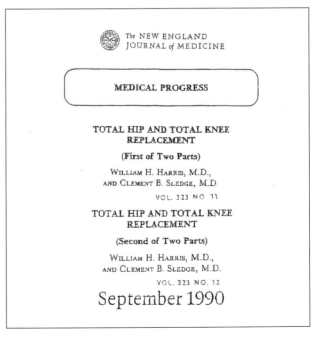

Title of Harris and Sledge's review article on total hip and total knee replacement in the *New England Journal of Medicine*. 1990; 323: 725.

Article in which Sledge and his colleagues reported their early research on radiation synovectomy. *Arthritis & Rheumatology* 1977; 20: 1334.

methacrylate (bone cement) and its associated bone lysis and the wearing out of the high-density polyethylene (the plastic used as the weight-bearing material) and the bone lysis associated with its particles. The second major development has been the vigorous efforts to improve the fixation of the components in order to increase the durability of total hip reconstruction...To eliminate bone cement, press-fit, porous coated, and threaded implants were developed. (Harris and Sledge 1990)

Synovial Joints

Sledge continued his research on articular cartilage with Sonya Shortkroff at the RBBH and expanded to include the synovium. With the RBBH's focus on the care of the patient with rheumatoid arthritis, he was influenced to expand his clinical and research interests into the field of preventive non-operative care, such as radiation synovectomy, in addition to total joint replacement. Over a 20-year period (1977–1998), he published about 15 papers on radiation synovectomy. He began with animal experiments in 1977 using dysprosium-165 (^{165}Dy) ferric hydroxide macroaggregate. The ferric hydroxide macroaggregate is a large, relatively inert carrier that minimized radionuclide leakage from the injected joint.

Seven years later, he published his first series of patients with rheumatoid arthritis treated by radiation synovectomy of the knee, which was 24 years after Kuhns and Morrison published their results using roentgenotherapy in the treatment of chronic arthritis at the RBBH (see chapter 45). He treated 53 knees in 44 patients with painful synovitis of the knee for longer than six months' duration; patients were followed for a least one year after treatment. Sledge et al. (1984) concluded that:

> The present study demonstrates that 80% of patients treated for chronic synovitis of the knee with ^{165}Dy-FHMA were improved at one year; nearly 90% of patients with Stage I roentgenographic changes had excellent, good or fair results. The ideal candidate...is a patient who is disabled by chronic knee effusions...beyond child-bearing years, has minimal roentgenographic evidence of joint destruction...resistant to conventional management [and] radiation leakage is at least one order of magnitude less than reported with other beta-particle emitting radiocolloids.

In 1987, Sledge and his coauthors reported on 111 patients with chronic synovitis of the knee treated with ^{165}Dy-FHMA, with a two-year follow-up in 59 of the treated knees. He wrote, "Of the twenty-five knees that had Stage-I radiographic changes, nineteen had a good result. Of the thirty-four knees that had Stage-II radiographic changes, twenty showed a good result. Systemic spread of the radioactivity from the injected joint was minimum" (Sledge et al. 1987).

In the early 1990s, Sledge collaborated with Dr. Jacquelyn C. Yanch and her colleagues at MIT using Boron Neutron Capture Synovectomy in excised samples of human synovium and cartilage with plans for future animal experiments. **Case 48.1** illustrates an example of a case from his research on synovitis in the hip with Dr. A. D. Boyd Jr. around the same time.

Case 48.1. Pigmented Villonodular Synovitis of the Hip

> "A 38-year old man reported a history of right groin pain that had been present intermittently for 14 years. The symptoms were related to a football injury that never completely resolved. No medical consultation was obtained at that time. The patient remained active in athletics and noted a recurrence of groin pain that usually resolved with rest. During the four months before evaluation, the patient noted a persistence of this pain in his groin in conjunction with stiffness and a limp. Review of systems and medical history were unremarkable.
>
> "On physical examination, the patient ambulated with a lurch to the right, which could be corrected voluntarily. The Trendelenburg test was negative. Range of motion of the right hip was painful at the extremes of motion with a range of 100° flexion, 0° extension, 5° internal rotation, 25° external rotation, and 45° abduction. The left hip was not painful and had a full ROM. There was no leg-length inequality and the remainder of the examination was normal. Laboratory studies and skin testing were also normal.
>
> "Plain roentgenograms of the pelvis revealed destructive lesions on both sides of the hip joint. Fullness of the right hip capsule was noted in addition to erosions of the acetabulum, femoral head, and femoral neck. These cystic areas appeared to have sclerotic margins suggesting a chronic process. Magnetic resonance imaging (MRI) revealed grapelike clusters of soft tissue throughout the right hip joint. A preliminary diagnosis of PVNS was made but other processes could not be ruled out.
>
> "A computed tomography (CT) scan was completed to evaluate the structural integrity of the femoral head and neck. Multiple views if the right hip showed destructive changes involving extensive segments of the femoral head and neck. Similar lesions were noted in the acetabulum with loss of portions of the articular surface. A three-dimensional reconstruction of the right hemipelvis was performed using computer-enhanced images from the CT scan to evaluate the usefulness of this technique in preoperative planning. This reconstruction demonstrated the severe erosive changes and thinning of bony structures throughout the acetabulum.
>
> "Because of the advanced destructive changes in the hip joint, it was believed that synovectomy and bone grafting alone could not provide adequate structural support of the femoral head and neck. Total hip arthroplasty (THA) was recommended and carried out through a standard posterior-lateral approach to the hip joint. At surgery the hip capsule was expanded with dark, hypertrophic synovial tissue under pressure.
>
> "A capsulectomy and complete synovectomy were performed thus requiring dislocation of the hip and curettage of multiple large cysts in the bony structures. Erosion of the articular surfaces with exposed bone was noted on the femoral head and in the acetabulum. The femoral head and neck were resected in preparation for THA, and all cystic areas were paced with allogeneic bone. An uncemented THA was then performed without complications. The postoperative course was uneventful, and the patient was discharged with orders for crutch ambulation and routine physical therapy. Evaluation of the patient at six and 12 months revealed a pain-free right hip, no limp, and a ROM equal to the left hip. Roentgenograms revealed no evidence of recurrent disease."
>
> (Boyd and Sledge 1992)

Establishing an Orthopaedic Biomechanics Laboratory

In 1980, Dr. Sledge recruited Peter Walker, PhD, to establish an orthopaedic biomechanics laboratory at the BWH and the West Roxbury VA Medical Center and to lead efforts to develop new designs of total joint implants. Their initial focus appears to have been on the tibial component fixation and also the patellofemoral joint while developing new total knee prostheses.

In 1981, Walker and his coauthors published their results on improving fixation of the tibial component. They stated:

> There are many designs of the non-linked condylar replacement type of knee prosthesis in use today. In virtually all of the clinical reports...

loosening of the tibial component has been cited as a significant complication. In a series of 500 polycentric knees followed for more than two years, there was 2.4 per cent loosening...geometric prostheses showed 8 per cent loosening, but 80 per cent of knees had radiolucent lines around the tibial component...Comparing unicondylar, duocondylar, and geometric prostheses, there was 12, 5, and 4 per cent loosening, respectively, and 60 per cent of the knees over-all had radiolucency...Sinking rather than loosening was given as the main problem in unicompartmental knees...No loosening was reported in 223 knees with the total condylar prosthesis...but 22 per cent had partial radiolucency, more than two millimeters thick in 3 per cent. The variable-axis knee prosthesis showed no loosening or radiolucency at all...There was a similar lack of problems for the intramedullary adjustable prosthesis...Both the variable axis and the intermedullary adjustable prosthesis used a metal backing for the tibial component.

[Walker, et al. studied] twelve different designs of tibial component: five pairs with one pair being all-plastic and the other being plastic encased in a metal tray, and two components made only of plastic...The compartmental components had two pegs...placed anteriorly and posteriorly. The anteriorly joined components had the same posterior pegs and an anterior blade below the cross-bridge. A one-piece component with a central peg, similar to the total condylar prosthesis, was made with and without a cut-out for retention of the posterior cruciate ligament. Finally, another one-piece component had posts...beneath the centers of the medial and lateral sides. Tests were carried out using six fresh tibiae...Two or three components were tested on the same bone, cemented under uniform and constant pressure...In order to carry out a larger number of tests on a consistent material, cylinders of Pedilen polyurethane foam were used...The femoral component consisted of a bicondylar roller...the components represented a prosthesis...A load sequence was devised whereby the components were subjected to compression; compression combined with anterior or posterior shear force; compression combined with internal or external torque; and compression combined with a varus or valgus moment...

Results in cadaver bone[:] The plastic and metal-tray compartmental components deflected similarly. For the one-piece components, the metal tray substantially reduced the deflections...An overall conclusion...the least attractive components were the compartmental ones. The one-piece metal-tray components with one or two posts were the best, together with one-piece plastic components with a post on each side. The presence of the posterior-cruciate notch in the single-post metal-tray design was not a disadvantage...the results... provide guidelines for current usage and future designs. (Walker et al. 1981)

Presented with a large number of patients at the RBBH with rheumatoid arthritis, Dr. Sledge and his colleagues continued to emphasize the importance of retaining the posterior cruciate ligament and the use of a minimally constrained prosthesis to protect the interface between the prosthesis and weak bone. They emphasized the importance of removal of a minimum amount of proximal tibial bone, the importance of "roll back" provided by the posterior cruciate ligament that allowed increased flexion, and the importance of ligamentous balance throughout flexion and preferred resurfacing of the patella to remove any remaining articular cartilage that would result in continued inflammation in the rheumatoid joint. The result of this thinking coupled with the biomechanical studies in the laboratory culminated in the development of the Kinematic knee prosthesis and its successors.

Orthopaedic surgeons at the BWH reported five-to-nine-year results in 192 kinematic total knee replacements in 1990:

The Kinematic-I total knee prosthesis...is conventionally cemented with methylmethacrylate. It has a metal-back tibial tray and a central stem for fixation...The posterior cruciate is preserved. The femoral component is anatomically shaped, so separate models are needed for the right and left knee. The all-plastic patellar replacement is symmetrical.

The long-term functional results were excellent and the rate of complications low... the postoperative arc of flexion averaged 109 degrees, and 65 per cent of the knees had an arc of flexion of 110 to 135 degrees...the rate of complications was acceptably low [35% with nonprogressive radiolucent lines, less than one millimeter wide]. Excluding the infected knees, only 4 per cent of the knees needed reoperation, and ultimately all had a satisfactory result. With the exceptions of one procedure that was done for a fracture of a tibial tray and four that were done for deep infection, all of the reoperations were done for patellar problems. The most common complication that necessitated reoperation was isolated loosening of the patellar component [especially in rheumatoid patients]...

There have been several reports on the results with cruciate-sacrificing models of prostheses at a minimum of five years after operation, as well as one [with] another model of posterior cruciate-preserving prosthesis [that] revealed...the results were satisfactory in the long term whether the posterior ligament cruciate [sic] was sacrificed or preserved...The only important difference was that cruciate-preserving models yielded a larger arc of motion of the knee than the cruciate-sacrificing devices... (Wright et al. 1981)

Sledge and his colleagues reported long-term successful outcomes with their ongoing clinical trials. They thus substantiated their original concepts: the importance of retaining the posterior cruciate ligament and careful soft tissue balancing with total knee replacement.

Report of 5–9-year results with the Kinematic Total Knee prosthesis at BWH. J. Wright et al., *Journal of Bone and Joint Surgery* 1990; 72-A: 1003.

American Academy of Orthopaedic Surgeons: President

Dr. Sledge was elected vice-president of the American Academy of Orthopaedic Surgeons (AAOS) in 1984 and president the following year. He had been encouraged by Dr. Barr (chief of orthopaedics at MGH) early in his career to become active in the academy. Beginning with an instructional course he continued to be active, emphasizing the need for every physician to be dedicated to life-long learning. When asked about his biggest challenge as president, he responded that the alienation between community and academic physicians and surgeons in orthopaedics was an obstacle that needed to be addressed. For Sledge, community orthopaedists focus on the economic issues faced by practicing physicians, whereas the academic orthopaedists were concerned mainly with teaching and education. Sledge wished that the academy could avoid such conflict. He contrasted that, however, by mentioning what he believed to be his greatest achievement: interweaving subspecialities into the academy's educational offerings. Finally, he described various crucial needs orthopaedic surgeons had to confront, including attaining and maintaining continuing medical education, learning new technologies, and cultivating practical skills.

In his first vice-president's address (1985), "Crisis, Challenge, and Credibility," Dr. Sledge predicted changes in the practice of medicine in the future at 10 years (1995). He said:

Crisis, challenge, and credibility.

Sledge, C B

The Journal of Bone & Joint Surgery: Apr 1985 - Volume 67 - Issue 4 - p 658-662

Title of Sledge's first vice president address to the AAOS.
C.B. Sledge, *Journal of Bone and Joint Surgery* 1985; 67: 685.

The over-all picture would be undesirable or intolerable to most of us...Origins of the crises...Foremost amongst the negative factors leading to our present situation [surgery reduced to piece work] is...an erosion of public credibility...the impression that physicians are overpaid and impersonal [that] technological advances increased the time costs of hospitalization...making healthcare costs a greater percentage of total national income [in spite of] the decade that has seen such enormous growth in the effectiveness of orthopaedic surgery...The physician is assumed, by public and government alike, to be responsible for hospital costs...Confusion regarding who is responsible for the escalating costs of medical care has contributed to the problem...There is also confusion in the public mind about who does what in health care [and] unreasonable expectations regarding the outcome of medical and surgical intervention...stimulated by media pronouncements regarding the "miracles of modern medicine," and we have often disregarded the ethics of clinical experimentation [and] loss of confidence in the profession...coincided with an oversupply of [less qualified] physicians and alternative providers...To gain the trust that the practice of medicine requires, physicians have had to assure the public of the reliability of their "product." If there is no boundary between the educated and the uneducated, the skilled and unskilled, there is a challenge to appropriate compensation and...to the physician's status as a professional rather than an employee [raising] the problems of credentialing and...testing...of competence [and] the pressure to be more economical in the provision of care will force physicians to make decisions that are contrary to the best interests of individual patients...The doctor's master must be the patient [and] another factor is the erosion of credibility in the public perception that "experimental" is a dirty word...Have we oversold [recent] advances and have we abused our privilege of investigation? Are we using unproven new operations without proper evidence of their potential for long-term success?...Ascribing excessive rates of failure to the "learning curve" must be discouraged, or at least the learning must be concentrated and taught in a few centers whose volume and experience will minimize the length of the learning period...

Some suggested solutions[:] Let me state categorically that I believe...innovation and research to be absolutely necessary. To maintain our credibility...trials must be appropriately controlled. Acting as the advocate for our patients, either we demand that there be hard evidence that a new procedure or device is safe and effective or we must undertake a carefully controlled study with the full understanding and agreement of the patient...to restore credibility...we can ensure that we continue to maintain our skills – technical and cognitive...We should let the public know what an orthopaedic surgeon is and what he or she does...This will require a public-awareness campaign...In addition, we must join our voices with other orthopaedic, surgical and medical organizations in a united effort to resist changes that diminish the quality or quantity of medical care. We must not let ourselves be compromised and our relationship with our patients diminished by being forced to ration medical care...Physicians should participate in the enumeration of...guidelines [with limited resources] to retain the traditional role of demanding the best possible care for each patient under his or her care. The most difficult step in restoring credibility…is to devise a system whereby we not only maintain our skills but demonstrate that maintenance to the public. (Sledge 1985)

Dr. Sledge, well-known as a clinical researcher, emphasized the importance of outcomes research and the importance of joint registries, following in the footsteps of Dr. E. A. Codman, whom he quoted in a guest editorial:

> E. A. Codman in 1934 said "every hospital should follow every patient it treats long enough to determine whether the treatment was successful and to inquire if not, why not." Our colleagues in internal medicine have long since embraced the concept of the randomized controlled trial for new drug interventions… There have been only a handful of such studies [in orthopaedics] for a number of reasons, which include the problem of surgeon bias in such studies. Rather than attempt to apply randomized trials…more important data can be gathered by using the techniques of outcomes analysis…Once the entry criteria have been established and assessment methods adopted, patients can be entered into the study and data gathered prospectively. At intervals after treatment, the various data elements are reassessed to determine which patients have benefitted… such as motion, pain, function and overall satisfaction. When other treatment methods are to be compared [an] honest comparison between the various treatments or no treatment [can be obtained]. (Sledge 1985)

Dr. Sledge had previously been elected president of the Hip Society in 1982, a position he held for one year. After he was elected president, he founded a total joint registry at the BWH and focused on funding that registry. The registry he founded was initially funded by his royalties and royalties from his colleagues at the BWH. Another past president of the AAOS noted, "He also failed [however], some 20 years later," because of lack of continuing financial support. After his retirement, his successor did not continue the funding for the registry; it was expensive, had about two to four staff members, and closed around 2000. On the national scene, the AAOS continued to voice support for a national joint registry, but funding remained a major barrier. As of 2005, spurred by the development of such a registry in Sweden, other groups, including the AAOS, have continued pushing for the creation of a total joint registry in the United States.

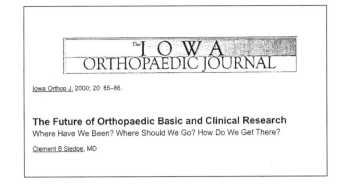

Title of Sledge's article discussing the future of orthopaedic basic and clinical research. *Iowa Orthopaedic Journal* 2000; 20: 85.

THE FUTURE OF ORTHOPAEDIC BASIC AND CLINICAL RESEARCH

In 2000, Dr. Sledge spoke about the future of orthopaedic basic and clinical research at the University of Iowa. He started by emphasizing the lack of such research—he had found fewer than a dozen articles describing clinical trials through an NLM search of the terms *orthopaedic* and *New England Journal of Medicine*, and most of those had been written by people who were not orthopaedists. This backed up his description of such orthopaedic research as being heavily "anecdotal." He went on to suggest how researchers in orthopaedics can take steps to develop high-quality and evidence-based studies: consider elements that have effects on outcomes, center studies around disease states and patients, apply clinical tools and methods that have been validated, and address and adjust for patient function before treatment and health care system-related factors. In those ways, Sledge believed, orthopaedics could expand its reach to non-orthopaedic journals and thereby a wider audience.

He did, however, point out two limitations of the evidence-based approach: lack of existing evidence, and a lack of consequence/relevance given to anecdotal evidence. For Sledge, clinical research should incorporate both anecdotal and clinical evidence, incorporating elements of both the condition and the patient in relation to treatments being studied—and in that way allowing orthopaedic research to move from the former toward the latter.

Dr. Sledge received many honors and distinctions during his career. A few that have not been mentioned in this chapter include the R. I. Harris Memorial Lecture (1986), given annually at the Canadian Orthopaedic Association's Annual Meeting, and two that are uncommon for orthopaedic surgeons: membership on the editorial board of Pharos (Alpha Omega Alpha Honor Medical Society) and election in 1992 into the Institute of Medicine.

CHAPTER 49

BWH
Other Surgeon Scholars: 1970–2000

The orthopaedic surgeons described in this chapter include some surgeon scholars—Harvard's name for these clinicians—who served at the Brigham and Women's Hospital after the Robert Breck Brigham Hospital (RBBH) and the Peter Bent Brigham Hospital (PBBH) merged with the Boston Hospital for Women in 1980. They may also have worked at the RBBH or the PBBH prior to or simultaneously with their work at the BWH. This chapter follows the trajectory of their careers between 1970 and 2000.

At the RBBH and the PBBH, these individuals made their contributions under the distinguished leadership of orthopaedic chief Dr. Clement Sledge (1970–1980). At the BWH, they were led by orthopaedic chiefs Drs. Sledge (1980–1996), Robert Poss (interim, 1996), and Thomas S. Thornhill (1997–). Many of these clinicians made contributions during a period of immense upheaval during the hospital merger as well as during a time of great change within the specialty.

Several of the individuals described in this chapter continue to publish at the time of the publication of this book. Data on the number and types of publications each surgeon scholar produced are included, however, research for each surgeon was completed over about a ten-year period and such information quickly becomes outdated. These data are representative of the breadth of their work. They may have written many more articles since that time. Those surgeon scholars covered in this chapter include:

Frederick C. Ewald	144
Robert W. Hussey	151
John E. Kenzora	153
J. Drennan Lowell	158
Lewis H. Millender	165
Robert Poss	169
Richard D. Scott	175
Barry P. Simmons	182
William H. Thomas	187

FREDERICK C. EWALD

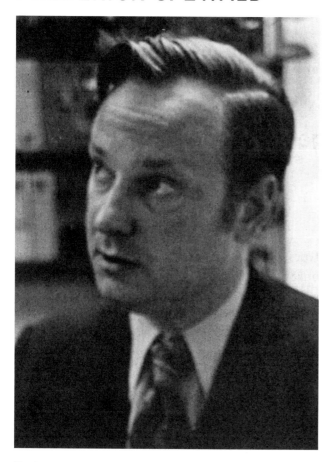

Frederick C. Ewald. Brigham and Women's Hospital Archives.

Physician Snapshot

Frederick C. Ewald
BORN: 1933
DIED: —
SIGNIFICANT CONTRIBUTIONS: Created the original design for the capitellocondylar total elbow prosthesis (1974); contributed to groundbreaking work in total knee replacement with Dr. Peter Walker and Dr. Clement Sledge, including the development of the kinematic total knee prosthesis; reported a new roentgenographic total knee arthroplasty-scoring system; founding member of the Society of Shoulder and Elbow Surgeons; founding member of the Knee Society and its sixth president (1989–1990)

Frederick C. Ewald was born in Detroit, Michigan on July 26, 1933. He received his BA degree in 1955 from Northwestern University and his MD degree from Northwestern University Medical School in 1962 (Beta Beta Beta 1958; Phi Kappa Alpha 1961). After an internship at the Wesley Pavilion of Northwestern University Hospital, Dr. Ewald was a resident in medicine at the University of Minnesota (1963–1964). He continued for an additional year at the university to complete his surgical residency for one year (1964–1965). Following a Helen Fay Hunter orthopaedic research fellowship at Children's Memorial Hospital in Chicago, he continued residency training in the Combined Boston Children's Hospital/Massachusetts's General Hospital Orthopaedic Program from 1966 until 1969.

Upon completion of his residency in Boston, Dr. Ewald returned to Chicago for about two years as director of the orthopaedic clinic at Children's Memorial Hospital and as an attending orthopaedic surgeon there and at Passavant Memorial Hospital. Initially an associate orthopaedic surgeon at Northwestern University Medical School, he was promoted to assistant professor the following year (1970–1971). While in Chicago, he published four different case reports in the *Journal of Bone and Joint Surgery* and the *Journal of Trauma*.

Early Research at the RBBH

In 1971, Dr. Clement Sledge recruited Ewald back to Boston. He asked Ewald to join the staff at the Robert Beck Brigham Hospital (RBBH) as an assistant surgeon, a position he held from 1971 until 1974. Ewald was also appointed consultant orthopaedic surgeon at the West Roxbury Veterans Administration Hospital and associate in orthopaedic surgery at the Peter Bent Brigham Hospital (PBBH), a position he held until 1980. That same year, Ewald was appointed clinical instructor in orthopaedic surgery at Harvard Medical School (1971–1977).

Dr. Ewald published about 60 articles throughout his career. Ewald's first publication after joining Sledge at the RBBH, "Effect of Distal Transfer of the Greater Trochanter in Growing

Animals," reported findings in five pedigree beagle puppies about three years after surgery. It was the culmination of research he had previously completed during his fellowship at Children's Memorial Hospital with Dr. Kenji Hirohashi. Ewald and Hirohashi reviewed growth changes in the proximal femur after trochanteric osteotomy—with implications for surgery in children with deformities secondary to a congenital dislocation of the hip. In their findings, they wrote, "No significant changes [resulted] in over-all growth of the femur, no change in the degree of anteversion of the femoral neck and no gross distortion in the configuration of the greater trochanter. There was, however, an 18 per cent decrease in diameter of the femoral neck" (Ewald and Hirohashi 1973).

In his 1971 annual report, Dr. Sledge stated that Ewald was "part-time at the Peter Bent Brigham Hospital doing major research in the management of arthritis with Dr. Sledge at the Robert Breck Brigham ("Annual Report, 1970–1971, Staff Booklet, Report of the Orthopedic Surgeon-in-Chief [Sledge]" 1971, 283). In his 1972 surgeon-in-chief's report, Sledge stated that Ewald was doing research on total knee development. In his CV, Ewald cited his three main areas of study as fixation of prostheses and the juncture between them and bone; joint motion and the effects of force over joints; and all aspects of the creation and appraisal of total replacements of ankles, knees, and hips.

Ewald was immediately active teaching anatomy and biomechanics of the knee joint to first- and second-year students; joint pain and arthritis to the third- and fourth-year students; and total knee replacement to the orthopaedic residents. By 1973, his research projects included three that were ready for clinical trials: a total knee prosthesis, a total elbow prosthesis, and a proximal interphalangeal joint prosthesis. The following year, he was promoted to surgeon at the RBBH, a position he held until 1980.

Total Elbow Prosthesis

Ewald had begun his original design for the capitellocondylar total elbow prosthesis by July 1974. In 1975, he published his first two papers from the Brighams, one on total elbow replacement and one on metal-to-plastic total knee replacement. That same year, Sledge reported that Ewald had enrolled 30 patients in a clinical trial of an unconstrained total elbow prosthesis (capito-condylar). Ewald's clinical trial expanded to a multicenter trial and after about one year, the prosthesis became available for general use (ca.1977).

In his first paper in which he described his nonconstrained total elbow prosthesis, the capito-condylar total elbow, he mentioned the disappointing results of radial head resection and synovectomy (47 elbows in 46 patients with rheumatoid arthritis) performed over almost 25 years at RBBH, with a mean seven-year follow-up. In those receiving a hinged total elbow prosthesis (G.S.B.), despite a 66% increase in range of motion after the procedure, failure occurred, or revision was required in almost one-quarter of the original procedures. Ewald noted that in hinge arthroplasty in the elbow or knee, the prosthesis often becomes loose, and sepsis and synovitis secondary to debris could occur.

He then described a non-hinged metal–polyethylene prosthesis designed for use in the elbow. Using wax, he created the articular surface of the metallic humeral portion. The ulnar component

---

Orthopedic Clinics of North America
Volume 6, Issue 3, July 1975, Pages 685-696

Total Elbow Replacement

Frederick C. Ewald M.D. (Clinical Instructor, Surgeon, Associate Orthopedic Surgeon, Orthopedic Consultant)

Title of Ewald's initial article on the capitellocondylar total elbow prosthesis. *Orthopedic Clinics of North America* 1975; 6: 685.

> ### Capitellocondylar total elbow arthroplasty
> Ewald, F C; Scheinberg, R D; Poss, R; Thomas, W H; Scott, R D; Sledge, C B
> The Journal of Bone & Joint Surgery: Dec 1980 - Volume 62 - Issue 8 - p 1259-1263

Ewald and colleagues' article reviewing their results with 69 total elbow replacements. *Journal of Bone and Joint Surgery* 1980; 62: 1259.

was made of polyethylene. Medial and lateral stability was provided by the trochlear groove and a medial lip on the ulnar component. The radial head was resected. Ewald thought that this construction, while allowing motion and avoiding torque and sheer at the interface of bone and cement, would distribute the forces to the collateral ligaments (which are retained during the procedure), the capsule, and the surrounding muscles. Although this was at the time still unproven and being tested in clinical trials, he mentioned that this prosthesis had been used in 17 patients—the first implanted in mid-1974—with ~10 months' follow-up. He listed two contraindications for its use: a history of joint sepsis or a history of resection of the capsule and collateral ligaments. By 1977, he and his coauthors published the results of their first 50 cases with at least a 2½ year follow-up.

Over the next decade, few design modifications were made to his capitellocondylar total elbow prosthesis and "the resurface geometry and the humeral component...remained unchanged." (Ewald and Jacobs 1984). The basic design endured, and, by 1978, they reported:

> the only major modification has been the addition of a metal boat and stem to the previously all-plastic ulnar component. A variety of sizes has been added as well. The concept of the three-point fixation for each component provides rotational control and may be one of the key factors, along with minimal constraint, in preventing loosening of the fixation of the prosthesis with time. (Ewald and Jacobs 1984)

Ewald and his colleagues published two papers with long-term results of the capitellocondylar total elbow replacement in patients with rheumatoid arthritis. In 1980, they reported on 69 implants in 64 patients with an average follow-up of 3½ years:

> Postoperative flexion and pronation were significantly improved, but no significant increase in postoperative extension or supination could be demonstrated. Based on a rating system evaluating pain and function, there were 87 per cent good or excellent results. The complication rate...was 39 percent. Eight patients required revision...four for dislocation of the prosthesis, two for sepsis, one for loosening, and one for fracture. Eight other asymptomatic patients showed minimum radiolucent lines adjacent to the ulnar component [none] adjacent to the humeral component...Most of the complications (ulnar nerve palsy, skin breakdown, and so on) have been minimized or eliminated by alterations in surgical technique. (Ewald et al. 1980)

In 1993, Ewald and his colleagues published the BWH's long-term results of 202 capitellocondylar total elbow replacements in 172 patients with rheumatoid arthritis with an average follow-up of 69 months:

> At the most recent follow-up examination, use of a 100-point rating score demonstrated an improvement from an average preoperative score of 26 points...to an average postoperative score of 91 points...The most improvement occurred in the categories of pain, functional status, and range of motion in all planes except extension. The improvements [including]

roentgenographic appearance...did not deteriorate with time...The roentgenograms showed a radiolucent line adjacent to eight humeral and nineteen ulnar components; most of the lines were incomplete and one millimeter wide or less. Revision of the prosthesis was necessary in three elbows because of loosening...and in three additional elbows because of dislocation of the prosthesis. Complications included deep infection in three elbows...problems related to the wound in fifteen...permanent, partial sensory ulnar-nerve palsy in five...permanent, partial motor ulnar-nerve palsy in one...and dislocation in seven...

There were three subsets in this study. The first consisted of fifty-six elbows that had been replaced by an all-plastic ulnar component through a posterior approach, from 1974 to 1977; the second, twenty-six elbows that had been replaced by a metal-backed ulnar component, through a posterior approach, in 1978 and 1979; and the third, 120 elbows that had been replaced by a metal-backed ulnar component, through a modified Kocher approach, performed from 1979 to 1987...In our experience, ligamentous instability in rheumatoid patients has not been a problem, nor is it a contraindication of resurfacing except in some elbows [where] the ligaments or capsule has been resected as part of a fascial arthroplasty...It appears that a more constrained prosthesis may be necessary when there is inadequate bone stock because there will not be enough bone for the surgeon to seat the prosthesis properly and thus to obtain three-point fixation in both the humerus and the ulna...However, two decades later, the concerns voiced in 1974 about long-term loosening of components, resorption of bone secondary to stress-shielding, polyethylene wear, and metal fatigue fracture continue to be problems. The difficulties related to the soft tissues can be solved by appropriate training and operative experience. (Ewald et al. 1993)

> J Bone Joint Surg Am. 1993 Apr;75(4):498-507
>
> **Capitellocondylar total elbow replacement in rheumatoid arthritis. Long-term results**
>
> F C Ewald [1], E D Simmons Jr, J A Sullivan, W H Thomas, R D Scott, R Poss, T S Thornhill, C B Sledge

Ewald and colleagues' article reporting their long-term results in 202 patients with a capitellocondylar total elbow replacement. *Journal of Bone and Joint Surgery* 1993; 75: 498.

In response to these concerns, other elbow designs became more popular—mainly because the operation was difficult using a non-hinged implant and recurrent implant subluxations and ulnar nerve symptoms often occurred. In the early twenty-first century, hinge elbow prostheses are commonly used but overall total elbows less so. This is largely due to breakthrough treatments using biologics to treat rheumatoid arthritis.

Total Knee Prosthesis

The same year that Dr. Ewald published his groundbreaking work on total elbow prosthesis, he also published his first paper on total knee prosthesis. **Case 49.1** provides an example of one of his case reports. Over the subsequent years, Ewald participated in many postgraduate courses and the academy's instructional courses. He frequently spoke about total knee replacement, in addition to total elbow and total ankle replacement.

In the 1970s, surgeons at the RBBH used a variety of knee implants, but under Sledge, they preferred a total knee prosthesis that retained the posterior cruciate ligament, if possible. Dr. Ewald with Dr. Peter Walker and Dr. Sledge (and later others) were instrumental in the evolution from the duocondylar to the duopatellar and then to the kinematic total knee prosthesis. Ewald et al. (1984) wrote:

The years of use of the all-plastic tibial component (1977–1981) and of the metal-backed tibial component (1978–1980) were about identical. However, most of the all plastic tibial components were eight millimeters thick, and bench-testing has shown these to be inferior to metal-backed plastic. (Ewald et al. 1984)

In 1981, Dr. Ewald, with Peter Walker and others, studied the fixation of 12 different tibial components including:

compartmental, anteriorly joined, posterior-cruciate retaining, and one-piece with one, two, or three fixation posts; all-plastic or with a metal tray...[They used an] apparatus [that] applied compressive load with anterior-posterior force, rotational torque, or varus-valgus moment. The relative deflections, both compressive and distractive, were measured between the component and the bone. The

---

Orthopedic Clinics of North America
Volume 6, Issue 3, July 1975, Pages 811-821

Metal to Plastic Total Knee Replacement

Frederick C. Ewald M.D. (Clinical Instructor, Surgeon, Associate Orthopedic Surgeon, Orthopedic Consultant)

Title of Ewald's article on the use of a metal and polyethylene total knee prosthesis. *Orthopedic Clinics of North America* 1975; 6: 811.

Case 49.1. Giant Cell Synovitis After Failed Patellar Replacement

"No. 1. A 67-year-old woman had experienced pain in both knees, more severe in the right than the left, for 20 years. The pain in the right knee was present at rest, awoke her from sleep at night, and she was unable to go up and down stairs. She took Codeine for pain, used crutches, and was essentially on a bed-chair regimen. There was no history of rheumatoid arthritis. Advanced destruction of the right knee joint was confirmed by physical and radiographic examination. The right knee flexed to 30° and extended to minus 10°. There was 12° of recumbent true varus and moderate medial collateral laxity. On March 1, 1972 the patient underwent a bicompartmental McKeever arthroplasty (3 mm lateral and 6 mm medial prosthesis) and replacement of the patellar articular surface with a polyethylene prosthesis. The patellar articular surface along with the femoral condyles and femoral patellar groove is shown. Post-operative radiographic examination showed satisfactory placement of the McKeever prosthesis and position of the patellar prosthesis. On the seventeenth postoperative day the right knee was manipulated to 70° flexion and fluoroscopy showed a posterior osteophyte blocking further flexion. Auscultation of the knee during flexion-extension revealed fine crepitus. The patient did well for approximately one year until she noted increasing pain in the right knee made worse by motion. She was unable to walk and the knee could not be extended past minus 20°. There was a moderate knee joint effusion and the knee was diffusely tender. At surgery on February 27, 1973, one year after the initial procedure, the synovium was inflamed and hypertrophied, and the capsule was thickened. The femur in the area of the notch was grooved longitudinally thorugh [sic] the subchondral bone. The patellar replacement remained firmly fixed, but the articular surface was extensively worn and grooved. The patellar prosthesis was removed from the bony patellar remnant with great difficulty and a synovectomy performed. The McKeever prostheses were removed, and the knee was converted to a hinged joint fixed with methacrylate.

"In addition, inflammatory tissue and polyethylene debris were seen histologically around the keel of the medial compartment McKeever prosthesis probably contributing to anterior dislocation of the prosthesis.

"Nineteen months following total knee replacement, the patient had 75° of the right knee motion and was walking without support."

(C. Ewald et al. 1976)

least deflections occurred with one-piece metal tray components with one or two posts and with one-piece plastic components with a post on each side. Compartmental components deflected the most. Clinical Relevance: The results are regarded as a screening method to provide guidelines for design and usage. (Walker et al. 1981)

Drs. Ewald, Sledge, and colleagues reported their results with the kinematic total knee prosthesis at two- to four-year follow-ups in 1984 and again in 1999 with a 10-to-14-year follow-up. At two-to-four-year follow-up of 124 knees:

> The average active postoperative flexion was 106 degrees (range, 94 to 120 degrees). Twenty-two knees (18 per cent) had incomplete, non-progressive radiolucent lines, less than one millimeter in width, at the tibial bone-cement interface…considered insignificant… less reaction at the bone-cement interface was found with the metal-backed kinematic tibial component…
>
> Evaluation of the tibial fixation is difficult and will require longer follow-up, although the two-to-four-year results are encouraging. Laboratory testing has demonstrated that the posterior cruciate ligament allows the transmission of significant sheer forces that would otherwise be borne by the bone-cement interface and capsular structures. The absence of clinical subluxation or dislocation after total knee replacement suggests that the posterior cruciate ligament is functional and that the soft-tissue length and tension can be restored. Other laboratory bench-testing has shown normal transmission of stress across the joint using a one-piece tibial component with a created peg and metal backing…
>
> Careful evaluation of the radiolucencies…showed several trends that may help surgeons to achieve better results. 1. In the patients with a preoperative varus deformity who had tibial zone-1 (medial) radiolucencies, the alignment was under corrected and the tibial components were placed in more varus angulation than the average. These errors can be corrected by better surgical technique. 2. In patients who had a proximal tibial defect filled with methacrylate, early postoperative radiolucencies developed. Recent evidence suggests that bone defects can be better treated with a custom-designed prosthesis, bone grafts, or reinforced methacrylate. 3. …some patients had a sclerotic subcondylar bone plate that was not completely resected [and] was associated with poor radiographic penetration of cement [which] could be improved by drilling the subchondral bone to allow penetration or by resecting the sclerotic area and using a custom-made prosthesis to replace the bone defect… (Ewald et al. 1984)

J Bone Joint Surg Am. 1984 Sep;66(7):1032-40.

Kinematic total knee replacement

F C Ewald, M A Jacobs, R E Miegel, P S Walker, R Poss, C B Sledge

---

Report of Ewald, et al.'s two–four-year results with the Kinematic total knee prosthesis. *Journal of Bone and Joint Surgery* 1984; 66: 1032.

J Arthroplasty. 1999 Jun;14(4):473-80

Kinematic total knee arthroplasty: a 10- to 14-year prospective follow-up review

F C Ewald [1], R J Wright, R Poss, W H Thomas, M D Mason, C B Sledge

---

Report of Ewald, et al.'s 10–14-year results with the Kinematic total knee prosthesis. *Journal of Arthroplasty* 1999; 14: 473.

In 1999, Ewald and his colleagues reported their experience with 306 primary procedures implanting the non-constrained kinematic total knee, a prosthesis that allows for the left or right femur to be replaced and preserves the posterior cruciate ligament, over 10 to 14 years (1978–82). They documented a 6.5% rate of revision, most often because of issues with the patella. Among those revisions, 10 (3.06%) were to fix a loosened patellar component and 2 (0.65%) were to resolve patellar subluxation. Because anterior knee pain was relatively common in those whose patellas were unsurfaced (21.8%) or replaced (11.2%), they concluded that replacement of the patella should ideally be avoided when using the kinematic total knee prosthesis.

Dr. Ewald was president of the Knee Society in 1989, when he reported a new roentgenographic total knee arthroplasty-scoring system:

> In addition to measurement of the knee alignment and component position, leg and knee alignment, and the prosthesis-bone interface or fixation…The knee is positioned in a standard manner…consensus [obtained] at two Knee Society Meetings…was that the number and location of the zones to be examined will be established by the prime developers of any particular knee design…The scoring system for each of the three components is determined by measuring the width of the radiolucent lines for each of the zones in millimeters for each [component]. The total widths are added for each zone for each of the three prostheses. This total produces a numerical score for each component…4 or less and nonprogressive is probably not significant; 5-9 should be closely followed for progression; and 10 or greater signifies possible or impending failure regardless of symptoms. (Ewald 1989)

Legacy

Dr. Frederick Ewald retired in 1999. Among his numerous publications, 31 were about total knee replacement outcomes, 14 on the capitellocondylar total elbow prosthesis, and 7 about outcomes after total hip replacement. From 1978 to 1980, Ewald served as vice-chairman of the medical staff at the RBBH. He also served on the joint conference committee at the BWH in 1980 and the BWH operations review committee in 1981. He served as the sixth president of the Knee Society (1989–1990) and was a founding member. He is a member of the following professional organizations: American Orthopaedic Association, Boston Orthopaedic Club, Massachusetts Medical Society, New England Rheumatism Society, American Academy of Orthopaedic Surgeons, Orthopaedic Research Society, New England Orthopaedic Society, International Society of Orthopaedics and Traumatology, American Medical Association, American Rheumatism Association, Eastern Orthopaedic Association; and a founding member of the Society of Shoulder and Elbow Surgeons.

ROBERT W. HUSSEY

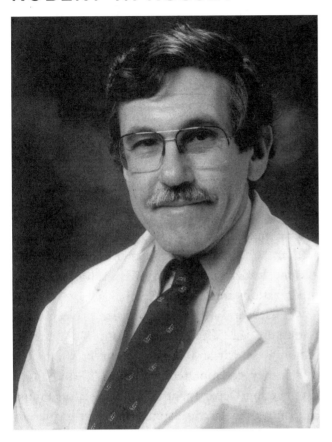

Robert W. Hussey. Courtesy of Tris Hussey.

Physician Snapshot

Robert W. Hussey
BORN: 1936
DIED: 1992
SIGNIFICANT CONTRIBUTIONS: Associate chief of the Spinal Cord Injury Service at the West Roxbury Veterans Administration Medical Center; chief of the Spinal Cord Injury Service at the VA Medical Center in Richmond, Virginia; president of the American Paraplegia Society 1983–1985

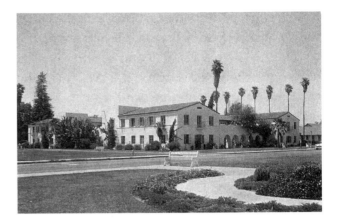

Rancho Los Amigos, mid/late-twentieth century.
Courtesy of Downey Historical Society and Rancho Los Amigos National Rehabilitation Center.

Title of Hussey and Stauffer's article identifying the essential muscles in the pelvis and lower extremities required for ambulation in spinal cord injured patients. *Archives of Physical Medicine and Rehabilitation* 1973; 54: 544.

Born and raised in Reading, Pennsylvania, Robert "Bob" William Hussey graduated as valedictorian from West Reading High School. He stayed in the area and attended Albright College, graduating cum laude in 1958. He then moved to Boston to attend Harvard Medical School (HMS); he graduated with an MD degree, also cum laude, in 1962.

During his time at Harvard, he was elected to Alpha Omega Alpha. He joined the US Navy in 1963 and spent two years serving as a medical officer on a submarine. After being discharged from the service, Hussey completed the Boston Children's Hospital/Massachusetts General Hospital residency program in orthopaedic surgery. He continued his training after that residency, spending 8 months studying spinal cord injury and working with patients with such injuries at Rancho Los Amigos in Los Angeles, California. His mentor, Dr. Clement Sledge, had recommended that Hussey specialize in spinal cord injuries.

After completing his fellowship at Rancho Los Amigos, Hussey was hired by Sledge at the Peter Bent Brigham Hospital (PBBH) and the West

Roxbury Veterans Administration Medical Center, and so he returned to Boston. He was awarded a teaching fellowship in 1970 and spent two years teaching orthopaedic surgery at HMS. Later he was named an assistant professor there.

Dr. Hussey, during his short career, published 16 articles, 7 of them while in Boston. After completion of his fellowship, he published his first paper, "Spinal Cord Injury: Requirements for Ambulation," cowritten with Dr. E. Shannon Stauffer. On the basis of results from 164 patients with SCI who had been treated at and discharged from Rancho Los Amigos, they noted that pelvic control was necessary for ambulation—in fact, it was one of the traits of patients who were able to ambulate at a community level. Other such traits, found among the 82 patients (50%) who ambulated at that level, included:

- good or fair hip flexor function
- good or fair quadriceps function (one or both legs)
- no braces or one short-leg/one long-leg brace
- no fixed deformity of any joint
- no extensive spasticity

He named three other categories of ambulatory ability—exercise, household, and nonambulatory—noting that those patients who only had pelvic control could not surpass the exercise ambulatory level, whereas those with no pelvic control could not ambulate (the nonambulatory category).

At the West Roxbury Veterans Administration Hospital, Hussey worked with Dr. Alain B. Rossier, chief of the spinal cord injury service and a specialist in spinal cord injuries who was a wheelchair user himself. Together they created a multipronged protocol for treating spinal cord injuries that included treatment of the immediate injury, rehabilitation, and follow-up in both an outpatient clinic and a Spinal Cord Injury Home Care Program. This program allowed veterans with SCI to receive ongoing care. Hussey and Rossier also created an SCI fellowship, and many former fellows became leaders in SCI services at hospitals and organizations across the US.

> Spine (Phila Pa 1976). Nov-Dec 1984;9(8):773-7
>
> **Forces in the halo-vest apparatus**
>
> P S Walker, D Lamser, R W Hussey, A B Rossier, A Farberov, J Dietz

Title of Walker, et al.'s article demonstrating the benefits of different pin designs in the halo-vest apparatus. *Spine* 1984; 9: 773.

Hussey and Rossier had other projects supported by the Veterans Administration Rehabilitation Research and Development Programs. In 1980, they collaborated with MIT's Mechanical Engineering Department to study functional muscle control by electrical stimulation of the afferent nerves. I was unable to locate any publications by Hussey and Rossier about this subject. With colleagues at the PBBH they also reported on six patients with severe spinal cord injury and cervical spine fractures treated early with corpectomy and a fibular strut graft. Although this condition was rare—occurring in only 6 of 62 patients—their goal was to secure the broken spine in a way that enabled the patient to move and ambulate, in contrast to placing the patient in traction, as was the usual practice.

Hussey published nine papers with Rossier and colleagues. With Dr. Peter Walker, they developed:

> a new program in clinical bioengineering within the Spinal Cord Injury Unit [which] was begun in the fall of 1980. An initial objective was to determine areas for research effort...relevant to the patient population of the unit...A problem which had received previous attention was how to devise a mechanical means for applying a reproducible "Closed Injury Lesion of the

Spinal Cord"...If a reproducible closed injury method can be found, this will be the model for studies on the effect of various treatments after injury. A second project dealing with the patient subsequent to an acute injury is entitled "Studies for the Design of a New System for Stabilization of the Acutely Injured Cervical Spine." ("Cervical Spine Injuries. Clinical Bioengineering Laboratory. VA Medical Center, West Roxbury, MA" 1981)

This latter study resulted in the publication "Forces in the Halo-Vest Apparatus" in which the authors concluded that sharply tapered pins would be able to be tightened in the bones of the skull more than those with a less extreme taper. They also noted that patients can affect the shearing forces of the pins in various ways: moving little when laying down or sitting; keeping the arms lowered; and not looking up, bending over, or turning to the side quickly. Hussey and his colleagues also believed that making the halo vest stiffer would help reduce movement that could affect pin placement, and they suggested further studies to determine the capacity of alternative vest designs and headpieces that are not anchored into the skull to maintain stability.

In 1981, Hussey resigned as associate chief of the Spinal Cord Injury Service at the West Roxbury Veterans Administration Medical Center to become chief of the Spinal Cord Injury Service at the VA Medical Center in Richmond Virginia and associate professor of orthopaedic surgery at the Medical College of Virginia. He was active on the VA Long-Term Care Panel and a member of the VA Liaison Committee. From 1983–1985 he served as president of the American Paraplegia Society.

Cancer forced Dr. Hussey to retire early, in 1991. Less than a year later, he died on September 2, 1992, in Richmond, Virginia. He was only 56 years old. Phyllis Ann, his wife, and their four children survived him.

JOHN E. KENZORA

Physician Snapshot

John E. Kenzora
BORN: 1940
DIED: —
SIGNIFICANT CONTRIBUTIONS: Recognized expert in osteonecrosis; received the Nicholas Andry Award with Dr. Melvin Glimcher; chief of the division of orthopaedic surgery at the University of Maryland and orthopaedic surgeon-in-chief at the University of Maryland Medical Center (1983–)

John Edward Kenzora was born on September 10, 1940, in Toronto, Canada. He graduated from the University of Toronto in 1961, and he received his MD from the University's medical school in 1965. While at the University of Toronto, he was in the Alpha Kappa Kappa fraternity, he played basketball and participated in track and field events. In his leisure time, he played golf and enjoyed hunting and fishing. After medical school, Kenzora interned (rotating) at Toronto General Hospital, 1965–1966.

He then moved to Boston where from July 1, 1966, to August 31, 1968, he was a research fellow under Dr. Melvin Glimcher at the Massachusetts General Hospital (MGH). While in medical school, he had worked in Glimcher's lab as a summer research fellow 1962—1964. On September 1,

Experimental Osteonecrosis of the Femoral Head in Adult Rabbits

J. E. KENZORA, M.D., R. E. STEELE, M.D., Z. H. YOSIPOVITCH, M.D. AND M. J. GLIMCHER, M.D.

Clinical Orthopaedics and Related Research
Number 130
January-February, 1978

Title of Kenzora, et al.'s article, "Experimental Osteonecrosis of the Femoral Head in Adult Rabbits." *Clinical Orthopaedics and Related Research* 1978; 130: 8.

1968, he entered the MGH/CHMC orthopaedic residency program; he spent the first nine months as an assistant resident at Boston Children's Hospital, the next 15 months as an assistant resident at the MGH, and the following eight months back at Boston Children's Hospital as an orthopaedic resident. In 1970 at MGH, his salary was $9,600 (in 2020 the equivalent was $65,516). From April 1971 through June 1971, he was a resident at the Robert Breck Brigham Hospital (RBBH). From July 1971 through September 1971, he was a resident at the Beth Israel Hospital, and from October 1971 through March 1972 (six months) he served as chief resident in orthopaedic surgery at the Peter Bent Brigham Hospital (PBBH).

During his two years in Dr. Glimcher's laboratory at MGH, Dr. Kenzora studied avascular necrosis of the femoral head in rabbits for which he and his colleagues later received the Kappa Delta Award in 1978. In their first paper, "Tissue Biology Following Experimental Infarction of Femoral Heads. Part I. Bone Studies," they wrote:

> Femoral heads were moved after osteotomy of the femoral necks in sixty mature rabbits and... then replaced and fixed in situ with threaded Kirschner wires. The animals were killed... between one hour and forty weeks after surgery...The earliest signs of avascularity and necrosis were autolysis of the marrow cells and osteoblasts and empty osteocyte lacuna, seen four days after surgery. Osteocyte viability was measured by autoradiograms...They were considered to be alive [for forty-eight hours postoperatively] even in the face of total infarction. Osteocytes that appeared morphologically intact for periods of infarction longer than forty-eight hours were considered non-viable.
>
> The distal marrow cavity provided the major source of the healing revascularizing connective tissue. While the osteotomy was uniting, the mesenchymal pool proliferated and filled the empty marrow spaces of the femoral head. One of the major biological functions of this invading tissue was of cellular modulation into osteoblasts with subsequent production of living bone on to dead trabecular surfaces. There was minimum evidence of preliminary bone resorption by osteoclastic cells. It was thought that this process...is more analogous to creeping apposition then to creeping substitution...Living woven bone and later living lamellar bone completely coated dead trabeculae and after many weeks, as new bone filled empty vascular spaces that tissue mass: volume ratio increased. Fully revascularized heads... became physically, roentgenographically, and histologically more dense. Revascularization was complete as early as six weeks and as late as sixteen weeks (average ten) following infarction. It was usually only after revascularization was complete that significant evidence of remodeling or removal of dead bone was seen. No sequential collapse was observed. (Kenzora et al. 1969)

Kenzora presented this research during his first year as an assistant resident in orthopaedics at Boston Children's Hospital. Three years later, while chief resident at the PBBH, he presented a second research paper, "The Osteocyte: Living, Dying, Dead. A Histologic, Functional Study," in which he observed the life span of osteocytes in rabbit femurs and humeri that were removed and stored at 37 degrees for up to four days. Samples of cortical and cancellous bone were incubated in solutions of H^3-proline and H^3-cytidine. Kenzora (1972) wrote, "At zero time, 6.5 per cent of all osteocyte lacunae incorporated isotope, 19 per cent did not, and 16 per cent were empty. At twelve hours only one-half as many cells were labeled. At twenty-four hours 8 per cent...By four days no cells were labeled. Sixty per cent of the lacunae were empty, and 40 per cent were filled with cells." That same year, he wrote a case report on a child with a heritable disease of connective

Case 49.2. Hydroxylysine-Deficient Collagen Disease

"A 12-year-old girl (born on October 3, 1958) was admitted to the Children's Hospital Medical Center, Boston, for surgical correction of kyphoscoliosis. She was the product of a full-term pregnancy manifested by lack of fetal movement, frequent spotting and premature membrane rupture at 3 months, forcing the mother to total bed rest. At birth the child weighed 2.27 kg and was noted to be quite floppy, with pectus excavatum and flexible kyphoscoliosis. She failed to cry spontaneously, sucked poorly and had many respiratory problems, including 3 bouts of pneumonia. Motor milestones were delayed: she sat at 1 ½ years and walked at 2-½ years. For many years she was thought to have amyotonia congenita. A Stanford-Binet test at the age of 5 revealed a low-normal IQ. An umbilical hernia present at birth corrected itself spontaneously. At one time or another she dislocated virtually every joint, shoulders and knees more other than others, which the mother was usually able to reduce. Skin bruises were commonly noted. When lacerations occurred, the skin edges retracted, with little bleeding, although wounds seemed to heal slowly. She complained frequently of leg cramps. She had not had blisters, broken bones or episodes of pneumothorax. At the time of admission, she was an average student in the 7th grade.

"Physical examination showed a girl who weighed 32.7 kg and was 148 cm tall, with an arm span of 150 cm (lower segment, 78 cm). The skin was pale, thin, velvety and apparently hyperelastic, with generalized, fine follicular hyperkeratosis accentuated on the extensor aspects of the extremities. There were no abnormal scars or molluscoid pseudotumors. Ophthalmologic examination revealed small corneas (10 mm) and scattered infiltrates in the anterior stroma. The lens and fundi were normal. The scleras were slightly blue, and there were no epicanthal folds. The palate was high arched, but the ears were normal. Examination of the heart revealed a widely split S2. Orthopedic examination showed mild pectus excavatum and kyphoscoliosis with a gibbus at the level of the 11th thoracic to 2d lumbar vertebras.

"Marked genu recurvatum and dynamic pes planus, were present. The joints were lax, and overall muscle mass appeared diminished. There was arachnodactyly, and the Steinberg thumb sign was present. The wrist sign was present, but the Gorlin tongue sign was absent. Hemogram, urinalysis and urinary amino acid analysis gave normal results, and a cyanide nitroprusside test for homocystine was negative. An electrocardiogram was normal. Roentgenograms of the skeleton revealed marked kyphoscoliosis. Pulmonary-function studies showed increased residual volume and mild airway obstruction, with a vital capacity of 2.44 liters (92 per cent predicted), a residual volume of 1.65 liters (190 per cent predicated), and a peak flow rate of 180 liters per minute (52 per cent predicted). At the time of surgical correction of the kyphoscoliosis, vertebral bone and lumbodorsal fascia were obtained for further examination. The skin appeared normal on routine histologic examination, as well as with special stains for elastic tissue and polysaccharide components...In vertebral bone from Case 1, the content of hydroxylysine was approximately 43 per cent of normal, and the ratio of hydroxylysine to lysine was 0.061 (normal, 0.145 0.036)."

(Pinnell, Krane, Glimcher, and Kenzora 1972)

tissue admitted for surgical correction of kyphoscoliosis (**Case 49.2**).

In 1978, Kenzora and his colleagues published an additional article on osteonecrosis of the femoral head in rabbits—an expansion of their original 1969 study that now included 250 adult rabbits. They studied the biologic changes in the cancellous bone and expanded to include the compact subchondral bone. They demonstrated osteonecrosis by the failure of the cells to incorporate H^3-cytidine. They wrote:

> Proliferation of capillaries and undifferentiated mesenchymal cells in the living bone marrow adjacent to the osteotomy site rapidly filled the marrow spaces of the necrotic femoral head... Eventually, fully differentiated and functioning osteoblasts covered the surfaces of the

> NICOLAS ANDRY AWARD
>
> **The Biology of Osteonecrosis of the Human Femoral Head and its Clinical Implications:**
> I. Tissue Biology
>
> MELVIN J. GLIMCHER, M.D. AND JOHN E. KENZORA, M.D.
>
> Clin Orthop Relat Res. Mar-Apr 1979;(139):283-312.
>
> **The biology of osteonecrosis of the human femoral head and its clinical implications: II. The pathological changes in the femoral head as an organ and in the hip joint**
>
> M J Glimcher, J E Kenzora
>
> Clin Orthop Relat Res. 1979 May;(140):273-312.
>
> **The biology of osteonecrosis of the human femoral head and its clinical implications. III. Discussion of the etiology and genesis of the pathological sequelae; commments on treatment**
>
> M J Glimcher, J E Kenzora

Glimcher and Kenzora's articles on the biology of osteonecrosis of the human femoral head.
Clinical Orthopaedics and Research 1979; 138: 284;
Clinical Orthopaedics and Research 1979; 139: 283; *Clinical Orthopaedics and Research* 1979; 140: 273.

dead trabeculae. New bone was laid down first on these surfaces and later...filled the spaces between the trabeculae. The resulting increase in bone mass per unit volume of tissue increased the radiodensity of the femoral head. The central cores of dead bone in the trabeculae were then resorbed and replaced by living bone...

The biologic response to death of the compact subchondral bone occurs much later because of its location at a distance from the site of initial repair. In contrast to coarse cancellous bone, the primary response here is bone resorption rather than bone formation. New bone formation fails to keep pace with bone resorption leading to the loss of bone mass subchondrally...penetration by capillaries and resorption of tissue continues into the cartilage, inciting a proliferative response of the cartilage cells and changes in the cartilage matrix similar to...osteoarthritis...a destructive synovial pannus forms [which] destroys the articular cartilage. (Kenzora et al. 1978)

Dr. Kenzora and Dr. Glimcher were recognized as experts in osteonecrosis. In 1978 and 1979 they published an abridged communication followed by a three-part series of articles on "The Biology of Osteonecrosis of the Human Femoral Head and Its Clinical Implications" for which they received the Nicholas Andry Award (see chapter 24). They stated:

> The weight of evidence in the literature and from the present in depth study of approximately 150 femoral heads strongly supports the conclusion that the series of events [of osteonecrosis]...is initiated by death of cells in bone as a substance, as a tissue, and as an organ, and may, therefore, reasonably and properly be grouped under the term "idiopathic osteonecrosis [I.O.]." The subchondral lucency (crescent sign) seen by x-ray in the early stages of the disease complex is a subchondral fracture through dead bone which occurs after the death of bone cells...[In] the case of subcapital fractures...or posterior dislocation of the hip we suggest...the term... "avascular necrosis" [Av.O.]...[In] those instances in which they etiology is not known or is obscure...it is best to use the term "idiopathic osteonecrosis"... The hallmark of the repair of the coarse cancellous bone is the formation of new, living bone on the surface of the dead trabeculae... The repair of dead cancellous bone consists of two distinct and apparently independent phenomena: (1) cell proliferation and spreading of the repair tissue throughout the femoral head; (2) differentiation of undifferentiated mesenchymal cells, initially to osteoblasts... which form new bone...and latter to osteoclasts...After a relatively short time [in idiopathic osteonecrosis] and after the new bone formed has extended only a few millimeters, differentiation of the mesenchymal cells to

osteoblasts ceases or slows very markedly so that the advancing "front" of the repair tissue consists of fibrous tissue and a loose accumulation of mesenchymal cells and capillaries. The repair tissue of coarse cancellous bone following Av.O. [avascular necrosis] usually spreads and forms new bone more rapidly and extensively than in [idiopathic osteonecrosis] once the repair tissue has crossed the subcapital fracture line...In contrast to the repair of course cancellous bone, the repair of compact bone of the subchondral plate in highlighted by bone resorption which far outdistances the relatively small amount of new living bone formed to replace the resorbed dead bone. This results in a marked loss of bone substance subchondrally. The repair process...continues unbridled into the calcified and uncalcified regions of the overlying articular cartilage...a repair response [that] contributes to the development of osteoarthritic changes in the articular cartilage...

The key event which initiates the fracture [subchondral] is the local weakness produced by the resorption of the peripheral portion of the lateral aspect of the subchondral plate and the overlying cartilage...In I.O. [idiopathic osteonecrosis] the fracture is propagated subchondrally as a result of shear stresses which are greatest at the junction of the compact subchondral plate and the spongy cancellous bone. In Av.O. [avascular necrosis] the fracture is propagated centrally within the femoral head at the junction between the dead bone and the living, repaired, compacted bone where the stress is concentrated due to differences in the elastic moduli and compliance of the dead coarse cancellous bone and the living, compacted, repaired bone tissue. (Glimcher and Kenzora 1978)

Dr. Kenzora joined the staffs of the PBBH and Boston Children's Hospitals after completing his residency. From 1972 to 1978, he was an instructor in orthopaedic surgery at HMS, assistant in orthopaedic surgery at Boston Children's Hospital, and until 1976 an assistant in orthopaedic surgery at the PBBH. He was promoted to associate in orthopaedic surgery at the PBBH in 1976. During medical school he published two papers; as an orthopaedic resident he published three papers; and while on the staffs of the PBBH and CHMC, he published 14 papers and two chapters. His clinical practice focused on foot and ankle problems, fractures of the hip and femur, and hip arthroplasty. He published more than 40 articles and made numerous scientific presentations.

In 1978, after six years in practice at the PBBH, Dr. John Kenzora moved to Baltimore as associate professor of orthopaedic surgery at the University of Maryland. He was on the staffs of the James Lawrence Kernan Hospital and Saint Joseph Hospital, and he served as orthopaedic surgeon-in-chief at the North Charles General Hospital (1981). From 1982 to 1983, he was acting chief of the division of orthopaedic surgery at the University of Maryland. In 1983, he was named chief of the division of orthopaedic surgery at the University of Maryland and orthopaedic surgeon-in-chief at the University of Maryland Medical Center.

J. DRENNAN LOWELL

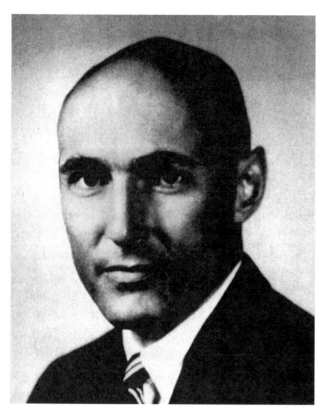

J. Drennan Lowell. C.B.S., "J. Drennan Lowell, M.D. 1922–1987," *Journal of Bone and Joint Surgery* 1987; 69: 1114.

> **Physician Snapshot**
>
> J. Drennan Lowell
> BORN: 1922
> DIED: 1987
> SIGNIFICANT CONTRIBUTIONS: Chief of the clinical services in orthopaedics at the Peter Bent Brigham Hospital (PBBH) (1970–1980); assistant chief of the department of orthopaedic surgery at the BWH (1980–1985); chairman of the orthopaedic section of the Massachusetts Medical Society (1970); president, Massachusetts Medical Society

James Drennan Lowell was born and raised in Worcester, Massachusetts. His spent his undergraduate and graduate years in Boston, graduating from Harvard College in 1944 and from Harvard Medical School (HMS) in 1946. He moved immediately into a year-long internship at Boston City Hospital. Following an internship, he served as a captain in the US Army for two years.

Early Training and Career

After two years as a general surgery resident at Emory University Hospital in Atlanta, Georgia, he applied for the Boston Children's Hospital/Massachusetts's General Hospital Orthopaedic Residency program under Dr. William T. Green. Included among his letters of recommendation from Emory was one from Dr. J. Hiram Kite. Dr. Kite stated:

> Dr. Lowell has had a rotating service at Emory and was on the orthopaedic service for a while. I saw little of his work except as he assisted in operations. He was always most cooperative and anxious to do everything to please that he possibly could and seemed to be very much interested in orthopedic problems. He has a nice personality and I take pleasure in recommending him to the Children's Hospital for training in orthopedics. (Barr 1955)

Dr. Robert P. Kelly (1950), chief of the division of orthopaedic surgery in the Department of Surgery at Emory, also wrote a recommendation. He said: "I am happy to recommend Dr. James Drennan Lowell for appointment as assistant resident in orthopedics at the Children's Hospital and the Massachusetts General Hospital...In making it, I am prompted by his qualities of integrity, industry, presence, and competence in dealing with his colleagues and patients." Lowell was accepted into and completed his orthopaedic residency at Boston Children's Hospital and Massachusetts General Hospital (MGH). As an assistant resident at MGH (beginning October 1, 1952), his salary was $500 per year (valued at $4,867 in 2020).

After completing his residency in 1955, he joined Dr. Otto Aufranc's private practice and through that became affiliated with MGH. In a letter to Dr. Dean A. Clark (the MGH General Director), Dr. Barr (1955) wrote: "Dr. Lowell will assist Dr. Aufranc in the care of private patients and will also care for his own private patients. He will also engage in teaching and in the work of the Orthopedic Clinic [beginning on July 1, 1955]." His appointment was assistant in orthopaedic surgery and his office was located at 266 Beacon Street.

For the next 15 years, Lowell remained on the active staff in the orthopaedic department at MGH primarily doing reconstructive surgery of the hip and trauma. Of his total of 20 publications, he published nine during this period. His first was a brief report of his experiences with the use of resin-impregnated plaster (water resistant) casts in the treatment of club feet, poliomyelitis deformities, scoliosis, and other conditions.

In 1966, Lowell's most significant publication was an extensive review of fractures of the hip, a two-part article in the Medical Progress section of the *New England Journal of Medicine*. He reviewed the history of the treatment of hip fractures, types of fractures, surgical procedures, postoperative management, and complications in detail. **Box 49.1** includes specific comments he made about the MGH's approach to treating hip fractures.

Box 49.1. Dr. J. Drennan Lowell on the MGH's Approach to Treating Hip Fractures

Is Operation an Emergency?

The question of whether or not a fractured hip is a surgical emergency is frequently raised. At the Massachusetts General Hospital, it is. At the moment before injury the patient is usually in his best state of health and the pain and obligatory immobility that are present in the interval between fracture and fixation serve only to increase the severity of associated medical conditions and slide him along a continuing path of deterioration.

Operative Procedure for Intracapsular Fractures

At the Massachusetts General Hospital, the Smith-Petersen triflanged nail continues to be effective and the simplest to use for the majority of patients. In selected cases pins of the Austin-Moore or Knowles type and collapsible nails are also being used…

Impacted Fractures

At the Massachusetts General Hospital, it is the practice of the Fracture Service to treat these patients on bed rest in traction for ten to fourteen days, If, at the end of this period, sensitivity has not left the hip joint, and active motion without pain has not been regained, the fractures are fixed in situ with a 3-flanged nail or pins. If the fracture is doing well, no operation is performed, and a total period of three to six weeks of bed rest is completed. Crutch protection until union is complete, usually four to six months follows…

Prosthetic Arthroplasty as Primary Treatment for Intra-capsular Fractures.

As reported by Barr, Donovan and Florence [MGH] use of the intramedullary prosthesis for fresh fractures or unsatisfactory unions produces a higher incidence of satisfactory results than its use for any other indication. Most authors report satisfactory results in 75 per cent of patients…Sepsis is disastrous, and in none of 26 infected hip prostheses seen at the Massachusetts General Hospital has the infection been cured without removal of the prosthesis…

Types of Trochanteric Fractures

At the Massachusetts General Hospital trochanteric fractures are subdivided into intertrochanteric, pertrochanteric and subtrochanteric, and further subdivided in accordance with presence or absence of comminution. Approximately 70 per cent of the Massachusetts General Hospital series are of the comminuted type. The most troublesome in his group are those with the lesser trochanter as a separate fragment, lying medially or proximately displaced, the 2 major fragments consist of the head and attached portion of the neck as 1 unit, and the upper end of the femoral shaft as the other. Often, there is a fourth, smaller fragment consisting of the greater trochanter. When the 2 major fragments are brought in contact with each other the very large defect remaining in the area from which the lesser trochanter has been displaced will lead to an unstable situation and to bending or breaking of the fixation device before the fracture is healed. In contrast to the intracapsular fractures, nonunion in trochanteric fractures is unusual, and aseptic necrosis does not occur. Nonunion, however, is reported, and malunion in a position of varus is frequent.

Operative Treatment

Although most members of the Fracture Clinic at the Massachusetts General Hospital employ a regular operating table for the treatment of intertrochanteric fractures, some prefer the use of a fracture table, fixing the affected limb in appropriate stirrups. In either approach, provision is made for obtaining radiographs in 2 planes, a tunnel cassette being placed beneath the pelvis for the anteroposterior film. The same protection is afforded the patient while anesthesia is induced as in the treatment of intracapsular fractures. If the fracture is minimally displaced or consists of a single line that can be reduced by traction, abduction and internal rotation, this is accomplished, and the knee is flexed to an angle of 90°, and the foot allowed to rest on a low stool beside the table. The reduction is revised or repeated as indicated by serial radiographs. If the fracture shows extensive comminution, and stable reduction cannot be obtained by manipulation, the leg is draped free so that it can be manipulated by the operator or his assistant during the course of the operation…For the comminuted intertrochanteric and subtrochanteric fractures in which good contact and apposition of the major fragments cannot be obtained with the nail plate combination alone either extra screws are placed at right angles to those holding the side plate or Parham bands are employed to secure larger fragments to the proximal shaft after the method of Boyd and Anderson, or the fracture is managed by the method of "displacement fixation"…

With the latter method the inferior neck spike, almost uniformly present on the proximal fragment, it levered into the open upper end of the shaft fragment after it is secured by a short tri-flanged nail 5.7 to 7.6 cm. in length. Care must be taken, however, as the major fragments are approximated, to avoid rotation deformity. Although 1.2 cm. or more of shortening results from this technic stability and good bone contact are immediately obtained. In three quarters of these cases the Fracture Clinic has employed a Jewett nail that has been specifically shortened for use with the displacement technic, and in the remainder, the McLaughlin nail-plate combination. To date there have been no cases of breaking of fixation devices, and union has generally been rapid.

After operation the patient should be protected in Russell's traction or in balanced suspension.

(Reprinted from Lowell 1966)

Author Recollections

As a resident at the MGH, I also recall being invited with other residents to a party at Dr. Lowell's home. His hobby was trains of all types and sizes. In addition to multiple trains in his basement, he had a larger train on tracks set up in his backyard that was large enough for an adult to sit on each one of the several cars while being pulled by the engine around a circuitous route. Everyone had a terrific time. Dr. Lowell was a real enthusiast for trains.

MEDICAL PROGRESS
ARCHIVE

Fractures of the Hip

J. Drennan Lowell, M.D.*

June 23, 1966

N Engl J Med 1966; 274:1418-1425

Lowell's medical progress report on hip fractures in the *New England Journal of Medicine*. New England Journal of Medicine 1966; 274: 1418.

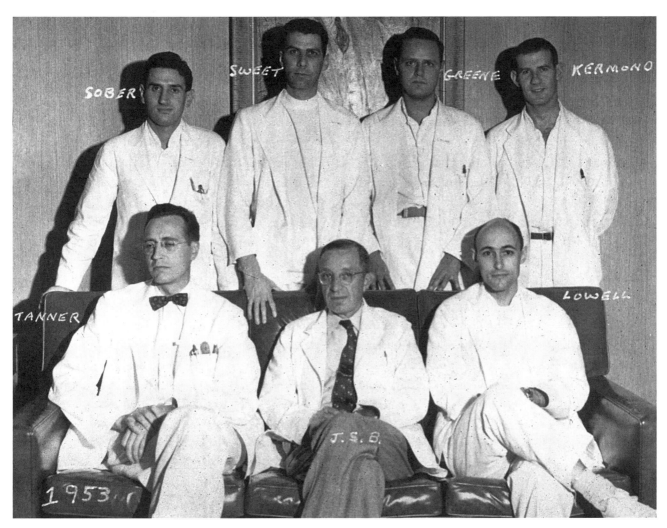

MGH residents with Dr. Barr, 1953. Dr. Lowell is in the front row, far right. MGH HCORP Archives.

Two years later, he coauthored a paper with Aufranc on the anterior approach to the hip joint originally described by Smith-Petersen in 1917. In the article, Lowell and Aufranc (1968) wrote that "Current modifications call for more extensive release of the abductors than he [Smith-Petersen] described, but less dissection of structures medially." When I was a resident on Dr. Lowell's service, I remember the long and extensive exposures to the hip that Dr. Lowell favored.

Chief of the Clinical Services in Orthopaedics at the PBBH

In 1970, Dr. Lowell was recruited by Dr. Clement Sledge to be chief of the clinical services in orthopaedics at the Peter Bent Brigham Hospital (PBBH), a position he held until for the next 10 years. Lowell's initial appointment at the PBBH was senior associate in orthopedic surgery. That year, he was also "appointed Dr. Sledge's principal assistant in conducting orthopedic affairs at the [PBBH]. Coincident with this change, Orthopedic Surgery [was] given department status" and Dr. Clement Sledge appointed orthopaedic surgeon-in-chief ("Annual Report, 1969–1970. Staff Booklet, Report of the Surgeon-in-Chief (Moore)" 1970, 202).

In Sledge's first report as orthopaedic surgeon-in-chief that year, he noted the full-time staff increases at the PBBH: Bill Thomas, Fred Ewald, Ed Nalebuff and Lew Millender (all from the RBBH) joined Dr. Lowell and Dr. William

Head. In addition, the orthopaedic staff included the Boston Children's Hospital orthopaedic surgeons and "a devoted group of part-time visiting surgeons" ("Annual Report, 1970–1971. Staff Booklet" 1971). At this time Dr. Lowell was chairman of the orthopaedic section of the Massachusetts Medical Society, secretary of the Boston Orthopaedic Club, and a representative for Programs in Orthopaedics of the American Medical Association.

Initially, an instructor in orthopaedic surgery at HMS at the MGH, Dr. Lowell was later promoted to assistant professor at the PBBH; and associate professor in 1975. He continued to research and publish, and **Case 49.3** includes an example of one of his case reports from this period. In 1977, he demonstrated his early interest in the use of ultraviolet light. He reviewed 1,200 total hip replacement cases at the RBBH in his support of the use of ultraviolet light in the operating room. In only three of those 1200 cases (0.25%) did the wound become infected.

The department of orthopaedic surgery at the PBBH continued to grow steadily over the next

Case 49.3. Bladder Fistula After a Total Hip Replacement That Used Self-Curing Acrylic

Two years prior to her first admission to Peter Bent Brigham Hospital, a 78-year old widow with diabetes and peripheral arteriosclerosis sustained a trochanteric fracture of the right hip. The fracture had failed to unite after nail and plate fixation and total hip replacement was selected as the most appropriate method of salvage. There had been no clinical evidence of wound infection during this period and preoperative cultures of the hip were negative.

As part of the reconstruction of the of the acetabular side of the joint, two holes were made in the dome and one each into the pubis and ischium to obtain secure fixation of the high density polyethylene component. No obvious problems were encountered during the procedure. Cultures obtained at operation showed no growth.

Over the next 5 weeks, several episodes of severe bleeding into the wound area occurred, ultimately requiring re-exploration and internal iliac ligation to control the source which appeared to be in the region of the greater sciatic notch. Repeated wound cultures prior to re-exploration were negative.

Four days later, however, *Escherichia coli* and *Serratia* were present and the wound became grossly infected. Proteus mirabilis was cultured at 14 days. Two extensive debridements without removal of the replacement components but accompanied by prolonged antibiotic therapy failed to resolve the problem. *Escherichia coli* which had been cultured from the urine at the time of hospitalization disappeared promptly with antibiotic therapy but had returned two months after iliac ligation. *Proteus mirabilis* was cultured from the wound 8 months later.

Following discharge from the hospital 4 months after the replacement procedure, the patient was able to get along at home with the use of a pick-up walker and with minimal drainage from one and occasionally two sinus tracts. A year later, increasing pain in the hip and frequency and dysuria required re-hospitalization.

At this time cultures of the sinus tract and of the urine showed *Proteus mirabilis* only.

A sinogram showed the dye reaching the hip joint, dissecting along the medial side of the iliac wing, into the retropubic space and possibly into the bladder. This prompted cystoscopy and a cystogram, delineating a definite fistula communicating with the same cavity previously outlined on the medial side of the ilium. There was a purulent cystitis and deformity of the lateral bladder wall.

At subsequent cystotomy, the fistula was found to be firmly adherent to a projecting mass of methylmethacrylate which had extruded through a small hole in the superior pubic ramus. This mass, visible on earlier films, had appeared to be innocuous.

With removal of the mass and closure of the fistula, the bladder problem ultimately resolved. Removal of the entire prosthetic replacement and conversion of the hip joint to a Girdlestone resection was necessary to control the joint infection.

(Reprinted from Lowell et al. 1975)

decade with clinical part-time staff. For example, in 1977, Dr. Lowell was listed as chief of the orthopaedic clinical services, reporting to Dr. Sledge, the Orthopaedic Surgeon-in-Chief. Associates in orthopaedic surgery included: Drs. Ben Bierbaum, Art Boland, Mike Drew, Hamish G. Gilles, Mel Glimcher, John Hall, Robert Hussey, John Kenzora, Jack McGinty, Lew Millender, Ed Nalebuff, Ted Riseborough, Bill Thomas, Art Trott, Hugh Watts, and Marvin Weinfeld. Junior associates in orthopaedic surgery included: Drs. Robert H. Arbuckle, St. George Tucker Aufranc, Stuart Cope, David W. Cloos, Lyle J. Micheli, Robert Poss, Robert K. Rosenthal, Richard Scott, William D. Shea, Lawrence R. Shields, Barry Simmons, Sheldon Simon, and William W. Southmayd. That year (1977–1978), Lowell was president of the PBBH staff, and he also became president of the medical staff at Brigham and Women's Hospital (BWH), a position he held for one year. Lowell was active in AAOS committees, including the OR Environment and Surgery Asepsis committee, and in various professional organizations (**Box 49.2**).

Box 49.2. J. Drennan Lowell's Professional Activities

Memberships

- American Academy of Orthopaedic Surgeons
- American Board of Orthopaedic Surgery
- American Orthopaedic Association
- American College of Surgeons
- Association of Bone and Joint Surgeons

Positions held

- President, Boston Orthopaedic Club
- President, Massachusetts Medical Society
- Chairman of the orthopaedic section of the Massachusetts Medical Society (1970)
- Secretary-treasurer and honorary president of the Hip Society (1981)

Assistant Chief of Orthopaedic Surgery at the BWH

After the merger of the three hospitals officially completed to form the BWH in 1980 (see chapter 47), Lowell transitioned from his role as former chief of the orthopaedic clinical services at the PBBH and was named assistant chief of the department of orthopaedic surgery at the BWH. Staff changes continued and orthopaedic surgeons included Drs. Boland, Drew, Ewald, Gilles, Hussey, Lipson, Millender, Nalebuff, Poss, Scott, Simmons, Simon, Thomas, Thornhill, and Weinfeld. Associates in orthopaedic surgery included Drs. Glimcher, Hall, McGinty, Riseborough, Trott, White, Cope, Emans, Micheli, Millis, Rosenthal, William Shea, and Ronald N. Chaplan. The junior associates in orthopaedic surgery included Dr. Shields, and the podiatrists included Dr. Bruce T. Wood.

In 1984, seven years after his earlier review of the use of ultraviolent light in the operating room, Lowell wrote about the then 14-year history of the orthopaedic service at BWH, which he began with Dr. Clement Sledge in the mid-1970s by incorporating the surgeons at PBBH and Robert Breck Brigham Hospital (RBBH). He noted that at the time of writing, total joint replacement was one of the main procedures the orthopaedic surgeons perform at BWH—probably outdone only by the Mayo Clinic, and Lowell referred to wound infection during recovery from that procedure

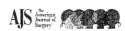

VOLUME 148, ISSUE 5, P575-577, NOVEMBER 01, 1984

The ultraviolet environment in a nutshell

J.Drennan Lowell, MD

Lowell's article reviewing use of ultraviolet light in the operating room. *American Journal of Surgery* 1984; 148: 575.

as a "disaster" (Lowell 1984). When the team at PBBH/RBBH began doing joint replacements, they experienced a 3% rate of deep infection despite taking all precautions to avoid it. Because laminar airflow technology was expensive—MGH installed such a system for $60,000 in 1970—and might soon be outdated, they began looking for alternatives. They learned about ultraviolet light used in operating rooms at Duke University's hospital from Carl Walter, and after a visit there and appropriate testing in orthopaedic operating rooms (ORs) at PBBH/RBBH, they found that ultraviolet light did indeed sterilize the ambient air in the rooms, reducing the amount of microbial particles in the air to almost zero while the UV lamps were turned on.

Lowell went on to describe the financial and surgical implications of the use of UV lamps in ORs for the hospital. Financially, with a cost of $1,500 for each UV setup (eight lamps in a single OR), the monetary outlay was substantially lower than that for a laminar flow system in just one OR. This reduced cost also applies to operations costs: each lamp uses just 40 watts of power and they do not heat up the room itself, and the UV light continually sterilizes the surgical instruments. Finally, these costs also equate to savings accrued by avoiding the costs of treating wound infections that occur postoperatively, which could be as high as $100,000. Surgically, the number of postoperative infections had declined significantly (**Table 49.1**). Lowell noted that the low overall infection rate achieved with UV light was similar to rates where other systems like body exhaust and laminar flow are used.

Dr. Lowell published three other papers and one letter to the editor about infection after joint arthroplasty and the benefits of ultraviolet lights in the operating room. During his 17 years combined at the PBBH and later the BWH, he published a total of nine articles; three were on ultraviolet radiation, four on total hip arthroplasty and its complications, and two on hip fractures.

Dr. J. Drennan Lowell was an associate professor of orthopaedic surgery at HMS from 1975 to 1987. After a long illness, Lowell died at his home in Winchester on January 13, 1987. He was 64 years old. He was survived by his wife (Ruth) and their four children.

Table 49.1. Infection Rates Before and After the Use of UV Light in ORs at BWH

	Before UV	After UV (beginning 1973)
Rate of deep wound infection		
Primary hip surgery	2.4%	<0.5%
Revision or repeat hip surgery	8%	<4%
Overall infection rate	ca. 3%	0.74%

Data from Lowell 1984.

LEWIS H. MILLENDER

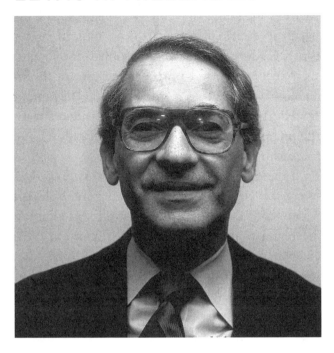

Lewis H. Millender. Digital Collections and Archives, Tufts University.

Physician Snapshot

Lewis H. Millender
BORN: 1937
DIED: 1996
SIGNIFICANT CONTRIBUTIONS: Assistant chief of the hand service at the Robert Breck Brigham Hospital; chief of occupational medicine at New England Baptist Hospital (NEBH) (1993–); coedited *Entrapment Neuropathies* (1990) with Drs. David M. Dawson and Mark Hallett; coauthored *Occupational Disorders of the Upper Extremity* (1992) with Dean Louis and Barry Simmons; the NEBH Occupational Medicine Center established the Lewis H. Millender Occupational Medicine Conference in his honor; the Combined Jewish Philanthropies (CJP) of Greater Boston established the Lewis H. Millender Community of Excellence Award in his memory; recognized in 1996 as an honorary member of the American Society of Hand Therapists for his role in elevating the status of hand therapy

Lewis H. Millender was born in Monroe, Georgia, in 1937. He attended Emory College and stayed on there to attend Emory Medical School. After preliminary surgical training at the Mt. Sinai

> J Bone Joint Surg Am. 1973 Jun;55(4):753-7.
>
> **Posterior interosseous-nerve syndrome secondary to rheumatoid synovitis**
>
> L H Millender, E A Nalebuff, D E Holdsworth

Article identifying rheumatoid synovitis of the elbow as a cause of the posterior interosseous nerve syndrome.
Journal of Bone and Joint Surgery 1973; 55: 753.

Hospital in Cleveland, Ohio, he served in the US Public Health Service. In 1966, he returned to Emory University for a three-year residency. He then went "to Boston to do a hip fellowship with Otto Aufranc at the New England Baptist. But in 1970, when Millender's fellowship was to start, Aufranc developed myasthenia gravis and could not take on the trainee. Nalebuff offered Millender a hand fellowship, launching what for Millender was to be a distinguished, though abbreviated, career as a hand surgeon" (Liang 2013). After completing his fellowship, he joined Nalebuff in practice at the Robert Breck Brigham Hospital (RBBH) and the New England Baptist Hospital (NEBH).

Early Career at HMS and the RBBH/BWH

In 1971, Millender was appointed clinical instructor in orthopaedic surgery at Harvard Medical School (HMS) and surgeon at the RBBH and the New England Baptist Hospital (NEBH). Dr. Millender published over 50 papers. About half addressed upper extremity problems in rheumatoid arthritis (17 coauthored with Dr. Nalebuff), five covered occupational related disorders, and the remainder were dedicated to other problems in the upper extremity. One of his first papers identified rheumatoid synovitis at the elbow as a cause of the posterior interosseous syndrome (see **Case 49.4**).

Case 49.4. Posterior Interosseous Nerve Syndrome in Rheumatoid Synovitis

> "[The patient], a sixty-five-year old woman, had a long history of moderately severe rheumatoid arthritis controlled with salicylates and prednisone. Three weeks prior to admission she noted increased weakness of the finger extensors and then inability to extend any of the fingers or thumb. An initial diagnosis of ruptured extensor tendons was made. However, on further evaluation, a history of pain in the elbow and radial-nerve neuritis was obtained. Examination showed antecubital fullness and tenderness, as well as inability to extend the fingers or the thumb. Dorsiflexion of the wrist was weak and was associated with radial deviation of the hand. The diagnosis of posterior interosseous-nerve syndrome was confirmed by electromyogram and direct muscle stimulation. Although she showed minimum recovery of thumb and index-finger extension over a six-week period, because of continued severe pain in the elbow and radial nerve neuritis, decompression of the posterior interosseous nerve and synovectomy of the elbow were carried out through an anterior approach. Twenty-four hours postoperatively she showed partial return of posterior interosseous-nerve function. Four days later she had recovery of all finger extension. Subsequently she underwent metacarpophalangeal arthroplasty for dislocated metacarpophalangeal joints."
>
> (Millender, Nalebuff, and Holdsworth 1973)

In 1973, he and Nalebuff participated in a Symposium on Interposition and Implant Arthroplasty published in *Orthopedic Clinics of North America*. They made a significant observation about the importance of release of contractures with arthroplasty—in addition to fixing any deformities and reorienting the affected finger/thumb—in treating patients with rheumatoid arthritis. The lack of full release of soft-tissue contractures and appropriate realignment can cause the deformity to recur, dislocation, or fracturing of the implant. Acknowledging that the silicone flexible implant had been in use since 1967, they discussed arthroplasty as performed at the RBBH—including its role in treating patients which severe rheumatoid arthritis, indications for the procedure in the metacarpophalangeal joint, their technique, and postoperative protocols for patient recovery and rehabilitation. They mentioned their scheme for assessing patients with rheumatoid arthritis before the procedure and forecasting its outcomes.

In another publication in the *Journal of Bone and Joint Surgery* in 1973, Millender and Nalebuff wrote that "Damage to the wrist joint is common in rheumatoid arthritis…2.7%. In addition, 95% [of patients] had bilateral wrist involvement. No standard of treatment…has been established[, but Millender and Nalebuff described] a modification of the surgical procedure for wrist fusion" using Clayton's method of a large intermedullary Steinmann pin to stabilize the wrist (Millender and Nalebuff 1973). They reported 70 arthrodeses in 60 patients at the RBBH.

They reported only two nonunions. Pleased with their results, they began to expand their indications to include patients with persistent, early loss of joint cartilage and those who failed conservative treatment. They stated: "The benefits of our modification of the methods of Clayton and Mannerfelt and Malmsten, with stable intermedullary rod fixation, have overcome many technical problems…Our method relies on a large Steinmann pin and staple…the internal fixation is sufficiently firm so that only a removable splint is needed" (Millender and Nalebuff 1973).

Six years later, in 1980, Millender, Nalebuff, and colleagues continued to report on their early experience with the flexible silicone rubber interposition implant for painful and deformed wrists in patients with rheumatoid arthritis. They reported results with 37 arthroplasties. Three prostheses fractured. For most patients with rheumatoid arthritis, they promoted wrist arthroplasty using a silicone prosthesis over wrist fusion. They did note particular signs indicating the appropriateness of wrist arthroplasty, and they cautioned that

> Orthop Clin North Am. 1973 Apr;4(2):349-71.
>
> **Metacarpophalangeal joint arthroplasty utilizing the silicone rubber prosthesis**
>
> L H Millender, E A Nalebuff

Title of Nalebuff and Millender's article describing their experience with use of the silicone implant MCP arthroplasty.
Orthopedic Clinics of North America 1973; 4: 349.

> J Bone Joint Surg Am. 1974 Apr;56(3):601-10.
>
> **Dorsal tenosynovectomy and tendon transfer in the rheumatoid hand**
>
> L H Millender, E A Nalebuff, R Albin, J R Ream, M Gordon

Article describing Millender and Nalebuff's experience in the surgical management of rheumatoid arthritis of the wrist.
Journal of Bone and Joint Surgery 1974; 56: 601.

the procedure is more painstaking for the surgeon than wrist fusion and that outcomes cannot be as easily forecasted.

During this period, he was also appointed surgeon at the Brigham and Women's Hospital (BWH) and lecturer at HMS. Dr. Nalebuff (2013) described him as having "contributed enormously to the understanding and treatment of patients with rheumatoid arthritis of the hand and wrist. Not only was he a meticulous surgeon, but he was a gifted teacher and helped train scores of hand surgeons now practicing throughout the U.S."

Later Career at Tufts and Assistant Chief of the Hand Service at the RBBH

In 1982, Millender was appointed clinical professor of orthopaedic surgery at Tufts University School of Medicine. Over the course of his career, he was also assistant chief of the hand service at the RBBH, on the staff of the Beth Israel Hospital and Children's Hospital Medical Center, and consultant in orthopaedic surgery at the West Roxbury Veteran's Administration Hospital.

In 1986, Millender and Brase reported findings from another series of patients using Swanson's silicone wrist implant while treated at the NEBH from 1976 until 1983. In their article, they noted that 20% of the silicone rubber wrist implants had fractured; 5% required revision for pain and deformity. On the basis of their findings, for joints with extensive deformity or instability they recommended wrist fusion, as wrist arthroplasty could result in a recurrent deformity with or without a fractured implant. They believed that wrist fusion obviates pain and fixes wrist alignment.

In 1991, Millender, T. O'Donovan, and A. Terrono made additional recommendations regarding wrist arthrodesis, which they referred to as the gold standard. Patients with rheumatoid arthritis achieved positive functional outcomes after the procedure, and the authors preferred it in patients requiring treatment in either one or both wrists. They noted that wrist arthroplasty was "helpful" in some cases, though they noted that wrist fusion and an opposite wrist arthroplasty would be most appropriate for patients with finger deformities and stiff PIP joints.

Chief of Occupational Medicine at NEBH and Later Legacy

Millender became ill and had to stop operating on patients in 1993. He instead moved into the position of chief of occupational medicine at the NEBH. He continued to actively contribute to the literature in his newly chosen field. Beginning with an editorial in 1992, Millender published five papers on work related disorders and injuries in three years in addition to a book. In the 1992 editorial, he predicted that occupational injuries,

> J Hand Surg Am. 1986 Mar;11(2):175-83
>
> **Failure of silicone rubber wrist arthroplasty in rheumatoid arthritis**
>
> D W Brase, L H Millender

Title of Brase and Millender's article reporting their nine-year experience of failed silicone wrist implants. *Journal of Hand Surgery* 1986; 11: 175.

most of which occur gradually, would dominate those treated during the rest of the 1990s. He noted the exponential increase in costs of such injuries for employers in only a relatively few years. Millender named three elements of occupational injuries that should receive attention: the legal component, psychological issues, and musculoskeletal issues. For Millender, orthopaedic (hand) surgeons should recognize the extensive effect of the psychological element when the physical (musculoskeletal) element does not resolve satisfactorily, i.e., they cannot identify a particular diagnosis or treatment does not work.

He coauthored the book *Occupational Disorders of the Upper Extremity* with Drs. Dean Louis and Barry Simmons, which published in 1992. In a 1993 review, Dr. Andrew H. Crenshaw Jr., of the Campbell Clinic, wrote: "This is not a surgical textbook, and it does not need to be. It outlines good, rational, conservative treatment, something that is lacking in many subspecialty textbooks...This book discusses all sides of this issue and approaches it from the standpoints of the employer, worker-patient, and physician or health care provider." Dr. Millender also coedited a second earlier book—entitled *Entrapment Neuropathies*—in 1990 with Drs. David M. Dawson and Mark Hallett, both of whom were neurologists.

Dr. Lewis H. Millender died in the Dana Farber Cancer Institute on November 21, 1996, at age 59. He was survived by his wife Bonnie (Cobert), two daughters, and a son. Evelyn J. Mackin, PT, wrote of the sadness felt among his colleagues, friends, and acquaintances, and reiterated Millender's place as a leader in the field of hand therapy. The Combined Jewish Philanthropies (CJP) of Greater Boston established the Lewis H. Millender Community of Excellence Award given annually in his memory. The NEBH Occupational Medicine Center honored him with a two-day Lewis H. Millender Occupational Medicine Conference.

Millender was heavily involved in elevating the status of hand therapy before the American Society of Hand Therapists was established in 1977, pushing hard for members of the existing American Society for Surgery of the Hand to support the organization. In 1996, the American Society of Hand Therapists named him as an honorary member, recognizing his dedication to the field of hand therapy and his "holistic" approach to patient care.

ROBERT POSS

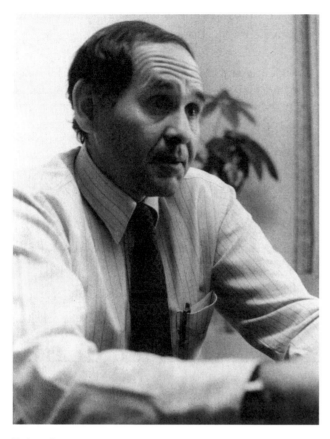

Robert Poss. Harvard Medical Library in the Countway Library of Medicine.

Physician Snapshot

Robert Poss
BORN: 1936
DIED: —

SIGNIFICANT CONTRIBUTIONS: Vice-chairman of the department orthopaedic surgery at the BWH (1985–1999); interim chief of orthopaedics at the BWH (1996); member of the Board of Directors of the American Board of Orthopaedic Surgery (ABOS) from 1992 to 2002; instrumental in the formation of the Total Joint Replacement Registry at the BWH; deputy editor for Electronic Media at the *Journal of Bone and Joint Surgery*

Robert Poss was born in New York City on October 26, 1936. At age 14, his family moved to New Jersey where he went to high school and graduated from Rutgers University with an AB degree in 1958. He received his MD degree from Upstate Medical Center in Syracuse, New York in 1962 and was elected into Alpha Omega Alpha (1961). Following a flexible internship and one year as an assistant resident in general surgery at Case Western University Hospitals, he served as a lieutenant in the medical corps of the US Navy for two years, from 1964 until 1966. After his discharge, Poss entered the Boston Children's Hospital/Massachusetts's General Hospital orthopaedic residency program from 1967 until 1970. Before beginning the clinical program, he had spent part of 1966 as an orthopaedic research fellow at Boston Children's Hospital.

Dr. Poss had a strong interest in research early in his career. Immediately after completing his residency and with the support of federal funding, he accepted a postdoctoral fellowship in biology in the Department of Biology at the Massachusetts Institute of Technology (MIT) from 1970 until 1973. His goal was to identify a possible virus as the cause of rheumatoid arthritis; a goal he did not achieve. He and his co-investigator Dr. Olaniyi Kehinde published their preliminary findings in the Proceedings of the Northeastern Regional Meeting of the American Rheumatism Association held in Newton, Massachusetts, in December 1974. They described their study of the role of genetics in rheumatoid arthritis, which they had investigated through the use of somatic cell hybridization in an amalgam of human tissue and murine cells with inactivated mouse parainfluenza virus type 1. They found no virus in the human tissue, which contradicted their hypothesis for a viral cause for rheumatoid arthritis. I was unable to find any further publications by the authors regarding a possible viral etiology for rheumatoid arthritis.

During the three-year period at MIT, Poss supported himself and his family by moonlighting in the practice of Dr. William Kermond at Winchester Hospital. He was able to maintain his orthopaedic surgical skills while working in the laboratory, and, in 1974, Dr. Clement Sledge hired him to work at the Robert Breck Brigham Hospital (RBBH). When I interviewed Dr. Poss in 2018, he described his experience at MIT as "wonderful." After discontinuing his research on a possible viral etiology of rheumatoid arthritis, he continued to collaborate with scientists at MIT over the next decade while practicing at the RBBH.

Poss's main clinical interest was arthritis of the hip and its treatment by total hip replacement or osteotomy. A year later he published his first paper as a new staff member; it was titled "Total Hip Replacement," and in it he reviewed 730 total hip replacements (314 in patients with rheumatoid arthritis) performed at the RBBH from 1969 to 1974. He also described the procedure surgeons at the RBBH were using at the time—the Gibson posterior approach with the patient in a lateral position. Poss listed seven aspects of the procedure that RBBH surgeons all apply, as well as the procedural steps; these are described in **Box 49.3**. He also outlined the methods used to avoid infection, including antibiotics (oxacillin and streptomycin) during and after the procedure, irrigation of the wound (Ringer solution with polymyxin and bacitracin), aspirin (not warfarin) before and after the procedure, salicylates preoperatively (only for patients with rheumatoid arthritis), and UV light in the operating room during the procedure. Overall, their main goal was to reestablish normal femoral anatomy so that the hip joint will achieve excellent function postoperatively. In this way, their patients had less pain postoperatively and recovered function, and the surgeons were able to correct deformities and achieve a low rate of postoperative complications.

Box 49.3. General Preferences of Surgeons Performing Total Hip Replacement at the RBBH in the Early 1970s

- Aufranc-Turner femoral head (32 mm)
- No trochanteric osteotomy
- Posteriorinferior approach with excision of external rotators and capsulectomy of the hip joint
- Do not apply forceful retraction on hip abductors
- Have one assistant and one nurse assist during the procedure
- Use a Mayo stand to position and stabilize the leg
- Restore normal proximal femur anatomy with optimal lengths of femur and muscles

Poss published more than 80 articles, of which 28 dealt with total hip replacement, including topics such as the use of trochanteric advancement for recurrent dislocation, revision total hip replacement, modern cementing techniques, impact of modularity, failure of the acetabular polyethylene liner components, and others. He also wrote many papers on complications and outcomes after total hip replacement, including topics such as the validity and reliability of a total hip outcome questionnaire, factors influencing infections, association

---

Orthopedic Clinics of North America
Volume 6, Issue 3, July 1975, Pages 801-810

Total Hip Replacement

Robert Poss M.D. (Clinical Instructor, Research Associate in Biology, Assistant Surgeon)

Title of article by Poss in which he reviewed five years of experience with total hip replacement at RBBH. *Orthopedic Clinics of North America* 1975; 6: 801.

J Bone Joint Surg Am. 1984 Jan;66(1):144-51.

The role of osteotomy in the treatment of osteoarthritis of the hip

R Poss

Title of article by Poss describing the role of osteotomy in the treatment of osteoarthritis of the hip. *Journal of Bone and Joint Surgery* 1984; 66: 144.

of hospital and surgeon volume with outcomes, incidence of dislocation and other complications, optimizing patient expectations, and others.

Poss continued to publish an occasional basic research paper while working at the RBBH (later the BWH) and publishing clinical results about adult hip and knee reconstructive surgery. In our interview, he referred me to one paper that he published in 1979 and described as "seminal": "Methylmethacrylate Is a Mutagen for Salmonella Typhimurium," which he cowrote with Professor William G. Thilly and D. A. Kaden. They used an assay called the Ames Test which determines if a chemical has the capacity to cause mutations in bacterial DNA, "as an index of its [i.e., methylmethacrylate] possible deleterious interaction with human DNA" (Poss, Thilly, and Kaden 1979). Concerned about the long-term effects of exposure to the monomer of methylmethacrylate they used the Ames assay to determine its toxicity and immunogenicity. In their conclusions they stated:

> 1. Methylmethacrylate monomer is mutagenic to Salmonella typhimurium. It is approximately 28 per cent as mutagenic as dimethylnitrosamine, a known mutagen and carcinogen of similar chemical structure. 2. Methylmethacrylate may have mutagenic and toxic effects on humans who are subjected to chronic exposure. 3. Persons at highest potential risk are those who are subjected to frequent exposure to methylmethacrylate: operating-room personnel and certain industrial workers. 4. Until the safety of this compound can be ascertained by new animal testing or continued uncomplicated use, it would seem prudent that human exposure be minimized through the use of proper ventilating and filtering techniques in operating rooms. (Poss, Thilly, and Kaden 1979)

Poss was promoted to assistant clinical professor of orthopaedic surgery at HMS from clinical instructor in 1981, and he was promoted to associate clinical professor of orthopaedic surgery in 1982. Two years later, he published a Current Concepts Review Article, "The Role of Osteotomy in the Treatment of Osteoarthritis of the Hip" in the *Journal of Bone and Joint Surgery*. He had a strong interest in the role of osteotomy of the hip in patients with osteoarthritis. After reviewing the literature on the evolution of osteotomy he concluded:

> The results of total hip arthroplasty are the benchmark with which osteotomy must be compared...The short-term results of this procedure [total hip] make it clearly the procedure of choice for...advanced arthritis of the hip. Its limitations...include uncertainty of the duration of results, particularly in younger active patients, and the difficulty of successfully revising failed implants with contemporary techniques. In contrast, osteotomy in properly selected patients offers a biologic alternative that can arrest if not reverse the disease process...Mueller estimated that two-thirds of patients with early arthritis and one-third to one-half of those with advanced osteoarthritis are suitable for some type of intertrochanteric osteotomy...that one can expect 80 per cent...a good long term result. Total hip arthroplasty and osteotomy are properly viewed as complementary rather than competitive procedures. The patient younger than 50...should be considered a candidate for osteotomy. The patient in the seventh decade of life is probably

---

J Bone Joint Surg Am. 1997 Oct;79(10):1529-38

Complications of total hip arthroplasty associated with the use of an acetabular component with a Hylamer liner

B J Livingston [1], M J Chmell, M Spector, R Poss

Article reporting the BWH's experience with the Hylamer acetabular liner. *Journal of Bone and Joint Surgery* 1997; 79: 1529.

better served by total hip arthroplasty...Careful observation of the results of...osteotomy will better define those patients for whom it is the procedure of choice. (Poss 1984)

From 1985 until 1999, he was vice-chairman of the department orthopaedic surgery at the BWH. During that time, he was also promoted to clinical professor of orthopaedic surgery at HMS in 1991; and, in 1993, after the merger of the for-profit Brigham Orthopedic Associates into the nonprofit Brigham Orthopaedic Foundation, he was appointed professor of orthopaedic surgery at HMS. In 1996, he also served as acting chief of the department at the BWH for three months between the retirement of Dr. Sledge and the appointment of Dr. Thornhill as chief of orthopaedics. While managing the responsibilities of these positions, Poss continued to publish about intertrochanteric osteotomy for osteoarthritis in two instructional courses and chapters on the same subject in three different major textbooks. He also published on the hip and in the Academy's Orthopaedic Knowledge Update on Hip and Knee Reconstruction.

With Ruben and others, he published two papers on the use of ultrasound to evaluate changes in the mechanical properties of bone after intensive physical activity and to measure osteopenia following immobilization. Some of his additional basic research papers included topics such as the mechanics of normal and arthritic hips, adaptation of bone to various loading conditions (Wolff's Law), and femoral stem designs to improve the fit of the stem in the femur.

In January 1991, surgeons at the BWH began using Hylamer metal-backed polyethylene acetabular components. Bradley et al. (1999) wrote:

> In an effort to improve the surface and wear characteristics of ultra-high molecular weight polyethylene, an enhanced... polyethylene (Hylamer) was introduced in 1991. It was anticipated that the wear characteristics of a Hylamer acetabular surface in combination with a ceramic modular femoral head would improve the long-term performance of prostheses in young, active patients.
>
> During our [BWH surgeons] routine clinical and radiographic follow-up at yearly intervals, we found radiographic signs of accelerated wear as early as one to three years postoperatively in some patients. [In 1996 Chmell and Poss] and colleagues found that six of the 143 hips...followed for at least two years had been revised because of accelerated wear. The mean rate of wear of the revised Hylamer liners was 0.48 millimeter per year...
>
> [A] review of a larger cohort of patients... evaluated at a minimum of two years, had a mean rate of wear of 0.27 millimeter per year compared with a 0.12 millimeter per year for a contemporaneous group of fifty acetabular cups with a conventional ultra-high molecular weight polyethylene liner...At a mean of 3.2 years, we found a significant difference... between the main rate of wear...when the Hylamer liner articulated with a...cobalt chrome femoral head...We concluded that the wear characteristics of the Hylamer liner in vivo are inferior to those of a conventional ultra-high molecular weight polyethylene liner. Also, the rate of wear of the liner is greater when the femoral head is from a [different] manufacturer...

J Bone Joint Surg Am. 2000 Oct;82(10):1506-9.

The value and promise of patient databases in orthopaedic surgery

J J Harrast [1], R Poss

Title of article about the BWH's experience with the hospital's Total Joint Replacement Registry. *Journal of Bone and Joint Surgery* 2000; 82: 1506.

Poss was a member of the Board of Directors of the American Board of Orthopaedic Surgery (ABOS) from 1992 to 2002. It was during this time that he developed an increased interest in applications of information technology, simulation in medical education, and computerized documentation, i.e., total joint registry. Regarding simulation, he was chairman of the ABOS research committee at the time board partnered with Boston Dynamics to develop a prototype arthroscopic knee simulator. The AAOS agreed to form a task force on virtual reality, composed of members of the ABOS, Boston Dynamics and members of the AAOS Council on Education. The task force collaborated with the Center for Human Simulation at the University of Colorado. Their goal was to create a graphic simulation that accurately portrayed the actual anatomy of the knee in order to eventually develop a simulator used in education (resident training) and as an evaluation tool for the arthroscopic skills of applicants for Part II of the ABOS examination.

Dr. Poss's personal interest in computerized documentation and the leadership of Dr. Sledge in the development of registries at academic medical centers led to the formation of the Total Joint Replacement Registry at the BWH. In 2000, Harrast and Poss wrote that, beginning in 1990, the registry:

> amassed a data-base with information on more than 15,000 patients and more than 20,000 joint replacement procedures...This database comprises patient demographics, histories, findings on physical examination, intraoperative findings, information on complications, patient outcomes, and patient-satisfaction data that were collected prospectively with informed patient consent. The annual operating budget of the registry...currently $350,000, with external grants accounting for $150,000 of the total... [generating] 110 publications as well as 140 presentations at the annual meeting of the American Academy of Orthopaedic Surgeons...In 1999, we decided to transfer the management of the Brigham Total Joint Replacement Registry to an offsite data management company... We realized immediate cost savings by relinquishing expensive rental space and reducing the number of full-time employees from 7.5 to three. We budgeted the total cost for the year 2000 to be in the same as that for 1998, but we anticipate...the cost...will be less because of outsourcing.

However, the leadership of the department at the time did not support the registry with royalty income, donations and grants, as the previous leadership had done; and it closed.

In 2000, Dr. Poss was also hired by Dr. James Heckman (editor of the *Journal of Bone and Joint Surgery* [*JBJS*]) as Deputy Editor for Electronic Media. In October 2000, he wrote his first editorial with Heckman about their plans for the *Journal* in the advancing electronic age:

> The Journal's website was introduced in November 1996. Current search capabilities include search by free text query, by subject, or by author as well as the capability to search a specific volume...Full text articles from 1996 to the present may be downloaded for free by subscribers...The next step in the development of our Web site is to use the audio, video, and text capabilities on the Internet to enhance the

> **The Journal of Bone and Joint Surgery**
> *American Volume*
> VOLUME 82-A, NO. 10   OCTOBER 2000
> Editorial
> The *eJBJS* (www.jbjs.org)
> *Robert Poss, M.D.*
> *Deputy Editor for Electronic Media*
> *James D. Heckman, M.D.*
> *Editor-in-Chief*

Editorial announcing the initiation of the *JBJS* website, *eJBJS*. *Journal of Bone and Joint Surgery* 2000; 82-A: 1371.

value of our printed articles...We view...time on the Web site as an opportunity to use [present] electronic supplements of related educational materials and resources. We seek...to attract new readers to a journal that is both print and Web based...eJBJS@www.jbjs.org.

We...will partner with HighWire Press of Stanford University...The new website will offer the following features: 1. Customization of the home page by orthopedic specialty interest...2. Capability to build unique subject files by collating searches from multiple sources...3. Article enhancements...4. Search capabilities...5. Interactivity...6. Online reviews...In *The Journal* we introduce a new feature of the Web site: The video Segment... Furthermore, we are proud to announce an alliance between *The Journal* and the *Video Journal of Orthopaedics* to produce monthly video segments and full-length videotapes to supplement articles... It is *The Journal's* function to provide the best and fullest presentation of new knowledge in the clearest and most educational formats to its readers. (Poss and Heckman 2001)

In his capacity as Deputy Editor for Electronic Media, Dr. Poss authored or coauthored another five editorials within four years updating the readers on new electronic developments at the *JBJS*. Regarding one of his favorite topics—outcomes data—he, along with Dr. Heckman and Dr. Charles Clark (Deputy Editor for Adult Reconstruction) developed "A Concise Format for Reporting the Longer-Term Follow-up Status of Patients Managed with Total Hip Arthroplasty." With the input of experts in the field and the deputy editors of the *Journal* this concise format eventually consisted of the "inclusion of certain outcomes data... specifically...the WOMAC (Western Ontario and McMaster University Osteoarthritis Index), a validated, patient-administered instrument that assesses the effect of arthroplasty on pain, stiffness, and function...Soon we will develop similar formats for reporting longer-term follow-up results of other reconstructive procedures" (Poss, Clark, and Heckman 2001).

Drs. Poss and Heckman supported dialogue between the authors and readers and encouraged letters to the editor, which in 2004 were made electronic, to shorten the prolonged interval between the publication of the article, the letters, and responses to the letters. His last *JBJS* editorial (2004) was coauthored with Drs. Thomas Bauer, deputy editor for research, and Dr. Heckman. They announced a policy change to the readers and authors regarding copyright. Because of "the potential of instant worldwide dissemination of new, possibly unvetted data [with] the electronic age [and] to protect its intellectual property and as an aid to authors...*The Journal* will require a copyright assignment at the time of submission of the manuscript [not after acceptance for publication] but will reconvey the copyright to the authors if that article is ultimately not accepted for publication" (Poss, Bauer, and Heckman 2004).

In addition to committee and administrative duties at the BWH and HMS, Dr. Robert Poss was active in national organizations. In the Academy, he chaired the Committee on Home Study (1987–1990) and the Committee on Electronic Media in Education (1989–1995). He was chairman of the Education Committee of the Hip Society (1992–1993), a member of the Arthritic Advisory Committee of the Food and Drug Administration in 1978–1979. He retired from clinical practice in about 2000 to spend his time with his wife Anita, their family, and to enjoy his favorite past time—sailing—in Marblehead Bay.

RICHARD D. SCOTT

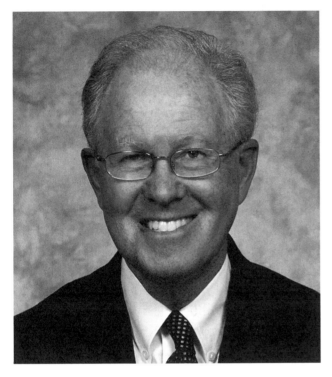

Richard D. Scott. Courtesy of Richard D. Scott.

Physician Snapshot

Richard D. Scott
BORN: 1943
DIED: —

SIGNIFICANT CONTRIBUTIONS: Developed a unicompartmental prosthesis with Dr. Peter Walker (1981); developed the PHC unicompartmental prosthesis with Dr. Thomas Thornhill (1990); developed the PFC Sigma prosthesis with Dr. Thomas Thornhill (1996); received the Ranawat Award from the Knee Society for the paper "Femoral Component Rotation During Total Knee Arthroplasty" with Dr. Christopher W. Olcott in 1999; published the text *Total Knee Arthroplasty* (2006);

Richard David Scott was born on March 28, 1943, in Philadelphia. He was raised in Philadelphia among a family of surgeons. His mother was Catherine Scott and his father, Michael Scott, was chair of neurosurgery at Temple University School of Medicine. His brother would go on to become a neurosurgeon as well. Scott "attended Williams College, receiving a Bachelor of Arts degree in biology in 1964, and Temple University, where he received a doctorate in medicine in 1968" (Mankin 1974). He had completed his medical education with distinction having been "elected to Alpha Omega Alpha in November 1966, and served as president of the Babcock Surgical Society, an honorary academic society" (Bucher 1968). While in medical school Scott had also shown a special interest in medical photography and received "honorable mention at the 9th Annual Medical Art Salon at Temple" (Butcher 1968).

Early Training and Career

Thereafter, he followed in his brother's footsteps by completing his general surgery internship at the Massachusetts General Hospital (MGH) where his brother was a neurosurgical resident (1968–1973). After his internship, Scott worked "as a research associate at the National Institutes of Health [1969–1971], doing work in cartilage metabolism. He returned to enter the Harvard Combined Residency Program," which he completed with "distinction" on June 30, 1974 (Mankin 1974). During his residency, Scott's salary was $10,700 per year ($66,693 in 2020).

Dr. Scott was appointed assistant in orthopaedics at the MGH in July 1974 upon the recommendation of Dr. Henry Mankin. He served as chief resident on the East Orthopaedic Service. After six months, he was promoted to clinical associate in orthopaedic surgery for one year in 1975, but he received no salary from MGH. Scott had two interests in orthopaedics at that time: pediatrics and hip and knee reconstruction. In a letter to Dr. John Hall, Scott (1975) wrote that he had a "safety valve association with Dr. Boyd and Dr. Huddleston (probably temporary)" Most likely he meant that he had a backup plan to stay in adult hip and knee reconstruction if he decided against specializing in pediatric orthopaedics or if didn't receive a position at Boston Children's Hospital. From January through June 1975, he had been a clinical fellow at the Robert Breck Brigham Hospital (RBBH). With strong support from Drs. Frederick Ewald and Bill Thomas he accepted a full-time position at the RBBH and Children's Hospital Medical Center in August 1975 and resigned from the MGH staff.

That same year, Scott was appointed an instructor in orthopaedic surgery at Harvard Medical School (HMS), and he co-authored five papers in 1975 and 1976 that demonstrated his interests in both pediatrics and adult reconstruction. Two articles were from Children's Hospital Medical Center: "Voluntary Posterior Hip Dislocation in Children" and "The Split Heel Technique in the Management of Calcaneal Osteomyelitis in Children." Two were about total hip replacement: "Femoral Fractures in Conjunction with Total Hip Replacement" and a brief note, "Avoiding Complications with Long-Stem Total Hip Replacement Arthroplasty."

Later Career: Adult Knee Reconstruction

Scott was promoted to assistant professor at HMS in 1980, and for the rest of his career his publications focused on adult reconstruction. He was a prolific writer and produced over 140 publications—40 about outcomes after total knee replacement, 35 on surgical techniques in total knee replacement, 23 papers concerned with unicompartmental knee replacement, 14 papers about total hip replacement, 3 about total elbow replacement, and one on total shoulder arthroplasty. He published more than 22 additional papers about specific and unique observations and problems associated with total knee arthroplasty. **Case 49.5** provides an example of one of his many case reports.

Partial Knee Reconstruction

In his book *Total Knee Arthroplasty*, Scott recalled creating, with Dr. Peter Walker at the RBBH, a unicompartmental prosthesis that they began implanting in 1974. It was a low congruence prosthesis with a titanium-backed tibial component and cemented in place. In 1981, Scott and Santore reported the results on the first 100 consecutive osteoarthritic knees treated with a unicompartmental prosthesis that resembled one half of a duocondylar prosthesis. They wrote:

> At follow-up [average: 3½ years], pain relief was good to excellent in 92 percent of the knees…average amount of flexion was 114°… Three failures had required revision. Radiolucent lines at the bone-cement interface were present around 8 percent of the femoral components and 27 percent of the tibial components. Two femoral components subsided in obese patients. There was no tibial loosening… The most common complication, pes anserinus bursitis, occurred in 12 percent…Surgical technique must be precise to prevent subluxation of the tibia on the femur…We usually reserve unicompartmental knee replacement for elderly patients with unicompartmental osteoarthritis.
>
> (Scott and Santore 1981)

The following year, his title at HMS was assistant clinical professor of orthopaedic surgery, and he was promoted to associate clinical professor by 1986. Scott and his colleagues published more than 20 papers on unicompartmental knee replacement over the next two decades, and by 1990 Scott and his colleague Dr. Thomas Thornhill

---

J Bone Joint Surg Am. 1981 Apr;63(4):536-44.

Unicondylar unicompartmental replacement for osteoarthritis of the knee

R D Scott, R F Santore

Scott and Santore's article reporting their experience with a new unicompartmental knee replacement prosthesis. *Journal of Bone and Joint Surgery* 1981; 63: 536.

Case 49.5. Metallic Tibial Tray Fracture After Total Knee Replacement

> "A seventy-four-year-old man with osteoarthritis had a total replacement arthroplasty of the left knee. He was 170 centimeters tall, and at the time of the operation he weighed ninety-six kilograms. The preoperative alignment at the knee was 17 degrees of varus angulation relative to the normal center of the femoral head and the center of the ankle. A large kinematic condylar prosthesis was used. The over-all thickness of the tibial plateau was eight millimeters. The alignment at the knee was corrected to 10 degrees of varus angulation. The patient was discharged from the hospital two weeks after the operation, at which time flexion of the knee was 85 degrees. He was instructed to use crutches for one month, but he discarded them after two weeks. Six months later, he had knee flexion to 105 degrees and no functional limitations. His weight was 100 kilograms. One year after surgery, while walking, he felt sudden pain on the medial side of the knee; this pain became constant and an effusion developed. Radiographs showed a fracture of the metal tray. At operation, the femoral component of the prosthesis was found to be solidly fixed, but it was removed for exposure. The central stem of the tibial component and the lateral plateau of the prosthesis also were rigidly fixed, but there was very little cement under the medial portion of the tray and there was poor penetration of the cement into the bone anteriorly. The bone beneath the fractured portion of the tray was deficient and had been replaced by fibrous tissue. Before implantation of a new component, the deficient area was built up with cement and two cancellous screws were used to supplement the cement. The tibial cut was adjusted to build some valgus angulation into the alignment of the knee. A sixteen-millimeter-thick tibial component was needed to restore stability, and a new femoral component was cemented in the original bed. A broken metal tray was returned to the manufacturer for evaluation. Based on the lot code, they determined that the prosthesis had been properly heat-treated and had been inspected radiographically for internal defects and by a fluorescent penetrant for surface flaws. It had also been visually and dimensionally inspected prior to insertion. The fracture surfaces were examined with a binocular microscope at magnification factors as high as forty. No metallurgical defects to which the failure could be attributed, such as shrinkage or microporosity, were observed. Examination of the fracture surfaces suggested that fatigued failure had originated at the corner of the posterior cruciate ligament cut-out and progressed transversely in the medial-to-lateral direction.
>
> "After the revision procedure the patient used crutches for three months and then used a cane for long walks. Six months after the revision he had no pain. The knee had 105 degrees of flexion and he could walk unlimited distances using a cane. His weight had decreased to eighty-eight kilograms."
>
> (Scott, Ewald, and Walker 1984)

developed another prosthesis, called the PFC unicompartmental knee. Six years later, they would evolve it further into the PFC Sigma prosthesis.

In 1991, they published the 8-to-12-year outcomes of the original 100 knees that Scott and Santore had reported on in 1981. They wrote:

> Survivorship analysis revealed 90% survivorship of the prosthesis at nine years, 85% at ten years, and 82% at 11 years...87% had no significant pain. The average knee flexion was 115°. Anatomic alignment average 3° of valgus for the knees with preoperative varus alignment and 8° of valgus for knees with preoperative valgus alignment...Sixty per cent had radiolucent lines [which] were incomplete in 96% of cases. (Scott et al. 1991)

In patients less than 60 years of age with unicompartmental osteoarthritis, Scott had continued to use the original McKeever tibial replacement prosthesis:

> Between December 1975 and December 19, 1990 [he] performed twenty-six consecutive McKeever hemiarthroplasties on twenty-four patients...While the indications for this procedure are limited [obese patients] are not

candidates for osteotomy [as well as patients who] are too young and active for joint arthroplasty...Its bone-sparing nature makes it an attractive option as a temporizing procedure for select patients with unicompartmental disease. (Springer et al. 2006)

He was promoted to professor at HMS around 2001, and the following year Drs. Deshmukh and Scott reviewed the first and second decades of results with a unicompartmental replacement prosthesis. They wrote:

Second decade results are less promising with studies often reflecting a rapid decline...The causes of late failure...include opposite compartment degeneration, component loosening, and polyethylene wear...From the initial implants used in the 1970s to the current designs, tibial aseptic loosening and polyethylene wear remain the most common causes of failed unicompartmental knee arthroplasty... Additional advances in prosthetic design have significantly reduced problems with prosthetic wear and aseptic component loosening. Mobile-bearing designs address these issues and could play a significant role in the future [and] improvements in the wear characteristics of polyethylene will enhance the performance of fixed bearings. (Desmukh and Scott 2002)

The rate of complications after a unicompartmental knee replacement increases the longer the implant is in place. Therefore, although their preference would indicate a less invasive procedure—such as a unicompartmental—because of the continued increase in problems with time, Scott believed that the unicompartmental knee arthroplasty was best suited for the octogenarian.

Total Knee Replacement

In 1982—one year after his seminal report on unicompartmental prosthesis—Dr. Scott

> Review   Clin Orthop Relat Res. 2001 Nov;(392):272-8.
>
> **Unicompartmental knee arthroplasty: long-term results**
>
> R V Deshmukh [1], R D Scott

Article reporting long-term results with the unicompartmental knee prosthesis. *Clinical Orthopaedics and Related Research* 2001; 392: 272.

> Orthop Clin North Am. 1982 Jan;13(1):89-102.
>
> **Duopatellar total knee replacement: the Brigham experience**
>
> R D Scott

Title of article, "Duopatellar Total Knee Replacement: the Brigham Experience." *Orthopedic Clinics of North America* 1982; 13: 89.

published his first paper on outcomes after total knee replacement, titled "Duopatellar Total Knee Replacement: The Brigham Experience." He briefly reviewed the history of knee arthroplasty at the RBBH and the various prostheses surgeons there used in the 1960s and 1970s (**Table 49.2**). Studies of the Duocondylar prostheses in 1974–75 showed that patellofemoral symptoms remained in 20% of patients undergoing knee replacement with the Duocondylar prosthesis (178 replacements) after two years. Outcomes with the duopatellar prosthesis are described in **Table 49.3**.

In patients with inadequate tibial bone stock who needed a total knee replacement, in addition to bone grafting or use of bone cement, Drs. Brooks, Walker, and Scott (1984) also investigated solid spacers in the laboratory. They wrote:

Use of a custom-made component that closely fitted the existing defect provided the most

Table 49.2. Evolution of Prostheses Used in Knee Arthroplasty at the Brigham Hospitals, 1960s–1990s

	Prosthesis	Materials	Procedure	Benefits
1960s	McKeever interpositional	Metal	Hemi-arthroplasty	Minimal bone loss
Early 1970s	Constrained hinge	Metal-metal	Arthroplasty	Knees with irreparable collateral ligament deficiency
	Modular	Metal-plastic	TKR	Improved wear characteristics Improved knee alignment
	Duocondylar		TKR	Restores medial-lateral stability
1973–74	Duopatellar		TKR	Tibial components provide intercondylar restraint and thereby reestablish mediolateral stability A flange provides a new interface between the patellofemoral joint and the femur Avoids excision/resection of the posterior cruciate ligament Relieves pain Provides alignment and stability
1980–1981	Brigham total knee system	metal-plastic		Allows for minimal to maximal restraint Variable sizing can be tailored to patient needs A deeper trochlear groove is aligned (7° valgus) to enhance patellar tracking Extended condyles allow the components to better engage over the full ROM The flat tibial component comprises a single piece with a stem in the center* Avoids excision/resection of the posterior cruciate ligament Provides maximal contact between bone and prosthesis to reduce loosening
	Kinematic knee system			Allows for minimal/maximal restraint Variable sizing can be tailored to patient needs Avoids excision/resection of the posterior cruciate ligament Provides maximal contact between bone and prosthesis to reduce loosening
1986–87	Omnifit knee			
Late 1980s	PFC modular knee revision system			Retained (or replaced) the posterior cruciate ligament
Late 1980s–1990s	Kinemax			Modular inserts Adjustable sizing Variable level of constraint Modular tibial and femoral components
	Kinemax Plus			
1996	PFC Sigma knee system			Mobile-bearing rotating platform Same design for both the patellofemoral and coronal femoral surfaces Can include or not intercondylar housing on the femoral side and an eminence on the tibial side

Data from Scott 1982, Springer 2006.
ROM, range of motion; TKR, total knee replacement.
*This single-piece component, now flat front to back, was adopted for use in 1978, replacing the two-piece tibial component.

Table 49.3. Outcomes with Duopatellar Prostheses in Knee Replacement at Brigham Hospitals in the Mid-1970s

First 747 Knees, 2- to 5-year follow-up	
Revision rate	2.8%
Patellar issues	50%
Aseptic loosening of two-piece tibial components	33%
First 100 replacements with one-piece flat, plastic tibial component	
Patients	
Rheumatoid arthritis	55%
Osteoarthritis	45%
Minimal or no pain at follow-up	95%
Postoperative ROM, mean	106°
Reoperations because of patellar button	2
Signs on radiographs	
Lines <1 mm thick, incomplete	74%
Involvement of radiolucent lines (n = 27)	
Only the medial plateau	50%
Lateral plateau	0%
Both plateaus	9%
Both plateaus and the central stem	19%
Issues with tibial component	
Drooping (varus alignment)	11%
Subsidence	2%

Data from Scott 1982.

rigid fixation. A metal wedge-shaped spacer was almost as rigid…Cement alone provided inadequate support…A central stem longer than normal, about 70 mm, carried about 30% of the axial load…a system of spacers that would enable the surgeon to match the needs of the individual patient [may be advantageous]. (Brooks et al. 1984)

Scott and his colleagues reported on the use of these metal tibial wedges in 20 patients with an average follow-up of 37 months in 1989. They noted:

There have been no failures of this technique and no loosening of tibial components. The incidence of nonprogressive radiolucent lines was 27%…No patient has had subsequent revision surgery…The wedge system is appropriate for defects of 20–25 mm or smaller… Larger defects [will need] a bone graft or a custom prosthesis. (Brand et al. 1989)

Orthop Clin North Am. 1989 Jan;20(1):89-95.

Press-fit condylar total knee replacement

R D Scott [1], T S Thornhill

Title of Scott and Thornhill's article on the PFC total knee prosthesis. *Orthopedic Clinics of North America* 1989; 20: 89.

In 1989, Scott and Thornhill reported the results of 500 procedures with the press-fit condylar knee (PFC), which allowed retention of the posterior cruciate ligament, over almost four years (November 1984–April 1988) at the New England Baptist Hospital and at Brigham and Women's Hospital (BWH) (**Table 49.4**).

Table 49.4. Results of 500 Total Knee Replacements with the PFC Knee Prosthesis, 1984–88

Cemented components	
All components	18%
Femoral component	22%
No components	4%
No or minimal pain	97%
Postoperative flexion	113°
Postoperative flexion contracture	1°

Data from Springer et al. 2006.

In 1999, Scott and Christopher W. Olcott received the Ranawat Award from the Knee Society for their paper "Femoral Component Rotation During Total Knee Arthroplasty." Scott and his colleagues continued to publish several other articles, reviewing 11- and 12-year results with the posterior cruciate retention total knee arthroplasty and two-to-four-year results with a hybrid press-fit

> J Bone Joint Surg Am. 2005 Mar;87(3):598-603
>
> **Modular fixed-bearing total knee arthroplasty with retention of the posterior cruciate ligament. A study of patients followed for a minimum of fifteen years**
>
> Michael C Dixon [1], Richard R Brown, Dominik Parsch, Richard D Scott

Article reporting Scott's long-term results with a posterior cruciate-retaining total knee prosthesis. *Journal of Bone and Joint Surgery* 2005; 87: 598.

uncemented femoral component posterior cruciate retaining condylar prosthesis. In 2005, he reported his own results in 139 consecutive total knee arthroplasties in 109 patients using a non-conforming posterior cruciate retaining prosthesis:

> Forty-five patients (fifty-nine knees) were examined at a minimum of fifteen years postoperatively...The patients were assessed clinically with use of the Knee Society clinical rating system, and...assessed radiographically. Survivorship analysis was performed... There were five reoperations, four...because of wear of the polyethylene insert. In addition, one loose cemented femoral component was revised at fifteen years. The survival rate without revision or a need for any reoperation was 92.6% at fifteen years. The mean Knee Society score and functional score at fifteen years were 96 and 78 points, respectively. The prevalence of radiolucent lines was 13%, with 2% around the femur, 11% around the tibia, and none around the patella. None of these lines were clinically relevant. There was no evidence of progressive radiolucent lines, and there was one case of asymptomatic femoral osteolysis. (Dixon 2005)

In another publication almost 25 years later after his original review of the history of knee arthroplasty at the RBBH, Scott described the main procedures and prostheses used from the mid-1980s to the late 1990s at Brigham hospitals (including the RBBH, PBBH, and the now merged BWH). Results are presented in **Table 49.2**. Drs. Sledge, Scott, and others at the Brigham hospitals strongly believed in the importance of preserving the posterior cruciate ligament, especially in patients with rheumatoid arthritis. Their continued development of improved total knee prostheses always included a design that allowed for preservation of the posterior cruciate ligament if possible.

Dr. Richard Scott continues to have a large clinical practice of patients with arthritis of the knees and hips. He operates mainly at the NEBH and the BWH. The following is a partial list of some of some of Scott's personal and unique observations that he published regarding his experiences with total knee replacement:

- Blood supply to the patella
- Bone loss in the distal anterior femur
- Metal induced synovitis
- Posterior polyethylene wear
- Popliteus tendon dysfunction after total knee replacement
- Management of periarticular fractures after total knee replacement
- Intraoperative test to predict postoperative range of motion
- Technical problems in Paget disease
- Synovial cyst compressing the peroneal nerve
- Kneeling ability after total knee arthroplasty
- Methods to determine femoral component rotation
- Rheology of joint fluid after total knee replacement
- Bony ankylosis after total knee arthroplasty
- Effect of patellar thickness on flexion
- Periprosthetic pseudo-osteolysis
- Magnitude of limb lengthening after total knee replacement

BARRY P. SIMMONS

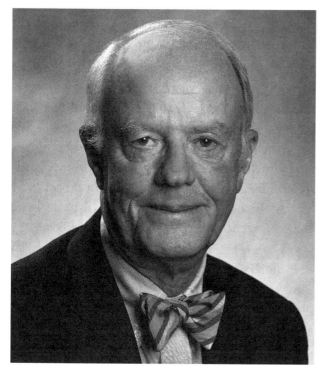

Barry P. Simmons. © Infinity Portrait Design 2018.

> **Physician Snapshot**
>
> Barry P. Simmons
>
> BORN: 1939
>
> DIED: —
>
> SIGNIFICANT CONTRIBUTIONS: Chief of the hand and upper extremity service at the Brigham and Women's Hospital (1982–2017); president of the Hand Study Society (1987); chairman of the Council of Musculoskeletal Specialty Societies of the AAOS (1994); coauthored *Occupational Disorders of the Upper Extremity* (1992) with Drs. Lewis H. Millender and Dean Louis; coauthored *Hands: Strategies for Strong, Pain-free Hands* with Joanne P. Bosch and Julie Corliss (2015)

Barry Putnam Simmons was born on December 18, 1939, in Boston, Massachusetts. After graduating with a BA from Harvard College in 1961, he received his MD degree from the Columbia College of Physicians and Surgeons in 1965. The next year he was an intern at Tufts New England Medical Center; followed by a year as a junior resident in surgery (1966–1967) at the University of California at San Francisco. At that time the war in Vietnam was active and Dr. Simmons spent two years in service there with the US Navy. Returning to the Boston area in 1969, he completed a research fellowship at Boston Children's Hospital in Dr. Judah Folkman's laboratory. Afterward he entered the Boston Children's Hospital/Massachusetts's General Hospital (MGH) orthopaedic surgery residency program. He coauthored an article on his research experience titled "Perfusion of the Isolated Rat Limb," which was presented at the 1970 Surgical Forum of the American College of Surgeons.

Simmons completed his orthopaedic residency in 1973 as chief resident at the West Roxbury Veterans Administration Hospital. His residency rotations are included in **Box 49.4**. He was then asked by Dr. Clement Sledge to join his group at the Peter Bent Brigham Hospital (PBBH). Following Dr. Melvin Glimcher's strategy, Sledge asked Simmons to complete a fellowship elsewhere. He chose hand surgery and did a six-month fellowship with Dr. Raoul Tubiana in Paris, France, from September 1973 until February 1974, followed by an AO trauma fellowship in Basil, Switzerland.

In 1974, Simmons was appointed associate in orthopaedic surgery at the PBBH, the Robert Breck Brigham Hospital (RBBH), Children's Hospital Medical Center (CHMC), and Beth Israel Hospital (BIH) as well as consultant in orthopaedic

Box 49.4. Residency Rotations for Dr. Barry P. Simmons

- Research fellow at Children's Hospital Medical Center (CHMC) from July 1, 1969, until December 31, 1969
- Assistant resident CHMC from January 1, 1970, until September 30, 1970
- Assistant resident at the MGH from October 1, 1970, until December 3, 1971
- Assistant resident and resident CHMC from January 1, 1971, until December 31, 1972
- Chief resident at Beth Israel Hospital (BIH) from January 1, 1973, until March 3, 1973
- Chief resident at the West Roxbury Veterans Hospital Medical Center from April 1, 1973, until June 30, 1973

surgery at the West Roxbury Veteran's Administration Hospital where he was director of the hand clinic (1974–1982). His appointment at Harvard Medical School (HMS) was clinical instructor in orthopaedic surgery. From 1974 to 1982, he was also on the staff of the Harvard Community Health Plan. In 1978, he became an associate in orthopaedic surgery at the New England Baptist Hospital (NEBH), upper extremity/hand consultant to the Harvard University Department of Athletics and orthopaedic surgeon to Harvard's University Health Service, and consultant to the Boston College Department of Athletics.

Dr. Simmons was appointed chief of the hand and upper extremity service at the Brigham and Women's Hospital (BWH) and assistant clinical professor of orthopaedic surgery at HMS in 1982. Six years later, he was promoted to associate clinical professor of orthopaedic surgery. Over the course of his career, he published more than 40 articles, authored or coauthored approximately 26 book chapters, and coauthored two books. He published *Hands: Strategies for Strong, Pain-free Hands* (2015) with Joanne P. Bosch and Julie Corliss, and a book on occupational disorders of the upper extremity with Drs. Lewis H. Millender and Dean Louis. The latter book was entitled *Occupational Disorders of the Upper Extremity* (1992). **Case 49.6** includes an example of one of his case reports. His publications have focused on carpal

Case 49.6. Focal Scleroderma of the Hand

"A three-month-old white boy, the first child of healthy parents and the product of a normal pregnancy and delivery, had a deformity of the left hand, noted at birth. There was a negative family history. On physical examination, the index finger of the left hand showed marked ulnar deviation. With gentle pressure, the ulnar deviation could be corrected; however, passive flexion of the metacarpophalangeal joint was limited. Tendon function could not be assessed. Both the index and long fingers were shorter and thicker than normal, and the soft tissues were firm and non-pliable. Radiographs confirmed the deformity. Manipulation and serial cast applications failed to correct the deformity. At the age of nine months, radial deviation of the left long finger developed, and a one by one-centimeter area of thickened skin had appeared on the dorsoradial aspect of the left hand. Also, there was a 10-degree valgus deformity of the left ankle, produced by a three by twelve-centimeter area of shiny, indurated skin that extended from the plantar aspect of the foot to the lateral aspect of the leg. All laboratory determinations included hematocrit, urinalysis, white-blood-cell count, erythrocyte sedimentation rate, antinuclear factor, and rheumatoid factor, were normal. Barium-swallow radiographs and the results of an electrocardiogram were normal.

"Through dorsal incisions, surgical exploration of the metacarpophalangeal joints and the dorsal apparatus of the index and long fingers revealed that the ulnar lateral band of the index finger and the radial lateral band of the long finger were thickened and fibrotic, and they were released. The extensor indicis proprius also was found to be thickened and was released. Capsulotomies of the metacarpophalangeal joints were performed and the extensor digitorum communis tendon of the index finger was centralized. The metacarpophalangeal joints were stabilized in a straight position and in 70 degrees of flexion with fine Kirschner wires. Four weeks later, the Kirschner wires were removed. A biopsy of the skin on the lateral aspect of the calf was also done and histological examination of the specimen demonstrated characteristic thickening and fibrosis in the subcutis and deep layers of the dermis. The patient was treated postoperatively with a splint worn on the left hand at night and with vigorous physical therapy for the left hand and leg.

"Two years postoperatively, the lesion on the dorsal aspect of the left hand had progressed to produce a severe contracture of the first web space and limited motion of the wrist. The index finger was not being used and remained in a straight position, with no motion of the joint. The long finger radially deviated 30 degrees and the motion of the metacarpophalangeal and proximal interphalangeal joints ranged from zero to 30 degrees. The ring finger had 20 degrees of radial deviation. Furthermore, the valgus deformity of the left ankle had increased, and focal areas of scleroderma had appeared on the abdomen."

(Lloyd, Simmons, & Griffin 1985)

> Arthroscopy. 1993;9(2):209-13
>
> **Endoscopic carpal tunnel release: a cadaveric study**
>
> J T Schwartz [1], P M Waters, B P Simmons

Simmons's article describing his cadaver research on endoscopic carpal tunnel release. *Arthroscopy* 1993; 9: 209.

> J Hand Surg Am. 1997 Jul;22(4):613-20
>
> **Patients' preferences and their relationship with satisfaction following carpal tunnel release**
>
> L Bessette [1], R B Keller, M H Liang, B P Simmons, A H Fossel, J N Katz

Article reporting patient preferences and satisfaction after carpal tunnel surgery, from the Maine Medical Assessment Foundation. *Journal of Hand Surgery* 1997; 22: 613.

tunnel syndrome (about one-third of his articles), of which the majority have focused on outcomes followed by open versus endoscopic techniques. He also published two papers related to outcomes in workers compensation patients His first article was on carpal tunnel, entitled "Endoscopic Carpal Tunnel Release: A Cadaveric Study." He later published three additional articles about technique in carpal tunnel surgery. His most significant contributions were his contributions to the outcomes movement in the last decade of the twentieth century, with a focus on carpal tunnel syndrome.

Publications on Carpal Tunnel Syndrome

Working with Dr. Jeffrey N. Katz (rheumatology) and others at BWH, Simmons was a member of a group in the Robert Brigham Multipurpose Arthritis and Musculoskeletal Disease Center in 1993 that developed a self-assessment questionnaire for the assessment of symptoms and function in patients with carpal tunnel syndrome. They wrote:

> The reproducibility, internal consistency, validity, and responsiveness…for the measurement of severity of symptoms and functional status were evaluated in a clinical study. The scales were highly reproducible…and internally consistent…Both scales had positive, but modest or weak, correlations with two-point discrimination and Semmes-Weinstein monofilament testing…In thirty-eight patients who were operated on in 1991 and…evaluated fourteen months postoperatively [and] twenty-six patients who were evaluated before and three months after the operation [who had similar improvement in symptom severity and functional status,] the scales for the measurement of severity of symptoms and functional status are reproducible, internally consistent, and responsive to clinical change, and that they measure dimensions of outcomes not captured by traditional measurements of impairment of the median nerve. These scales should enhance standardization of measurement of outcomes in studies of treatment for carpal tunnel syndrome…
>
> There is broad consensus that rigorous outcomes research is needed to distinguish interventions that are effective from those that are not. This task requires standardization, patient-centered measures that can be administered at a low cost; have proved reliability, validity, and responsiveness; and can be compared across studies. (Levine et al. 1993)

He also collaborated with Dr. Katz, Dr. Robert Keller (see chapter 27), and others in clinical research regarding carpal tunnel syndrome. Simmons and Keller were former residents and colleagues in the Harvard teaching program. In 1997, they used the Maine Carpal Tunnel Syndrome Study to further their research. In the early 1980s, the Maine Medical Assessment Foundation was organized by physicians practicing in the state of Maine. They created eight groups, each for a particular specialty, which evaluated disparities and differences in practice patterns of that specialty's clinicians throughout the state. On the basis of the collected data, the groups helped to increase quality of care and reduce overutilization of healthcare-related resources. Keller was executive director of the Maine Medical Assessment Foundation and also had frequent collaborations with Dr. John Wennberg, the director of the Center for Evaluative Clinical Services at Dartmouth Medical School.

The study data included 404 patients—250 of whom completed a presurgical questionnaire about why they elected to have surgery and which among 10 areas they most hoped to see improvement, and they reported on the preferences of and satisfaction with the results of treatment for the condition. The main reasons for having the procedure was to reduce pain during the day (13%) and at night (37%), and to alleviate numbness (21%). On the basis of an association between a patient giving a higher rating to strength as an area of hoped-for improvement postoperatively and lower satisfaction six months after the procedure, they suggested that surgeons recognize and address any unrealistic expectations that patient might have.

The following year—the same year Simmons also became an associate in orthopaedics at Faulkner Hospital—the group published the "Maine Carpal Tunnel Study: Outcomes of Operative and Nonoperative Therapy for Carpal Tunnel Syndrome in a Community-Based Cohort." That study included 429 patients with carpal tunnel syndrome within the state of Maine; the investigators evaluated symptom severity and functional status in those patients at three time points after enrollment (6, 18, and 30 months). Scores increased by 23% to 45% across the 30 months in patients who had undergone surgery, whereas scores changed very little those who did not. Although patients who were receiving workers compensation experienced poorer results after surgery, just over half were well satisfied with their results at the 30-month follow-up.

> J Hand Surg Am. 1998 Jul;23(4):697-710
>
> **Maine Carpal Tunnel Study: outcomes of operative and nonoperative therapy for carpal tunnel syndrome in a community-based cohort**
>
> J N Katz [1], R B Keller, B P Simmons, W D Rogers, L Bessette, A H Fossel, N A Mooney

Article reporting outcomes of patients with carpal tunnel syndrome treated operatively and non-operatively. *Journal of Hand Surgery* 1998; 23: 697.

In 2002, Drs. Katz and Simmons wrote an article on carpal tunnel syndrome in the *New England Journal of Medicine* Clinical Practice series. The authors followed the clinical guidelines of the AAOS and similar guidelines from the American College of Occupational and Environmental Medicine:

Patients with discomfort of the hand and wrist... should be evaluated with a detailed history...and a physical examination...Findings on such examination have limited diagnostic value...If carpal tunnel syndrome seems likely, conservative management with splinting should be initiated...We suggest that patients reduce activities at home and work that exacerbate symptoms. Although the effects of nonsteroidal anti-inflammatory medications on carpal tunnel syndrome have not been well studied, we generally suggest a trial of these agents if there are no contraindications. We do not recommend use of vitamin B6...or oral corticosteroids...We generally screen for and treat common underlying disorders – specifically, diabetes and hypothyroidism.

If the condition fails to improve, we recommend referral to a specialist...If the diagnosis appears secure, the clinician should discuss the options of corticosteroid injection and surgical therapy...Injection is especially effective if there is no loss of sensibility or thenar muscle atrophy and weakness and if symptoms are intermittent rather than constant. We perform electrodiagnostic studies if the diagnosis is uncertain, particularly if surgery is contemplated. For surgically treated patients, we favor the limited open incision for carpal tunnel release. (Katz and Simmons 2002)

In 2006, after coediting a special report from the Harvard Medical School, Simmons was asked about carpal tunnel syndrome in the workplace with the increased use of computers. He voiced his belief that development of the syndrome is not related to one's occupation or computer use, as many health conditions can cause it, including, among others, arthritis, diabetes, thyroid disorders, obesity, and pregnancy. He also blamed 50% of the cases of carpal tunnel syndrome on genetics. Normal aging and female sex also increase one's risk of developing it. For Simmons, hand and wrist pain with computer use is overuse syndrome, not carpal tunnel.

Leader in the Outcomes Movement

Simmons was also active in the outcomes movement, and he served on committees in the American Academy of Orthopaedic Surgeons (AAOS) and the American Society for Surgery of the Hand (ASSH). In 1987, while president of the Hand Study Society, he was a member of the outcomes committee of the ASSH. From 1992 until 1995, he served on the clinical guidelines committee for ASSH. As a member of the Academy's Board of Directors and for six years (1995–2001), he served on the Academy's outcomes committee.

In 1994, he was elected chairman of the Council of Musculoskeletal Specialty Societies (AAOS). In this role, Simmons was active in the academy's development of the Musculoskeletal Outcome Data Evaluation and Management System (MODEMS) during the mid-1990s. The MODEMS compiled both various validated instruments that measured patient-reported outcomes (PRO) and newly developed methods of doing so in subspecialty fields, with the goal of bolstering their use by orthopaedic surgeons. At the time, the academy also started determining the mean scores on the various instruments among general populations; making such values available to practicing physicians and surgeons in order to allow them to evaluate their own patients' scores against the standard mean. In 2000, however, various barriers precluded the continuation of the MODEMS and its study—lack of financing, of methods for data reporting, and of the necessary high-level technology (electronic medical systems and patient portals), as well as poor compliance.

During this period, Dr. Simmons also collaborated with Dr. Katz in his contributions to the outcomes literature. For example, in patients with carpal tunnel syndrome who were receiving workers' compensation, they reported that instruments measuring health-related quality of life are valid and reliable, and they suggested their use by researchers investigated occupational injuries and illnesses.

Teaching and Honors

Dr. Barry P. Simmons led a fellowship program for two positions per year for 35 years, from 1982 until 2017. In his personal statement on his CV, he emphasized his enthusiasm for and investment in teaching. In national organizations, he contributed to the development of a national matching program in orthopaedic fellowships, including an electronic application form for orthopaedic resident applicants. Dr. Peter Waters (2013), who in 1988 had been one of Simmons early fellows, wrote in a dedication to Dr. Simmons: "The ebb and flow of calmness, humor, and connection that defines the temperament of Barry's service results in high quality care and has helped attract many Harvard residents to careers in hand surgery." Some of Simmons additional professional honors include the Sir Robert Jones Lecturer at New York University Hospital for Joint Diseases (2002), the Stromberg Memorial Lecture for the Chicago Society for Surgery of the Hand (2005), the 17th Annual Richard J. Smith Lecturer at MGH (2006); and he has been an invited presenter at numerous meetings, grand rounds, and postgraduate courses.

WILLIAM H. THOMAS

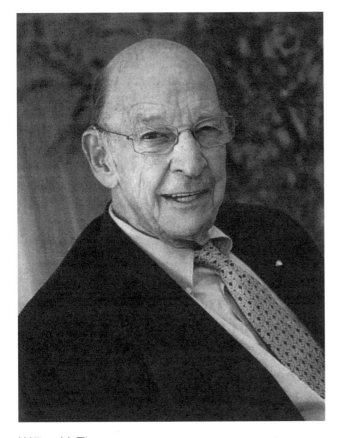

William H. Thomas. Courtesy of Sue Thomas Macleod.

> **Physician Snapshot**
>
> William H. Thomas
> BORN: 1930
> DIED: 2011
> SIGNIFICANT CONTRIBUTIONS: Began the first foot clinic at the RBBH in 1969; the Orthopaedic Department at Brigham and Women's Hospital named the William H. Thomas Award for a graduating orthopaedic resident in his honor

William H. Thomas, born in 1930 into a medical family (his father Charles was a physician), was known as "Bill" to friends and family. He was raised on Lookout Mountain in Chattanooga, Tennessee. During his formative years he attended the McCallie School, a boys-only prep school in Chattanooga, and the Choate School. He went on to Dartmouth College for his undergraduate education, but he spent only two years there before being accepted into the US Naval Aviation Cadet program. He put his education on hold, spending four years as a bomber pilot and instructor. He then returned to Dartmouth to complete his junior and senior years, moving on then to Dartmouth Medical School and Harvard Medical School (HMS).

After graduation from HMS, he was an intern and a resident in surgery at Strong Memorial Hospital in Rochester, New York (1961–1963). He trained in orthopaedic surgery in the Boston Children's Hospital/Massachusetts's General Hospital (MGH) program from 1963–1967; served as chief resident at the Peter Bent Brigham Hospital (PBBH) and the West Roxbury Veterans Administration Hospital from April 1966 to April 1967. From April 1967 to October 1968, he was a hip fellow at the MGH with Dr. Otto Aufranc. During this experience, Thomas coauthored three papers in the *JAMA* Fracture of the Month series: "Fracture of the Acetabulum with Dislocation of the Hip and Sciatic Palsy," "Dislocation of the Elbow with Fracture of the Radial Head and Distal Radius," and "Radial Neck Fracture in a Child." This series was led by Dr. Aufranc and in addition to Dr. Thomas these three papers were coauthored by Dr. William N. Jones and Dr. Roderick H. Turner.

That same year, he did an arthritis fellowship at the Robert Breck Brigham Hospital (RBBH) with Dr. Theodore Potter. After completing his fellowship, Thomas was appointed assistant in orthopaedic surgery at HMS when he joined the staff at the RBBH in private practice. He remained at RBBH, which would soon join with PBBH to become Brigham and Women's Hospital, throughout his almost 35-year career.

In 1969, Thomas was secretary of the medical staff at the RBBH. After his arrival at the Brighams in 1970, Dr. Clement Sledge stated: "Because of the enlarged scope of my duties, greater responsibilities have fallen to Drs. William Thomas and Marvin Weinfeld here [at the RBBH] and to Dr. J. Drennan Lowell at the PBBH" ("Annual Report,

1970, Surgeon-in-Chief's Report [Sledge]" 1970, 18). These responsibilities included teaching and patient care. Numerous lectures to students and residents were given by Drs. Sledge, Thomas, Ed Nalebuff, and Lew Millender. In 1970, Thomas was promoted from assistant in orthopaedic surgery to associate physician at the RBBH. That same year he started the first foot clinic for rheumatoid patients at the RBBH. In his chief's report, Sledge wrote: "A milestone in surgery of the rheumatoid knee has been reached this year; Drs. Potter, Thomas and Weinfeld have completed their review of knee arthroplasties with metallic prostheses. Their review will establish this procedure, now not widely appreciated, in its rightful place in the surgical armamentarium" (Annual Report, 1970, Surgeon-in-Chief's Report [Sledge]" 1970, 18).

Dr. Thomas published 36 papers; he was the lead author on 14 of those, including 8 on the foot. By 1975, he had published two papers on the rheumatoid foot and was promoted to clinical instructor in orthopaedic surgery at HMS. In the first, on metatarsal anatomy, he noted that surgeons at the RBBH had long used metatarsal head excision to treat metatarsalgia. One patient, however, changed that practice: the surgeons could not proceed with the planned excision surgery because of another injury to the foot, ecchymosis distally and a fracture of the second metatarsal. They treated this injury with an elastic bandage and no weight bearing (the patient used crutches), and after 10 days the patient was pain free and the fracture had healed. Surprisingly, however, the angle at which the bone healed precluded the need for the excision surgery.

Thomas went on to describe a subsequent literature review that found a 1916 publication in which Roland O. Meisenbach described using osteotomy for a condition such as Thomas's patient had. After that find, RBBH surgeons began to use Meisenbach's osteotomy procedure to treat metatarsal pain with non-severe deformity (they still used excision when the metatarsophalangeal joint was dislocated). To support this, Thomas highlighted their 96% success rate—pain relief was achieved after 69 of 73 metatarsal osteotomies over four years of follow-up.

> Orthopedic Clinics of North America
> Volume 6, Issue 3, July 1975, Pages 831-835
>
> Surgery of the Foot in Rheumatoid Arthritis
>
> William H. Thomas M.D. (Clinical Instructor in Orthopedic Surgery, Surgeon)

Title of Thomas's article on surgical treatment of the rheumatoid foot. *Orthopedic Clinics of North America* 1975; 6; 831.

In addition to publishing two articles on the use of CT scans of the hindfoot, he coauthored papers in 1976 and 1997 on the management of the rheumatoid hindfoot. The 1997 paper was a review that included the RBBH's experience in treating rheumatoid patients with hindfoot pain and planovalgus deformity (1976) in adult rheumatoids or a varus hindfoot in juvenile rheumatoids with additional patients added in a review presented in 1982. They "reported on 104 isolated talonavicular fusions in which more than 95% of patients obtained good or excellent pain relief with only a 5% nonunion rate. Follow up [averaged] 52 months and…no patient has required revision to a triple arthrodesis for progressive valgus deformity" (Kindsfater, Wilson, and Thomas 1997).

Dr. Thomas wrote or cowrote articles in Surgical Clinics, Orthopedic Clinics, and Radiology Clinics and was a main coauthor on two papers on the use of McKeever and MacIntosh prostheses for the knee in rheumatoid arthritis. Both were long-term follow-up studies, the first published in 1972 (MacIntosh and McKeever protheses) and

> Clin Orthop Relat Res. 1997 Jul;(340):69-74
>
> Management of the rheumatoid hindfoot with special reference to talonavicular arthrodesis
>
> K Kindsfater [1], M G Wilson, W H Thomas

Title of Thomas's article reviewing the RBBH's experience on the surgical treatment of the rheumatoid hindfoot. *Clinical Orthopaedics and Related Research* 1997; 340: 69.

the second in 1985 (McKeever prothesis). In the first, Thomas, Potter, and Weinfeld wrote:

> In our series of ninety-six rheumatoid knees, the results (56 per cent good to excellent ratings) are only slightly better than the previously reported average results, and are not nearly as good as the results in some of the smaller series. Results in our osteoarthritis patients, on the other hand, compare quite favorable with those in previous studies. If our two groups are combined, the over-all results were good to excellent in 62 percent...Patelloplasty...in twenty-one patients...did not have a deleterious effect of knee arthroplasty...Secondary surgical procedures were performed...in twenty-one of the knees evaluated. Twelve...necessitated by complications...Posterior capsulotomy or supracondylar osteotomy is likely to be required when the preoperative flexion deformity is more than 30 degrees...Hip disease had a definite deleterious effect on the results of knee arthroplasty...From these findings it is concluded that knee arthroplasty of the type described when performed in properly selected patients is an effective method to relieve pain and restore function.

In the second paper on the McKeever prosthesis in unicompartmental degenerative arthritis, Thomas, along with Richard Scott, Michael Joyce and Frederick Ewald, reported the long-term results (average eight years) from the RBBH:

> Forty patients with forty-four unicompartmental McKeever metallic uncemented hemi-arthroplasties were followed five to thirteen years...Thirty-nine had a medial and five, a lateral arthroplasty...At the final follow up, 70 per cent of the knees were rated as good or excellent...Six knees (14 per cent) had required revision to either a unicompartmental or a bicompartmental total knee replacement. The average preoperative and postoperative knee flexion did not change, but knees with initially poor motion improved...Complications were rare...The McKeever...arthroplasty... [is] an attractive surgical alternative in a knee with unicompartmental degenerative arthritis when proximal tibial osteotomy is contraindicated or has failed and the patient is too young, too heavy, or too active to consider total knee replacement. (Scott et al. 1985)

After he retired in the late 1990s, Thomas spent much of his time working as a pilot with the Florida Civil Air Patrol in the southwest region. He also continued to enjoy his favorite outdoor activities like camping, fishing, and skiing. He, along with his wife, Margaret (known to her friends as "Dickey"), were also involved in wildlife conservation. After over a decade of enjoying retired life, Thomas received a diagnosis of cancer. He died soon after, on November 18, 2011. Dickey and their two daughters survived him.

In recognition of his personal skills as a physician and a role model for residents, the faculty at the BWH annually present the William H. Thomas Award to the graduating orthopaedic resident who "best exemplifies excellence in orthopaedics, devotion to patient care, collegiality and teamwork" ("2010 Harvard Combined Orthopaedic Surgery

Residency Program Graduation Reception and Dinner" 2010). All winners from the inception of the award in 1996 through 2020 are listed in **Box 49.5**.

Box 49.5. William H. Thomas Award Winners

- 1996 Rajendra Kadiyala, MD
- 1997 Deryk Jones, MD
- 1998 Peter Kloen, MD
- 1999 Christopher Chiodo, MD
- 2000 Lisa Taitsman, MD
- 2001 Upshur Spencer, MD
- 2002 Donald Bae, MD
- 2003 James O'Holleran, MD
- 2004 Brandon Earp, MD
- 2005 John Abraham, MD
- 2006 Nicholas Avallone, MD
- 2007 George Dyer, MD
- 2008 Mark Price, MD, PhD
- 2009 Coleen Sabatini, MD
- 2010 Arnold Alqueza, MD
- 2011 Olivia Lee, MD
- 2012 Conor Kleweno, MD
- 2013 Eric Black, MD
- 2014 Xavier Simcock, MD
- 2015 Stephen Huffaker, MD
- 2016 Youssra Marjoua, MD
- 2017 Shaun Patel, MD
- 2018 Erik T. Newman, MD
- 2019 Hai Le
- 2020 Brian Schurko

CHAPTER 50

BWH's Modernization and Preparation for the Twenty-First Century

After the tremendous achievement of the highly complex, 20-year merger process, Dr. Clement Sledge continued as chief of orthopaedics at the newly established Brigham and Women's Hospital (BWH) (see chapters 47 and 48). Sledge had served as chief for both previous hospitals, the Robert Breck Brigham Hospital (RBBH) and Peter Bent Brigham Hospital (PBBH). On November 12, 1980, Orthopaedic Grand Rounds resumed for the first time in the new location. They continued at 5 PM each Wednesday and were held in the 16 B conference room until September 1981 when they were then moved to the main amphitheater on the Pike at 7:30 AM for an hour and a half. A resident's conference was begun at 5:30 PM on Wednesdays, in the 16 B conference room; alternating weekly with a fracture conference. In December 1980, an acute rehabilitation service had opened at the BWH, in pods C and D on the 14th floor. For the first three months, they had 10 beds (medical and surgical), but, in 1981, they expanded to 25 beds. The unit was opened seven days a week. The medical director was Dr. Sheldon Simon.

After the final merger, Dr. Sledge had established the Brigham Orthopedic Associates (BOA) and the Brigham Orthopaedic Foundation (BOF) (see chapter 47). By the late 1990s,

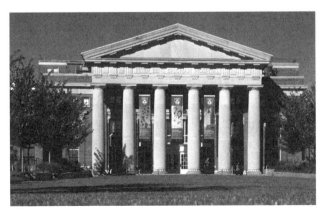

Administration Building, PBBH (BWH). Brigham and Women's Hospital.

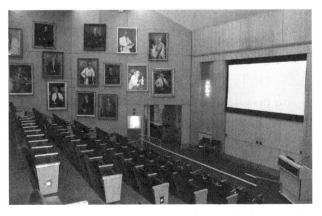

Main amphitheater (Bornstein Family Amphitheater), main pike (2nd-floor hallway). © Lee Hoy.

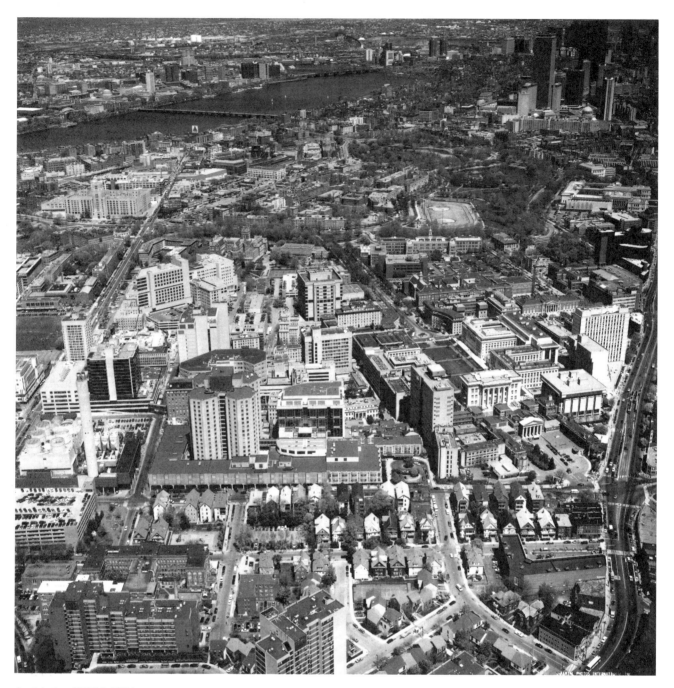

Aerial view BWH, 1994. Brigham and Women's Hospital Archives.

at the hospital's direction to reform its organization and governance, the "for-profit BOA [was incorporated into] the not-for-profit BOF. The final transition occurred in 2001 as the Brigham Orthopaedic Foundation joined the Brigham and Women's Physician Organization (BWPO), whose sole corporate member, like the MGH Physician's Organization, is Partners Healthcare" ("Chief's Report. Brigham and Women's Hospital" 2003). At that time the BOF orthopaedic staff became full-time faculty at HMS.

Dr. Sledge slowly expanded the staff by providing hospital appointments to many physicians in private practice and to those at Boston Children's Hospital, in addition to the geographic full-time staff, many of whom remained on staff for short periods; those who worked full-time at Boston Children's remained on the BWH staff. Some of these physicians included the following as associates in orthopaedic surgery: Drs. Benjamin Bierbaum, Michael Drew (chief of orthopaedics at the Harvard Community Health Plan), Jack McGinty, Hamish G. Gilles, Arthur Boland; from Children's Hospital: Drs. Arthur Pappas, Melvin Glimcher, John Hall, Edward Riseborough, Arthur Trott, and Hugh Watts. The following were junior associates in orthopaedic surgery: Drs. Robert R. Arbuckle, William Head, Donald Riley, St. George Tucker Aufranc, Stuart Cope, David W. Cloos, William W. Southmayd; and Lyle Micheli, Robert K. Rosenthal, Frank Bates, Robert Keller, Panos Panagakos (all from Children's Hospital). Inactive emeritus staff included: William A. Elliston and Franklin G Balch, Jr. The podiatrist was Bruce T. Wood. By 1981, Drs. Gus White, Mike Millis, John Emans, and Ronald N. Chaplan were listed as staff.

Sledge remained chairman of the department at BWH for 26 years, until June 30, 1996. The May 3, 1996, issue of the *BWH Bulletin* published a brief article about him at his retirement:

> [He] leaves behind [a] legacy of Excellence and Caring...The first chief of fledging three–MD Department located in a small trailer in the parking lot of the Peter Bent Brigham (PBB) Hospital. More than 25 years later, the retiring chief leaves behind scores of grateful patients and a renowned department of 75 physicians, which is listed annually among the best of the best in the US News and World Report survey...While Sledge is retiring, he does not plan to give up medicine, but will continue to play an important role as chairman of the newly established BWH organization.

Dr. Robert Poss was then appointed interim or acting chief (July 1, 1996–September 30, 1996), until Dr. Thomas Thornhill was chosen by the leadership at the BWH, on October 1, 1996, to become the second chairman of the department of orthopaedic surgery. The following year, I was appointed chairman of the department of orthopaedic surgery for Partners Healthcare, the parent organization of the BWH and the MGH. Initially Thornhill began to recruit needed faculty: "Dr. Charles Brown...Chief of Sports Medicine, Dr. Tamara Martin, recruited...in the areas of foot and ankle, and sports medicine, [and] Dr. Richard Ozuna...with fellowship training in spine surgery" (Thornhill 2003). Other members of the department in 1998–1999 included: Drs. Robert Poss, Richard Scott, Barry Simmons, Gregory W. Brick, Jonathan L. Schaffer, Dan M. Estok II, Mark J. Koris, Scott D. Martin, Tom Minas, John E. Ready, Michael G. Wilson, and R. John Wright. In 2002, Dr. James Ioli was named chief of the podiatry division of the foot and ankle program.

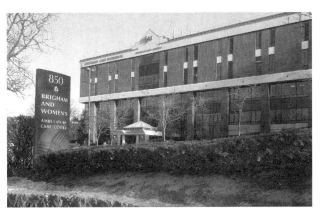

Ambulatory building in front of hospital towers, ca. 1988. Brigham and Women's Hospital Archives.

Brigham and Women's Ambulatory Care Center, 850 Boylston Street, Chestnut Hill, MA. Len Rubinstein.

When I received the financial commitment of Partners Healthcare in 1998 for recruitment of new faculty at both the BWH and the MGH, I collaborated with the chief of the orthopaedic surgery in each hospital to recruit outstanding faculty in needed areas. At the BWH, with Dr. Thornhill, this included Drs. Jon P. Warner, Mark Vrahas, Christopher Chiodo, Peter Millet, Wolfgang Fitz, Philip Blazar, and Mitchel Harris.

By 1999, the leadership of the BWH had collaborated with Harvard Vanguard Medical Associates, offering services of the hospital to their patients and staff privileges for their physicians. The group's orthopaedic surgeons at that time included: Drs. Robert Chernack, John A. K. Davies, Jerry L. Knirk, Robert Miegel, Mark Steiner, and Craig Stirrat.

Sledge had previously recruited Myron Spector, PhD, as director of orthopedic research at the BWH in 1987. Spector remained director until 2002, when he became director of tissue engineering at the VAMC in Boston. Other members of the orthopaedic research laboratories during the transition in 1998 included: Julie Glowacki (skeletal biology), Hu-Ping Hsu (joint biomechanics), Schuichi Mizuno (collagen regeneration), Anuj Bellare (polyethylene wear), and Sonya Shortkroff. In 2000, I recruited Dr. Chris Evans and Dr. Steve Ghivizzani to the BWH to establish a Center for Molecular Orthopaedics. Dr. Thornhill hired Dr. Mark Brezinski, a cardiologist and expert on optical coherence tomography (OCT), to study in vivo articular cartilage imaging.

Major initiatives to increase the Brigham's clinical footprint also began in 1999. The orthopaedic facilities included: The Brigham and Women's Ambulatory Care Center (850 Boylston), which focused on sports medicine and rehabilitation, the merger with the Faulkner Hospital which housed the Foot and Ankle Center (Dr. Mike Wilson was chief of orthopaedics), a new consolidated unit of the Orthopedic and Arthritis Center at Braintree HealthSouth Hospital (rehabilitation), and a few years later the Brigham and Women's/Mass General Health Care Center in Foxboro (clinic and ambulatory surgery center), next to the Patriots Gillette Stadium.

In 2003, Dr. Thornhill briefly summarized the department's growth in the *Orthopaedic Journal at Harvard Medical School*:

> The Department's volume of office visits and surgical procedures has grown considerably, particularly in the area of ambulatory surgery. Total office visits from FY 98 through FY 02 increased 31%. While 97% of these visits took place at the Ambulatory Building at the BWH in FY 98, the Department's ambulatory practice is now spread across five locations—the BWH campus, 850 Boylston, Braintree,

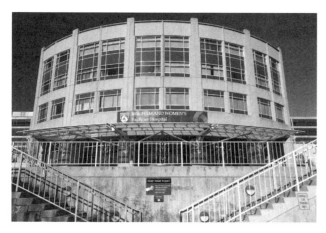

BWH: Faulkner Hospital, 1153 Centre Street, Jamaica Plain, MA. Len Rubinstein.

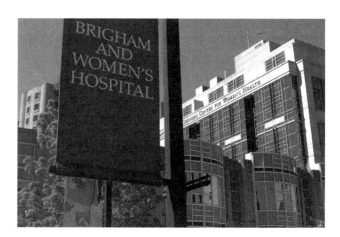

BWH: Facility built in 1994 was renamed the Mary Horrigan Conner's Center for Women's Health in 2002. Brigham and Women's Hospital.

Faulkner Hospital and the New England Baptist Hospital, with BWH visits representing an estimated 80% of total visits... The total number surgical procedures performed increased by 39% from FY 98 through FY 02. The increase in inpatient procedures over this period was just 6.4% indicative of a saturated inpatient infrastructure [similar problem three decades before at both the RBBH and PBBH], while the number of outpatient surgical procedures doubled from a relatively small base in FY 98... in FY 98 outpatient surgery represented only 28% other department's surgical procedures as compared to 43% in 2002... We have had substantial growth at these satellite locations... Of significant concern to the growth of our surgical practice is the availability of OR space at the Brigham for both inpatient and outpatient procedures... clearly an escalating problem given the shift to ambulatory surgery as a standard for many procedures. Beginning in February 2002, the Hospital reached an agreement with New England Surgicenter to utilize its facilities. Our surgeons did 554 outpatient surgeries... [there] from February through September 2002, compared to 1188 for the full year at Faulkner Hospital and FY 02.

BWH hired excellent clinical surgeons (see **Box 50.1**) to provide cutting-edge musculoskeletal care and surgery as well as clinical research. They established a broad base of basic science

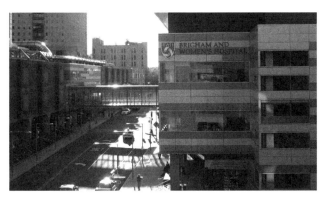

BWH: Bridge to the Carl J. and Ruth Shapiro Cardiovascular Center; opened in 2008. Brigham and Women's Hospital.

Box 50.1. Clinical and Research Faculty

Professorships at BWH

- John Ball and Buckminster Brown Professorship:
  - Robert W. Lovett 1915–1924 (Boston Children's Hospital)
  - Robert B. Osgood 1924–1931 (Boston Children's Hospital)
  - Frank R. Ober 1937–1946 (Boston Children's Hospital
  - Joseph S. Barr 1947–1964 (MGH)
  - Clement B. Sledge 1978–2000 (BWH)
  - Thomas S. Thornhill 2000–present (BWH)

- Robert W. Lovett Professorship:
  - Christopher H. Evans 2001–2008
  - Elena Losina 2018–present

Research Laboratories/Centers

- Musculoskeletal (MSK) Research Center
- Orthopaedic and Arthritis Center for Outcomes Research. Director: Jeffrey N. Katz; Co-Director: Elena Losina
- Skeletal Biology Laboratory. Director: Julie Glowacki
- Center for Molecular Orthopaedics. Director: Christopher H. Evans
- Cartilage Repair Center. Director: Thomas Minas
- Tissue Engineering Laboratory, VA Medical Center. Director: Myron Spector

Clinical Faculty (at the turn of the twentieth century)

Thomas S. Thornhill (Chairman), Robert Poss, Richard Scott, Barry P. Simmons, Gregory W. Brick, Jonathan L. Schaffer, Charles H. Brown Jr., Daniel M. Estok II., James H. Herndon, Jon J.P. Warner, Mark J Koris, Scott D. Martin, Tamara L. Martin, Tom Minas, Richard M. Ozuna, John E. Ready, Michael G. Wilson, R. John Wright, James P. Ioli

Harvard Vanguard Medical Associates: Robert Chernack, John A. K. Davies, Jerry L. Knirk, Robert E. Miegel, Mark E. Steiner, Craig R. Stirrat

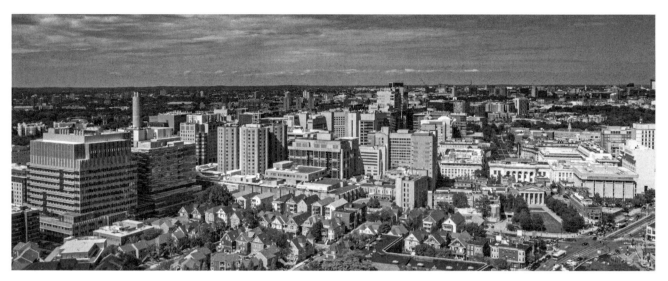

Aerial view of BWH. Jim Rathmell.

research laboratories focusing on biology and molecular biology of musculoskeletal tissues, and they had hired preeminent orthopaedic chairmen to lead these efforts (**Box 50.2**). The Department of Orthopaedic Surgery at the BWH is well-prepared to continue its clinical practice and research as well as its modern educational programs through the remainder of the twenty-first century.

Box 50.2. Brigham And Women's Hospital Orthopaedic Chairmen

RBBH

- Charles F. Painter, ca. 1912–1917
- Loring T. Swaim, ca. 1917–1938
- John G. Kuhns, 1939–1962
- Theodore A. Potter, 1962–1969
- Clement Sledge, 1970–1980

PBBH

- William T. Green, 1951–1968
- Henry H. Banks, 1968–1970
- Clement Sledge, 1970–1980

BWH

- Clement Sledge, 1980–1996
- Robert Poss, 1996 (interim)
- Thomas S. Thornhill, 1997–

Section 7

Beth Israel Deaconess Medical Center

"And whoever saves a life, it is considered as if he saved an entire world."
—Mishnah Sanhedrin 4:9, *Yerushalmi Talmud*, Tractate Sanhedrin 37a.

"There are in round numbers in the United States 50 Jewish hospitals. It seems surprising that New England, the first permanently settled portion of the United States and always one of the most thickly populated and maintaining the traditions of the best culture and the keenest public spirit, would be without a similar institution and our surprise is intensified when we realize that Boston is one of the four leading ports of entry for Jewish immigrants into this country, and that within 50 miles of the State House live nearly 5% of all the Jews in the United States. It cannot therefore be explained by lack of numbers. It cannot be for lack of funds, for some of the best hospitals mentioned are supported by annual subscriptions of from twenty-five cents to five dollars. It cannot be for lack of usefulness, for in spite of the fact that Boston has plenty of other hospitals, Jewish patients flock to our humble doors, until we can treat no more because we have reached the limit of our capacity. The fact that many of our patients come from surrounding towns and often-times from a considerable distance effectually and practically answers the question of whether the institution is needed"
—**Report of the Superintendent,** *Annual Report, Mount Sinai Hospital 1912*. Boston, MA.

CHAPTER 51

Beth Israel Hospital
The Beginning

At the time of their establishment, Mt. Sinai and Beth Israel hospitals primarily treated Jewish patients, and they paid special attention to non-discrimination in care. During the late-nineteenth century, medical care was limited and "only a few Jewish doctors practiced in Boston" (Linenthal 1990). Furthermore, Jewish doctors were often not allowed to practice in some institutions (including house staff). Care for Jewish patients was available from some private physicians, hospitals, and dispensaries; nevertheless, they often had trouble accessing that care or would avoid it because many Jewish patients spoke only Yiddish, would eat only kosher food—refusing to stay in hospitals without it—and no provisions were made for observance of the Sabbath. Others, however, did seek hospitalization, rarely and reluctantly. Jewish leaders tried several times to affect protocol at Boston City Hospital and the Massachusetts General Hospital; for example, they tried to have separate wards established in the hope they could be cared for by Jewish nurses and be served food in accordance with their religious beliefs. That attempt failed.

> The Jewish physician and the Jewish hospital must be one and inseparable. There exists between a Jewish hospital and the Jewish physician a definite relationship which neither the institution nor the physician can ignore or repudiate, and which must be accepted by both as the only means by which a Jewish hospital may be successfully operated in the interest of those who come to it for relief.
> —Drs. M. E. Barron, B. E. Greenberg, and S. H. Rubin (Committee on Arrangements) to "The Jewish Physicians of Boston." December 3, 1923
> (Quoted in Linenthal 1990, 226)

Surges of immigrants had flooded the northeastern United States throughout the 1800s; large cities like Boston grew even larger as newcomers jostled for space. Many immigrants, strangers in a strange land, clung to the religion and culture of their homeland even as they attempted to assimilate into their new home. The late 1800s saw an influx of Jewish immigrants from eastern Europe, e.g., Poland, and in the 15 years between 1880 and 1895, the Jewish population in the United States increased by 250%. Although many Americans initially viewed these new immigrants as a danger to the US way of life, in the latter half of the century—particularly after the Civil War, in which many Jews served, fighting for the Union—they began to gain acceptance, both politically and socially.

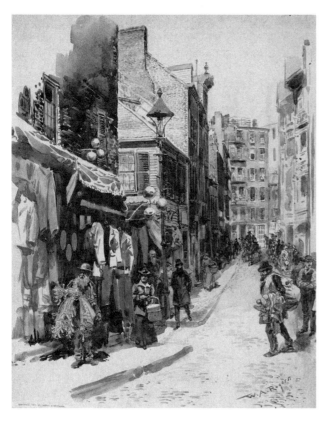

The Jewish Quarter, Boston. Painted by William Allen Rogers, ca. 1899. Street scene in Boston showing crowded street with shoppers, busy shops, and street vendors.
S. Baxter, "Boston at the Century's End," *Harper's Magazine* 1899; 99: 845. Library of Congress.

In the heavily Protestant Boston, however, some groups—mainly Jews and Irish Catholics—had to fight hard to find a balance between their "Americanness" and their religion and culture. Even toward the end of the nineteenth century, they still had not achieved widespread acceptance into American society. In Boston, "most of the new, Jewish immigrants crowded into [the] West End, called the 'Jewish Ghetto,' and into the North End" (Linenthal 1990). But they continued to establish themselves: they began small businesses as tailors, in the shoe and textile arenas, and as doctors, builders, shopkeepers, and lawyers as they also founded charitable organizations, schools, synagogues, and hospitals. This economic spread created a "dynamic ethnic marketplace" (quoted in Dwyer-Ryan 2016) and allowed many Jews to build both reputations and wealth.

The Jewish community also developed numerous humanitarian organizations in the city, including homes for the elderly, orphanages, and, of course, hospitals.

MT. SINAI HOSPITAL

By the summer of 1896, a group of physicians, businessmen, and religious leaders met to begin discussions and planning for a Jewish hospital in Boston. Other cities were opening Jewish hospitals because inpatient care for Jews was difficult and limited and because non-Jewish hospitals would not hire Jewish physicians as members of staff or as private physicians in hospitals. The group appealed for support from the Federation of Jewish Charities, but their proposals were rebuffed. Apparently, the community was not ready for such an endeavor. In November 1897, the physician group formed their own society—the Boston Medical Society—for Jewish and non-Jewish physicians. Their goals were to foster harmonious relations amongst doctors and to support continuing education. They continued attempts to improve medical care for Jewish immigrants.

The number of Jewish physicians continued to slowly increase in Boston, but by 1898 there were still only 36 out of a total of 1550 physicians practicing there. Some had attended medical school in Europe; others graduated from medical schools in New York City. The physicians educated in New York were familiar with the Mt. Sinai Hospital there, which was the first Jewish Hospital in the United States. They were very supportive of establishing a similar hospital in Boston. Jewish physicians and a group of wealthy Jewish leaders next formed "Mt. Sinai Hospital Society of Boston" in November 1901. According to their early records:

> A Hebrew hospital is in contemplation in Boston. In a discussion recently held by the Mt. Sinai Hospital Association, one of the reasons brought forward for the establishment of

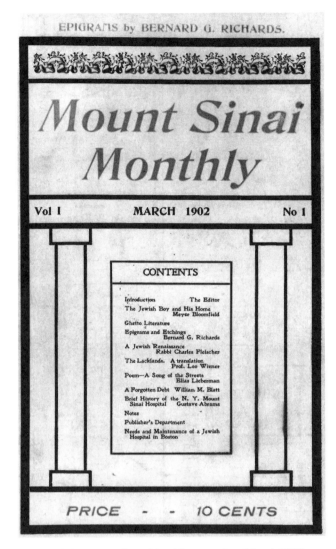

Cover of the *Mount Sinai Monthly* magazine, March 1902.
First a Dream: The History of Boston's Jewish Hospitals by Arthur J. Linenthal. Boston: Beth Israel Hospital in association with the Francis A. Countway Library of Medicine, 1990. The Ruth and David Freiman Archives at Beth Israel Deaconess Medical Center.

Box 51.1. Mt. Sinai Hospital: Chambers Street and Compton Street

> "The Chamber Street rooms consist of the basement and street floor. The street floor is divided into 7 rooms, medical apothecary, surgical, women's department, eye and ear, and nose and throat, also a large waiting room. The basement will be used for storage. The rooms are fitted with the latest improvement in instruments and other needed appliances…The surgical department is also fully equipped, but no major operation will be attempted there for the present…One of the few departures undertaken…is the distribution of literature printed both in Hebrew and English…to assist mothers unused to the care of little ones [and] to tubercular patients consisting of…rules to prevent infection and instruction [of] exercises for the lungs to prevent the progress of the disease…The labels and instructions on all the bottles of medicine…will be printed in Hebrew as well as English to prevent any accident… as has been the case in many instances in [Boston] as other cities on account of the ignorance of the patients of all other languages but their own. The department on Compton Street is also fully equipped…The medical staff…consists of 36 physicians divided between the two places…The physicians of the two departments [West End and South End] will make calls at the home of the patient and the treatment and medicine will be free. Nurses will also be provided in all cases where they will be needed…no charge will be made for medicines and care…an institution of this kind in needed in this city…much relief will be afforded the public institutions which have been patronized until the present time… The physicians who have worked so hard for the success of the institution have not only given their time, but have in many instances given instruments and other useful appliances."
>
> ("For Jew and Gentile Alike" 1902)

such a hospital was the strict adherence of the Hebrews to the laws of diet, which could not be granted them at a public institution. ("Medical Note" 1901)

The official purpose of the Mt. Sinai Hospital Society of Boston was to provide "medical and surgical aid and nursing to sick or disabled persons of any creed or nationality" (Linenthal 1990). It was intended for "the poor and is strictly nonsectarian" ("For Jew and Gentile Alike" 1902). Dr. Thornton Brown, in his Osgood lecture (ca. 1983), commented on the Mt. Sinai Hospital in Boston and noted that it also gave

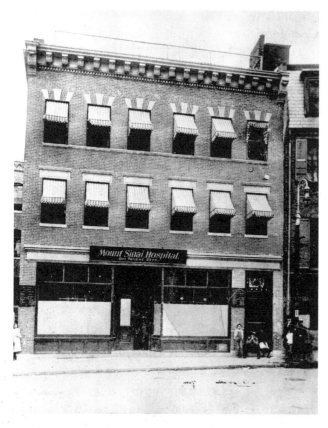

Mt. Sinai Hospital on Chambers Street, West End.
The Ruth and David Freiman Archives at Beth Israel Deaconess Medical Center.

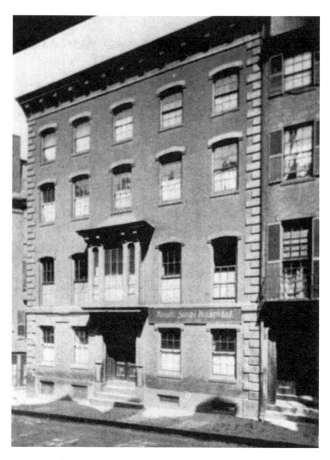

Mt. Sinai Hospital on Compton Street, South End.
The Ruth and David Freiman Archives at Beth Israel Deaconess Medical Center.

Jewish physicians a place to practice. Fundraising was started, planning for a small hospital with 20 beds. The major source of money was to be received from a monthly magazine, *Mount Sinai Monthly*, via membership dues and donations. In the summer of 1902—starting with an outpatient dispensary—the Mt. Sinai Hospital Association opened the hospital at two sites: in rented space at 105 Chambers Street in the West End and at 23 Compton Street in the South End. **Box 51.1** provides a description of the hospital from early records.

As expected, the hospital was very busy. After only one year in operation, the Chambers Street facility became too small, and the hospital moved to a four-story brick building at 17 Staniford Street. The following year, the dispensary started an orthopaedic clinic in 1904. Three years later in 1907, Mr. H. Morrison—a fourth-year student at Harvard Medical School (HMS)—highlighted the impact of stress on illness among Jewish patients as well as misinterpretation of pain symptoms they described. He studied 51 patients with a condition called "Hebraic debility" at the Massachusetts General Hospital. The symptoms of the patients were vague pains, sometimes localized and other times generalized. **Box 51.2** addresses some of Morrison's findings.

By 1910 the medical staff established bylaws, including procedures for new appointments, staff meetings, requirements for new departments and other organizational issues. The secretary of the medical staff at the time was Dr. Albert Ehrenfried (see chapter 52). Ehrenfried, a leading surgeon in Boston who made many contributions to orthopaedic surgery, was a member of the recently formed Boston Medical Society and the American

Box 51.2. Morrison's Description of "Hebraic Debility"

In his findings, Mr. H. Morrison (1907) noted that:

"The history of one of these patients has been summed up as follows: 'She complains of back-ache and everything else.' One of the physicians at the hospital was inclined to think that such symptoms were peculiar to Jews, that they were more than neurasthenic [today considered chronic fatigue syndrome] It has been supposed by some that the adjectives 'brennend' and 'stechend' are peculiar to the symptoms of these Jewish patients, that people of other races do not describe their pain sensations in such terms. I find, however, that they are used idiomatically in Yiddish. Moreover, I have heard not infrequently [that] others than Jews describe their sensations of pain as 'burning' or 'cutting.' Another error due to misinterpretation comes in the localization of the pain. The great majority of these patients speak of 'pain in the heart,' – 'es brennt nicht es stecht nicht mich ins Herzen.' Often this may be translated literally into 'heart-burn.' Much more frequently, however, the term 'heart' covers a larger region, including the whole chest and upper abdomen" (Morrison 1907).

Morrison (1907) continued:

"1. Debility is a common condition among the Jewish patients coming to the Massachusetts General Hospital; as a rule, it is temporary, but is apt to recur.

"2. The prevalent symptoms are pain, constipation and apprehension.

"3. The etiology of these debilitated conditions is to be traced to the peculiar circumstances under which the Jews have lived and still live in eastern Europe. Here in America the economic strain during the early years after arrival is an important factor.

"4. Debility is especially common among the Jewish women of the immigrant class, because the economic strain weighs heavily on them. With them, also, imitation and tradition and the case which medical advice can be obtained are factors to be considered."

He also noted that in addition to this economic stress, issues with communication—understanding and being understood—can complicate the health problems Jewish patients experience. Morrison (1907) concluded that:

"5. These debilities are peculiar not to the Jew, but to the abnormal conditions under which he has been living. As soon as he is relieved from these conditions his symptoms are not different from those of other races.

"6. Finally, in the treatment of these cases considered it is well to bear in mind the importance of the old sentiment, 'not the disease only, but also the man.'"

Jewish Committee. Ranks of the staff included visiting surgeon, assistant visiting surgeon, and graduate assistant.

A STUDY OF FIFTY-ONE CASES OF DEBILITY IN JEWISH PATIENTS.
FROM THE OUT-PATIENT DEPARTMENT, MASSACHUSETTS GENERAL HOSPITAL.
BY H. MORRISON,
Fourth-Year Student at the Harvard Medical School.
BOSTON MEDICAL AND SURGICAL JOURNAL
Vol. CLVII 1907

Title of Morrison's article on debility in Jewish patients.
Boston Medical and Surgical Journal 1907; 157: 816.

Growth in Outpatient Care

Financial troubles had persisted for Mt. Sinai Hospital. By 1905, leaders were concerned whether the dispensary could survive or not, let alone build an inpatient facility; however, over the next decade patient outpatient visits and staff numbers continued to increase. Specialty clinics also increased because of demand. Private specialty physicians charged high fees. Orthopaedics was one of the early specialty clinics opened. By 1908 there were 23 clinics, including a children's clinic, that were staffed by physicians who worked on average in three-month blocks, seeing patients in clinics three times per week. Surgery was performed under ether in multipurpose rooms that were overcrowded. Surgeons complained about unsanitary conditions. It was here that Ehrenfried successfully used an old skin grafting method, called the Reverdin or stamp grafting technique. Fees at the time were 10 cents for an initial or subsequent visit and 50 cents for an operation with ether. That same year, the first teaching service started at Mt. Sinai: an obstetrical service affiliated with Tufts with newly appointed house officers.

Despite promises of support for a new hospital in Mt. Sinai's 1911 annual report, the dispensary's debts precluded the board of directors from moving forward with any such plan. The board decided to wait until it could ensure appropriate funding and support before taking on the development and construction of a contemporary hospital for the city's Jewish population. Despite these obstacles, outpatient visits increased by more than four times between 1905 and 1914, from 6,592 visits to 27,680 visits. Staff grew from 31 in 1906 to 65 by 1916. There were over 120 physicians on staff at various times, of which about 74 were not Jewish. Over half of the physicians had HMS appointments and about 30% had faculty appointments at Tufts School of Medicine. In 1916 the board raised the fees for an initial visit to 25 cents. The community response was a decline of 45% of outpatient visits. Throughout this initial ten years of the dispensary's operation, physicians complained about the lack of inpatient beds.

Orthopaedics

Although we cannot know for sure, it is possible that Dr. Frederic J. Cotton was surgeon-in-chief between 1908 and 1912 at Mt. Sinai. He is described as surgeon-in-chief during those years at Beth Israel Hospital in several obituaries written by Lund and others. However, Beth Israel Hospital did not open until 1917, and I suspect that these comments were about Mt. Sinai Hospital and not Beth Israel Hospital.

Orthopaedic surgeons on staff (all appointed "visiting surgeon, orthopedics") included Dr. Edward A. Tracy (1905–1913), Dr. John D. Adams (1908–1916), and Dr. Louis A. O. Goddu (1913–1916). Clinical educational meetings held in orthopaedics during this period included:

- "Functional Spine" on March 13, 1910 led by John D. Adams with Ehrenfried and others
- "Mechanism of the Dislocation of the Peroneal Tendons" on March 15, 1911, by E. A. Tracy
- "Osteomyelitis with Bone Transplantation" on February 18, 1912 led by F. A. Hamilton with Ehrenfried

Drs. Adams, Ehrenfried, and Goddu also each published one paper on orthopaedics, and Dr. Tracey published four papers on orthopaedics. Orthopaedic treatments had increased since 1904 (**Table 51.1**).

Table 51.1. Orthopaedic Treatments at Mt. Sinai Hospital, 1904–1913

Year	Treatments, n
1904	15
1905	23
1906	12
1907	68
1908	85
1909	196
1910	122
1911	178
1912	205
1913	175

Advocacy for Inpatient Care and the Shuttering of Mt. Sinai

Conventional wisdom held that Boston had sufficient hospital beds to meet the needs of the community, but the Beth Israel Hospital Association, founded in 1911, pointed out that observant Jews needed a hospital where they could get kosher food, respect other relevant traditions, as well as experience an atmosphere that was not hostile to their needs or even frankly antisemitic. Physicians, as always, wanted a total Jewish hospital with inpatient beds and outpatient clinics. Ehrenfried was very involved, both as secretary of the medical staff and as chair of the executive committee of the Federated Jewish Charities. He was aware of the need for a total hospital, but he knew that raising the necessary money would be difficult. The hospital's board was also aware of the community's desire for a complete hospital: "The cry has been louder and more insistent than ever for the establishment of a Jewish Hospital in Boston" (Linenthal 1990). The board was supportive, but took no action, year after year.

Financial difficulties had continued for Mt. Sinai Hospital. In May 1915, the board voted to close it. The fire department also condemned its building. By 1916, the Welfare Committee reported to the board that "investigation…had disclosed 'errors and defects in management and administration' and considerable 'time, labor and earnest thought' had been given to devising a remedial plan" to cover the hospital's debt and continuing expenses (Linenthal 1990). The dispensary closed in 1916 as well, transferring all of its furnishings to the Beth Israel Hospital Association.

BETH ISRAEL HOSPITAL

The Beth Israel Hospital Association was established in 1911, four years before the Mt. Sinai Hospital was officially closed. It raised $8,000 between 1911 and 1915 from doctors and other donors. Incorporated on December 6, 1915:

> Certificate of Incorporation [was] issued by Commonwealth of Massachusetts to 204 women and 27 men who had associated themselves with the intention of forming a corporation under the name The Beth Israel Hospital Association, for the purpose of establishing, supporting and managing an institution to be known as the Beth Israel Hospital, and the affording medical and surgical aid and nursing to sick or disabled persons of any creed or nationality. (Dana 1950)

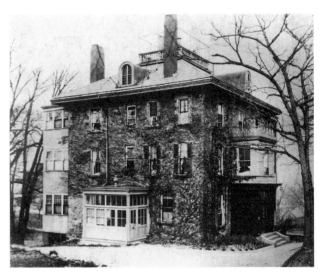

Original BI Hospital on Townsend Street, 1917. The Ruth and David Freiman Archives at Beth Israel Deaconess Medical Center.

The Association then purchased the old Dennison estate at 45 Townsend Street in Roxbury, which was on the edge of an area with a large Jewish population. The Association converted the house to a 45-bed hospital and opened in 1917. The mortgage had been previously paid off in March 1916 with the assistance of Dr. Ehrenfried who "had acquired considerable experience in the construction and administration of hospitals, was largely responsible for the final design and layout of the institution" (Dana 1950).

On February 4, 1917, the Beth Israel Hospital admitted its first patient. This was approximately eight months after Mt. Sinai Hospital closed, ending any significant competition for Beth Israel. The Jewish population in the area had also grown to 80,000 (10% of the total population). The new hospital ensured a focus on the main nonmedical needs of Jewish patients—namely, helping them adjust to customs and language, and providing

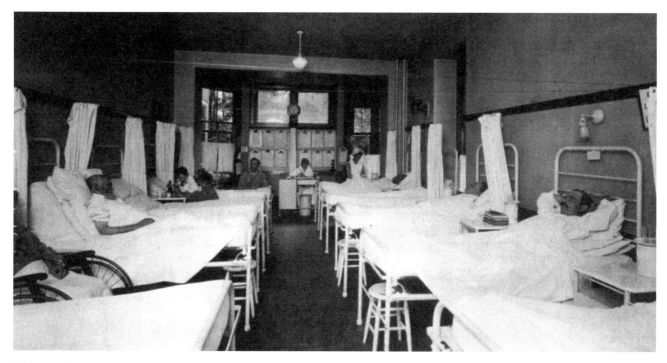

Male ward in the BI Hospital on Townsend Street. The Ruth and David Freiman Archives at Beth Israel Deaconess Medical Center.

Kosher food. In turn they received thanks from patients, who were "happy...to have been in a hospital among their own people" (quoted in Vogel 1980).

Leadership and Staff

The new hospital was busy from the day it opened the doors. Dr. Isidore D. Bronfin (from New York's Beth Israel Hospital) was named the new superintendent (administrative head of the hospital) and resident physician (supervised medical conduct). He was an ex officio member of the medical executive committee; Dr. Ehrenfried had been elected chairman. The first meeting of the staff (49 members; 25 had been on the staff of Mt. Sinai Hospital) took place at the Elysium Club on June 25, 1917. Dr. Ehrenfried opened the meeting with the following remarks:

> This meeting place will bring to many of us here, pleasant recollections of the Clinical Meetings of the Staff of the old Mount Sinai Hospital, a lobby of devoted and loyal men who labored for years to establish a Jewish hospital in Boston. It is to be hoped that the present staff organization will carry on this project with the same devotion, the same loyalty, and the same high idealism. (Linenthal 1990)

After three years, the staff included the best of the Jewish physicians in Boston. Dr. Ehrenfried—a busy surgeon (who performed 303 operations under ether in one year) and a teacher and writer (who taught anatomy and surgical technique at HMS)—had accepted one of the top three positions on the surgical staff at the new Beth Israel Hospital. Ehrenfried "had been an active laboratory and clinical investigator. A reviewer of his 1915 translation of a German surgical text-book had characterized him as 'a young man of ability and tireless activity.' His bibliography numbered 22 publications. Two were books: as junior author with Dr. [LeRoi] Crandon" (Linenthal 1990).

Beth Israel Hospital

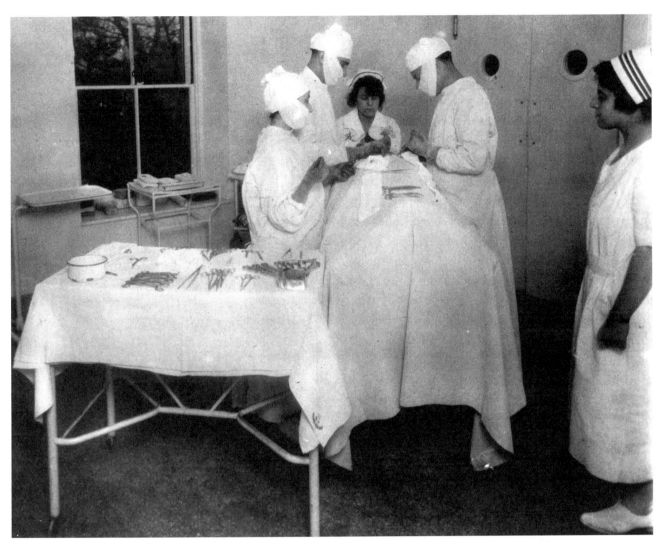

Sole operating room in the BI Hospital on Townsend Street. The Ruth and David Freiman Archives at Beth Israel Deaconess Medical Center.

Two other candidates were selected from Boston City Hospital: Drs. LeRoi G. Crandon and David D. Scannell. Each was appointed visiting surgeon-in-chief in 1917. Another surgeon considered was Dr. Frederic J. Cotton (appointed consultant surgeon in 1920). A medical advisory board of 12 physicians (including Dr. Ehrenfried) wrote the staff bylaws and copied the department organizational structure from Mt. Sinai. In April 1918, an executive committee of four members was formed. Dr. Ehrenfried was a member "with authority to name consultants and assistants" (Dana 1950). His office was in the Back Bay. There were also two resident house staff.

Early Facilities and Departments

The new hospital had 45 beds with a staff room, an operating room, ether and recovery rooms, an x-ray department, a laboratory, and a sun parlor for convalescent patients. Mt. Sinai Hospital's equipment that was "not being used, such as furniture, drugs and surgical apparatus, was turned over to the Beth Israel Hospital" (Dana 1950). Just two years after admitting its first patient, "the inadequacy of the remodeled main building had become apparent...At the end of 1918, the medical executive committee reported that the structure was 'already outgrown[and a] new, adequate, well-ventilated ward building' was essential and space was desperately needed for an out-patient department [but] sufficient money was a problem..." (Linenthal 1990).

The surgical departments at the time included surgery; diseases of the eye; and diseases of nose, throat and ear. Outpatient surgical clinics included surgery, genitourinary, and gynecology. There were no orthopaedic departments, outpatient clinics, or orthopaedic committees. However, a board of consultants was also approved—to include other specialties in medicine and surgery. Orthopaedics was one of the specialties. The first orthopaedic consultant appointed was Robert W. Lovett in 1919 (1919–1923). **Box 51.3** includes a list of the orthopaedic surgeons at Beth Israel Hospital appointed between 1919 and 1928.

Ehrenfried urged the medical staff to organize and work collaboratively with the executive committee for the benefit of the hospital. A period of reorganization then took place. Bronfin founded a nursing school where Jewish women could study to become nurses, providing a new career option for them. He also established a social service department. A real visionary, he urged that the hospital affiliate with a medical school as a teaching hospital. Medical schools had begun requiring a one-year internship in a recognized hospital as a requirement for receiving an MD degree; he appreciated the importance of Beth Israel becoming a hospital that medical students desired to work in as interns. The new Beth Israel Hospital was inspected by the American College of Surgeons, receiving a "Grade A" classification; meaning that they could participate in Surgical Congresses.

In 1920, "a system of staggered appointments of the two house officers" (see **Box 51.4**) was established and continued until 1928 (Linenthal 1990). That same year, continuing education meetings were started. On February 28, 1922, Drs. Torr W. Harmer, Arthur W. Allen, and Carl Bearse lectured on traumatic surgery and infections

Box 51.3. Orthopaedic Surgeons Appointed Between 1919 and 1928

Consultant, Orthopedics

- Robert W. Lovett 1919–1923
- Elliott G. Brackett 1928–
- Robert B. Osgood 1928–
- Charles F. Painter 1928–

Orthopedic surgeon, Out-Patient

- Maxwell H. Bloomberg 1928–
- Samuel L. Marnoy 1928–

Orthopedic surgeon

- Armin Klein 1923–1928

Assistant visiting orthopedic surgeon

- Armin Klein 1928–
- Myron A Strammer 1928–

Visiting orthopedic surgeon

- Mark H. Rogers 1928–

(Linenthal 1990)

in the hand. Dr. Carl Bearse held an operative clinic on early locomotion after leg amputation. During this period, Ehrenfried also arranged a program, including operative clinics, which was acceptable to the college (which approved and suggested) that Beth Israel's staff meetings be more "analytical...[that] the goal of the organized Staff, and indeed, the aim of the standardization program, is the analysis of the hospital's results." The staff meeting was considered the "pivot upon which the success or failure of hospital standardization turns..." (Linenthal 1990). By early 1923 Dr. Ehrenfried was appointed chairman of the monthly meetings.

Box 51.4. House Officers at Beth Israel

"During the first six months, the house officer was the 'Junior' and had charge of the medical cases. He examined the patients, did…special tests, and kept the medical records. He was also responsible for the medical cases when the visiting physician was not in the hospital. If his service was satisfactory, he was promoted to 'Senior' for the second six months. Then, in addition to doing the regular examinations and tests, he kept the surgical records and was responsible for the surgical cases when the visiting surgeon was not present. He also directed preoperative preparations and postoperative treatments, assisted in major operations, and performed minor surgery. According to the American College of Surgeons, each house officer was expected to gain experience in 'performance of circumcision, tonsillectomy, paracentesis for acute suppurative otitis media, empyema and ascites, herniotomy, appendectomy and treatment of varicose veins, varicocele, hydrocele, burns and fractures and skin grafting, venesection, intravenous administration of saloarsan, transfusion and hypodermoclysis and regulation of a Murphy drip.'"

(Linenthal 1990)

Continued Growth and the Establishment of New Facilities

In 1919—only two years after the hospital had admitted its first patient—relations of the medical staff and Dr. Bronfin, as well as with the Board of Directors, were strained. Dr. Bronfin was frequently absent from medical staff meetings and the medical staff were upset that the board "never invited the Medical Executive Committee to cooperate with it on the problems of the hospital… there was no one qualified to advise the Board, though the Medical Executive Committee [has] intimate knowledge of such matters [and] the situation has consequently become intolerable to us" (Linenthal 1990). Beginning in 1918, Dr. Ehrenfried had previously submitted his resignation on at least three occasions (see **Box 51.5**).

Box 51.5. Dr. Albert Ehrenfried's Attempts at Resignation

First Instance of Resignation

"The first instance was in April 1918 soon after he and three other doctors had been asked to help reorganize the hospital…Dr. Ehrenfried had wanted the board to appoint a chief of medicine and a chief of surgery. The board…decided not to do so."

Second Instance of Resignation

"The second occasion had involved differing ideas about the hospitals' long-range goals. In 1921 [he and three other physicians] had been asked to recommend such goals and to develop plans for the hospital's expansion. When they reported early in 1922, Dr. Ehrenfried wrote a minority report. Unlike the three other doctors, he did not identify research as an important hospital function, he argued against affiliation with a medical school, and he thought that the expansion should be on Townsend Street rather than in the Longwood area. The board… accepted the majority report…"

Third Instance of Resignation

"[T]he third occasion had involved the question of 'seniority' on the various services…Ehrenfried thought that a 'seniority system' was needed before…provisions for teaching could…be made. [The board] felt…that Dr. Ehrenfried's interpretation of seniority had 'no place in the Hospital at the present time,' [that there was] no connection between the issue of seniority and the question of teaching…'if any member of the staff has an opportunity…to teach in the Beth Israel Hospital, it would be the duty of the Medical Executive Committee to make provisions for the same, no matter how great the sacrifice…because…that was one of the justifications for the existence of a Jewish hospital.'"

(Linenthal 1990)

"From the outset of the reorganization, Beth Israel had had about twice as many surgical as medical patients," and throughout these tumultuous circumstances, the hospital experienced a period of tremendous growth in overall patient volume (Linenthal 1990). According to Linenthal (1990):

> Even in the early 1920s, the number of surgical patients and the number of operations increased so as to tax the facilities of the hospital. The proportion of private patients also increased... Despite the medical executive committee's [chairman: Dr. Ehrenfried] early plea...a second operating room was not constructed.

Simultaneously, in 1920, "the capacity of the hospital was 'taxed to its utmost limits' and there was a long list of patients waiting to be admitted" (Linenthal 1990). The following year "a subcommittee consisting of Drs. Ehrenfried, Linenthal, Rosenau and Solomon was appointed to recommend definite plans [for a new hospital]" (Linenthal 1990). **Box 51.6** details their reports. The board accepted the majority report and began a major fund-raising campaign: "Agreement was reached on the number of beds... about 150 beds: 90 (60%) for ward patients, and 60 (40%) for private patients [plus] a maternity unit [with] a total of 350...seen as a future goal" (Linenthal 1990).

During this period, Ehrenfried offered his final (and fourth) resignation on December 31, 1923. In November, he had resigned from the building committee, which "had signaled a lessening of his intense interest in the hospital...The committee was to meet with the architects [about the proposed new buildings]...Although Dr. Ehrenfried had been very much interested in just such details, and had even worked with an earlier architect to develop such plans, he resigned from the committee on the day before the meeting" (Linenthal 1990). When Ehrenfried submitted his final resignation, he "was almost forty-years old, had been a major figure in the Jewish hospital movement since 1907, and was the outstanding Jewish surgeon in Boston...[The board asked him to meet with a special committee, but

Box 51.6. Subcommittee Reports for the Establishment of a New Hospital Location

> "After nine months of study, this subcommittee presented two reports early in January 1922: a majority report...and a minority report by Dr. Ehrenfried. The majority report reaffirmed the primary purpose of the hospital...'to care for the sick.' In addition...the doctors identified other valuable hospital functions...that Beth Israel 'stimulate investigation and research' and 'offer facilities for the teaching and training of medical students and physicians. To facilitate these activities, and for various other reasons, the majority [report] recommended that the hospital move to the 'Medical Center [in] the vicinity of the Harvard Medical School'... In his minority report, Dr. Ehrenfried disagreed with the other [three] doctors about these important issues. He did not identify research as a hospital function that should be developed; he did not mention medical student teaching, although he supported the training of 'graduates in medicine – as house officers;' and he thought that the new buildings should be on Townsend Street."
>
> (Linenthal 1990)

he] declined [stating] 'I refuse to be a party in any argumentative debate on hospital policy'" (Linenthal 1990).

"On February 13, 1924, the board appointed a committee to purchase sufficient land for new buildings in the Longwood area" to fulfill their dreams of a modern facility (Linenthal 1990). In less than three weeks, they bought "333,000 square feet of land...on Brookline Avenue, extending south to within 300 feet of the corner of Longwood Avenue (Linenthal 1990). Following the purchase, the 'Breaking of Ground' [occurred] on Sunday afternoon, October 5 [and actual] work at the site started about one month after the ceremonial ground breaking" (Linenthal 1990).

Meanwhile, because "none of the patients paid the full cost of care...about $6 per day in

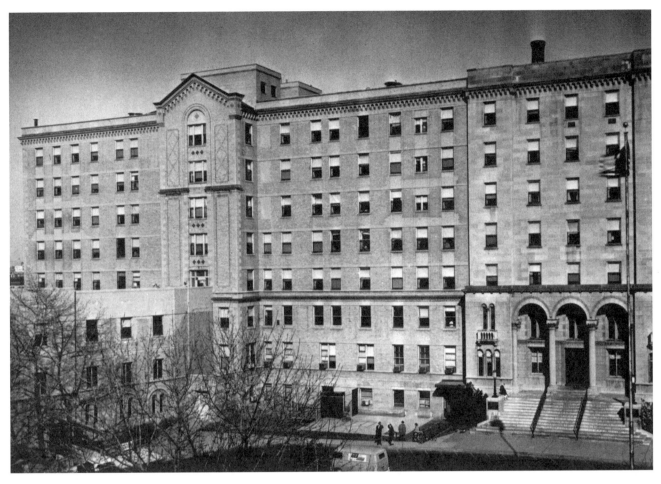

Beth Israel Hospital at its new location on Brookline Avenue, 1928. The Ruth and David Freiman Archives at Beth Israel Deaconess Medical Center.

1924 [$83 in 2014]" the hospital's financial solvency became problematic (Linenthal 1990). At the time, "Approximately seventy percent [of patients] were 'ward' patients [who] occupied beds in the two large wards, their care was the responsibility of doctors on the visiting staff or associate staff who received no compensation for this service…About forty percent paid nothing…approximately thirty percent…were 'private'" (Linenthal 1990).

Three years after the groundbreaking ceremony, a committee was appointed to begin "the formal process of organizing a medical staff for the larger hospital" (Linenthal 1990). That committee determined that "the Out-Patient Department shall not be a separate entity, but shall be cared for by the staff of the hospital" (Linenthal 1990).

They also reversed the decision of the 1918 reorganization and began the process of appointing chiefs of service, and thereafter "the medical executive committee recommended the 'single chief system'…one Chief of the Medical Service…One Chief of the Surgical Service [and] two or more visiting surgeons and a suitable number of visiting specialists…also…assistant visiting…surgeons as well as assistant visiting specialists…" (Linenthal 1990).

The first chief of the new surgical service was Dr. Wyman Whittemore. There were two surgical specialty services: urology as well as nose and throat. Orthopaedic surgery was not mentioned. By August 1928—the date Beth Israel opened to patients at its new location on Brookline Ave– there were 163 physicians on the staff at Beth

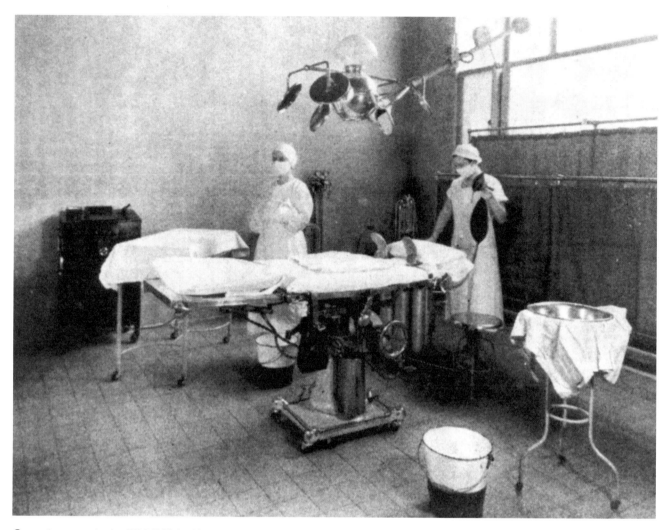

Operating room in the BIH 1928 building. The Ruth and David Freiman Archives at Beth Israel Deaconess Medical Center.

Israel Hospital and 14 house staff positions. Many had been on the staff of Mt. Sinai Hospital. The age limit for medical staff was 62 years.

On April 16, 1928—about two months after Beth Israel moved—the Roxbury Ladies' Bikur Cholim Association purchased the original Townsend Street property and named the 42-bed hospital the Greater Boston Bikur Cholim Hospital. This new hospital "provided medicine, money, prayer and support to those who lacked medical care…the hospital was primarily a custodial institution accepting patients other hospitals were no longer able to keep" ("Guide to the Records of the Jewish Memorial Hospital and Rehabilitation Center" 2017).

In 1937, the Greater Boston Bikur Cholim Hospital changed its name to the Jewish Memorial Hospital. Over the next six decades the hospital's services continued to expand, and in 1992 the hospital's name changed again—to the Jewish Memorial Hospital and Rehabilitation Center. As the 1990s continued the center experienced ongoing financial losses, and it was eventually bought out by Radius Management Services; under the new management the organization had 207 beds for patients with chronic conditions and those who needed rehabilitation (Rowland 2005). Despite the new management, the hospital (then called Radius Specialty Hospital) remained unprofitable and closed in 2014.

Beth Israel Hospital

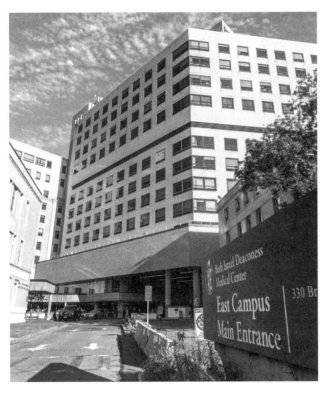

BIDMC East Campus. Kael E. Randall/Kael Randall Images.

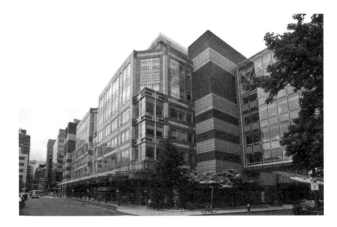

BIDMC West Campus. Bruce R. Wahl/Media Services, Beth Israel Deaconess Medical Center.

Affiliation with Harvard Medical School and Tufts College Medical School

Early in its founding, the leadership at Beth Israel Hospital strongly desired to have the hospital become a teaching hospital of HMS. Dr. David L. Edsall had become part time dean at HMS after Dr. Edward Bradford retired in 1918. (Although Edsall became dean when the medical school was in deficit, some ten years later he had balanced the budget.) He was named a consultant at Beth Israel shortly thereafter, and he began a series of discussions over the next decade with the leaders at Beth Israel. He believed "that 'a medical school should have more than one university hospital and should make every effort to have as much clinical material available as it could...The strength of Harvard', he maintained, 'lay in having several very good hospitals'" (Linenthal 1990).

Four years later and at the same time they had purchased land for a new facility, Beth Israel wanted "to stimulate investigation and research" and "to offer facilities for the teaching and training of medical students" (Linenthal 1990). Another five years later:

> the hospital agreed to provide a salary for a full-time doctor in charge of such research and teaching; to provide space and financial support for his research department, to provide an office and examining room where he could see private patients, to permit him to keep the fees from these patients, to make the wards and out-patient department available for teaching, and to work "conjointly...with the University authorities" in appointing the staff to carry out these functions. (Linenthal 1990)

That year orthopaedics was listed for the first time as an outpatient clinic in the new hospital. The 1928 Harvard Medical School catalogue contained the following description of Beth Israel Hospital:

> The Beth Israel Hospital – This is a newly completed general hospital with a capacity of 180 beds, 102 [sic] of which are available for teaching. The institution is located on Brookline Avenue around the corner from the Harvard Medical School. The hospital is equipped for teaching and research, having a medical

research and pathological laboratory, each under the direction of a full-time physician who is associated with the Faculty of the Harvard Medical School There are also electrocardiograph and basal metabolism laboratories, animal research equipment, and an extensive X-ray department. There are eighteen pediatric beds. An out-patient department, capable of serving over twenty thousand patients per year, will have the following clinics: medicine, surgery, pediatrics, gynaecology, dermatology, genitourinary diseases, ophthalmology, otolaryngology, neurology and orthopedics. (Linenthal 1990)

Also in 1928, Beth Israel Hospital completed an affiliation agreement with Tufts College Medical School (**Box 51.7**). The plan proposed by the Dean at Tufts was accepted by Beth Israel with three provisions, including: "Assignment of teaching positions are understood not to be exclusive in the department as against appointees from other schools if in the judgment of the hospital, it is felt advisable to extend the teaching concurrently with other schools" (Linenthal 1990).

Today Beth Israel Deaconess Medical Center (created from the merger of Beth Israel Hospital and New England Deaconess Hospital [see chapter 56]) remains a major teaching hospital of HMS with the hospital's physician practice group, Harvard Medical Faculty Physicians (HMFP). It provides patient care, teaching, and research services through 13 departments, each under the leadership of a chairperson. It also remains affiliated with Tufts University School of Medicine mainly through its affiliate, the New England Baptist Hospital. Future affiliates included the Winchester Hospital and the Lahey Hospital and Medical Center.

Box 51.7. Beth Israel's Affiliation Agreement with Tufts College Medical School

> "On February 23, 1928, Dean Albert Warren Stearns [dean of Tufts College Medical School, 1927–1945] wrote to Mr. Louis E. Kirstein [chairman of both the executive committee of the board, BIH, and the committee on medical school affiliations]: At the present time, Tufts College Medical School wishes to avail itself of teaching privileges in the following departments: Medicine, Surgery, Pediatrics, Urology and Orthopedics…Our present plan is to appoint one man in each of these departments (preferably the head of the department) to the staff of the Medical School. This man will have entire charge of teaching in his department…We should suggest that, in the event of future vacancies in those teaching positions, no appointments be made except by the mutual consent of the Trustees of Beth Israel Hospital and Tufts College Medical School… At the present time, we wish to appoint the following members of the staff of the Beth Israel Hospital to serve as teaching heads at the hospital…Dr. Mark Homer Rogers – Orthopedics…"
>
> (Linenthal 1990)

CHAPTER 52

Albert Ehrenfried

Surgeon Leader at Mount Sinai and Beth Israel Hospital

Albert Ehrenfried was born in Lewiston, Maine, on February 9, 1880; he was "the son of George and Rachel (Blauspan) Ehrenfried" ("Albert Ehrenfried Papers. Manuscript Collection No. 28," n.d.). He graduated from Boston Latin School in 1898 "after his family moved to Boston in 1895" ("Albert Ehrenfried Papers. Manuscript Collection No. 28." n.d.). He later graduated cum laude in 1902 with an AB degree from Harvard and in 1905 received his MD from Harvard Medical School (HMS). He moved immediately into a position as a house officer on the surgical service at Boston City Hospital, and two years later he became a surgeon in the sanitorium division there. He had also become affiliated with Mount Sinai Hospital in 1907, and joined the Jewish Memorial Hospital as a consulting surgeon and Boston Children's Hospital as an assistant surgeon.

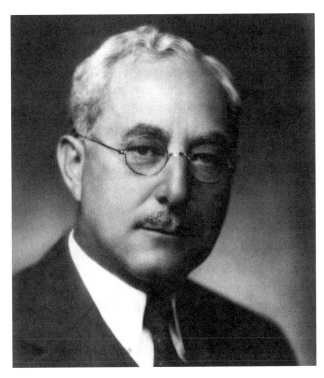

Albert Ehrenfried. The Ruth and David Freiman Archives at Beth Israel Deaconess Medical Center.

EARLY ORTHOPAEDIC CONTRIBUTIONS

Dr. Ehrenfried lived at 33 Centre Street, Brookline; his office was at 362 Commonwealth Avenue. During his experience as a surgeon of the sanitorium division of Boston City Hospital, Ehrenfried cared for patients with active pulmonary tuberculosis, and he also reported on his personal experience with phrenicectomy and his development of an insufflation anesthesia apparatus in 1911. Krause and Heymann (1917) wrote:

> **Physician Snapshot**
>
> Albert Ehrenfried
> BORN: 1880
> DIED: 1951
>
> SIGNIFICANT CONTRIBUTIONS: Innovative surgeon; reported on Ehrenfried's disease (hereditary deforming chondrodysplasia); reintroduced with Dr. Frederic Cotton the Reverdin method of skin grafting; coauthored with Dr. Le Roi G. Crandon *Surgical After-Treatment: A Manual of the Conduct of Surgical Convalescence*, a textbook on the postoperative management of patients; wrote *A Chronicle of Boston Jewry: From the Colonial Settlement to 1900*

The intratracheal insufflation method of anesthesia originated by Meltzer and first employed on human beings by Elsberg of New York, and Ehrenfried of Boston, has many advantages...for intrathoracic surgery, for which it was first devised. The chief difference between this method and that of Kuhn consists in the fact that a single thin lisle or soft-rubber catheter replaces the larger but shorter metal tube...The apparatus of Ehrenfried represents the earliest simplified form of apparatus. It consists of a Wolff bottle with three necks, sitting within a copper waterjacket, which is filled with hot water, and a foot bellows. By means of cocks on the outside of the jacket, the stream of air from the bellows can be carried either through the hot water, over the top of the ether (contained in the Wolff bottle) or can be made to bubble through the ether when a particularly strong vapor is desired...Air and ether can be mixed in any proportion.

In 1909, at the Laboratory of Comparative Physiology at HMS, Dr. W. T. Porter allowed two young physicians, Dr. Ehrenfried and anesthesiologist Dr. Walter M. Boothby, to perfect the technique of vascular anastomosis. They used the abdominal aorta in cats as their model. Dr. E. H. Nichols of the Department of Surgical Pathology assisted in studying the anastomosis in the sacrificed animals. They chose the cat abdominal aorta because it is just slightly larger than the brachial artery and slightly smaller than the femoral artery in humans. They perfected their technique of a continuous running suture (the Carrel method), concluding that extensive practice on animals is necessary in order to master the procedure of end-to-end arterial anastomosis. They then briefly reported the successful use of this method in a patient with a lacerated femoral artery by Drs. L. R. G. Crandon and Ehrenfried.

Early in his career Ehrenfried published several significant papers, including topics addressing club feet, the Reverdin method of skin grafting, the design of an insufflation anesthesia apparatus, and the technique of end-to-end arterial anastomosis. His contributions on club feet (two papers) included his experience in nonoperative treatment, which he presented at the 1909 annual meeting of the American Orthopaedic Association. He concluded:

1. Practically all cases of congenital club foot are curable without operation if taken in hand before the child is six weeks old.

2. The younger the infant at the time of instituting treatment the better.

3. The results are better than if treatment is postponed until operation becomes necessary.

4. The routine treatment consists of manipulation, followed by a plaster bandage, every two weeks, progressively overcorrecting the foot; as soon as the foot offers no resistance to overcorrection and maintains the normal position naturally, continued manipulation, a tin splint to be worn at night, or a brace if the child is old enough to walk.

5. Relapses are bound to occur under any form of treatment if the aftercare is neglected; the patient should be kept under close observation for one year after apparent complete recovery. (Ehrenfried 1909)

Dr. Ehrenfried and Dr. Frederic Cotton (see chapter 59) reintroduced the Reverdin method—a method of using small pinch grafts—in America. Dr. Jaques-Louis Reverdin, a Swiss surgeon, while he was an intern under Guyon in Paris in 1869, had previously observed that "small bits (of about 1 sq. mm.) of epidermis lifted from the skin...and held in place [over granulation tissue]...took root and from them...the epithelium spread to the margin of the [wound]" (Ehrenfried 1909). He called

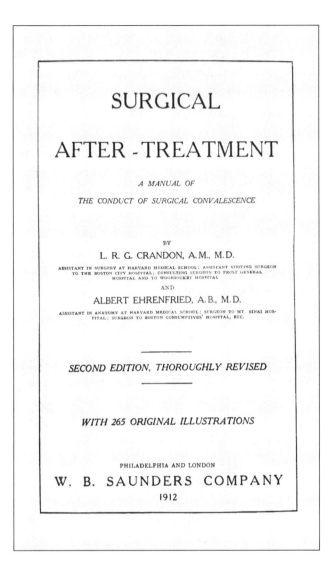

Crandon and Ehrenfried's book about the care of patients after surgery. Philadelphia and London: W. B. Saunders Company, 1912. Author's photo.

this "epidermic grafting" (Ehrenfried 1909). Cotton and Ehrenfried wrote:

> The method...of Reverdin...like many another procedure of demonstrated value...has fallen gradually into disuse, so that, with few exceptions, textbooks...mention it disparagingly, or not at all. More brilliant and complicated methods...have arisen and have occupied the center of the stage until their deficiencies became evident...Now, when ingenuity seems at least to have exhausted itself, it is worthwhile to consider the peculiar advantages of the original and more practically discarded method...[In support of the Reverdin method they summarized:]...It is essentially a minor operative procedure...The procedure is simple and may be performed by one person upon a patient in his bed at home...It entails no involved source of preparation...involves no additional disfigurement of the patient or sacrifice on the part of the patient's family or friends...The after-care is not irksome[and] the likelihood of distressing complications arising is small. (Cotton and Ehrenfried 1909)

The following year, Ehrenfried coauthored a textbook with Crandon on the postoperative management of patients titled *Surgical After-Treatment: A Manual of the Conduct of Surgical Convalescence*. Two years later, a 1912 review of the book's second edition in the *American Journal of Orthopedic Surgery* stated:

> This volume is prepared especially for the use of house-surgeons in hospitals and general practitioners in communities which are not surgical centers. Though the metropolitan surgeon often operates in smaller towns, he leaves the care for after-treatment in the hands of the town physician...This book is written for this man...an elastic, but detailed, set of directions, [for] the handling of patients after surgical treatment...This volume...is to be a guide to... proper methods and to prevent certain mistakes. ("Book Reviews" 1912)

LATER ORTHOPAEDIC CONTRIBUTIONS

Later Ehrenfried became third assistant visiting surgeon at Boston City Hospital in 1913. He was also a visiting surgeon, on the staff of Mt. Sinai Hospital with Cotton (who was in charge of orthopaedics). During this period, Ehrenfried was appointed assistant in anatomy and surgery at HMS and "an instructor of army surgeons during World War I" (S. K. 1951). By 1915, he was appointed first assistant visiting surgeon at Boston City Hospital.

Ehrenfried made his most significant contribution to orthopaedics in the middle of World War I. He reported on hereditary deforming chondrodysplasia, which was a name he gave to a condition previously called multiple cartilaginous exostoses also now known as Ehrenfried's disease. He reported his first case in 1915 (see **Case 52.1**), and he wrote "with the permission of Dr. Lovett, I investigated the case clinically and roentgenologically, and removed a strip of bone from across the affected epiphysis for pathologic study" (Ehrenfried 1917). In his first paper of 1915, he discussed the pathologic findings:

> I have been fortunate...to get a specimen from across the epiphyseal line in a young patient, and this has received careful study at the hands of Dr. Ash of the pathologic department of Harvard. There is no specimen of just this sort, I believe, on record...Under the microscope the resemblance to chondroma is striking. This extends for some distance up the shaft, so that

Case 52.1. Cartilaginous Exostoses in Heredity Chondrodysplasia

> "History – [The patient], white, aged 11, entered the Children's Hospital, November 6, 1914. She was born in Beverly, Mass. Father a French Canadian. Father, mother and six other children living and well. Detailed family history not obtained. She was an 8 months' baby, fourth child and very diminutive. Had breast milk for nine months followed by cow's milk and general table diet. She has always been a weak child. Began to walk at 19 months. Whooping cough the only disease of childhood. The deformity of forearm was first noticed at 6 months; it has become more and more prominent with time. The flatfoot has been noticed since the child began to walk.
>
> "Local: Patient stands with slight left dorsolumbar scoliosis, with both shoulders thrown forward, a mild degree of knock knee on each side, and the feet everted. She walks with a rather uncertain gait, throwing her weight on the inner side of the feet, especially on the right. The face is symmetrical, and shows no deformities. Motions at the right shoulder joint normal. The outline of the right elbow is distorted. The forearm can pronate, supinate, flex and extend normally, but the head of the radius is subluxed outward and is greatly increased in size over normal. Muscle power is good, however. Joint motions are free and there are no contractures. Both bones of the forearm are unusually short and to palpation feel thicker than normal. At the wrist, motions are free. There are no contractures and muscle power is good. The styloid process of the ulna is, however, at least 1 inch above the styloid of the radius and there is a distinct gap below the end of the ulna and wrist joint. The lower ends of both bones are oversize and there is a slight inward bowing of the ulnar at about its lower third. The left arm shows free motions at the shoulder, good muscle power and no contractures. At the elbow the outline of the joint is distorted. The head of the radius is subluxed externally and posteriorly, and is greatly increased in size. The motions of flexion and extension, pronation and supination are free, and there are no contractures. The forearm shows considerable bowing of both bones. At the wrist the ulna is short, the styloid process being at least 1 inch above the radial styloid; the lower ends of both ulnar and radius are increased in size. Muscle power is good in all groups, and there are no contractures. The hands are rather small, and the fists cannot be more than half clenched, on account of the obstruction offered by the enlarged extremities of phalanges and metacarpals. At both hips the trochanters are on Nélaton's line, joint motions are free and muscle power good. At the knees muscle power is good. There are no contractures, and joint motions are free. At the right ankle the internal malleolus is unduly prominent and the whole foot is held everted; joint motions are free, and muscle power good in all groups. There are no contractures. The left ankle is held

the end is usually ballooned out, with a thin irregular cortex, and in the roentgenogram is greatly rarefied, so that it has much the same appearance as a cyst. The cartilage, of course, casts no shadow, and what little ossification there is shows up in fine strands running up and down and obliquely across the irregular cystic space. The Roentgen ray shows the epiphysis to be small or misshapen, the intermediary cartilage narrow, irregular, oblique or zigzag, and sometimes prematurely ossified. Scattered along in the thickened and hyperactive periosteum of the end of the shaft are to be found clumps or nests of cartilage cells, persisting uncalcified where they were left in the process of growth. These groups may develop later into cartilaginous exostoses or chondromas. (Ehrenfried 1915)

> MULTIPLE CARTILAGINOUS EXOSTOSES
> —HEREDITARY DEFORMING CHONDRODYSPLASIA
> A BRIEF REPORT ON A LITTLE KNOWN DISEASE *
> ALBERT EHRENFRIED, M.D.
> Fellow of the American College of Surgeons
> BOSTON
> JOUR. A. M. A.
> MAY 15, 1915
> VOLUME LXIV
> NUMBER 20

Ehrenfried's article in which he first describes multiple cartilaginous exostoses. *Journal of the American Medical Association* 1915; 20: 1642.

---

somewhat in the same position as the right. The internal malleolus is abnormally prominent. There are no contractures and muscle power is good in all groups. Reflexes: Knee jerks present on both sides. No clonus, Babinski, nor Oppenheim. Right arm: acromion to internal condyle 9 ⅛ inches. Left, 9 ¼ inches.

"Left leg: length, 28 ⅛ includes. Circumference: thigh, 12 ¾ inches; calf 8 ¾ inches.

"Roentgenologic Examination: Cranium negative; stella turcica of normal size. Thorax free, except for slight irregularities in lower ribs. Marked lateral curve in lumbar spine. Slight irregularities about sacro-iliac articulations. Both ilia show a peculiar series of radiating striations about the crests. Clavicles and scapulae are free, and the humeral heads show slight thickening. The lower third of the shafts of the humeri show some deviation from normal contour. The circumference is lessened, and the bone is bent. The humeral condyles show mottling. The ulnae are relatively short, bowed concave forward, and at the lower end present a large irregular bulbous enlargement, in which the epiphyseal line is lost. The radii are straight, with the upper end dislocated outward and upward, so as to form a marked projection at the level of the outer condyle. The lower end presents a similar irregular cystic-like enlargement, but the epiphysis is present intact, though relatively small. The entire carpal articulation is carried on the radius. The distal ends of all the metacarpals and the proximal ends of the first two rows of phalanges show the globular striated enlargements referred to. The femoral heads are squat and thick, with flat epiphyses and prominent trochanters. There is mild genu valgum in both legs, and the diaphyseal extremities of tibiae and fibulae are widened and irregularly striated; the fibulae are relatively short, so as to destroy the ankle mortise, and the tarsus is offset outward to create an extreme pes valgus. The heads of the metatarsals, and the proximal metaphyseal extremities of the first phalanges show the globular vacuolated enlargements already seen on the fingers. On the left foot the first and third digits show comparatively slight involvement and are accordingly relatively longer than the other digits.

"The deformities in this case consist in a scoliosis, shortening and bowing of the forearms, ulnar deviation of the hands, dislocation of the heads of the radii, moderate knock knee, extreme tarsal valgus, irregularity in length of toes, and shortness of stature. There are no exostoses, few hyperostoses, and the deformities are symmetrical

"The roentgenograms were taken at the Children's Hospital."

(Ehrenfried 1917)

In his last paper on hereditary deforming chondrodysplasia (published in 1917), he commented that he had seen a total of 22 personal cases and that there were 77 cases reported in the literature (total of 99 cases in the US.). He focused on two issues: heredity and differential diagnosis. He wrote:

> The question of ancestry has definite interest...we find...26 of Dutch origin [,]18 of German[,] 3 of Irish origin, 2 negroes and 1 each Italian, Austrian, English, French-Canadian, and mixed French-Canadian and English. In most of the remaining 45 cases, no statement as to ancestry is made...As to heredity, we can now add two interesting families to those already known. Montgomery's family presents five cases in three generations, and the family...I have reported presents eight cases in three generations...the question of differential diagnosis has arisen. Hereditary deforming chondrodysplasia should not be confused with the developmental exostoses (epiphyseal exostoses, "exostoses de croissance," "Wachstumsexostosen"), which are fairly common, but so little recognized...One is inclined to believe that developmental exostoses represent an abortive type of chondrodysplasia...where the diagnosis is in question, roentgenograms of the entire skeleton should be made. (Ehrenfried 1915)

One year prior to the publication of this last paper, he had joined the staff at BIH as a senior visiting surgeon when it opened in 1916. (Although Dr. Fred Lund, in his obituary of Dr. Cotton, stated that Cotton was chief surgeon at Beth Israel Hospital (BIH) during the years 1908 to 1912, he probably was referring to the Mt. Sinai Hospital. I could find no reference to another chief of orthopaedics after Cotton in 1912 at Mt. Sinai Hospital nor at BIH, although Ehrenfried was one of four doctors on the executive committee of BIH when the medical board reorganized, and the hospital changed management in 1918; a decade later, in 1928, Dr. Mark H. Rogers became chief of the orthopaedic service. There was one reference to an early orthopaedic clinic at Mt. Sinai, but in 1928 when BIH moved to Brookline Avenue in the Longwood area, 11 specialty clinics were opened, including orthopaedics.)

Over his career Ehrenfried had published 15 articles, including six on orthopaedics, two books and edited/translated a third book. Late in his career, he wrote *A Chronicle of Boston Jewry: From the Colonial Settlement to 1900*, which was privately printed in 1963—twelve years after his death—by his daughter Fredrika and her husband Irving Bernstein. The book also focuses on Ehrenfried himself and describes the extent of his civic and professional engagements, examples of which are listed in **Box 52.1**. In a 1965 review of the book, Jacob Neusner explains that according to Albert Ehrenfried's son (George), his father wrote the book to highlight the Jewish people's achievements throughout the twentieth century. Neusner notes Ehrenfried's "graceful" and "careful" writing that moves from describing early Jewish impact in Massachusetts, to their participation in the Revolutionary War, to their movement into other areas of the New England region. Neusner appreciates the book's in-depth treatment of Jewish community and altruistic organizations in Boston as well as its deep dive into the spiritual and intellectual life of a Jew living in Boston in the early twentieth century, which, for Neusner, can be extrapolated to help understand Jewish American life in general at that time.

In late July 1951—the midst of the Korean War—Ehrenfried, as one of the editors of the *Norfolk Medical News*, wrote to the editor of *JAMA* about the lack of physician volunteers for the military. He noted the statistic that by the end of the previous summer (August 1950) only 1 in 3000 physicians not currently in active duty had volunteered to serve, and by April of 1951 only half of those physicians drafted agreed to serve. For Ehrenfield, much of this lack of initiative to

Box 52.1. Albert Ehrenfried's Civic and Professional Engagements

- Examining Committee member, Boston Public Library
- Trustee, Boston Medical Library
- Fellow, American Association for the Advancement of Science
- Fellow, American College of Surgeons
- Counselor, Massachusetts Medical Society
- President, Norwood Medical Society
- Honorary life-president and trustee, Temple Sinai Memberships
- American Genetics Association
- American Eugenics Association
- Bostonian Society
- American Jewish Community
- Phi Rho Sigma medical fraternity
- Tau Epsilon Phi (originally a Jewish fraternity)
- American Medical Association
- Brookline Town meeting
- Boston Medical Library
- American Jewish Historical Society
- Old South Historical Society
- Harvard Club
- Boston Society

serve has been inculcated by deferment programs and spans the entire continuum of the medical field—medical school faculty and instructors; hospital trustees and department and service chiefs; residents, interns, and students; and physicians and surgeons. He emphasized that all needed to share the burden of military service, and that such people should want to serve despite the apparent financial and professional benefits obtained by those who defer. To this end he made three suggestions:

1. allow physicians up to age 55 to be drafted
2. draft more physicians toward the high end of the acceptable age (45–55 years)
3. allow those at medical schools and health care organizations like hospitals time off to serve and a rotation of service

That was Ehrenfried's last publication. He died just two months later, on September 25, 1951, "at Baker Memorial Hospital after a long illness" (S. K. 1951). He was 71 years old. His wife had died six years earlier, in 1946, but he was survived by their three children.

CHAPTER 53

Beth Israel Hospital
Orthopaedic Division Chiefs

Beth Israel Hospital (BIH) was founded in 1911, four years before Mt. Sinai Hospital officially closed. In the beginning (after opening in 1917), it primarily treated Jewish patients and provided more inclusive care than many other hospitals at the time. When Mt. Sinai Hospital shuttered (1916), BIH received many of the dispensary's furnishings and also welcomed many of its physicians to its staff (see chapter 51). Dr. Robert Lovett was the first orthopaedic consultant appointed at BIH, in 1919, but orthopaedics was not listed as a division separate from surgery until 1928. Dr. Mark Rogers served as its first chief of orthopaedics.

The orthopaedic surgeons described in this chapter include those leaders who served as orthopaedic division chief between 1928–1978, followed by a section on Dr. Louis Meeks, who served as acting orthopaedic surgeon-in-chief from 1990 until 1992. Prior to Dr. Meeks, Dr. Augustus White had served as the first orthopaedic surgeon-in-chief of the newly established orthopaedic surgery department from 1978 until 1991 (see chapter 54). Today, BIH has been incorporated into Beth Israel Deaconess Medical Center (see chapter 56). Dr. Stephen Lipson, who served as chief of orthopaedic surgery at BIH from 1992–1996 and then as chief of the department at BIDMC until 2001 is discussed in chapter 55. The orthopaedic chiefs covered in this chapter include:

Surgeon-in-Chiefs	
Mark H. Rogers	224
Armin Klein	231
Meier G. Karp	240
Robert Ulin	242
Seymour Zimbler	245
Harris S. Yett	250
Louis W. Meeks	254

MARK H. ROGERS

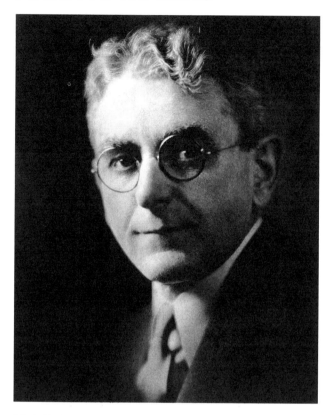

Mark H. Rogers. "Centennial Celebration of the *JBJS* 1903–2003," *Journal of Bone and Joint Surgery* 2003: 10.

Physician Snapshot

Mark H. Rogers
BORN: 1877
DIED: 1941
SIGNIFICANT CONTRIBUTIONS: Orthopaedic division chief at Beth Israel Hospital 1928–1941; first editor of the *American Journal of Orthopaedic Surgery*; orthopaedic chief at MGH on two separate occasions; professor and chairman of the orthopaedic division at Tufts University School of Medicine; convinced that tuberculosis of joints initially began in the synovium followed by the bone and not vice-versa, which was commonly believed at the time

Mark Homer Rogers was born in South Sudbury, Massachusetts, on May 21, 1877, and he went to the Boston Latin School in the city. He later attended Williams College in Williamstown, Massachusetts, graduating with a bachelor of arts degree in 1900. He returned to Boston to attend and graduate from Harvard Medical School, receiving his MD degree in 1904.

Early Training and Career

Immediately after graduation, Rogers accepted an internship at Corey Hill Hospital (1904–1905). Corey Hill was located in Brookline, Massachusetts; Dr. Joel Goldthwait had established it in the early 1920s in order to provide care to private patients (chapter 33). While at Corey Hill Hospital, Rogers decided to be an orthopaedic surgeon and after his internship he collaborated with Charles Painter while both were practicing at the Carney Hospital, which Painter left in 1913. While at Carney Hospital, Rogers coauthored his first publication with Painter in 1907 on neoplasms presenting to a chronic joint clinic. During this period, Rogers also began his career affiliated with Massachusetts General Hospital (MGH), where he continued learning the specialty from Goldthwait and Painter. From 1905 to 1924, Rogers was an assistant orthopaedic surgeon to outpatients at the MGH. His office was located at 418 Beacon Street.

It was in his position at MGH that he developed an interest in tuberculosis, publishing seven papers over a 16-year span. His first paper from MGH in 1911 was about psoas abscesses in tuberculosis (see **Case 53.1**). That same year he published a follow-up of 23 cases of tuberculosis of the ankle joint over a seven-year period. He concluded:

> A complete operation, a radical removal of the focus, should be performed before there is much involvement of the various joint-surfaces and it should not be undertaken only because fixation has failed…Amputation has been necessary in over 50% of these cases…when the process has invaded several joint surfaces especially posterior to the astragalus…The results of amputation are good from the patient's point of view and an artificial leg is much preferable

Case 53.1. Psoas Abscess in the Lumbar Retroperitoneal Lymph Glands

> "[The patient], aged twenty-two. In August, 1910, she had an erosion of a tuberculous process of the patella, from which she was making a good recovery. About a month after leaving the hospital the right leg became flexed and there developed a psoas abscess which was not painful nor tender. There was no evidence of any kyphos and careful X-ray examination failed to show any bone lesion. At no time was there any temperature. The abscess cavity was opened by an incision just above Poupart's ligament, and was found to extend along the psoas muscle. A culture on blood serum gave us no growth, but inoculation into a guinea-pig caused tuberculosis. The incision healed readily and the flexion of the leg came down without traction. Examination afterward showed no evidence of spinal lesion."
>
> (Mark H. Rogers 1911)

PATHOLOGY OF TUBERCULOSIS OF JOINTS. A STUDY FROM
THE CLINICAL STANDPOINT.*

BY MARK H. ROGERS, M.D., BOSTON, MASS.

JBJS, 1922, Volume 4, Issue 4

Title of Rogers's article in which he identifies synovium as the primary source of tuberculosis infection in joints and not bone as was previously believed. *Journal of Bone and Joint Surgery* 1922; 4: 679.

to long-continued dressings and sinuses. The length of treatment should be diminished to within two years. (Rogers 1911)

Four years later, Dr. Rogers published a series of 100 patients with tuberculosis of the knee treated at the MGH. Sixty-seven of the cases underwent surgery. He followed the article with one on tuberculosis of the spine. In that article, he referred to his previous two papers, on the ankle and the knee, stating: "The general conclusions arrived at were that in both conditions the method of conservative treatment which is generally used in children was not sufficient to obtain a good result in adults…we could not base our prognosis on what we know as regards children" (Rogers and Foley 1917).

Rogers was also named one of four members of the advisory board of Trumbull Hospital, a new hospital that opened in 1921 in Brookline. The following year, he was invited to become a member of the associate staff of the New England Deaconess Hospital, along with other physicians and surgeons, including Dr. Z. B. Adams. He was also orthopaedic surgeon for the Boston and Maine Railroad. That same year, in 1922, using his earlier work as a foundation, he expressed his opinion regarding the primary focus of tuberculosis in joints:

> In the decade of 1890–1900, there was…a great deal of controversy concerning the question of synovial and bone tuberculosis, but the teaching was toward considering the bone as the primary focus and the joint as being involved secondarily. The conception that primary synovial tuberculosis is anything more than a rarity was evidently disputed and to a large extent discarded after the pathological work done by Nichols in 1898…Nichols…in the department of Surgical Pathology of the Harvard Medical School, studied a series of 120 cases of tuberculosis of the joints…material…from operations and largely from autopsies…As part of his conclusions, he states that…he is of the opinion that the primary focus is in the bone and that the involvement of the joint is a secondary process…the evidence as published is distinctly that tuberculosis of the joint arises from a focus in the bone and that the joint structure is involved as a secondary infection. (Rogers 1922)

Dr. Rogers then referred to Dr. Nathaniel Allison's paper published in 1921 in which Allison also concluded: "the evidence points towards a bone focus as the starting point. He [Allison] states that he agrees with Nichols" (see chapter 36). Dr. Rogers, however, had observed:

> that a considerable percentage of cases of tuberculosis of joints as seen at the Massachusetts General Hospital clinic could be classified as the synovial type, especially if [they] are seen within the first year of the onset of the symptoms...during the third year after the onset then they are generally classified as tuberculosis affecting the bone...After a study of Nichol's and Allison's work, I [Rogers] am not convinced that their conclusions...should be accepted as absolute fact...A policy at the [MGH] clinic [is] to perform an arthrotomy on cases of suspected tubercular knees...first for diagnostic purposes, and second, to make an attempt with iodoform-oil to affect the tuberculosis [method of Dr. E. G. Brackett] ...None of these cases showed any evidence of bone involvement that could be detected by careful x-ray studies or by operative inspection. [However] these same cases...later developed definite bone changes... and if the material were studied four years after the onset of symptoms, would, I believe, coincide with Nichol's and Allison's results.
> (Rogers 1922)

Later studies supported Rogers's opinion; in his 2006 book titled *Pathophysiology of Orthopaedic Diseases*, Dr. Henry Mankin noted that tuberculosis of the bone began in synovial joints, mainly indicated histologically by the presence of various cell types (epithelioid and Langhans giant cells and lymphocytes) and necrosis. It eventually evolved into bone erosion. Dr. Rogers continued to publish about a variety of orthopaedic conditions—about 20 articles, most while at the Massachusetts General Hospital. He held various positions at MGH, Harvard Medical School, and Tufts throughout the 1920s (**Box 53.1**).

Box 53.1. Mark Rogers's Positions at MGH, HMS, and Tufts in the 1920s

- Associate in orthopaedic surgery, Harvard Medical School (1915–24)
- Assistant professor of orthopaedic surgery, Tufts Medical School, (1915–24)
- Chief of orthopaedics, Massachusetts General Hospital (1918 and 1922)
- Professor and chairman orthopaedic division, Tufts University School of Medicine (1925–41)
- Chief of orthopaedic surgery, Beth Israel Hospital (1928)

World War I and Editor of the *American Journal of Orthopedic Surgery*

In between his publications on tuberculosis at MGH, Dr. Rogers was appointed as the first editor and business manager of the *American Journal of Orthopedic Surgery* (later named the *Journal of Bone and Joint Surgery*) in 1916. He replaced a three-man editorial committee. At the time, "the journal was moved to Boston [from Philadelphia, where it had been published by Blakiston's Son and Company] and published by Ernest Gregory" (Cowell 2000). Until 1914, the journal was published quarterly; in 1915 it began to be published monthly.

During this period, he also served during World War I, completing his active duty in the United States and not overseas (details are unknown); he simultaneously joined the staff of the Burrage Hospital that year as a consulting surgeon. The hospital opened in 1916 on Bumpkin Island in Boston Harbor; other consulting surgeons included Drs. Charles Painter, Robert Osgood, Lloyd T. Brown, and Harry C. Low. A Boston philanthropist, Albert Burrage, opened the Burrage Hospital every summer on the island for children with physical disabilities. The hospital burned down in 1946.

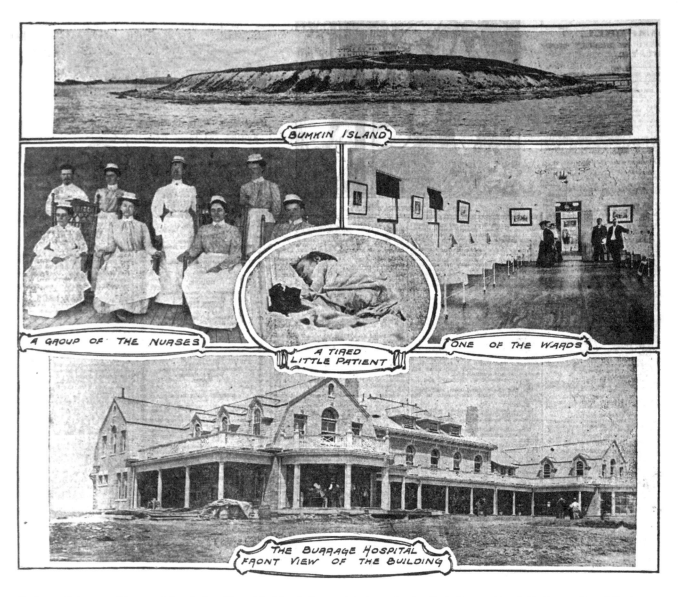

Collage of photos of Burrage Hospital on Bumpkin Island, Boston Harbor. "Begins Work: Burrage Hospital is Thrown Open," *Boston Globe*, July 15, 1902: 7.

The following year, as World War I continued into its third year in 1917, Rogers remained in the US Army Medical Corps with the rank of major. By the end of the war, he had been promoted to lieutenant colonel. Upon being discharged he stayed in the Medical Reserve Corps.

Rogers proposed a resolution at the 1918 American Orthopaedic Association meeting, which was adopted at that meeting. One historian writing about the association referred to it as the AOA's most impactful decision related to orthopaedics worldwide within the first two decades of the century. Two years after he had taken the helm as editor of the journal, he:

> presented the following resolutions: "Whereas, There has recently been formed an association in the specialty of Orthopaedic Surgery in Great Britain, Be it resolved, that the American Orthopedic Association express its general approval of offering the use of the official organ, the *American Journal of Orthopedic Surgery*, as the official organ of the newly formed association of Great Britain…" (Coventry 1977)

Rogers resigned as editor that same year.

Orthopaedic Division Chief at Beth Israel Hospital

When Rogers became chief of orthopaedic surgery at Beth Israel Hospital in 1928, orthopaedic surgery was encompassed under the division of surgery. Including Rogers, the orthopaedic staff comprised only five orthopaedists. Robert Osgood was, at the time, an orthopaedic consultant. When Rogers came on as chief, Beth Israel Hospital and Boston City Hospital took over teaching duties for students at Tufts Medical School.

While professor and chairman of orthopaedics at Tufts and during his transition from the MGH to chief of orthopaedics at the Beth Israel Hospital, Rogers published a paper on the teaching of orthopaedics to medical students. He had presented it at the 1927 annual meeting of the American Orthopaedic Association:

> This Association harbors a good many teachers of orthopaedic surgery...I am presenting certain principles in regard to teaching orthopaedic surgery to undergraduates. It is a fact that the primary function of such a course is to furnish a general knowledge of bone and joint conditions on the basis that the student is to be a general practitioner...It has been stated to me by men who also have been out of school for some years that what they were taught in a course of orthopaedic surgery and what they could read in orthopaedic textbooks did not take in the most important conditions that they meet in practice...In 1917 within a few months after declaration of war, there was established a course...in orthopaedic surgery. In this the author was associated with the late Dr. Lovett. It was necessary to determine what should be taught in such a course...it was necessary to outline a course that would fit the needs of the students rather than...embrace all the points of advanced orthopaedic surgery. I believe the same principle should hold true for teaching undergraduates...the chief emphasis was placed on certain principles...first, on physical diagnosis and physical examination; second, on constant review of anatomy of bones and joints, especially as regards function; third, on the effect of disease and injuries. (Rogers 1927)

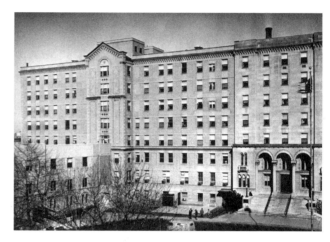

Beth Israel Hospital, Brookline Avenue, 1928. The Ruth and David Freiman Archives at Beth Israel Deaconess Medical Center.

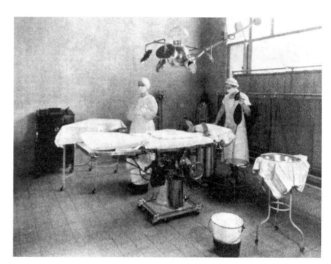

BIH operating room that Dr. Rogers used while chief of orthopaedics. The Ruth and David Freiman Archives at Beth Israel Deaconess Medical Center.

After discussing several common musculoskeletal conditions, he summarized his current teaching methods. He emphasized using the case method with smaller groups of students (using actual cases) and starting the session with a short lecture while giving an overview of the topic.

He then stressed the importance of the physical exam. During the session he always focused on the importance of anatomy and function. The exercise also included discussion and questions. He preferred not to give the students specific details of treatment, especially complex surgical procedures. He wrote:

> The course at Tufts Medical School is divided into four parts: the didactic lecture, the clinical lecture, case teaching, and group teaching. There is a tendency in present-day teaching to omit the didactic lecture. It would be a good thing...to substitute for this lecture sufficient reading of textbooks...but I do not believe it is practical for undergraduates. In this lecture there should be a general survey...of a given subject on which they can pin their knowledge obtained by reading...The clinical lecture is the most valuable as well as the best liked method of teaching...the first emphasis is placed on a definite method of examination...Then naturally will follow a discussion of diagnosis and treatment which will be based on actual facts already obtained...It seems to me that a very important part of our teaching comes in what we call case teaching. This takes the place of what we used to call recitation. It is the time when subject matter at hand is reviewed, opportunity is given for questions to be asked, and discussion of the various points is taken up. [Finally] section work consists of a limited number of exercises to small groups using actual cases as a basis. The tendency in teaching is towards small group teaching...The purpose... is to emphasize the importance of teaching principles...leaving the details of more complicated subjects to post-graduate work. (Rogers 1927)

During his 13 years as chief of orthopaedics at the Beth Israel Hospital, he published three articles: "Diabetic Neuritis with Paralysis" with Dr. Howard F. Root, a case report "Giant-Cell Tumor of the Sacrum," and "Fractures in Paget's Disease," cowritten with Dr. Robert Ulin. Many of his later staff positions and professional leadership roles are listed in **Box 53.2**. Dr. Henry Banks wrote of Rogers's faithful involvement in the weekly conferences at Boston City Hospital, where other physicians and residents greatly

Box 53.2. Mark Rogers's Later Professional Roles and Memberships

- Associate surgeon, VI Surgical Service (Bone and Joint Service), Boston City Hospital
- Associate in orthopaedic surgery, Harvard Medical Graduate School
- Orthopaedic consultant, US Public Health Hospital (Brighton, MA)
- Consultant to the medical staff, Evangeline Booth Home and Hospital
- Consultant in orthopaedic surgery, Joseph H. Pratt Diagnostic Hospital

Honorary staff member

- Cambridge Hospital
- New England Baptist Hospital
- Salem Hospital
- Massachusetts General Hospital
- Hospital Cottages for Children (Baldwinville, MA)
- Norwood Hospital
- Advisory board member, Household Nursing Association

Member

- American Medical Association
- Massachusetts Medical Society
- American Academy of Orthopaedic Surgeons
- Boston Orthopaedic Society
- Fellow, American College of Surgeons
- Member, American Legion

respected and appreciated his guidance and input. Rogers was on the staff of the Bone and Joint Service as an associate surgeon at Boston City Hospital (although it is not clear from the historical record whether he was employed there). He appears to have been active at Boston City Hospital throughout much of his career at Beth Israel Hospital. Banks (1999) called Rogers a "kind" and "modest" man who was a "superb" practitioner and academician.

Legacy

Dr. Mark Rogers, a well-regarded educator, remained involved in his teaching roles until his sudden death in 1941. At age 64, he experienced a heart attack and died in Belmont. At that time, he was survived by his wife Emily (Ross) and a son, daughter, and two grandchildren.

While chief of orthopaedics at the Beth Israel Hospital, in addition to his many other hospital and consulting commitments, Dr. Rogers oversaw a monthly clinic for handicapped children, in Gardner, for the Commonwealth of Massachusetts from 1937 to about the time of his death in 1941. His obituary honored him with the following words:

> His wide interests were evidenced by the large number of societies and institutions with which he was associated in different capacities… Known to his friends in the medical profession as one on whom they could depend, he was called to fill places where considered council was needed. To few men have come the opportunities for such service as was shown for the long list of hospitals to which he was consultant or an active member of the staff. His many medical friends realized that the same quality was expressed in other fields and he was interested in many others than his medical duties. In his hometown of Belmont, Massachusetts, for many years he was Chairman of the Playground Committee, and it was through his vision and guidance that the town has some of the best facilities and best planned policies for playground and recreational opportunities. His interest in the development of the youth was not confined to his town alone, for up to the time of his death his interest in his Alma Mater was unflagging. He was a constant attendant at the reunions and assemblies of the Alumni, and his associates always looked forward to meeting him at these gatherings for they appreciated his intellectual, gracious and conservative qualities.
>
> Another side was his love of music. He had shown particular fondness and talent for music in college, where he had taken part in the musical activities. He was organist for the College Chapel Choir, Manager of the Musical Association, and a member of the College Glee Club. For many years he was organist at All Saints' Church in Belmont. He also served his church as vestryman. As Choirmaster of this church came another opportunity for the expression of his love of music. It was a touching tribute to him that at the memorial services most of the original choir he had trained returned to sing.
>
> To him came the satisfaction of having carried on to the end the chosen work of his life and to his friends in all spheres of life he has left memories of work well done and a life well lived. ("Mark Homer Rogers, 1877–1941" 1942)

ARMIN KLEIN

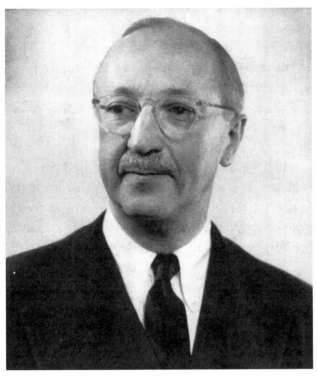

Armin Klein. "Armin Klein 1892-1954," *Journal of Bone and Joint Surgery* 1954; 4: 886.

Physician Snapshot

Armin Klein
BORN: 1892
DIED: 1954

SIGNIFICANT CONTRIBUTIONS: Orthopaedic division chief at Beth Israel Hospital 1941-1954; director of the posture clinic at MGH; member of the team that completed the Chelsea Survey of body mechanics in 1708 children; member of the White House Conference on Child Health and Protection Subcommittee on Orthopedics and Body Mechanics under the Committee on Medical Care for Children; chairman of the U.S. Department of Labor's Committee for Investigation and Research on Scoliosis; lead author of the monograph, *Slipped Capital Femoral Epiphysis*; originator of Klein's Line to identify a SCFE on frontal x-rays of the hips and pelvis

Armin Klein graduated from Harvard University in 1914 and three years later from Harvard Medical School. It was there that "his superior mental attainments proved him to be a scholar of the highest grade and proficiency" ("Obituary. Armin Klein. 1892-1954" 1954). Afterward, he took on a year-long (1917-18) surgical internship at Boston City Hospital, and in 1918 he was admitted to the Massachusetts Medical Society. He spent the next two years as a lieutenant in the US Army Medical Corps.

Early Career

After discharge from the US Army in 1920, Dr. Klein started his private practice and was assistant orthopaedic surgeon to the outpatient department at the Massachusetts General Hospital (MGH). His office was located at 483 Beacon Street. Originally living in Chelsea, in 1925, he moved to Brookline, and later to Newton.

> In addition to being on the staff at the MGH, Dr. Klein also joined the staff at Beth Israel Hospital when it opened on Brookline Avenue in 1928. He began at Tufts Medical School as an assistant in orthopaedics, and he held a faculty appointment at Harvard Medical School as an instructor early in his career as well. Although referred to as humble and unassuming, when engaged Klein was a clever and good-natured raconteur. He was well liked by colleagues and students alike, loved teaching, and was a gifted surgeon.

Scoliosis

Dr. Klein published two papers on the treatment of scoliosis between 1922 and 1924; "early [in his] career, he became associated with Dr. Robert Osgood [Orthopaedic Chief at MGH, 1919-1922] in the study of scoliosis and later became Chairman of the United States Department of Labor's Committee for Investigation and Research on Scoliosis" ("Obituary. Armin Klein. 1892-1954" 1954). Both papers were based on his experiences treating patients in the scoliosis clinic at MGH. He stated the aim of the clinic was:

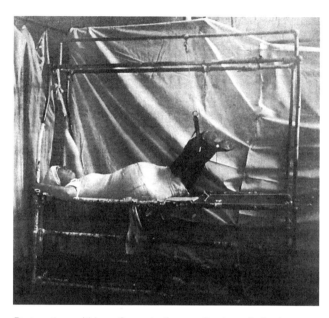

Patient in an Abbott frame before application of a body cast. Klein used the Forbes method—rotating the shoulders toward the thoracic curve's convexity while rotating the lower spine and pelvis in the opposite direction, with the use of a pelvic swathe. Begun at MGH by Z. B. Adams, the method had been used at the MGH for 10 years.

A. Klein, "Subsequent Report on the Treatment of Structural Scoliosis at the MGH," *Journal of Bone and Joint Surgery* 1924; 6: 864.

to improve the symmetry of the severe scoliotic, so that after the maximum amount of correction has been obtained, the muscles may become, with proper training, adequate to compensate for the remaining deformity. The methods followed are: first, carefully supervised exercises to mobilize the contracted muscles and ligaments and to acquire complete control over the respiratory muscles, the importance of which had been previously demonstrated by Bucholz. When this control is obtained, and this mobilization accomplished, the patient is placed in the Abbott frame and a fenestrated corrective jacket is applied, the pelvic girdle being rotated on a shoulder girdle as a fixed point in a direction similar to that employed by Forbes. Felt padding is applied once a week between the posterior convexity of the ribs and the cast, and the cast itself changed when it is no longer effective, the series being interrupted by exercise periods and split or hinged casts... As soon as the maximum amount of correction by cast has been obtained, the patient resumes muscle strengthening exercises and is fitted with a light retaining brace, the essential feature...is an accurately fitting pelvic base. The general condition of the patient is checked [frequently]...throughout the course of treatment, which...the patients agree to continue for at least two years. (Osgood et al. 1923)

In 1924, Klein published his second paper on scoliosis. He reported a longer follow-up on his patients treated in the clinic at MGH, up to 3½ years, because of an increased focus in the country on early fusion of the spine. He wrote:

some authorities have claimed that though these cases [structural scoliosis] might be actually somewhat improved, that this improvement could be maintained only by a corrective jacket, and that any brace would allow a certain amount of relapse. Because of this difficulty of retention, and to shorten the period necessary for treatment...they have advocated fusion operations of the spine. (Klein 1924)

He did not accept this premise and reported longer follow-up on some of his patients who worked and functioned well in a brace. He argued again for treatment using:

a combination of the exercise and corrective plaster jacket methods...The pelvis and the thorax are rotated on each other so as to warp the trunk over to the side of the concave deformity...augmented by intensive exercise and... by direct pressure on the posterior convexity of the ribs...for correction of the deformity... All this seems the natural thing to do...to straighten a twisted spine. Untwist both ends of the spine in opposite directions while separating these ends, and then force at the center...The method...is safe, ambulatory, and causes very little discomfort to the patient...The brace is [then] used to retain any correction obtained...

There has been a great swing of the pendulum toward the operative treatment of structural scoliosis. It is, therefore, timely to show some results of the conservative treatment and to stress the advantages of the method. (Klein 1924)

Dr. Klein presented this paper at the 1924 annual meeting of the American Orthopedic Association. The discussion was both challenging and remained controversial. Dr. A. Mackenzie Forbes (1924), an orthopaedist from Montreal, remarked: "Dr. Lovett treats scoliosis by lateralization [to correct rotation] as opposed to rotation. On the other hand, Dr. Klein attempts to treat by rotation [by untwisting both ends of the spine in the opposite direction]." Dr. Armitage Whitman (1924), from New York City, stated:

> I cannot see that the principles of his [Klein] treatment differ in any degree from those we have been applying at the Hospital for the Ruptured and Crippled [Hospital for Special Surgery] for the past nine to ten years. I am always impressed when I go to Boston with the control that the physicians in Boston exercise over their patients. I think Dr. Klein's principles are sound... In New York I am sorry to say, we cannot get a large number of patients to attend the clinic with the same degree of regularity. We cannot get them to come to exercises every other day...in the summer [the patients will not] wear this jacket...If the patients are willing to follow Dr. Klein's jackets and exercises for a period of five or six years...it is fine, but in our cases, if they will not continue the treatment, we resort to operation...we can accomplish by six to eight weeks in the recumbent position on the convex stretcher frame all that can be gained by two or three years of [wearing a] corrective jacket.

Posture

Posture has been a major topic of interest since the earliest writings of Nicolas Andry in 1743. It wasn't until the early twentieth century, however, that "serious" research and investigation on the subject began, led by the likes of Goldthwait, Klein, and Osgood. The term *body mechanics* replaced *posture* because it referred to not only the positioning of the body when standing but also how various systems—the skeletal, muscular, and neurological systems—worked together to make the body move (see chapter 33). The widespread negative effects of peoples' sedentary habits, especially among children, validated such study.

In 2012, Beth Linker, a historian at the University of Pennsylvania, highlighted one source that referred to 75% of US schoolchildren as "defective" as of 1925. Their "defects" included caries and tooth decay (in 50%), poor vision (in 25%), and tuberculosis (in 5%). A full 20%—that is, ~4 million schoolchildren—were judged to have orthopaedic deformities. Linker ties these health issues to guidance from the US Children's Bureau that public schools perform a physical examination of each student twice during the school year.

James T. Sullivan, in 1927, wrote an article in the *Boston Globe* about proper posture and the special clinic developed at the MGH. His interest had been piqued by a conversation with Klein. Sullivan harkened back to 1914, when Lloyd T. Brown and Joel Goldthwait began the posture clinic at MGH after recognizing patients' poor posture as they "slouched along" (Sullivan 1927). Statistics also showed that almost half of the men drafted to fight in World War I were denied because of conditions that with proper posture could have been avoided. Brown, Goldthwait, and others had begun to "[preach] the gospel of posture" at meetings and through their publications, attracting the interest of physicians, nurses, and the public nationwide (Sullivan 1927). Sullivan also described Goldthwait's 1915 Shattuck Lecture in which he discussed poor posture and its negative effects on health. The surprising thing, for Sullivan, and for patients at the clinic, was being prescribed exercises instead of medicine. The patients' results led to Brown and his Harvard colleague, Dr. Roger

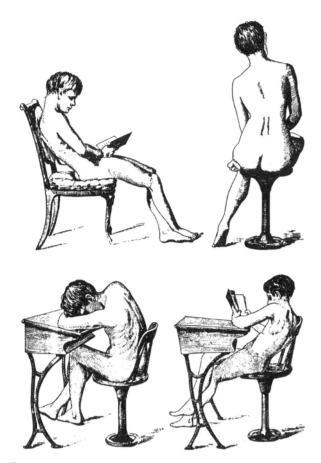

Poor sitting posture in school children demonstrated in this drawing.
Treatise on Orthopedic Surgery, Second Revised Edition, by E. H. Bradford and R. W. Lovett. New York: William Wood and Company, 1899.

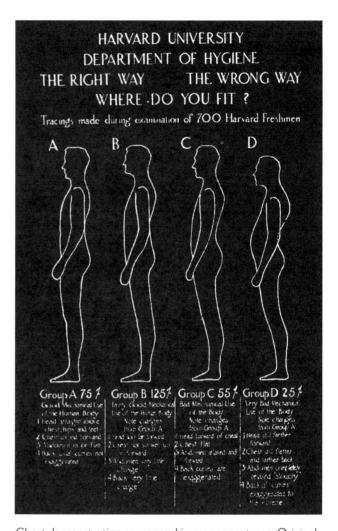

Chart demonstrating proper and improper postures. Original from R. Lee and L. T. Brown's study of 700 Harvard freshmen. "A New Chart for the Standardization of Body Mechanics," *Journal of Bone and Joint Surgery* 1923; 5: 754.

Lee (professor of hygiene), instructing all new students at the university on posture. Other universities and even the US government also expressed interest in the Harvard posture program as well.

Dr. Klein, after a couple of years on the staff at MGH, became director of the posture clinic. In 1923, he was a member of a team that studied 1,708 children (ages 5 to 18 years) in Chelsea, Massachusetts, through what became known as the Chelsea Survey (funded by the US Department of Labor). The investigators found that a majority of youth—between 75% and 80%—showed deficient body mechanics. For this team, the extent of the problem portended negative effects on health for a large swath of the nation's children and adolescents. Potential problems included poor metabolism, insufficient weight gain, lethargy, decreased oxygenation through the lungs, and reproductive issues (in girls). These could lead to, among other things, emotional problems and high rates of school absenteeism. Klein and his colleagues reported that fixing a child's posture seemed to help chronic conditions get better and improved school attendance.

In 1926, Klein authored two reports for the Children's Bureau of the US Department of Labor: "Posture Clinics. Organization and Exercises," Bureau Publication No. 164 and "Posture Exercises. A Handbook for Schools and Teachers of Physical Education," Bureau Publication No. 165. In the first publication, after defining poor

Klein and Thomas report on "Posture and Physical Fitness" for the Children's Bureau of the U.S. Department of Labor. The report contained their results from the "Chelsea Survey," 1923. Washington, DC: United States Government Printing Office, 1931. University of Minnesota/Google Books.

Klein and Thomas report on "Posture Exercises" for schools and physical education teachers. Washington, DC: United States Government Printing Office, 1926. University of Michigan/Google Books.

posture and its ill effects, he described how a posture clinic should be organized and methods of teaching proper posture to children. In the second publication he included drawings of posture standards, graded from "excellent" to "bad," for children, referring to three different body types: stocky, intermediate, and thin. These body types had been approved by the Children's Bureau of the United States Department of Labor (**Table 53.1**). Klein also provided detailed descriptions of numerous specific exercises. For Klein, the main thing children should be taught was to identify the extent of poor posture or curvature, from "normal" to "exaggerated." Normal curvature comprised slight convex curves at the shoulders, torso, and buttocks, whereas exaggerated curves were more extensive in the spine, causing a slumped or hunched stance and a low, forward-thrusting chin.

President Herbert Hoover held a White House Conference on Child Health and Protection in 1932. A Subcommittee on Orthopedics and Body Mechanics under the Committee on Medical Care for Children included Dr. Robert Osgood (chair), Dr. Lloyd T. Brown, Dr. John B. Carnett (vice dean

Table 53.1. Posture Associated with Thin, Intermediate, and Stocky Body Types of Children

Grade	Rating	Posture
A	Excellent	Head up and balanced above shoulders, hips, and ankles; chin in
		Chest up, with the breastbone farthest forward
		Flat lower abdomen, pulled in
		Back curves within normal limits
B	Good	Head forward slightly
		Chest lowered slightly
		Lower abdomen in, not flat
		Back curves slightly increased
C	Poor	Head forward
		Chest flat
		Abdomen relaxed and farthest forward
		Back curves exaggerated
D	Bad	Head markedly forward
		Chest depressed, sunken
		Abdomen fully relaxed, protruding
		Back curves extremely exaggerated

Data from Armin Klein, "Posture Standards," in *Posture Exercises: A Handbook for Schools and for Teachers of Physical Education* [Washington, DC: US Department of Labor, 1926], Figs. 3–8.

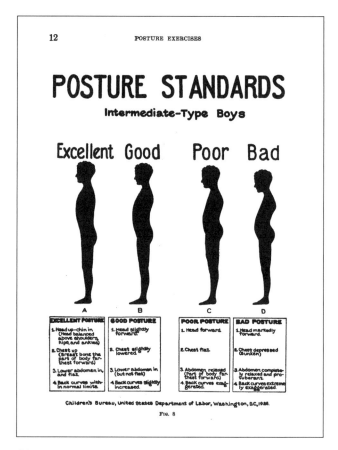

Chart demonstrating posture standards for boys; contained in Klein and Thomas report on "Posture Exercises. A Handbook for Schools and Teachers of Physical Education."
Washington, DC: United States Government Printing Office, 1926. University of Michigan/Google Books.

and professor of surgery at the Graduate School of Medicine, University of Pennsylvania), Dr. Armin Klein, and Leah C. Thomas (assistant professor of hygiene and physical education at Smith College). In their final report, the subcommittee recommended requiring postural instruction in all US schools. The subcommittee emphasized that "body mechanics should be made the basic principle of all physical education" (quoted in Gorman 2006). Dr. John B. Carnett wrote of his hope that US schools will soon require children to pass not only academic requirements but also physical requirements pertaining to posture and body mechanics to move to the next grade.

Orthopaedic Chief at Beth Israel Hospital and Later Contributions

By 1932, Dr. Klein was listed as an assistant professor of orthopaedic surgery at HMS; four years later, he was promoted to clinical professor of orthopaedics at Tufts Medical School in 1936. By 1941, he was named chief of the orthopaedic service at Beth Israel Hospital; a position he held until his death in 1954. He followed Dr. Mark Rogers. Dr. Klein also remained on the staff at MGH during this period.

Dr. Carter Rowe noted Klein's pragmatic attitude and his aptitude for delving to the bottom line of an issue. Rowe referred to Klein's attitude with, "Away with the phony, let's have the facts!" (quoted in Rowe 1996). Interns and residents alike appreciated Klein's approachable manner and the "paternal interest" he expressed, which they "not only appreciated but loved" ("Obituary. Armin Klein. 1892–1954" 1954). They found that he:

was never too busy to listen to their problems, their troubles, their mistakes, and to sympathize with them, yet to give sound advice… with unswerving truth…his house staff never hesitated to come to him for help…knowing that they would receive wise counsel and the absolute truth…he had a tolerance of others and was, above all, intellectually honest…he was extremely loyal to them…One of his most admirable qualities was his ability to overlook the weaknesses in others, even when he himself was badly hurt and grieved by them…by nature he was a very sensitive person [with] exceptionally fine character. ("Obituary. Armin Klein. 1892–1954" 1954)

Slipped Capital Femoral Epiphysis

In addition to his contribution on posture, Dr. Klein's had a second main area of interest in slipped capital femoral epiphysis. From 1943 to 1952, he published four papers with his colleagues at the MGH (Drs. Robert Joplin, John Reidy, and Joseph Hanelin, a radiologist). In 1943, Klein et al. noted some negative outcomes among 39 patients who had been treated over eight years (1924–32) with manipulation and fixation in a plaster cast by Dr. J. Albert Key, or with open reduction and plaster fixation by Dr. Philip D. Wilson. Patients who had undergone open reduction with the use of a triflanged nail and mobilization soon after the procedure showed improved outcomes. The triflanged nail, which Marius Smith-Petersen had introduced in 1925 (see chapter 37), allowed surgeons to achieve normal anatomic positioning and stabilization of the bone, which allowed mobilization sooner after the procedure and earlier gains in function. This, in turn, avoided the need for plaster fixation and reduced the incidence of arthritis.

They divided the 36 hips treated at MGH during the previous ten years into three groups: a group with different treatments, a group treated by open reduction and nailing, and a third group treated by lateral nailing in situ. In three cases, osteotomies were performed for severe slippage of the epiphysis. They identified overall poor results—37.4% of normal—in all three cases on the basis of a modified Ferguson-Howorth "index of motion" score. With hip arthrotomy, epiphyseal repositioning, and fixation with the triflanged nail, however, resulted in better function—76.8% of normal. Hip arthrotomy with lateral nailing, however, provided the best results—94.8% of normal—when only minimal epiphyseal slippage occurs.

Following this report, the standard method of treating slipped capital femoral epiphysis at MGH was lateral nailing in situ for minimal slips and by arthrotomy, repositioning of the displaced epiphysis, and fixation of the head with a Smith-Petersen nail. In 1948, Klein, Joplin, and Reidy published their second paper on 45 patients with 51 slips. Nailing in situ was appropriate for ~28 of those patients (62%), but the other 17 (38%) required arthrotomy and reduction first. The authors reported no aseptic necrosis. All patients used crutches for three months postoperatively. The authors concluded that in situ nailing should occur as early as possible, as early nailing provides as much as 90% of normal hip motion and 96% of normal hip function. On the other hand, when arthrotomy is necessary, hip motion only recovers to ~85% of normal, whereas hip function might be only 92% of normal.

Various physicians commented in the discussion of this paper. Dr. H. R. McCarroll called out the authors for not including absorption of the femoral neck as an indication of aseptic necrosis after surgery. Dr. Joseph Barr recalled his and his colleagues' previous negative outcomes, which upon reevaluation indicated the need for a new perspective in treatment. He confirmed both that Klein, Joplin, and Reidy's results had been evaluated and vetted by the staff at MGH and that aseptic necrosis had not occurred in any of the patients reported, though he qualified that finding by recognizing the small sample size.

Drs. Klein, Joplin, and Reidy were then joined by coauthor Dr. Joseph Hanelin—their radiologist collaborator—in presenting their series of patients with slipped capital femoral epiphysis to the Joint Meeting of the American, British, and Canadian Orthopaedic Associations' meeting in Quebec in 1948. It was a roentgenographic survey of the cases they treated at MGH. They wrote:

> The roentgenograms taken at the end of a seven-year follow-up period...in which nailing was done in situ, traumatic arthritis or aseptic necrosis of the femoral head has not occurred... Sixteen patients...were treated with arthrotomy, osteotomy through the epiphyseal plate, replacement of the head to its anatomical position...and lateral nailing for fixation. After an average follow-up period of thirty-three and one-quarter months...We should...like to emphasize that there are two additional basic requirements necessary to obtain [good] results...First, the hip should be approached through an incision [Smith-Petersen] that gives sufficient exposure to permit replacement of the head. Second, the hip joint should be entered through an incision...across the capsule, over the anterior portion of the epiphyseal plate. This spares the ligamentum teres and the posterior, superior, and inferior portions of the visceral capsule...These details minimize the possibility of damage to the circulation of the head...In this series, traumatic arthritis has been encountered in only two cases. (Klein et al. 1949)

In 1953, Drs. Klein, Joplin, Reidy, and Hanelin published the book *Slipped Capital Femoral Epiphysis*, a monograph on roentgen diagnosis in the American Lecture Series. In their introduction, they reaffirmed the overall results that they had reported earlier: positive results with open reduction but less so with nailing in situ. Early treatment with nailing, especially before extensive slippage occurred, provided the best outcomes, thus emphasizing the need for both early identification of slippage and a gold standard for comparison. The book mainly consists of x-rays of normal hips, various degrees of slips, and the results of treatment.

I recall a conversation with Dr. Clement Sledge (see chapter 48) about avascular necrosis after open reduction of the femoral head in cases of displaced slipped capital femoral epiphyses. He stated that he had reviewed many of the cases of Drs. Klein, Joplin, and Reidy from their series. At long-term follow-up, he recalled that many of the patients had developed avascular necrosis (unpublished).

Klein's Line

Klein and his colleagues presented their thoughts on the disabling effects of slipped capital femoral epiphysis and the vital importance of early diagnosis to the American Academy of Orthopaedic Surgeons in 1951. The resulting terminology—Klein's Line—became the standard method to identify an early or minimal SCFE. It is a line drawn on the superior border of the femoral neck on a frontal x-ray of the hips and pelvis. The cephalad portion of the line should pass through the proximal epiphysis. If it does not, it is an indication of a SCFE. In their later publication, Klein and his coauthors (1952) wrote:

> patients frequently do not appear for diagnosis and treatment with early complaints and signs but wait until the epiphyseal slipping is so marked that they are noticeably crippled. This is undoubtedly true in some instances, but many of our patients...were cases of "missed diagnosis"...Another factor in delayed diagnosis and treatment has been the failure of even those alert to the possibility of slipping to recognize the early stigmata roentgenographically.

Klein et al. also reported contralateral involvement in 20% of cases, but after longer follow-up they revised that figure to 40%. With a standard protocol for anteroposterior and frog-leg lateral

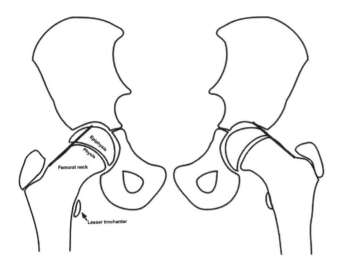

Drawing of Klein's line. On the left is a normal hip with Klein's line passing through the epiphysis. On the right is an abnormal hip with Klein's line not passing through the epiphysis—suggesting the presence of a SCFE.

E. J. Rebich, S. S. Lee, and J. A. Schlecter, "The S Sign: A New Radiographic Tool to Aid in the Diagnosis of SCFE," *The Journal of Emergency Medicine* 2018; 54: 836.

x-rays, the authors examined over 100 children from birth to maturity. They observed:

> In the anteroposterior view, at the age of three, the head overhangs the neck so that prolongation of the superior neck line proximally transacts a portion of the head. This relationship persists into adult life…In the later phase of slipping…the proximal part of the neck at its juncture with the epiphysis was left bare superiorly and anteriorly over an area equivalent to the amount of slipping. (Klein et al. 1952)

In the discussion of Klein's paper, Dr. Robert W. Johnson Jr. (1952) of Baltimore closed: "I think that Dr. Klein and his associates, in bringing a phase of our ever-present diagnostic and therapeutic problem so clearly and graphically before us, have rendered a real service to the Academy, especially to its younger and less experienced members." In 2009, Daniel Green and his associates studied the reliability and efficiency of Klein's Line and a modification of Klein's Line that measured the width of the epiphysis lateral to Klein's Line. They found a classic Klein line in only 40.3% of slipped epiphyses. Their modification allowed an almost 80% sensitivity for identifying slipped epiphysis when the epiphysis and the hip were separated by 2 mm.

Legacy

Dr. Armin Klein continued in his position as chief of orthopaedics at Beth Israel until he died on April 3, 1954, at 62 years old. He was survived by his wife, three children (two sons and a daughter), and five grandchildren. Klein was an active member of various professional organizations (**Box 53.3**) throughout his career. Although "he had been given a warning some months previously by a heart attack that his life might be interrupted at any time…he did not allow this to interfere with his regular daily life ("Obituary. Armin Klein. 1892–1954" 1954). In response to a recommendation that he take it easy:

> he replied, "I shall cooperate in every way, but I will not reduce my work"…he looked forward willingly to his day's work; and on the day before his death, he was at his usual place in the Orthopaedic Clinic at the Massachusetts General Hospital…his death was a shock because he appeared to be in good health. He arose from his bed on the morning of April 3 in a happy frame of mind and was actually joking, with a smile on his lips, at the moment death called him. ("Obituary. Armin Klein. 1892–1954" 1954)

Box 53.3. Armin Klein's Professional Memberships

- American Board of Orthopaedic Surgery
- American Academy of Orthopaedic Surgeons
- American Orthopaedic Association
- American Medical Association
- Harvard Club
- Boston Orthopaedic Club (president in 1940)
- Greater Boston Medical Society (chairman in 1951)

MEIER G. KARP

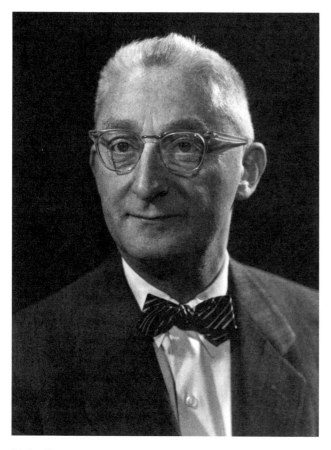

Meier Karp. The Ruth and David Freiman Archives at Beth Israel Deaconess Medical Center.

Physician Snapshot

Meier G. Karp
BORN: 1904
DIED: 1962
SIGNIFICANT CONTRIBUTIONS: Orthopaedic division chief at Beth Israel Hospital 1954–1962; orthopaedic surgeon-in-chief at the US Army Thayer General Hospital in Nashville, Tennessee during World War II

Meier Goldstein Karp graduated from the University of Virginia School of Medicine in 1931, and continued surgical training at an unknown location. On September 1, 1935, he completed a chief residency at Boston Children's Hospital where "his service was satisfactory on all counts" ("Annual Report [63rd], Boston Children's Hospital, 1935" 1935). He was succeeded by Dr. Paul Hugenberger. At the time, he held the appointment of assistant in orthopaedic surgery at Harvard Medical School and lived on Yarmouth Street in Brookline. He started a private general practice in orthopaedics, caring for his patients at Beth Israel Hospital; he was admitted to the Massachusetts Medical Society in 1937. Karp was a member of the staff at both Boston Children's Hospital and the Peter Bent Brigham Hospital. He was also a consultant to the Veterans Administration Hospital in Roxbury.

Dr. Karp was an excellent clinician but lectured and published little. He published two papers: "Köhler's Disease of the Tarsal Scaphoid" (1937) and a paper coauthored with Dr. A. H. Brewster, "Fractures in the Region of the Elbow in Children" (1940). In the former, he reviewed 45 cases of Köhler's disease treated at Boston Children's Hospital, concluding:

> This syndrome occurs predominantly in male children between the ages of two and one-half and seven and one-half years...manifested by pain, a limp, swelling and localized tenderness...It is more frequently unilateral [with] a characteristic x-ray picture...unrelated to duration of symptoms or to treatment. Complete regeneration of the involved bone takes place in an average of two and three-fourths years, and a normal foot is the usual end result.
> (Karp 1937)

Three years later, in his second paper coauthored with Brewster, they "examined eight cases of cubitus varus deformity and found that clinical measurements of the lengths of the outside of the arm exceeded those of the inside by one-quarter to three-quarters of an inch in six" (Smith 1960). They went on to conclude it was:

> caused by stimulation of the external epicondylar and capitellar epiphyses. [Dr. Lyman Smith twenty years later stated] this explanation seems most unlikely, as it has been

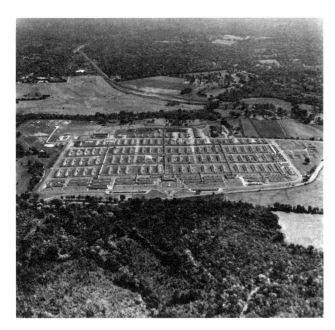

Aerial view of U.S. Thayer General Hospital, White Bridge, TN. U.S. National Library of Medicine.

demonstrated in this study that simple medial tilt of the distal fragment gives the same appearance. Furthermore, it is difficult to explain the deformity on the basis of a pure growth disturbance in view of the overwhelming predominance (ten or more to one) of varus deformities…growth disturbance is a rare complication and seldom is the cause of a change in the carrying angle. (Smith 1960)

Not long after these early publications, Karp served as a US Army major during World War II. He was stationed at Thayer General Hospital in Nashville, Tennessee, where he served as the orthopaedic surgeon-in-chief. He most likely spent most of the war located there. I found evidence of only two presentations: "Shoulder Girdle Pain of Cervical Nerve Root Origin (Radiculitis)" given at a meeting of the Greater Boston Medical Society at Beth Israel Hospital in 1951; and "Orthopedic Problems in General Practice," given with Drs. Carter Rowe and Thomas Quigley at a meeting of the Norfolk District Medical Society in 1955.

The previous year, he replaced Armin Klein as head of the orthopaedics department at Beth Israel Hospital in 1954. That same year he was promoted to instructor in orthopaedics at HMS. He was also a member of the American Academy of Orthopaedic Surgeons, the American College of Surgeons, the Massachusetts Medical Society, the American Medical Association, and Alpha Omega Alpha.

Dr. Meier Karp was head of the division of orthopaedic surgery at Beth Israel Hospital for eight years, until his death on Thursday, September 13, 1962. He was 58. His wife, Evelyn (neé Gerstein) and their three sons mourned his death.

ROBERT ULIN

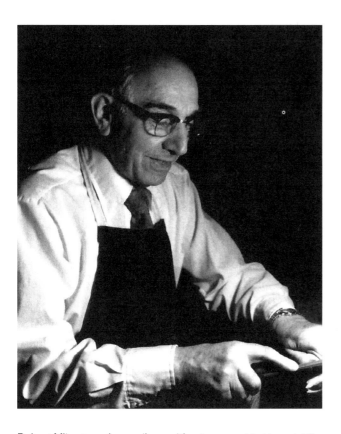

Robert Ulin at work as a silversmith. Courtesy of Dr. Kenneth Ulin.

Physician Snapshot

Robert Ulin

BORN: 1903

DIED: 1978

SIGNIFICANT CONTRIBUTIONS: Acting chief of orthopaedics at Beth Israel Hospital 1962–1966; chief of orthopaedics at the General Hospital in the Philippines and at Lowell General Hospital at Fort Devens in Massachusetts during World War II; expert silversmith

Robert Ulin was born and raised in Boston, attending the English High School in the city. He stayed in the area for college, graduating in 1924 with a bachelor of science degree from Harvard College and then with an MD degree from Harvard Medical School in 1928. He completed his surgical internships and his residency at Boston City Hospital, working closely with Drs. Frederic Cotton, Otto Hermann, and Joseph Shortell. He began a private practice at 485 Commonwealth Avenue in Boston. In 1932, he was appointed assistant orthopaedic surgeon to the outpatient department at Beth Israel Hospital and assistant surgeon to the fracture outpatient department at Boston City Hospital with a faculty appointment at Tufts as a teaching fellow.

It was during his first few years in practice that Ulin published two papers: the first on "fender fractures" at Boston City Hospital (see **Case 53.2**) and the second on fractures seen in Paget disease, cowritten with Dr. Mark H. Rogers from the Beth Israel Hospital. In his twentieth-century history of orthopaedics at Tufts University, Banks wrote of Ulin as an example of the type of orthopaedic surgeon who was essential to the advances and achievements of orthopaedic educational programs—knowledgeable and talented surgeons who work tirelessly to provide high-quality care to their patients and to teach would-be surgeons all they need to know. Ulin did just that at Boston City Hospital (see chapter 60) and at the Boston VA Hospital. He was also on the staff of Faulkner Hospital.

Ulin joined the US Army during World War II and was stationed at a hospital in the Philippines, practicing as an orthopaedic surgeon until 1944,

Case 53.2. Fender Fracture With Unusual Cause

"[The patient] aged 51, while crossing the street, about to step on the curbstones, missed the curbstone, missed the curb, twisted his ankle and fell. As he was falling he felt a snap and sharp pain in his knee and was unable to walk.

"Examination at the hospital three days later showed knock-knee deformity, edema of thigh and leg, effusion into the knee joint, ecchymosis in the popliteal space with tenderness over upper end of tibia, and especially the external condyle. Motions were painful and there was abnormal lateral mobility. X-ray [showed a fracture of the external condyle]. All laboratory tests to rule out pathological basis for fracture (including biopsy at open reduction) were negative" (Robert Ulin 1934).

when he was promoted to the hospital's chief of orthopaedics. Two years later, he returned to the US to take on the same position at Lowell General Hospital at Fort Devens in Massachusetts. Upon his discharge in 1947, he went back to Boston and picked up where he had left off in his private practice.

In 1951, he gave a talk on subdeltoid bursitis at a meeting of the Greater Boston Medical Society (the only lecture I could find given by Dr. Ulin) and published a paper on recurrent subluxation of the ankle with Drs. Mack Clayton and Arthur Trott (at the Veterans Administration Hospital). His fourth and final paper, "Slipped Proximal Femoral Epiphyses," was published in 1965. He wrote:

> At the Boston City Hospital from 1947 to 1957, 35 hips with minor degree of epiphyseal slipping were, in all cases but 1, treated with a narrow triflanged cannulated nail. One hip was treated by the Howorth procedure. The results in all were excellent or good...Among 28 hips with mild or moderate slip during the years 1960 to 1964, only 9 were nailed, 16 were treated with 1 or 2 screws, 1 with Hagie pins and 2 by epiphysiodesis...The results to date in these also have been uniformly good. The problem of the marked gradual slip [>1 cm] still presents the most serious difficulties in treatment and the highest incidence of early or late disabling joint changes. Encouraged by the high percentage of good results obtained by Klein, Joplin and Reidy [ORIF] this technique was followed at the Boston City Hospital...in 16 hips from 1947 to 1957...If no complications ensue, correction of the deformity at the site of pathology produces better anatomic and functional hip than by other methods of treatment. However, the results in 5 of the 31 cases were unsatisfactory, due to avascular necrosis and for degenerative changes. This discouragingly high percentage of unsatisfactory results has been the reported experience of most other surgeons...Because of this, during the years 1960-1964, a somewhat more pronounced degree than 1 cm. of slipping was considered to be acceptable for fixation without replacement...For the most part, the reported results of wedge osteotomy of the femoral neck...are about as discouraging as those of replacement of the head...[In summary] the treatment is operative to prevent further slipping...the method a matter of personal preference, whether fixation with screw, threaded wires or epiphysiodesis. The hazards of the use of the triflanged nail make this generally the least desirable...in the already advanced stage, open reduction of the displaced epiphysis or cervical osteotomy have given a large percentage of good results in the hands of some surgeons, but most have a high incidence of avascular necrosis of the head. A safer procedure is that of osteoplasty...combined with epiphysiodesis. For residual deformity with restricted abduction and internal rotation, trochanteric osteotomy provides a satisfactory means of improving the range of motion. (Ulin 1965)

From 1962 to 1966, Ulin was acting chief of orthopaedics at Beth Israel Hospital. During his

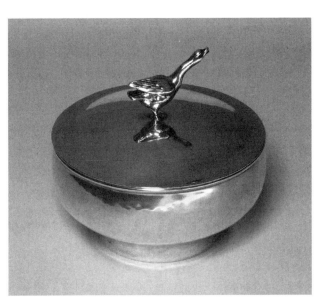

Handwrought Box with a cast finial. Courtesy of Dr. Kenneth Ulin.

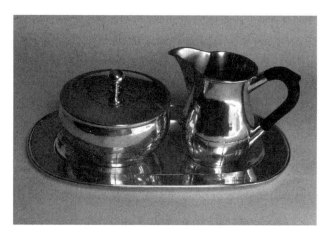

Chased silver sugar and creamer. Courtesy of Dr. Kenneth Ulin.

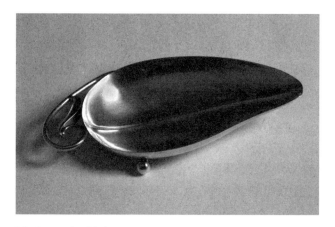

Modernist leaf dish. Courtesy of Dr. Kenneth Ulin.

time as chief, medical students from Tufts University's medical school stopped rotating through Beth Israel Hospital's orthopaedic service, which at the time did not work with orthopaedic residents either. Dr. Ulin was promoted to clinical professor orthopaedic surgery at Tufts College of Medicine in 1969, and he was also an assistant in orthopaedic surgery at Harvard Medical School. He was a popular figure at Tufts; liked by his coworkers, his patients, and his residents and students for his empathy and kindness. Dr. Ulin was a member of the Massachusetts Medical Society (admitted 1932), the American Academy of Orthopaedic Surgeons (admitted 1940), the American Medical Association, the American Physicians Fellowship and the New England Orthopedic Society.

Ulin had cultivated an unusual hobby, silversmithing, beginning early in his career and continuing throughout his life. He began taking classes from Edwin Leinonen, a noted silversmith in the city, in the early 1930s. Over the course of about 45 years (and until his death), he continued those classes and crafted a variety of items, from spoons to coffee pots and cups, working from a studio at his home and applying his own maker's mark to his pieces. He eventually helped Leinonen teach the classes. Ulin passed his interest in silversmithing on to his son, Kenneth, who continued the practice as well as the use of his father's mark.

He was 74 years old when he died at home in Jamaica Plain on June 21, 1978. He had been honored the prior year by the Beth Israel Hospital for 45 years of service in 1977. His wife, Dorothy (neé Lewenberg), had predeceased him in 1967. They had two children, a son and a daughter.

SEYMOUR ZIMBLER

Physician Snapshot

Seymour Zimbler
BORN: ca. 1932
DIED: 2021
SIGNIFICANT CONTRIBUTIONS: Orthopaedic division chief at Beth Israel Hospital 1966–1970; primary interest in pediatric orthopaedics; chief of pediatric orthopaedics at New England Medical Center

Seymour "Zeke" Zimbler graduated from the New York State College of Medicine in Syracuse in 1958. Following a surgical internship and a year of surgical residency at Boston City Hospital on the Tufts service, he entered the Combined Boston Children's Hospital/Massachusetts General Hospital orthopaedic surgery residency program in 1960. His first six months were spent in the research lab at Boston Children's Hospital under Dr. Jonathan Cohen. Zimbler later remembered:

> The lab work was not really basic science. There were a couple of projects that we [residents] picked up that were kind of clinical things that we did ourselves…Like the one that I worked on was actually on septic arthritis where we collected synovial fluid from people…on antibiotics and we were trying to measure the levels of antibiotics in the synovial fluid. And that was pretty tough. We kept it in a freezer, but the whole thing failed. My basic science [research] failed. (Zimbler, interview with the author, 2009)

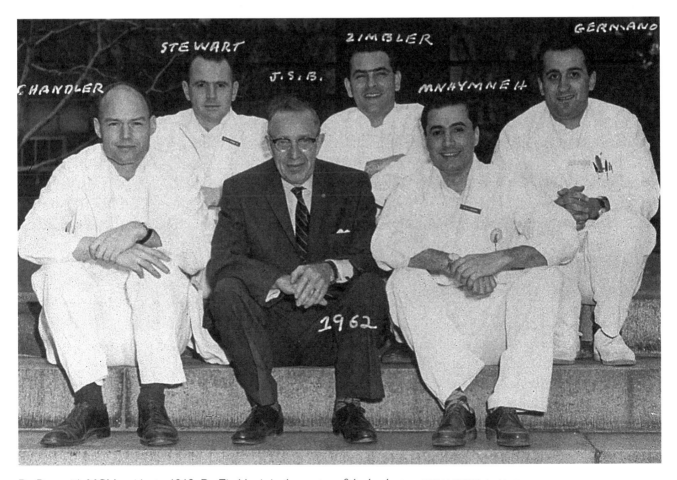

Dr. Barr with MGH residents, 1962. Dr. Zimbler is in the center of the back row. MGH HCORP Archives.

While in the lab, he was also responsible for giving anatomy lectures to the physical therapy students at Simmons College. After his six months in the laboratory, his orthopaedic residency program rotations included: one year at Boston Children's Hospital, one year at Massachusetts General Hospital (MGH), six months at the Peter Bent Brigham Hospital, and 12 months as senior resident at Boston Children's Hospital. As a resident at Boston Children's, Dr. Zimbler received no salary. He had a family with two children and another on the way. He was forced to borrow $100K to support his family. At MGH, his salary was $120/month, plus laundry. Upon his return to Boston Children's as a senior resident, he received a salary of $75–$95 per month plus laundry. When on call at MGH, he recalled that residents could eat all the ice cream they wanted.

Upon completing his residency, Dr. Zimbler was drafted into the Vietnam War. He entered the navy for two years in 1964. With his interest and extra training in pediatric orthopaedics, the navy was interested in sending him to the San Diego Naval Center, which had a large pediatric service. Dr. Al Crawford headed the pediatric orthopaedic service and was leaving. Dr. William Stryker, a captain and chief of the orthopaedic service, wanted Dr. Zimbler to come to San Diego. Zimbler remembered, "At the last minute I got a call from the navy…you are a very valuable person…but you have three children and because we have to send you across the country, we want you to volunteer for an extra year. We want you to stay three years in San Diego" (Zimbler, interview with the author, 2009).

Because of his debts, he refused the extra year in the navy. After discussion, he was eventually sent to the Charleston Naval Hospital in South Carolina, a 250-bed hospital with a children's ward. At the time, he recalled that the Vietnam War was not official, but the United States was engaged, and wounded soldiers were being returned to the United States. His hospital received about 15 wounded soldiers each week. Later when the war became official, he observed that all military physicians/surgeons on the west coast who treated trauma patients were sent to Vietnam.

Zimbler served two years at the Charleston Naval Hospital, completing his military obligation there in 1966. He published one paper while in the navy on the use of intravenous regional anesthesia in treating children with fractures of the upper extremity. While in Charleston, he had made a couple of return visits to Boston. He spoke to Dr. Green, who offered him a staff position at Boston Children's:

> I wanted to come back to Children's but I really didn't want to be a super resident…I didn't like the way [the staff] were treated. They were not colleagues…Dr. Green was president of the American Board, the American Academy of Cerebral Palsy [and the American Academy of Orthopaedic Surgeons] during that time and was away a lot [the staff had to take care of his patients] they had to do everything; they were on the phone to him all the time. There were no cell phones, no computers so it was difficult…they had to ask [him] about everything…the simplest things on up, plus make major decisions, plus run the program when he was not there. (Zimbler, interview with the author, 2009)

About the same time, Beth Israel Hospital expressed plans to hire more staff and expanding their clinical services:

> I knew some of the people that were administrators at the Beth Israel. There was…Jack Caston, who was an assistant administrator and the chief of surgery was Jake Fine…He contacted me and said we'd like you to be the chief of orthopaedics…I said OK, but I don't really want to give up my pediatrics…can I go to a clinic at Children's all year and be an attending at Children's? So, they said yeah, you can do that…I had an office at the Beth Israel and I was an attending [teaching service] about

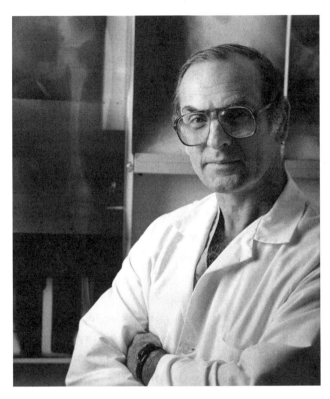

Seymour "Zeke" Zimbler. James Koepfler/Boston Children's Hospital.

six months a year...and every week I came [all year] and did a whole clinic...so I was like the club foot guy, the way it worked out. (Zimbler, interview with the author, 2009)

After being discharged he became a staff member at both Boston Children's Hospital and Beth Israel Hospital. In 1966 he also applied for membership in the Massachusetts Medical Society. At the time, he lived at 28 Gay Street, Newtonville, Massachusetts. The orthopaedic staff at Beth Israel were all private practitioners, including Dr. Robert Ulin who had been acting chief of orthopaedics before Dr. Zimbler. Other staff included Drs. Joe Copel, Bob Dines, Marv Weinfeld, and Ralph Bender. There were also consultants, including Dr. Osgood and Dr. Goldthwait and others from MGH.

Dr. Zimbler was a private physician at Boston Children's Hospital and fulltime at Beth Israel as chief of the division of orthopaedic surgery. He had a Harvard Medical School faculty appointment through Beth Israel. As chief of the service, he received a salary of $1,200 per year from Harvard, about $10,000 per year from Beth Israel, and he was permitted to have a private practice. Zimbler recalled the orthopaedic service at the Beth Israel in the late 1960s:

[Being chief] was a dubious honor. We had general surgeons that rotated on the service; there were no orthopaedic residents initially. General surgery residents rotated with us...usually one or two. There was little trauma at the Beth Israel...Officially, the BI had an open emergency room and they wanted it to be more active because they were not known for anything complicated [to manage]. They always transferred the patient out...Around the time I started, the general surgeons...wanted a more active emergency room. So, I went back to [the] group of adult attendings and said we're going to have to cover the emergency room. And so, what they said was we refuse; we won't do it. They all had offices on Beacon Street or Brookline Avenue, and they didn't need the emergency room. And, of course, at that time it was a certain percentage of drunks and people without insurance, so they didn't want them...they actually refused. And so, I didn't make a big deal about it. I said well, okay, if you won't do it, then I'll do it myself...you won't believe this, but for three years, I covered the BI emergency room myself, day and night [1967–70]. (Zimbler, interview with the author, 2009)

Dr. Zimbler published only one paper during his busy three years as chief of orthopaedics at Beth Israel Hospital. It was a case report on a patient with two primary cancers, carcinoma of the breast and a chondrosarcoma of the femur (see **Case 53.3**). He also made a significant contribution to the Harvard Combined Orthopaedic Residency Program. In discussions with Dr. Melvin Glimcher, it was agreed that residents would begin a six-month rotation at Beth Israel Hospital,

Case 53.3. Breast Carcinoma and Chondrosarcoma

> "[The patient was a] 25-year old unmarried Caucasian woman, a university instructor, was a native of Costa Rica. She was admitted to the Beth Israel Hospital for the first time on July 16, 1967 with a chief complaint of a "tumor" in the right breast. The patient had been well until March, 1967 when she noted a mass in the upper outer quadrant of the right breast. This was tender to touch. She consulted a physician in Costa Rica and a biopsy was performed on July 9, 1967. Microscopic sections were interpreted as 'comedo carcinoma.' The patient was told that further surgery would be necessary. At the urging of her family, she then came to the Boston area to seek further medical therapy.
>
> "Past medical history revealed that the patient had typhoid fever on 2 previous occasions. Review of systems and family history were unremarkable.
>
> "Physical examination on admission showed a well-developed well-nourished Caucasian woman in no acute distress. Her blood pressure was 118/60, pulse 72, respiration 14 and temperature 98°. Examination of the head, neck, eyes, ears, nose and throat was unremarkable. The chest cage was symmetrical and nontender. Her lungs were clear to percussion and auscultation. The heart was not enlarged and showed no murmurs. The right breast showed a healing surgical incision in the upper outer quadrant. There was some induration and fullness within the incision in the right breast but there was no fixation of tissue to the skin or chest wall. The left breast showed a fine nodularity but no definite masses. No nodes were palpable in either axilla or supraclavicular area. Abdominal examination showed no masses or tenderness and no enlarged organs. Pelvic examination was within normal limits as was the rectal examination. Examination of the musculoskeletal system was recorded as negative. Neurologic examination was normal. Laboratory work on admission included a hematocrit of 40, a white count of 10,900, platelet count 252,000, corrected sedimentation rate of 9; normal prothrombin time, FBS, BUN, calcium phosphorus, alkaline phosphatase and total protein. Urinalysis was also normal.
>
> "Following review of the slides of the biopsy from Costa Rica, a diagnosis of 'ductal cell carcinoma' of the right breast was made. On July 17, 1967, a right radical mastectomy was carried out. Pathologic examination of the mammary tissue showed 42 axillary lymph nodes which were free of tumor. There was some infiltration of the breast tissue in the region of the original breast biopsy. Postoperatively, the patient did well and the wound healed primarily. She was discharged from the hospital on July 27, 1967. Follow-up chest roentgenograms and metastatic survey have been completely negative.
>
> "While convalescing from the radical mastectomy, the patient began to notice a sensation of pain in the left lateral calf and also in the left buttock. In August 1967 she noted a smooth firm mass in the posterior left distal thigh. A physician was consulted who obtained roentgenograms which revealed a lesion in the posterior distal left femur. The patient was then seen in orthopedic consultation and admission advised. There had been no other symptoms except for occasional discomfort over the medical aspect

covering general orthopaedics and trauma. Initially they worked only with Dr. Zimbler, but in 1970 he was joined by Dr. Harris Yett, first as a fellow and then on the staff as Dr. Zimbler's assistant. The service grew and eventually the hospital designated one floor to orthopaedics. For over one year, Zimbler had all the patients on the service, 30 to 35 patients and all were fracture cases. He noted, "All of a sudden I had a gigantic adult practice plus the pediatric practice [at Boston Children's Hospital]. So, I was pretty busy, and I kept it up because it supported the BI. That was the reason and that was what the residents learned. At times it was pretty difficult" (Zimbler, interview with the author, 2009).

In July 1970, Zimbler became an associate professor of orthopaedics at Tufts Medical School and vice-chairman of the Division of Orthopaedics. He really wanted to limit his practice to pediatric orthopaedics and felt he was

> of the left clavicle. The patient had a 10-lb weight loss since June 1967.
>
> "The patient was readmitted to the Beth Israel Hospital on November 27, 1967. At that admission, the general physical examination was unchanged. The right radical mastectomy incision was well healed. Abdominal examination showed no abnormality and the chest remained clinically clear. Examination of the left lower extremity showed a 5 x 5-cm firm mass in the region of the left distal thigh. This appeared to be just beneath the tendon of the biceps femoris. The deep tendon reflexes were equal and active in both lower extremities and motor power was completely normal. The left knee flexed to 140° while the right flexed to 150°. Extension of both knees was to neutral. Laboratory work on admission showed a hematocrit of 37, white count 9400, BUN 11, serum phosphorus 3.3, total protein 7.7 Calcium and alkaline phosphatase were also within normal limits.
>
> "A complete metastatic survey including roentgenograms of all long bones showed no bony abnormality other than the femoral lesion and an irregularity of the medial aspect of the left clavicle. Roentgenograms of the left distal femur showed a mass extending from the distal posterior femur. This appeared to have a narrow sclerotic base and spotty calcification within the lesion.
>
> "On November 29, 1967, under general anesthesia, a posterior exploration of the left distal femur and popliteal area was performed. Dissection revealed a firm encapsulated mass (5 x 5 cm) extending from the left distal femur in its posterolateral aspect. The base was 2 cm in diameter and appeared to arise from the periosteum of the distal femur. It was not adherent to the surrounding tissues in any area. It was noted at the time of surgery that the common peroneal nerve lay directly over the mass itself. Drill holes were made in the cortex of the distal femur and the entire mass was removed, including the cortex from posterior distal femur. The excision extended well into the medullary canal of the distal femur.
>
> "The excised mass was measured 7 x 5 x 5 cm in size. Its external surface was bosselated but was generally smooth, glistening and translucent. The color was mainly white with some pink-red to yellow areas. Cut surface of the lesion showed a translucent gray-white tissue which was slightly gelatinous and included opaque white hard flecks. There was one area of cyst formation with necrotic material within it.
>
> "Microscopic examination revealed lobulated cartilaginous tissue within which were binucleated sarcoma cells in lacunae.
>
> "Postoperatively, the patient was maintained in a long leg plaster splint and she gradually progressed to active exercises and partial weight-bearing on crutches. The wound healed primarily and the patient regained full range of motion of the left knee within 3 weeks of the time of surgery.
>
> "At the present time, the patient has returned to Costa Rica. At last examination (February 2, 1968) she showed a full range of motion of the left knee and a normal gait. She was completely asymptomatic and on full activities."
>
> (Zimbler 1968)

doing too much adult work at Beth Israel. He left Beth Israel Hospital, stopped his clinic at Boston Children's Hospital, but remained on the staff. He continued teaching at Tufts, however, and was promoted to professor of orthopaedics in 1974. He was named associate orthopaedic surgeon-in-chief at New England Medical Center the same year. This was followed, in 1978, by his appointment as chief of the Division of Pediatric Orthopaedics. Six years later, in 1984, Dr. Zimbler became the acting chairman of the department and acting chief of orthopaedic surgery at the New England Medical Center. When he left the New England Medical Center for private practice in 1987, his appointment was changed to clinical professor. Dr. Zimbler remained a very busy clinician, a true workaholic. "Jim [Kasser] tells stories of Zeke Zimbler making rounds at Tufts with a flashlight after midnight" (Emans 2009).

Dr. Zimbler published about 40 articles and chapters on the spectrum of pediatric orthopaedics while at Tufts. They varied from numerous articles on the spine, tumors, cerebral palsy, arthrogryposis and trauma to a few on myelodysplasia, congenital abnormalities, foot deformities, hemophilia and others. He was a member of the Legg-Perthes Study Group.

In 1991, the *New York Times* published an article about shoes for children. It noted that although Dr. Lynn Staheli, then the director of orthopaedics at the Seattle Children's Hospital (in an article from the *Journal of Pediatrics* that same year) recommended that children go barefoot, their shoes should flex easily, be lightweight, take the shape of a quadrangle, with no arch support or stiffness. The *New York Times* article then quoted Zimbler as saying that Staheli had a "vendetta" toward shoes worn for correction, and that, "With some mild deformities, I believe a shoe with some correctives has an ability to help, but it's difficult to prove" (quoted in Angier 1991).

Dr. Henry Banks wrote of Zimbler as an example to leagues of orthopaedic residents, who would have done well to emulate Zimbler's "zealous" care for his patients. Zimbler was also known as a top-rate practitioner and an excellent educator. I remember Dr. Zimbler as an attending at Boston Children's Hospital. He was a dedicated teacher, well-liked by the residents, extremely dedicated to patients, and hardworking. He was always available to the residents. After entering private practice, he worked at both the MGH and Boston Children's Hospital. By 2009, he had retired from surgery, but he continued to see patients, especially those with neuromuscular problems, at Boston Children's Hospital.

HARRIS S. YETT

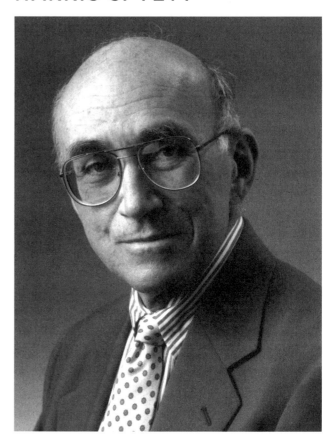

Harris S. Yett. The Ruth and David Freiman Archives at Beth Israel Deaconess Medical Center.

Physician Snapshot

Harris S. Yett
BORN: ca. 1934
DIED: N/A

SIGNIFICANT CONTRIBUTIONS: Orthopaedic division chief at Beth Israel Hospital 1970–1978; president of the Massachusetts Orthopaedic Association 1991; president BIH staff council 1983–1985

Harris S. Yett was born in Barre, Vermont. He attended Tufts University, graduating with a BS degree, *magna cum laude*, in 1955. In 1964, he received his MD degree from Tufts University School of Medicine. After an internship in surgery (1964–1965) and a year of residency in surgery (1965–1966) at Boston City Hospital, Dr. Yett entered the Combined Boston Children's Hospital/Massachusetts General Hospital residency program in orthopaedic surgery. In 1969, he was a chief resident at the Massachusetts General Hospital (MGH). That same year, Dr. Yett was appointed a clinical instructor in orthopaedic surgery at Harvard Medical School.

After completing his residency program, Yett did a six-month fellowship in orthopaedic surgery at the Beth Israel Hospital (BIH). Dr. Seymour Zimbler was chief of the division of orthopaedic surgery at the time, and he had preliminary discussions with Dr. Melvin Glimcher about developing a rotation for orthopaedic residents at the BIH. It apparently was planned for Dr. Yett to join the staff following his fellowship in preparation for including the BIH as a clinical rotation in the Combined Boston Children's Hospital/Massachusetts General Hospital orthopaedic residency program. Beginning in 1970, BIH welcomed orthopaedic residents from Harvard, and those rotations continue today. These residents are able to attend to many older adults in whom fracture and joint diseases such as arthritis are prevalent and who often have multiple comorbidities.

In 1970, Dr. Yett, an associate orthopaedic surgeon, became chief of the division of orthopaedic surgery at BIH. Active in the teaching program of house staff and students rotating there, Yett was honored in 1975 by the initiation of an annual "Harris S. Yett Prize in Orthopedic Surgery." It is given in recognition for a particular resident's dedication to quality in orthopaedic surgery—the one who best emulates Yett through their practice. The award was made possible by a gift from one of Dr. Yett's former patients.

Dr. Yett remained in his position as chief of orthopaedics at BIH for eight years until 1978. Since 1978, he has held the appointment of orthopaedic surgeon at BIH. He has also been on the courtesy staff of Boston Children's Hospital, a staff physician at Brookline Hospital, and a consultant at the Hebrew Rehabilitation Center in Roslindale, Massachusetts, and at Mt. Sinai Hospital in Stoughton, Massachusetts. The Boston Orthopaedic Group was the name of his clinical practice,

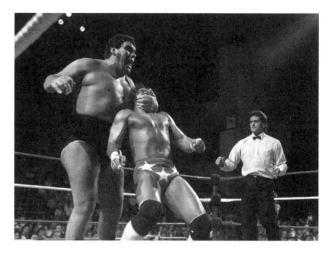

André the Giant. Pictorial Press Ltd./Alamy Stock Photo.

located at 330 Brookline Avenue, Shapiro 2, at Beth Israel Hospital. Other members of the group included Drs. H. Glick, T. Gerhart, and S. Kim.

The same year he stepped down from his position as chief at BIH, he spoke at the Summer Review Course at Colby College in Waterville, Maine. His topic was fractures of the hip and pelvis. Dr. Yett also coauthored four publications and authored or coauthored three letters to the editor. In a letter to the editor of the *New England Journal of Medicine* in 1978, Yett, Skillman and Salzman wrote:

> Between December, 1976, and March, 1977, 17 patients with fractures of the hip were entered into a randomized study to compare the effectiveness of a combination of aspirin and heparin to heparin as prophylaxis for deep vein thrombosis…of the 12 patients treated with aspirin and heparin, eight had serious bleeding complications…In these small groups of patients, there was no difference in the rates of venous thrombosis. Because of the excessive number of serious bleeding complications…the study was stopped after 12 patients were admitted to this group…the combination of heparin and aspirin…is dangerous and should not be used for prophylaxis.

(Yett, Skillman, and Salzman 1978)

Thirteen years later, Dr. Yett and his colleagues reported the results of a randomized controlled trial comparing a low-molecular-weight heparinoid (Lomoparen) with Warfarin for deep vein thrombosis in patients with fractured hips. They "concluded that low-molecular-weight heparinoid…is a safe, convenient, effective antithrombotic agent for the prevention of venous thrombosis after an operation for fracture of the hip" (Gerhart et al. 1991).

Dr. Yett had a unique patient care experience after being in practice only 11 years. André Roussimoff, known as "André the Giant," a professional wrestler, had previously come to the United States from France in 1972. He was billed as being 7'4" tall and weighing 420 pounds. After many successful matches around the world, Vince McMahon, head of the World Wide Wrestling Foundation, took charge of his career and named him "André the Giant." On May 2, 1981, while wrestling "Killer Khan" (6'5") from Mongolia, Khan fell on André's left ankle, fracturing it. They were wrestling in Rochester, New York. He came under the care of Dr. Yett, who told me that he had to use two tourniquets to wrap around André's massive thigh. Yett used two special enormous screws and he recalled making the biggest cast that he had ever seen. André required a special nine-foot bed

Case 53.4. Renal Transplant Infarction During Total Hip Arthroplasty

"A 58-year-old woman with chronic renal failure secondary to rapidly progressive glomerulonephritis underwent cadaver renal transplant to the right iliac fossa on September 17, 1975. Vascular anastomoses were end-of-renal-artery to side-of-right-external iliac-artery, and end-of-renal-vein to side-of-right-external-iliac-vein. Following one mild and easily reversed rejection reaction at two months, she was maintained on immunotherapy of 150 mgm of Imuran and 10 mgm of prednisone a day. In 1977 she developed right hip and then left hip pain. Aseptic necrosis of the hips was diagnosed both clinically and radiologically. Because of progressive symptoms, she underwent a right total hip arthroplasty on May 15, 1979. Although arthroplasty of the left hip was planned for the same admission, it was delayed due to bleeding in the area of the first hip surgery. Renal function remained stable with creatinine levels ranging from 1.3 to 1.7. She was readmitted on June 17, 1979, for a left hip arthroplasty. A creatinine level of 1.8 had been recorded one week prior to this admission and on admission her blood urea nitrogen was 30. Her hematocrit was 36, and white blood cell count 4,900. Urinalysis showed some bacteria, but no white cells. Otherwise her health was stable.

"On June 19, 1979, the patient underwent a total left hip arthroplasty in the standard right lateral decubitus position. The surgery progressed uneventfully with no recorded hypotension. However, on the night after surgery, she was notably pale. Her hematocrit had fallen from 34 to 26, prothrombin time was 14.6/12.1 and a platelet count was 175,000. She received two units of packed cells again without an interval of recorded hypotension and without any clinical transfusion reaction. She also complained immediately after surgery of some discomfort over the cadaver renal transplant area of the right lower quadrant. She was "incontinent" through this first night of small amounts of urine and on the following morning, was catheterized for 200 cc. She had a temperature reading of 99°–101° for the first 48 hours. She passed no urine on the morning after the catheterization (June 20) and developed exquisite graft tenderness. On June 21st she underwent angiography, which demonstrated occlusion to flow in the renal artery just after its takeoff from the right external iliac artery. Because a catheter, introduced into the orifice of the renal artery at its anastomosis with the external iliac artery, revealed the former to be clotted throughout its full length, no angioplasty was possible, and surgery for this infarcted organ was not recommended. Tenderness decreased gradually over the ensuing week. The patient subsequently made no further urine, and chronic hemodialysis was reinstituted on this admission. On August 12, 1979, the patient underwent a second successful cadaver renal transplant to the left iliac fossa. The infarcted graft was not disturbed."

(Zimmerman and Yett 1982)

in the hospital. Special crutches had to be made; the largest size available was too small for André. During his first interview after the operation on June 8, 1981, André mentioned that his cast was to be removed the next day. Apparently, the fractures healed. On July 20, 1981, 2½ months after his fracture, André returned to the ring in Madison Square Garden. His opponent was "Killer Kahn." Kahn was knocked unconscious, but both wrestlers were disqualified after a very brutal match.

Yett continued to publish, and in 1982 he and Dr. C. Zimmerman reported a case of infarction of a kidney transplant during a total hip procedure (see **Case 53.4**). A transplanted kidney is usually placed in the lower anterior abdomen and the diseased kidneys are left in place. In the case, they reported a steel support bar, i.e., kidney rest, was placed on each side of the patient to keep the patient in a lateral decubitus position. The anterior kidney rest or bar obviously compressed the transplanted kidney for the duration of the operation—resulting in a thrombosed artery and the need for a repeat kidney transplantation. Harris and Zimmerman published this case to warn other surgeons to avoid the problem. In their discussion they concluded:

> The standard support system for the lateral decubitus position in total hip arthroplasty in potentially hazardous to a renal allograft in the typical iliac position when the allograft is on the opposite side of the operated hip…curved metal supports ("kidney rests") that attach to the table…exert pressure precisely over the area where the kidney graft resides…the pressure was sufficient to cause a compression in the renal artery…to allow irreversible clotting…An awareness of this potential problem should lead to alternate methods of supporting the patient [such as] the vacuum-activated "bean-bag" support [or] an anterolateral approach, with the patient resting in the supine position. (Zimmerman & Yett 1982)

Since the founding of the Massachusetts Orthopaedic Association (MOA) in 1981, Dr. Yett has been a member of its board. In 1991, he was elected president of the MOA and in 2015 was named "Orthopaedist of the Year" in acknowledgment of his dedication to patient care, resident and student education, and excellence in orthopaedic practice. Yett was extensively involved in helping to amend and improve the commonwealth's Workers' Compensation program.

Yett has been very active on the staff at BIH, serving on many committees, as vice-president of the staff council and later president of the staff council from 1983–1985. Since 1991, he has been a trustee of the hospital. Dr. Yett continues to see patients and teach at the Beth Israel Deaconess Medical Center.

LOUIS W. MEEKS

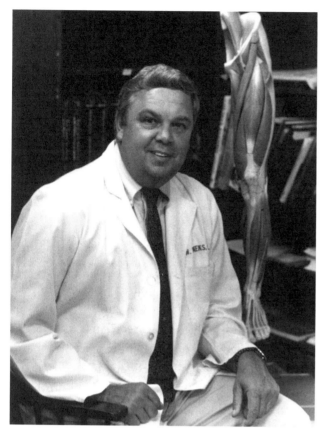

Louis W. Meeks. The Ruth and David Freiman Archives at Beth Israel Deaconess Medical Center.

Physician Snapshot

Louis W. Meeks
BORN: 1937
DIED: 2015
SIGNIFICANT CONTRIBUTIONS: Chief of Sports Medicine at Beth Israel Hospital; acting orthopaedic surgeon-in-chief at Beth Israel Hospital 1990–1992; first surgeon to perform outpatient arthroscopic ACL reconstructions at Beth Israel Hospital; recipient of the orthopaedic residents' Golden Apple Teacher of the Year Award 2001

Louis (Louie or "Papa Lou") Walter Meeks was born the second of four children. He was raised on their family farm in Michigan, and "his early childhood was typical of that life with early morning chores. During these years his strong work ethic and discipline were forged. He says of that time 'the sun never caught Louie Meeks in bed'" (Zilberfarb 2008). Louie graduated with a BA in biology in 1959 from Albion College, which was a small private liberal arts college in Albion (a town in south central Michigan equidistant from Kalamazoo to the west and Ann Arbor to the east). While at Albion, he had played football and was in the marching band, where he played trumpet.

In 1963, he graduated from the University of Michigan School of Medicine, and, after a rotating internship at the University of Michigan Medical Center, completed a year of residency in surgery. His training was interrupted by the Vietnam War; he was drafted into the US Army in 1966. He spent one year of military service "in Vietnam as Commanding Officer for the southern half of South Vietnam (Dr. Gus White [see chapter 54], another Michigan alumnus, was the Commanding Officer for the Northern half of South Vietnam). He relates that this was by far the busiest, most educational and most emotional period in his career" (Zilberfarb 2008).

Early Orthopaedic Contributions

After his discharge from the army in 1967, Meeks returned to the University of Michigan Medical Center where he completed his residency training in orthopaedic surgery (becoming board certified in 1972). In Ypsilanti and Ann Arbor, Michigan, he started a private practice (see **Case 53.5**) specializing in sports injuries three years later. It was during this period that:

> along with Lanny [Johnson] he developed one of the first arthroscopic courses in America… Throughout his long career, he has especially enjoyed mentoring medical students and residents, and has inspired many residents to specialize in Sports Medicine. Asked why he enjoys teaching so much he'll tell you "when you teach a little bit of yourself lives on…I have always thought of myself as a teacher first." (Zilberfarb 2008)

His numerous awards support his insights: in 1974 he was voted the outstanding instructor by the graduating medical class of the department of surgery at the University of Michigan Medical Center; in 2000, he later received the Daniel Federman outstanding clinical educator award at Harvard Medical School; and in 2001 he received the Golden Apple Teacher of the Year award from the graduating class of the Harvard Combined Orthopaedic Residency Program.

Chief of Sports Medicine and Acting Orthopaedic Surgeon-in-Chief at BIH

In the late 1980s, Beth Israel Hospital President Dr. Mitchell Rabkin was searching for a new chief of sports medicine. He impressed Meeks, who agreed to leave his position at the University of Michigan for Boston. Meeks was 52 years old. He threw himself into life in Boston, and his love for sports grew to include the Boston and New England teams. As chief of sports medicine, he was the first surgeon at the Beth Israel Hospital to perform outpatient arthroscopic ACL reconstructions.

In 1990, he was asked by Dr. Gus White (see chapter 54) to serve as acting surgeon-in-chief of orthopaedics, a position he held until 1992. The residents during this period called their rotations at BIH the "penalty box" because they had poor educational experiences. Dr. Meeks reversed that on the sports service, which became a favorite rotation of the residents:

> In 1994 the residents presented him with a plaque thanking him for taking them "out of the penalty box" with the new Sports Rotation at the B.I. Since then this rotation has been consistently ranked at or near the top for all resident rotations in the Harvard program. In 1996 he left the academic group to open a very busy private practice on Beacon Street in Brookline.
> (Zilberfarb 2008)

Dr. Meeks was not a prolific writer; he published only five papers over his career. In 2000, he was asked to write a current review of the status of orthopaedic surgery for the *Journal of the American College of Surgeons*. He discussed researchers' incorporation of biomaterials into treatments that allowed quicker wound healing, creation of prosthesis and matrices, and tissue regeneration. Meeks cited the work of several Harvard faculty, describing in particular studies of gene therapy to treat rheumatoid arthritis and tissue engineering.

Dr. Louis Meeks was involved with various community organizations; these are listed in **Box 53.4**. He and Berneda, his wife, also helped the community close to home, particularly through the philanthropic groups Second Step and the 2Seeds Network. He had a large family, including five children and 11 grandchildren, whom he loved spending time with. Meeks, who suffered

---

Case 53.5. Vertebral Osteophytosis and Dysphagia

"[The patient], a sixty-six-year-old farmer's wife, was referred to University Hospital in 1969 with a six-month history of progressive painless dysphagia and a sixteen-kilogram weight loss. She was able to swallow only pureed foods and liquids and had recently noted the onset of intermittent aspiration and mild hoarseness. Physical examination disclosed tipping of the larynx and hoarseness, as well as moderate loss of forward neck flexion. Roentgenographic studies, including barium swallow, showed hyperostosis at the second, third and fourth cervical vertebrae, and also at the sixth cervical vertebra compressing the esophagus. The diagnosis of ankylosing vertebral hyperostosis was established by plain roentgenograms of the cervical and thoracic spines. Additional studies, including endoscopy, revealed no evidence of neurological disease or neoplasia. The patient was treated by surgical excision of the hyperostosis through an anterolateral cervical approach. Immediate relief of the dysphagia was accomplished and three years after the surgery, the patient was asymptomatic."

(Meeks and Renshaw 1973)

from chronic obstructive pulmonary disease, died on September 14, 2015. His daughter Laura noted that they would "miss his kindness, compassion and sense of humor" (quoted in "In Memory of Dr. Louis W. Meeks" 2008).

Box 53.4. Louis Meeks's Community Involvement

- Board member, Wang Center
- Board member, New England Conservatory
- Member, Sports Museum of New England
- Member, Boston Symphony Orchestra Business Fund Committee
- Overseer, New England Conservatory of Maine
- Council member, Brookings Institute (Washington, DC)

CHAPTER 54

Augustus A. White III

First Orthopaedic Surgeon-in-Chief at Beth Israel Hospital

Augustus "Gus" A. White III was born and raised in Memphis, Tennessee. Although his nuclear family was middle class—his father was a physician and his mother a librarian—his grandparents had been enslaved. As Gus grew up in the late 1930s and 1940s in the South, the evidence of segregation surrounded him, and he and his family lived it daily—attending all-Black churches and theaters, using water fountains and bathrooms designated only for use by Black people, and, for Gus, going to a segregated school. When Gus was eight years old, his father died and he and his mother moved in with his aunt and uncle, a pharmacist.

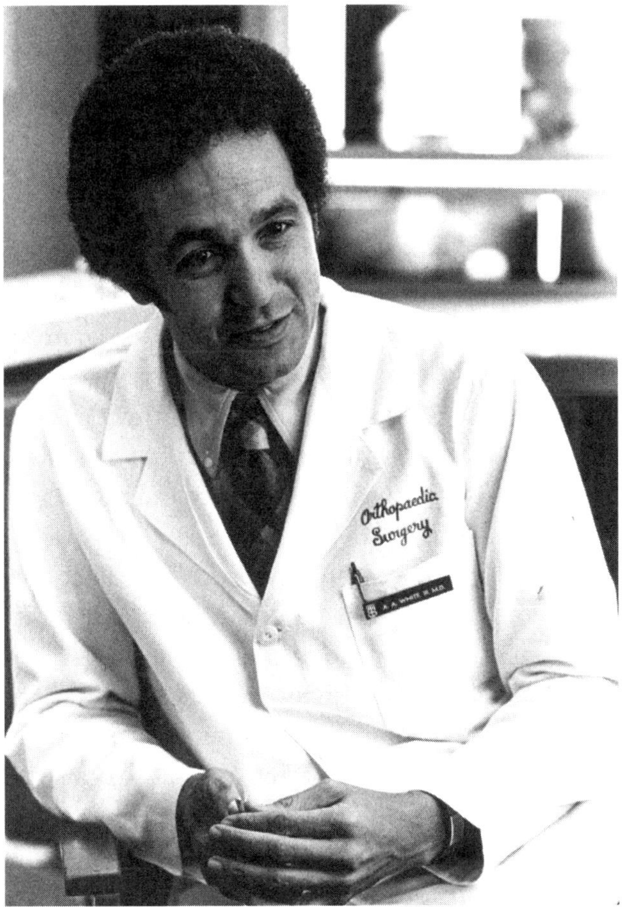

Five years later, in 1953, White was sent to Northfield, Massachusetts, where he began attending Mount Hermon School. What began in 1879 as a girls' school and extended to a separate boys' school two years later, founded by the Protestant Dwight Moody, accepted students who lacked

Augustus A. White III shortly after arrival at BIH. The Ruth and David Freiman Archives at Beth Israel Deaconess Medical Center.

Physician Snapshot

Augustus A. White III

BORN: 1936

DIED: —

SIGNIFICANT CONTRIBUTIONS: First orthopaedic surgeon-in-chief of the newly established orthopaedic surgery department at Beth Israel Hospital; president of both the Cervical Spine Research Society and the Federation of Spine Associations; Ellen and Melvin Gordon Professor of Medical Education at HMS; chair of the Provost's Interfaculty Council on Health Care Disparities at Harvard; director of the Oliver Wendell Holmes Society; chair of the founding committee of the AAOS J. Robert Gladden Orthopaedic Society and served as its first president; published *Seeing Patients: Unconscious Bias in Health Care* with David Chanoff

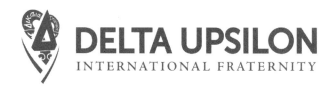

Delta Upsilon Fraternity logo. Courtesy of Delta Upsilon International Fraternity.

social and financial advantages—the sons and daughters of enslaved Africans as well as Native Americans and immigrants. The girls' and boys' schools eventually merged in 1972 as Northfield Mount Hermon. White worked odd jobs to pay for his Northfield tuition, and he excelled there: he was a member of the choir and did well in his classes. White was also captain of the wrestling team and was later elected into the school's Athletic Hall of Fame.

Upon graduating from Northfield, White matriculated at Brown University—one of just five Black students in the class of 1957—where he played football (both offensive and defensive end) and focused on (and excelled in) premed studies. While on the football team at Brown, he began to consider a career in the field of sports medicine, rather than becoming a psychiatrist as he had originally intended. He was the first Black member of the Delta Upsilon fraternity, both at Brown and nationwide; he became chapter president during his junior year. As president, he was expected to attend the fraternity's Undergraduate Convention with other chapter presidents, to be held in Vermont the following year (1956). However, numerous chapters at schools in the South made it clear they would boycott the convention if White attended, and the hosting chapter—because of "circumstances beyond its control" (Schwartzapfel 2011)—decided to reschedule the convention until 1957. White's brothers continued to support him, and because of the cancellation and other issues, it renounced its membership in the national fraternity. It wasn't until the late 1980s that the international leadership of Delta Upsilon formally apologized to White and awarded him the Award for Outstanding Achievement. By doing, so the fraternity fulfilled its motto: "Justice, Our Foundation." In light of this, the Brown chapter reassociated itself with the Delta Upsilon fraternity. With this apology, White wrote: "I can tell you that the delivery and celebration of justice does feel good to all concerned. No matter how long you might have to stick around to see it" (Schwartzapfel 2011).

White also acted as secretary for the class of 1957 student council. He joined the Sigma Xi fraternity and was awarded the Class of 1910 Trophy, given to the senior football letterman who had the best grades. In 1957, he graduated with a bachelor of arts degree in psychology, with distinction.

Beginning in Tennessee, then moving to Massachusetts and Rhode Island, White's education took him away once again—this time to California, where he attended Stanford Medical School. During his time there he cultivated an interest in back pain. He graduated in 1961 and was the medical school's first Black student to do so. Afterwards, Dr. White was off to Michigan, and then back again to California: from 1961 to 1962, he was a rotating intern at the University of Michigan Medical Center, followed by a year as an assistant resident in surgery at Presbyterian Medical Center in San Francisco. In 1963, he went back to the East Coast for a three-year-residency program in orthopaedic surgery at Yale University, where he studied back pain under Wayne Southwick. With this residency he achieved another first, this time as the first Black surgical resident at the Yale teaching hospital.

Another move came upon the completion of his residency—this time, around the world. White was drafted during the Vietnam War and served in-country with the US Army Medical Corps beginning in 1966. He held the rank of captain and received a Bronze Star for his work with Vietnamese patients with leprosy and his selfless efforts during a medical rescue mission. He wrote: "Being in orthopaedic surgery…I was able to be of special service to the patients, most of whom, of course, had trouble with their hands and feet. The patients tended to be most grateful and sometimes our staff would sit and talk and then wonder who was helped most by our efforts[:] the patient or the doctor" (quoted in Brown University Office of the Curator, n.d.). He reflected further: "On the bumpy jeep ride out to the leprosarium…I was seeing the worst that man can do to man, then I go down the road to see the worst that nature can do…Man's inhumanity to man and nature's cruelty to man – both of them an absolute bitch" (Schwartzapfel 2011). After one year in Vietnam, White returned to the United States—back again to California—to complete his military obligation of a second year, as chief of the orthopaedic surgery service, at the Fort Ord US Army Hospital in Monterey.

EARLY ORTHOPAEDIC CONTRIBUTIONS

After his discharge from the army in 1968, White became a National Institute of Health Orthopaedic Trainee in the Orthopaedic Section of Yale University School of Medicine. He earned a doctorate of medical science in orthopaedic biomechanics under Professor Carl Hirsch at the University of Goteborg in 1970. His thesis was entitled, "Analysis of the Mechanics of the Thoracic Spine in Man. An Experimental Study on Autopsy Specimens" and published in *Acta Orthopaedica Scandinavica*.

In the introduction to his dissertation, White quoted Dr. Robert Lovett's 1905 work, "The Mechanisms of the Normal Spine and Its Relation to Scoliosis":

> It is as if one undertook, for example, to investigate a railroad accident solely from a study of the wrecked cars. Much could be learned as to the effect and direction of the destructive forces, the amount of force expended, and the kind of damage done, but more could be learned and future accidents could be better prevented by a study of the normal running time of the trains, their proper relation to each other at the time of the accident, and by an investigation of the signal system and the routine precautions adopted. (Lovett 1905)

Dr. White's doctoral thesis. Published in *Acta Orthopaedica Scandinavica*. 1969; 127: 1.

For White, Lovett's previous work makes clear the need to study not only how trauma affects the thoracic spine but also the normal function of the thoracic spine. White proposed to answer six questions with his thesis research, related to (1) extent of extension and flexion, (2) extent of bend and rotation laterally, (3) alterations in the preceding two elements when considering them cephalocaudally, (4) connection of axial rotation (and its direction) with lateral bend, (5) locations of centers of motion, and (6) whether vertebrae move differently if posterior components are missing.

For the first three topics, he would evaluate how vertebrae move relative to each other in two dimensions under controlled loads. For the latter three, he intended to investigate groups of thoracic vertebrae in motion in three dimensions. White applied such study to 27 autopsy specimens and found extensive differences in vertebral motion between specimens and within the same specimen. Various data on degrees of flexion and extension at the interspaces and motion such as bending and rotation at the various levels of the spine led him to conclude that age and amount of motion were not correlated.

White also noted that rotation of a vertebral body along one axis is constantly associated with rotation of the vertebral body along another axis (i.e., the concept of coupling). Lovett's previous observations on coupling had included:

- Noting that a lateral curve (scoliosis) in the cervical spine and upper thoracic spine, as well as in the lumbar spine and lower thoracic spine, is associated with axial rotation of the vertebral bodies to the concavity of the curve
- But, with a lateral curve (scoliosis) in the mid-thoracic spine, the axial rotation of the vertebral bodies is the reverse—to the convexity of the curve
- With removal of the posterior elements of the spine, motion is increased in flexion, extension, and rotation.

White analyzed the axes of rotation in the frontal, sagittal, and horizontal planes. He reported that flexion occurred below the disc, extension above the disc, and lateral bending at or near the disc to the contralateral side of the bending. White (and Panjabi), with the use of 3-dimensional studies, introduced the concept of the helical axis of motion of the spine: helical or twist axis is a line that is simultaneously in the axis of rotation and the axis of translation of a vertebral body. He found that little motion occurred in the vertebral bodies of the thoracic spine and that the helical axis is a useful tool to describe the 3-dimensional kinematics of the spine.

Dr. Manohar M. Panjabi was studying in Sweden during this same period in a graduate school program at the Chalmers University of Technology in Gottenberg. Dr. White acknowledged in the foreword to his thesis the important help Panjabi gave him related to engineering and applied biomechanics issues. In a first of many future publications together, Panjabi and White published the article "A Mathematical Approach for Three-Dimensional Analysis of the Mechanics of the Spine," in which they found it possible to quantify kinematics of the spine by measuring the helical axis of motion. The kinematics are measured vis a vis the motion of the spine on an axis—for example, with flexion, extension or lateral bending. In the introduction, they quoted Kelvin, who wrote in 1891, "I often say that when you can measure what you are speaking about and express it in numbers you know something about it; but when you cannot measure it, when you cannot express it in numbers, your knowledge is of a meagre and unsatisfactory kind."

After completing his doctorate thesis, White returned to Yale as an assistant professor of orthopaedic surgery where he remained for about ten years, eventually being promoted to full professor in 1977. He also subsequently published three papers with Professor Hirsch on biomechanics: two on the thoracic spine and one on the load-bearing capacity of iliac bone graft. Panjabi joined him on the faculty at the medical school where they established a small biomechanics research laboratory. Together they were successful in receiving public health grants to study biomechanics of the cervical spine and biomechanics of fracture healing and published over 23 papers the next ten years on these and other biomechanical issues.

Drs. White, Southwick and Panjabi's article in which they reported a checklist for evaluating stability of the cervical spine following injury. *Spine* 1976; 1: 15.

Based on their studies, White and Panjabi, along with Dr. Wayne Southwick, published an important paper on instability of the lower cervical spine in 1976. They developed a widely accepted checklist that surgeons could use to evaluate instability of the lower cervical spine. The checklist gave two points to each of six elements—anterior and posterior components that did not work or had been damaged beyond repair, translation >3.5 mm and rotation >11° in the sagittal plane, a positive result on the stretch test, and damage to the spinal cord—and one point to each of three elements: damage to the nerve root, atypical narrowing of the disc, and the potential for precarious loading. A total point score exceeding five indicated spinal instability, although surgeons are meant to use their clinical judgement when interpreting this score in light of the loads a patient's spine might be required to support; for example, occupationally, loads would differ for a seamstress and a professional football player. White, Southwick, and Panjabi also highlighted particular ways surgeons could evaluate each of the elements in the checklist; these varied from a history and physical examination, to radiography, to measurement of lateral projections on the posteroinferior and

Case 54.1. Nonunion of a Hangman's Fracture and Late Cord Compression

"A fifty-one-year-old woman, was in an automobile accident as she drove the vehicle through an intersection. She sustained a brief loss of consciousness and had symptoms in the chest, the left shoulder and the neck. The roentgenograms of the cervical spine were normal, and the patient was treated for a pneumothorax. She was released after eight days of hospitalization and had no pain in the neck at the time of discharge. At no time did she have a neural deficit. The patient returned four months later complaining of intermittent pain in the right side of the neck and she noted 'shocky electrical' sensations in all four extremities whenever she tried to bend over. Roentgenograms of the cervical spine revealed a hangman's fracture with non-union and with an anterior subluxation of the second on the third cervical vertebra of four millimeters.

"The patient was hospitalized. A cervical myelogram showed a step-off at the second and third cervical vertebrae with an anterior extradural defect behind the second cervical vertebra close to the level of the interspace. The root sheaths of the sixth and seventh cervical vertebrae on the right side were encroached on. A computerized axial tomogram revealed no significant anteroposterior compromise of the canal. Because the patient reported paresthesias and weakness on forward flexion, no flexion-extension roentgenograms were made. Because the patient's symptoms fit established criteria for the diagnosis of clinical instability, we elected to do a spine fusion.

"The bodies of the second and third cervical vertebrae were fused using the modification of the Bailey-Badgley procedure. Post-operatively, the patient was kept in traction with two kilograms of pull maintained until the third postoperative day. A prefabricated halo jacked was then applied and the patient was allowed to walk. Ten days later, she was discharged home. Evaluation of the patient at subsequent clinic visits showed no further subluxation. Twelve months postoperatively, there was evidence of healing of the fusion. The patient was free of symptoms at the time of writing, fifteen months postoperatively."

(White and Moss 1978)

posterosuperior angles, to clinical evidence of disc space narrowing or damage to the spinal cord. Two years later, Drs. White and H. L. Moss published a case report (see **Case 54.1**) on an injury to the cervical spine.

In 1978, White and Panjabi published their popular and famous book, *Clinical Biomechanics of the Spine*. In his foreword, Professor Alf Nachemson wrote that the authors provide a broad evaluation of existing knowledge of the spine and how it moves—both as a whole and its components. For Nachemson, White and Panjabi's text matches the level of the then-classic (and 45-year-old) German treatise *Dis Gesunde and die Kranke Wirbelsäule im Röntgenbild und Klinik*, published in 1932 by Georg Schmorl and Herbert Junghanns

In their preface to the book, White and Panjabi wrote of the benefits of their teamwork—one an orthopaedic surgeon, the other a mechanical engineer—to fully incorporate knowledge of both mechanics of and problems in the spine with the theory and practice of engineering. White dedicated the book to his family, Martin Luther King, Jr. and Mohandas Karamchand Gandhi.

FIRST ORTHOPAEDIC SURGEON-IN-CHIEF AT BETH ISRAEL HOSPITAL

After 10 years on the faculty at Yale University School of Medicine, Dr. White was recruited in 1978 to Boston's Beth Israel Hospital (BIH) as orthopaedic surgeon-in-chief of the newly established Department of Orthopaedic Surgery. Dr. William Silen was chief of surgery at the time. White was also appointed Professor of Orthopaedic Surgery at Harvard Medical School. Although Panjabi remained at Yale, becoming the director of the biomechanics research laboratory, he continued to collaborate with White. White also began to collaborate with Dr. Wilson (Toby) C. Hayes, who had been working in the research laboratory at BIH since 1976 and, after White's arrival, was named director of the Orthopaedic Biomechanics Laboratory at BIH in 1979.

White remained orthopaedic surgeon-in-chief for 13 years, until 1991. During that time, he wrote nine annual reports of the department. In his first year (1978–1979), he focused his efforts on research and organizational issues of patient care, education, and academic productivity. The staff included Dr. George Lewinnek, a Harvard Combined Orthopaedic Residency Program graduate who returned to BIH after two years at Northwestern, and 12 part-time physicians—including Drs. Harris Yett, Hyman Glick, Lewis Millender, Robert Davies, Barry Simmons, Joseph Copel and others. About 100 patients were seen weekly in the orthopaedic clinics. Teaching conferences included chief's walk rounds; some specialty conferences; and a combined conference with Boston Children's Hospital, the Peter Bent Brigham Hospital, and the Robert Breck Brigham Hospital on Friday mornings. White instituted clinical research protocols in spine. Hayes's laboratory was funded by the National Institutes of Health with focuses on spine biomechanics, fracture healing, and knee joint mechanics.

In his second report (1979–1980), White wrote that the research protocols were in place, the newly renovated outpatient clinic was now seeing 150 patients each week, and he listed the department's presentations and publications. The research program grew in 1980. It included five post-doctoral students, six MIT undergraduates and research teaching conferences for the staff were held weekly. In his fourth report (1983–1984), the staff had increased to 14, including Drs. Jerry Knirk, Tobin Gerhart, and Timothy Hosea. Two fellows were selected and Thomas Edwards, PhD, from MIT began research in spine biomechanics. Dr. White organized a Board of Consultants, which included Drs. Henry Banks, Melvin Glimcher, Paul Griffin, John Hall, Henry Mankin, and Clement Sledge and started a back-pain school. The orthopaedic biomechanics lab began its own annual report.

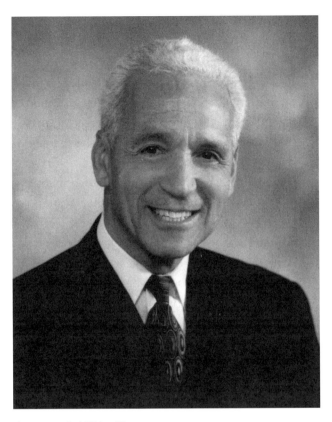

Augustus A. White III. Courtesy of Dr. Augustus A. White III.

In 1983, Mr. Daniel E. Hogan, a lawyer, businessman, and friend of Dr. White, donated $235,000 to endow the spine fellowship program. White headed this program from 1983 to 2003. By 1985, two more PhDs were added to the research laboratory. There were only two professors in the department, Drs. White and Hayes. Five part-time instructors included Drs. Ed Cheal, John Davies, Tom Edwards, Tobin Gerhart, and Jerry Knirk. Two clinical instructors included Drs. Harris Yett and Hyman Glick. The teaching program expanded to include specialty conferences in addition to the combined grand rounds (Boston Children's Hospital, Brigham and Women's Hospital, and Beth Israel Hospital) and participation in the residency core curriculum held Saturday mornings (8:30 AM to 10:30 AM) at MGH. The department also held its first CME conference on new management strategies for patients with low back pain and sciatica. White reported that the full-time physicians had formally organized as the Harvard Community Health Physicians at Beth Israel Hospital.

The sixth report (1986–1987) contained more changes. Dr. Gerhart was named deputy chief of the department focusing on research activities; and hand surgeon Dr. Hillel Skoff was hired. The outpatient volume had plateaued to about 3400 visits per year. The chief residents and full-time staff were reported to have operated on slightly less than 400 cases per year. The 1987–1988 report marked the tenth anniversary of the Department of Orthopaedic Surgery at Beth Israel Hospital. An evening celebration followed a program that included visiting professor Maurice Mueller from Switzerland, who later endowed a research professorship for the department.

Dr. White wrote in his eighth annual report that the board of consultants was reduced to Drs. Banks, Glimcher, Mankin, and Sledge. Both Drs. Cheal and Dr. Gerhart were promoted to assistant professors. The first BIH/Camp International Visiting Lecture was held on January 11, 1989; given by Dr. Arthur H. White of the Spine Care Medical Group in Daly City, California. In his last department annual report (1989–1990), Dr. White had asked Dr. Mark Bernhardt, who just completed his spine fellowship, to care for the spine patients for the next six months while he went on sabbatical. Dr. Hayes became the first recipient of the newly endowed Mueller Professorship. In January 1990, Dr. Louis Meeks joined the full-time staff as clinical director of the department of orthopaedic surgery with an appointment at Harvard Medical School as clinical instructor of orthopaedic surgery.

The year 1989 had been a significant one for Dr. White. He was selected from among 20 contenders in a nationwide search to become president of the University of Maryland Health Center—again the first Black man to do so. This prestigious appointment, with an annual salary of $245,000, gave White power over six of the state's healthcare-related schools, a graduate school with more than 4,500 students, and a quarter-million-dollar budget. White accepted the position in June 1989, with the intention of starting in January 1990. Two months later, however, the Maryland Board of Regents Chair Peter O'Malley told him that the university intended to move the schools of law and social work from Baltimore to other campuses. Despite being the new president, White had not been involved in this decision, an oversight he called "personally and professionally objectionable and intolerable" (quoted in Sharfstein 1989), and he subsequently resigned the position before it had even begun and went back to Boston. White's withdrawal from the position of president left the University of Maryland hanging, what university leadership called a "firestorm" that had "blown across the very top of the structure, at the planning level, which has now been thrown into disorder" (Daniels 1989).

Over the next decade, White, Hayes, and others continued to publish over 20 articles on biomechanics and clinical issues involving the spine, including three articles with Dr. Jennifer Kelsey and the major publication, "The Impact of Musculoskeletal Disorder on the Population of the United States" in 1979. White stepped down as orthopaedic surgeon-in-chief in 1991 at age 55. He continued to provide patient care and conduct his research at BIH.

BIAS, DIVERSITY, AND CULTURALLY COMPETENT CARE

In 1999, Dr. White began to change the focus of his publications from biomechanics and spine problems to issues of diversity with two publications: "Compassionate Patient Care and Personal Survival in Orthopaedics; a 35-Year Perspective" and "Justification and Need for Diversity in Orthopaedics." Two years later, he retired from operating at 65 years old, continuing to dedicate his time to furthering diversity initiatives in orthopaedics. He presented the 2002 Alfred R. Shands, Jr. Lecture, "Our Humanitarian Orthopaedic Opportunity," stating:

> We, as physicians, can be society leaders in facing racism clinically, not emotionally, but rationally, objectively, and constructively…I think that we can extend [our] skills to the management of racism…Our Humanitarian Orthopaedic Opportunity is to eliminate disparities in the care of the musculoskeletal system… Here are some things we can do. First of all, we can achieve more diversity in our profession…Second, we must make the challenging administrative and policy changes necessary to solve the financial, insurance, and other access problems, and we need to establish control systems to evaluate and monitor progress. Third, we must recognize the usefulness of educating minority patients…We need to remind minority patients that they can do something immediately to improve their health…Fourth, we must teach all physicians to provide culturally competent care…Implicit in this is the elimination of conscious and unconscious bias against any patient…In summary, health-care disparity for minorities in the United States today is a problem, which includes racial bias. That bias is intimately woven into the fabric of our medical culture…It is not our fault, but it is our responsibility to correct this unconscionable reality. (White 2002)

At the time he gave the AOA Alfred R. Shands Jr. lecture, White had become Director of the Oliver Wendell Holmes Society and the Ellen and Melvin Gordon Professor of Medical Education at Harvard Medical School; a position he held until 2006. He continued to speak and write about bias and racial and ethnic disparities. At Harvard Medical School, he was a member of the Executive Council on Diversity (1998–2000) and for several years was chair of the ad hoc committee for cross-cultural education, the initial chair of the culturally competent care education committee

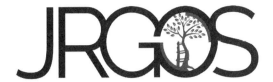

Logo of the J. Robert Gladden Orthopaedic Society. Courtesy of the J. Robert Gladden Orthopaedic Society.

and chair of the Provost's Interfaculty Council on Health Care Disparities at Harvard University. He served on numerous other institutional and organization committees, including Brown University Presidents' Advisory Council on Diversity, Chair of the Visiting Committee on Diversity at Brown University, the NIH National Advisory Council of the National Center on Minority Health and Health Disparities, and many others. He was chair of the founding committee of the AAOS J. Robert Gladden Orthopaedic Society and served as its first president. In 2011, he published his last book, *Seeing Patients: Unconscious Bias in Health Care*, with coauthor David Chanoff.

LEGACY

Dr. White has received numerous academic and organizational awards for his contributions in the field of spine care, biomechanics, diversity, bias and culturally competent care. He served as president of both the Cervical Spine Research Society (1988) and the Federation of Spine Associations (1998). In 2004, the BIDMC orthopaedic department began a yearly Augustus White III Symposium on the spine in his honor (**Box 54.1**). A few of his awards include the Kappa Delta award for outstanding research (1976), the AAOS Diversity Award in 2006, the AOA Distinguished Clinician Educator Award in 2007, and the AAOS William W. Tipton Jr., MD Leadership Award in 2010. He was honored by the Harvard Law School in 2013 which awarded him the Justice Award, Charles

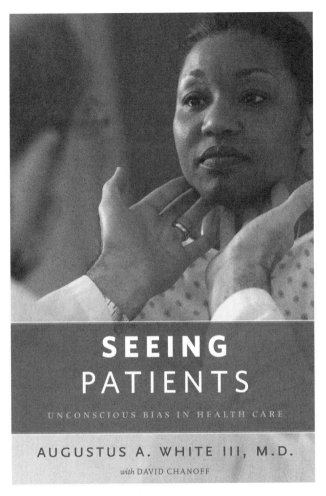

White and Chanoff's book, *Seeing Patients: Unconscious Bias in Health Care*.

Seeing Patients: Unconscious Bias in Health Care by Augustus A. White III, M.D. and David Chanoff, Cambridge, Mass.: Harvard University Press, Copyright © 2011 by Augustus A. White III, M.D. and David Chanoff. Used by permission. All rights reserved.

Hamilton Houston Institute for Race and Justice; by Brown University in 2014 when the alumni awarded him the Joseph M. Fernandez Award; and by Stanford University where he was inducted into the Multicultural Alumni Hall of Fame in 2014. White has long pushed for diversity in medicine, and he compares the struggle to attain diversity to a musical composition: "There are variations on the same theme. Melodies are expressed in many different ways, and there are improvised variations, but the theme is recurrent. It shows up everywhere" (Kahn 2006). He noted that despite hardships and some failures, he wouldn't be where he is without "tremendous help from stalwart allies, both black and white" (Kahn 2006).

Today Dr. White remains at Harvard Medical School as the Ellen and Melvin Gordon Distinguished Professor of Medical Education. While a graduate student in Sweden, he had met and married Anita Ottemo. They have three children.

Box 54.1. White Symposium Keynote Speakers 2004–2020

- 2004   Alvin Crawford, MD
- 2005   Louis Sullivan, MD
- 2006   Oheneba Boachie-Adjei, MD
- 2007   Gunnar B.J. Anderson, MD
         James N. Weinstein, DO
- 2008   Henry H. Bohlman, MD
- 2009   William Toby
- 2010   Alan S. Hilibrand, MD
- 2011   Kevin J. Bozic, MD
- 2012   Todd J. Albert, MD
- 2013   _____
- 2014   _____
- 2015   Thomas R. Oxland, PhD
- 2016   Mary I. O'Connor, MD
- 2017   Alvin H. Crawford, MD
- 2018   Claudia L. Thomas, MD
- 2019   Gary Friedlaender
- 2020   Cato T. Laurencin, MD, PhD

CHAPTER 55

Stephen J. Lipson

Chief of Orthopaedics at Beth Israel Hospital and Beth Israel Deaconess Medical Center

Stephen Jay Lipson was born on September 25, 1946. After being raised in Staten Island, New York, he matriculated at Yale University. He received his undergraduate bachelor's degree cum laude in 1968. He then went to Harvard Medical School (HMS), from which he earned an MD in 1972. Dr. Henry Mankin (see chapter 41) described Lipson's educational experience:

> His interest in biology was well established during his time at Yale...his honor's thesis in the Department of Chemistry investigat[ed] certain aspects of cytochrome B2 [at] Harvard Medical School [and] because of his excellent preparation [at Yale] Stephen...was excused from certain courses and assigned to Dr. Glimcher for a tutorial reading period his first year [at HMS]. Stephen worked closely with Dr. Glimcher in the field of connective tissues, and it was quite clear from the beginning that he had unusual intellectual abilities. He did an outstanding job in the elective... (Mankin 1977)

From 1972 to 1973, Lipson was an intern at Massachusetts General Hospital (MGH) in general surgery. He spent the following year as a surgical resident there. From July 1, 1974, through June 30, 1977, he was a resident in the Harvard Combined Orthopaedic Residency Program. He spent the next six months as chief resident at the MGH.

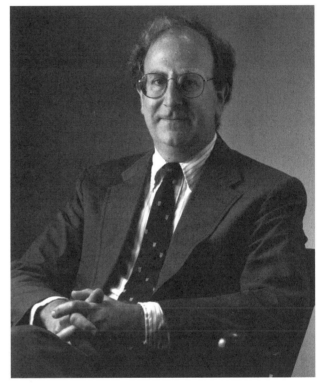

Stephen J. Lipson. The Ruth and David Freiman Archives at Beth Israel Deaconess Medical Center.

Physician Snapshot

Stephen J. Lipson
BORN: 1946
DIED: 2013

SIGNIFICANT CONTRIBUTIONS: Received the Volvo Award in Basic Science from the International Society for the Study of the Lumbar Spine for his research with Dr. Helen Muir; chief of orthopaedic surgery at Beth Israel Hospital and later at Beth Israel Deaconess Medical Center

EARLY ORTHOPAEDIC CONTRIBUTIONS

During his residency and as early as 1976, Dr. Lipson had applied for a Berg-Sloat Traveling Fellowship for research after completing his residency. In his letter of support, Dr. Mankin (1977) wrote that Lipson was "very interested in basic science as it applies to orthopaedics and particularly in studying various aspects of the biochemistry and immunology of cartilage and, more specifically, the cartilage which is present in disc tissue. He has a number of very good ideas in this area and has a good enough background in biochemistry to pursue this further." While Lipson was a senior resident, Mankin also wrote a strong letter to Dr. Helen Muir in England supporting Lipson for a research position in her laboratory.

After completing his chief residency, Lipson completed a research fellowship with Dr. Muir in the Kennedy Institute of Rheumatology in Hammersmith, London. He published three research papers with Muir on experimental disc degeneration and proteoglycan changes. In 1980, his research with Muir, supported by an NIH grant, received the Volvo Award in Basic Science from the International Society for the Study of the Lumbar Spine. In rabbits, they surgically caused a vertical herniation of two-to-three lumbar discs, leaving the remaining discs as controls. The injury led to changes similar to disc degeneration. They highlighted the occurrences of metaplasia that caused the disc space to become fibrocartilage, osteophytes on the vertebrae, collection and saturation of proteoglycans as degeneration began, and a reduction in the amount of hyaluronic acid in the discs. For the authors, these changes seemed to represent a failed attempt at repair rather than deterioration subsequent to proteoglycan changes. **Case 55.1** highlights an example of a patient case Lipson reported that same year.

Following his year of research, Lipson joined the full-time staff at the Peter Bent Brigham Hospital, a position he held for about 14 years. He

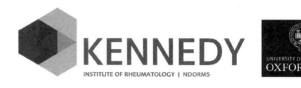

Logo of the Kennedy Institute of Rheumatology, which in 2011, became an independent institute within the Nuffield Department of Orthopaedics, Rheumatology and Musculoskeletal Science at the University of Oxford.
Courtesy of the Kennedy Institute of Rheumatology.

published more than 15 articles during this time on a variety of clinical problems of the spine, including rheumatoid arthritis of the cervical spine, spinal stenosis, C1–C2 fusion with bone graft, wires and metal mesh and stabilized with methyl methacrylate, and perioperative airway management in rheumatoid arthritis patients undergoing posterior cervical spine fusion.

CHIEF OF ORTHOPAEDICS AT BETH ISRAEL HOSPITAL

At age 45, in 1992, Dr. Lipson was chosen to succeed Dr. Augustus White (see chapter 54) as chief of the orthopaedic department at Beth Israel Hospital. He held this position for four years, followed by chief of the orthopaedic department at BIDMC for an additional five years until he retired in 2001. Lipson continued with his interest in adult spine disorders; his clinical research focused on degenerative spinal stenosis and rheumatoid arthritis of the cervical spine. He wrote another 15 papers and seven book reviews for the *New England Journal of Medicine* and the *Journal of Bone and Joint Surgery*, and he coauthored a research paper demonstrating increased spine fusion rates in rabbits with the use of direct current electrical stimulation alone or in connection with the use of coralline hydroxyapatite.

In 1995, Dr. Lipson wrote a "Point of View" for *Spine*. He referred to an unpublished paper he

Katz, Lipson, et al.'s article on long-term outcomes after decompression laminectomy for lumbar spinal stenosis.
Journal of Bone and Joint Surgery 1991; 73: 809.

and his coauthors presented at the Cervical Spine Research Society in December 1993. The topic was predictors of preoperative neurological deficits and postoperative outcomes in rheumatoid patients with subaxial cervical spine involvement. They named four main elements that can indicate neurologic effects after surgery: reduction in cervical height (which they referred to as the cervical height index), largest amount of subluxation, additional lordosis, and the extent of signs and symptoms indicating neurological issues.

Most of his papers dealt with degenerative spinal stenosis; seven of these were cowritten with Dr. Jeffrey Katz and others at the Peter Bent Brigham Hospital. They demonstrated "long-term outcome of decompressive laminectomy is less favorable than has been previously reported, and that co-morbidity and a single-interspace laminectomy are risk factors for a poor outcome" (Katz et al. 1996). In a seven-to-ten-year-outcome study of decompressive surgery for spinal stenosis, they reported that among the almost one-quarter of patients who required a second surgery, just about one-third reported severe back pain. In light of

Case 55.1. Spinal Stenosis Due to Epidural Lipomatosis in a Patient with Cushing Syndrome

"A 53-year-old woman with Graves' disease, euthyroid after radioiodine therapy, had infiltrative opthalmopathy with optic-nerve involvement. When she was treated with prednisone, 150 mg per day, cushingoid features developed rapidly. Two months after the initiation of therapy, with the prednisone tapered to 100 mg per day, the patient reported a low-back ache that radiated to the and thighs. The pain worsened over months, was exacerbated by walking, and showed a claudication pattern. After six months the prednisone had been tapered to 50 mg per day, and the patient was able to walk only a few steps. She could sit comfortably, could extend her spine to only 20 degrees of flexion with further flexion to 80 degrees, and could tolerate the supine position only very briefly. Straight leg raising reached 90 degrees bilaterally. The lumbar spine was nontender, and the sciatic notices and nerves were tender to palpation. The findings of neurologic examination of the lower extremities were unremarkable except for the absence of deep-tendon reflexes in spite of reinforcement.

"Electromyographic findings in the lower extremities included chronic, bilateral denervation in the L4 and L5 distribution. Radiographs of the lumbosacral spine revealed diffuse osteopenia without evidence of collapse. A lumbar metrizamide myelogram revealed a complete extradural block at L4-5 with ventral indentation at the disk space and a prominent epidural space posterior to the body of L4. Computed tomography of the lumbar spine failed to reveal metrizamide below L4-5. The bony canal and foramina were of normal dimensions and the intracanal soft-tissue density measured – 80 to 0 Hounsfield units, indicative of fat density.

"A lumbar bilateral laminectomy was performed at the L4 and L5 levels. Copious epidural fat herniated through the incision in the ligamentum flavum. Abundant epidural fat was found throughout the area exposed. The L4-5 disk appeared normal and the L5-S1 disk had a diffuse degenerative bulge. Histologic examination of the fat revealed normal adult adipose tissue. After operation, the patient had immediate relief of buttock and thigh pain and was able to walk, to extend her spine fully, and to lie supine."

(Lipson et al. 1980)

this, Katz et al. identified a correlation between spinal symptoms and lessened functional ability. In another paper they concluded that patients' satisfaction with surgical outcomes of surgical treatment for lumbar spinal stenosis with related degeneration is significantly lower when they have back pain before surgery, high comorbidity, poor function, or a combination of these. In 1999, they reported that among patients operated on for spinal stenosis (decompressive laminectomy with or without arthrodesis), after two years the occurrence of severe pain was reduced by 50%. Having "good" or "excellent" health and having few cardiovascular issues before the procedure were related to positive surgical results.

That same year, Harvard Medical School published a "Family Health Guide" written by Harvard faculty. Lipson advised adults with low back pain who are considering surgery to avoid it if possible. His reasoning for this was the responsiveness of back pain to noninvasive, less extreme measures such as pharmacologic treatments, rest, and exercises. For Lipson, back surgery should be performed only if necessary to relieve severe back pain in patients whose pain does not respond to the aforementioned methods, and when the benefits of the procedure are certain to outweigh the risks.

Lipson had simultaneously continued with his research while providing steady leadership during a period of seismic change in the department. He was the chief of the orthopaedic department at Beth Israel during the financial and disruptive changes and the merger of the Beth Israel and Deaconess Hospital beginning in 1996 (see chapter 56), and he remained as chief of the department in the new Beth Israel Deaconess Medical Center (BIDMC). He wrote two chief's reports (BIDMC) for the *Orthopaedic Journal at Harvard Medical School* in 1999 and 2000. In 1999 he wrote:

> The Department of Orthopaedic Surgery at Beth Israel Deaconess Medical Center has grown and developed since I came here as orthopaedic surgeon-in-chief in July 1992... The recent merger of the Beth Israel and the New England Deaconess Hospitals in 1997 has brought about much pressure and continued evolution in the Beth Israel Deaconess Medical Center. The majority of orthopaedic activities remain at the East Campus (the new name for the old Beth Israel Hospital). The clinical activity involves a range of adult orthopaedics and is centered on the full time academic staff and the private 'Beacon Street' practitioners...Dr. Donald Reilly remains very active and is pursuing clinical investigation in joint replacement surgery...Don's vigorous and enthusiastic teaching continue to be a hallmark of the Beth Israel Deaconess experience. New additions...include Drs. Robert G. Davis, Gregory T. Altman and Michael Vostrejs. Dr. Robert G. Davis, a graduate of the Harvard Orthopaedic Residency Program and Dr. Lyle Micheli's sports medicine fellowship, is...pursuing sports medicine...Dr. Gregory T. Altman completed his orthopaedic training at Hamot Medical Center in Erie, Pennsylvania. He then completed fellowships in trauma surgery with Dr. David Lhowe at Massachusetts General Hospital and Dr. Chip Routt at Harborview in Seattle. Greg joined the Department...in 1998 and pursues trauma surgery, sports medicine, and general orthopaedics...Dr. Michael Vostrejs was educated at New York Orthopaedic Hospital, Columbia Physicians and Surgeons. He completed a knee surgery fellowship with Dr. John Siliski at Massachusetts General Hospital and then a spine fellowship at the Brigham and Women's Hospital. He joined us this year to pursue general practice orthopaedics with an emphasis on spine surgery... The private practitioners provide constant input of clinical care with geriatric orthopaedics always one of the characteristics of the Beth Israel Deaconess Medical Center...Dr. Paul Glazer concentrates on spinal disorders

and is a valued resource and teacher for the residents. In the recent past he has helped care for the majority of the traumatic spine injuries and runs our Tuesday morning Spine Conference...he is very active in the Orthopaedic Biomechanics Laboratory...the Musculoskeletal Medicine Unit, functioning in the orthopaedic unit of the Shapiro Clinical Center has provided an excellent interaction over regional musculoskeletal disease problems. The Unit is currently staffed by a rheumatologist...The Orthopaedic Biomechanics Laboratory has been in transition since Dr. Wilson C. (Toby) Hayes left for Oregon in 1998. Dr. Bryan Synder...of Children's Hospital has been acting director while a Harvard Medical School search committee searches for a new lab director. (Lipson 1999)

In his chief's report of 2000. Dr. Lipson wrote:

Most of the orthopaedic activities remain on the east campus...but will ultimately be moving to the west campus (the old New England Deaconess) when emergency service facilities are renovated and opened there. The Medical Center remains as a Level I trauma center and is a source of such activity and a resource for the chief resident and faculty who participate in trauma call...The coordination of the third-year Harvard Medical Students rotating on their surgical rotation at the Medical Center, where an orthopaedic/musculoskeletal medicine 2-week rotation occurs, is accomplished by Kathryn MacDonald and undertaken by all members of the orthopaedic faculty. It was developed into and remains a significant component of the surgical rotation in the third year. Dr. Donald Reilly...teaches with enthusiasm that is recognized as a strength of the BIDMC rotation by the orthopaedic residents...Dr. Altman has coordinated trauma conferences along with Dr. Mark Vrahas, Chief of Orthopaedic Trauma Services for Partner's Orthopaedics. (Lipson 2000)

While orthopaedic surgeon-in-chief at the Beth Israel Deaconess Medical Center, Dr. Lipson had developed multiple sclerosis. Because of progression of the disease, he had to stop operating and stepped down as chief in 2001. He kept seeing patients at Harvard Vanguard clinics, and he continued to teach at HMS and maintained his involvement in the school's alumni activities. He also worked on the editorial staffs of the *New England Journal of Medicine* and three specialty journals—*Perspectives in Orthopaedic Surgery*, *Spine*, and *Journal of Spinal Disorders*—and he continued to engage with the AAOS and the Cervical Spine Research Society. In 2004, he wrote a brief article for the *New England Journal of Medicine*, "Spinal-Fusion Surgery – Advances and Concerns." He briefly reviewed the modern technological advances of instrumentation with pedicle screws and plates or rods, intervertebral cages, and substitutes for autologous bone grafts (frozen or freeze-dried allografts, hydroxyapatite, tricalcium phosphate and collagen sponges with bone morphogenic protein). He concluded that "The advances in spinal-fusion surgery are exciting but they continue to provoke questions about the appropriate clinical place for this complex surgery" (Lipson 2004).

LEGACY

Dr. Stephen Lipson's disease worsened, however, and on December 17, 2013, he died peacefully at his home. His wife, Jenifer (neé Burns), and their two children and two grandchildren survived him. His obituary in the *Boston Globe* recalled his personal interest in his patients, his love of teaching, and his humorous and optimistic personality. In honor of Dr. Lipson, the Department of Orthopaedic Surgery at the Brigham and Women's

Hospital sponsors an annual Stephen J. Lipson, MD Orthopaedic and Spine lectureship (**Box 55.1**).

Box 55.1. Stephen J. Lipson, MD Orthopaedic and Spine Lectureship

- 2015   Zoher Ghogawala, MD
        (Lipson Inaugural Speaker)
- 2016   Charles A. Reitman, MD
- 2017   Robert F. Heary, MD
- 2018   David A. Wong, MD, MSc, FRCS(C)
- 2019   Ziya L. Gokaslan, MD
- 2020   *canceled due to Covid*

CHAPTER 56

Beth Israel Deaconess Medical Center

A History of New England Deaconess Hospital and Its Merger with Beth Israel Hospital

New England Deaconess Hospital (NEDH) was originally established on February 5, 1896, as an extension of the Deaconess Home and Training School, which had been incorporated under the name the New England Deaconess Home and Training School seven years earlier. (See **Box 56.1** for a history of the term "Deaconess.") The hospital was opened at an adjacent property at 691 Massachusetts Avenue; it was "a 14-bed hospital [where] the religiously trained Deaconesses continued the transition towards becoming...highly trained...medical nurses...this early hospital [was a] tall, narrow, five-story building [that] had no elevator [and] a small operating room with gaslight illumination" (McDermott 1995).

The goal of the Deaconess leadership was to make all patients, rich and poor alike, feel like they were being cared for in their homes. Some, however, actually were: those who could afford it paid a caregiver or nurse to come to their home or received in-home care directly from the hospital's physicians. In 1900, four years after the hospital opened:

> an Association report set forth the goals for the undertaking: "The object of the New England Deaconess Hospital is to afford those who need and desire it an opportunity to avail themselves of the skill of the most eminent physicians and surgeons in New England, and at the same time enjoy the comforts of a home where the very atmosphere seems laden with that warmth and sweetness of devotion which makes pain more easily borne, and which hastens the return of health." The second aim...was to "train young women" who would give their lives to nursing, "especially as deaconesses, either in the hospital...or in district nursing among the poor."
> (Brauer 1995)

Original NEDH at 692 Massachusetts Avenue, 1896.
The Ruth and David Freiman Archives at Beth Israel Deaconess Medical Center.

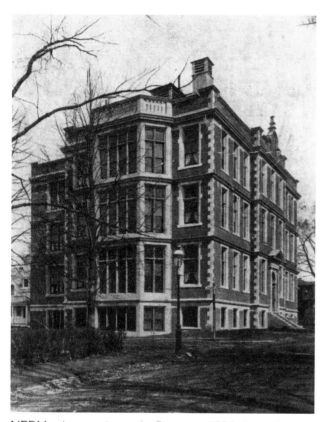

NEDH at its new site on the Riverway (175 Bellevue Street) in 1907. It contained 50 beds. The Ruth and David Freiman Archives at Beth Israel Deaconess Medical Center.

Box 56.1. Revival of the Term "Deaconess"

> "The term 'Deaconess' [servant] was revived in 1836, when a Lutheran pastor named Fliedner and his wife developed a Deaconess training program in Kaiserswerth, Germany...a forerunner of what later developed in the Methodist Church as a school of nursing... Interestingly...Florence Nightingale was a student at the Reverend Theodor Fliedner's Deaconess Home in Germany. Deaconesses from Fliedner's training program first appeared in the United States at Pittsburgh in 1850, where they established the Passavant Hospital."
>
> (McDermott 1995)

The hospital leadership and the staff all came to consensus regarding how the hospital would set itself apart, opting to create a niche by focusing on medical and surgical (sub) specialties, thereby treating mostly middle- and upper-class patients and avoiding patients presenting with the broad and common ailments treated at other all-encompassing hospitals in the city. At that time, growing demand had led to a paucity of hospital beds and the Deaconess was able to attract:

> a number of leading practitioners...Heading the list was Maurice Howe Richardson, a renowned [abdominal] surgeon at Massachusetts General Hospital...Moseley Professor of Surgery at Harvard [who was] frustrated by the paucity of private beds at MGH as well as by that hospital's policy, which prohibited doctors from collecting professional fees from patients...Richardson was a warm individual, sometimes playing hymns and songs for patients and deaconesses alike. He also brought freshly caught fish to the nurses...Richardson's young assistant, Daniel Fiske Jones, who was fond of wearing a carnation in his lapel, was also remembered for his warmth and general concern for patients...Among the hospital's young physicians was Joel E. Goldthwait, a thirty-year-old orthopaedic surgeon who had held a minor staff position at Children's Hospital for three years. In 1922 Goldthwait would write the doctor's bible on posture. Another promising doctor was the young Elliott P. Joslin, who began to practice medicine in 1898... Consistent with what was occurring nationally, a large majority of patients admitted were surgical, not medical. (Brauer 1995)

Little is known about orthopaedic surgery in these early years of the NEDH. In what was described as a typical operative week, July 1–8, 1920, Charles Scudder, one of the hospital's practicing orthopaedic surgeons at the time, operated only once to treat a glenohumeral joint dislocation in a patient with bone cancer. (Scudder had stepped down as chief of both the fracture service and the East Surgical Service at MGH that year.

Beth Israel Deaconess Medical Center

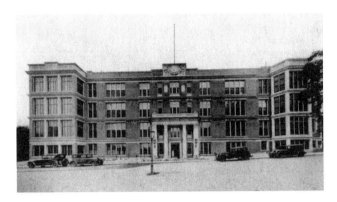

NEDH in 1923 included an expansion on the 1907 building. It contained 175 beds. The Ruth and David Freiman Archives at Beth Israel Deaconess Medical Center.

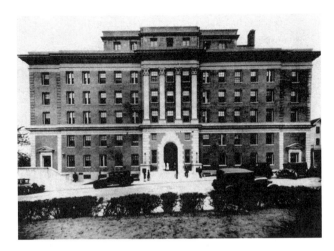

Palmer Memorial Hospital on Pilgrim Road, 1927.
George Brayton/The Ruth and David Freiman Archives at Beth Israel Deaconess Medical Center.

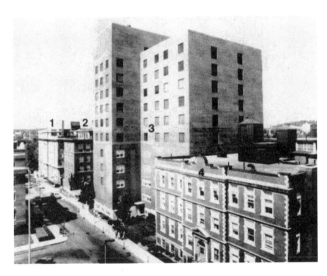

Aerial view of NEDH, 1971. Palmer Memorial Hospital (1), George P. Baker Building (2), Farr (Central) Building (3), Deaconess Building (4). The Ruth and David Freiman Archives at Beth Israel Deaconess Medical Center.

He remained a consultant at MGH with operating privileges at NEDH. See chapter 31.)

A brief timeline of the early history of the NEDH is outlined in **Table 56.1**. After Richardson's death at age 61, Jones was named surgeon-in-chief (1912–1927). In 1927, Frank Lahey took over that position and Jones became surgeon-in-chief at Palmer Memorial Hospital. Lahey had trained and then taught at Harvard—he became a professor of clinical surgery at Harvard Medical School (HMS) and the director of its Fifth Surgical Service at Boston City Hospital in 1922—Lahey cut ties with the school and its affiliated hospitals in 1923, potentially because of personal or professional differences with Dr. David Edsall, then dean at HMS. That year he started the Lahey Clinic (a multispecialty group practice), and for more than 55 years the Clinic's patients received most of their care at NEDH, which at that time had no affiliation with Harvard. The Clinic was also later affiliated with Baptist Hospital and other hospitals.

In 1927, the Cullis Consumptive Home (Hospital for Tuberculosis) moved from Blue Hill Avenue in Roxbury next door to the NEDH, becoming part of the New England Deaconess Association as the Palmer Memorial Hospital. The two remained separate but closely affiliated. Palmer was a new building that had 75 beds in private rooms and wards, three operating rooms, a sun room on every floor, a large solarium, and a library on the roof. It was dedicated to the care of cancer patients. In 1951, the Deaconess medical staff and the Palmer medical staff reorganized into one medical staff of the NEDH.

Lahey held the position of surgeon-in-chief at NEDH until 1947, when Richard B. Cattell, who had been Lahey's assistant, stepped into the role. (Lahey's thoughts on the relationship between NEDH and Palmer Hospital appear in **Box 56.2**.)

Table 56.1. Early History of the New England Deaconess Hospital (NEDH)

Year	Event
1896	NEDH opens with 14 beds
1899	Fundraising begins for a new three-story building in the area near Fenway, which would hold 50 beds
1901	NEDH and the Home and Training School are combined into the New England Deaconess Association
1907	On April 8, the new facility for NEDH is opened with 50 physicians on staff
1912	Surgeon Maurice Howe Richardson dies (age 61) Daniel Fisk Jones named surgeon-in-chief
1927	Cullis Consumptive Home (Hospital for Tuberculosis) becomes part of the New England Deaconess Association as the Palmer Memorial Hospital and opens next door Daniel Fisk Jones becomes surgeon-in-chief at Palmer Memorial (a position he held until 1931) Frank H. Lahey becomes surgeon-in-chief at NEDH
1932	Leland McKittrick succeeded Jones at Palmer Memorial Hospital
1947	Lahey stepped down (voluntarily because of age) as surgeon-in-chief of Deaconess Hospital
1951	New England Deaconess Association combined NEDH and Palmer Memorial Hospital; both staffs merged into NEDH McKittrick became single surgeon-in-chief of the newly merged NEDH
1966	Cornelius E. (Neil) Sedgwick succeeded McKittrick as surgeon-in-chief at NEDH
1980	William McDermott succeeded McKittrick as surgeon-in-chief of NEDH
1985	Glenn D. Steele succeeded McDermott as surgeon-in-chief at NEDH
1996	Merger of NEDH and BIH to become Beth Israel Deaconess Medical Center (BIDMC) Stephen J. Lipson becomes chief of orthopaedics at the newly merged BIDMC (a continuation of his role as chief of orthopaedics at Beth Israel Hospital)

Data from Suh 2005.

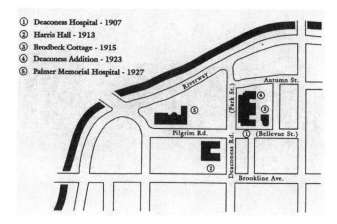

Map of the NEDH, 1929. The Ruth and David Freiman Archives at Beth Israel Deaconess Medical Center.

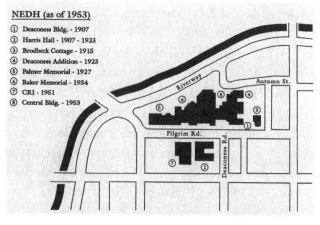

Map of the NEDH, 1953. The Ruth and David Freiman Archives at Beth Israel Deaconess Medical Center.

Cattell also became director of the Lahey clinic six years later, when Lahey died unexpectedly. Meanwhile, at the Palmer Memorial Hospital, Leland Sterling McKittrick came on as surgeon-in-chief in 1932, after Jones's tenure in the position ended. McKittrick had previously advanced the procedure of transmetatarsal amputation.

The two surgeons-in-chief ran their separate hospitals and staffs (though both were overseen by the NEDA) until 1951, when the NEDA decided to combine them. McKittrick became the single surgeon-in-chief handling all operations—with both hospitals now merged as NEDH—and held the position into 1966. In 1966, Cornelius Sedgwick was named as the new surgeon-in-chief at NEDH, a position he held for almost 15 years, stepping down in 1980. (Sedgwick had graduated from Cornell Medical School in 1940 and interned at Roosevelt Hospital, New York City. He had practiced as a general surgeon at the Lahey Clinic in Burlington, Massachusetts.)

Box 56.2. Lahey's Letter to Shields Warren

> "The strength of Dr. Lahey's feelings for independence was emphasized in a letter he wrote to Shields Warren about six years after the reorganization, in which he specifically stated: 'it should be made clear that Dr. McKittrick is Surgeon-in-Chief at the Palmer Memorial Hospital, while I am Surgeon-in-Chief at the Deaconess General Hospital.' Thus, the die was cast, and the staffs would remain separate and inviolate until final fusion in 1964. Clearly, this was not a satisfactory structure with which to pursue moves into the future, but it was not entirely unusual in the Boston area. The Massachusetts General Hospital had two distinct services – the East and the West – with a separate Chief of Service on each visit until 1950, when they were coordinated into a single surgical service."
>
> (McDermott 1995)

In the 1960s and early 1970s, Robert "Don" Lowry, the Executive Director of the NEDH and a seasoned executive, pursued a goal of forming a collaborative relationship with HMS (academic affiliation in 1973) and to unify the medical staff which consisted of "the separate units of the Palmer Memorial, the Deaconess Hospital, the Joslin Clinic, the Overholt Clinic and the independent staff…After a period of thoughtful review and a logical…presentation…a unified staff at the hospital was created" (McDermott 1995). The beds at the hospital were allocated to, and the physicians who practiced there were affiliated with, these institutions (**Table 56.2**). "In addition, the Lahey [Clinic] was responsible for more than 45 percent of patient days, and constituted at least half of the Deaconess's total staff in…orthopaedic surgery…and other specialties" (Brauer 1995).

The Lahey Clinic "approached Deaconess management in 1970 about a possible merger" (Brauer 1995). Such a merger proved more tumultuous than they initially imagined and, although initially approved, it was rescinded within just two weeks. Thereafter, a study was commissioned to review future planning for Deaconess in Boston (see **Box 56.3**).

Table 56.2. Bed Allocation and Affiliations of Physicians Practicing at NEDH, 1970

Bed allocation (%)	
Lahey Clinic	40
Joslin Clinic	25
General staff	35
Physicians' other affiliations (n)	
None/private practice	119
Lahey Clinic	84
Joslin Clinic	15
Overholt Clinic	4

Data from Brauer 1995.

William McDermott and the Harvard Service would not have moved to NEDH had it not been for Sedgwick, who had been McDermott's classmate at Harvard during medical school. McDermott (who at the time was the director of the Harvard [Fifth] Surgical Service at Boston City Hospital and David W. and David Cheever Professor of Surgery at HMS) handled the educational and teaching activities at the hospital, and Sedgwick, still surgeon-in-chief, retained control of the clinical side. McDermott remembered:

> In early 1973, a series of what proved to be extraordinarily fortuitous events took place. First of all, the political furor at the Boston City Hospital, which had been brewing for some months, came to a head, and Mayor White pulled a rather astute, albeit, political, maneuver, insisting that one medical school should run the hospital…these events from the point of view of the Deaconess' staff and administration [were described by Dr. Neil Sedgwick]…at the time that the Harvard Service was planning to leave the Boston City Hospital, first Mr. Lowry and then a small group of the Trustees spoke to me about the possibility of the Harvard Service

coming to the Deaconess Hospital. I felt at the time that this was a great opportunity for the Deaconess, that we could accomplish in one bold stroke something that would take years to develop. However, many of the general surgical staff did not agree, and felt that the Deaconess was sort of a special place to bring special patients. (McDermott 1995)

The Trustees, BIDH leadership, and the physician staff all "understood that bringing McDermott to the Deaconess would effectively give the Department of Surgery full status at Harvard instantaneously; under the Harvard system, McDermott, as a full, tenured professor in the academic faculty, had considerable authority in recommending appointments to Harvard's clinical faculty" (Brauer 1995). Not everyone supported "strengthening the relationship with Harvard," however, and Sedgwick worked to address these concerns among several independent surgeons and the general surgical staff (McDermott 1995).

The staff physicians were concerned that they would lose their independence and would be influenced or forced to become full-time salaried employees. There were also concerns that "they might somehow have less access to operating rooms…In addition, the fear remained that patient care would devolve to residents once academic surgeons arrived on the scene" (Brauer

Box 56.3. Planning for the Future of Deaconess in Boston

"[A] merger seemed a natural consequence since the Deaconess knew all about running a hospital and the Lahey Clinic knew all about operating a group practice…[Dean] Ebert's imprimatur suggested that the old animosity between Harvard and the Lahey Clinic had dissipated…

"In early September 1971, the Deaconess Executive Committee recommended to the full board of trustees a consolidation with the Lahey Clinic…Within hours after these recommendations had been disclosed, however, an agitated general staff began to organize meetings in opposition. Although the independents were all going to be 'grandfathered' in, they nevertheless were frightened by the prospect of a Lahey takeover. All the traditional disdain by independent physicians toward 'corporate medicine' and group practice came rushing to the fore…doctors discussed getting rid of Lowry [Executive Director of NEDH]…As it happened, many independent staff members had hospital trustees as patients and in many cases, they had been their patients for a long time. These doctors quickly organized a series of visits, often going in pairs to see individual patient-trustees…at their homes at night. These 'house calls' proved highly effective. Although the Executive Committee had voted unanimously in favor of a merger, it soon became evident that the idea did not command a majority of the fifty-one trustees. Consequently, within two weeks of approving the merger…the Executive Committee reversed itself and decided to defer action.

"Following the denouement of the Lahey merger…the Long-Range Planning Committee authorized a study by the Cambridge Research Institute to examine trends in the hospital industry and the Deaconess's position in the Boston area. The consultants presented a number of options for the hospital's future…(1) becoming a community hospital; (2) remaining a specialty-referral hospital while strengthening ties to Harvard Medical School; or (3) moving toward a contractual relationship with a health maintenance organization (HMO) or even forming the nucleus of an HMO…Evolving to a community hospital was not promising…since both Beth Israel and the Peter Bent Brigham were fulfilling that role already in the Longwood section of Boston [and] health maintenance organizations were still too experimental [and] would entail significant risk for the Deaconess [because] HMOs depended on primary-care physicians, not the legion of specialists who constituted the vast majority of the Deaconess staff… Strengthening the hospital's position as a specialty-referral center while moving closer to Harvard thus became the underlying strategy of Deaconess management."

(Brauer 1995)

1995). In response, Sedgwick even "went to see Dr. George Dunlop in Worcester, who at the time was head of the Blue Cross/Blue Shield professional advisory committee, and he agreed that the residents could "do cases, as long as the attending surgeon was in the operating room" (McDermott 1995). Ultimately, McDermott's "move to the Deaconess promised to strengthen the hospital's surgical residency program…the Fifth Harvard Surgical Service…which in 1973 had forty residents [and] would be based at the Deaconess" (Brauer 1995).

> At the time of the transition, McDermott felt that there was a shortage of orthopaedic clinical cases and lack of enough orthopaedic surgeons for an adequate teaching program for students and surgical residents. In the short term, having MacAusland's group of orthopaedic surgeons open an office on the BIDH campus provided a group of active orthopaedists who were on the clinical faculty of HMS. He wrote, "This specialty [orthopaedics] presented a major problem which was temporarily solved by the move of Dr. William MacAusland and members of his group to headquarters in the Medical Office Building." (McDermott 1995).

Sedgwick retired in 1980, at which time McDermott took over the clinical services in addition to the academics, managing both aspects of the hospital's operations until his retirement five years later, in 1985. The same year that Sedgwick retired at NEDH, "Lahey Clinic Medical Center opened its own 200-bed hospital in Burlington [on November 24, 1980] and, as a result, reduced its daily bed utilization" at Deaconess (Brauer 1995). The resulting empty beds at NEDH "were largely filled by the general surgical and medical staffs, including the Joslin and Overholt Clinic members [and by] September 1981…the hospital had, remarkably enough, achieved a 94.9 percent occupancy, based on the 472 beds that were then open" (Brauer 1995). New staff were recruited and the patient rooms and operating rooms were renovated.

By the mid-1980s, "admissions and occupancy began to decline slightly" and "by 1985 the presence of energetic young heads of medicine and surgery, Robert Moellering and Glenn Steele, respective, each with mandates to increase their staffs and expand research activities…required that the Deaconess examine how well its physical plant was meeting both current and future needs" (Brauer 1995). After "inpatient utilization in the Commonwealth declined by 27 percent between 1983 and 1991 [and]…Anticipating the winds of change, in the late 1980s and early 1990s Deaconess Hospital began developing a strategy to strengthen its position as a specialized tertiary-care facility" (Brauer 1995). Meanwhile, in his review of the surgical departments, McDermott wrote that the division of orthopaedic surgery:

> was reorganized in 1991, with Dr. Frank Rand becoming the Director of Orthopedic Programs. Dr. Rand will continue to build an ongoing relationship with the neurosurgical division in the formation of the final reconstruction program designed to evaluate complex spinal problems related to tumors, deformities and instability. Drs. Edward Fink and Paul Pongor have continued to be active members of his unit, which is so important in treating the skeletal problems affecting our patients. (McDermott 1995)

Dr. Rand was an instructor of orthopaedic surgery at HMS.

Orthopaedic spine fellows at the Baptist rotated on both the orthopaedic and neurosurgery services at the Deaconess. Plans were developed for the establishment of a foot and ankle service in the division of orthopaedics to work with podiatry, which was also in the department of surgery. Clinical instructors of orthopaedic surgery at the Deaconess in 1991 included Drs. Leonard Dabuzhaky, Michael A. Drew, and Edward Fink. In 1992,

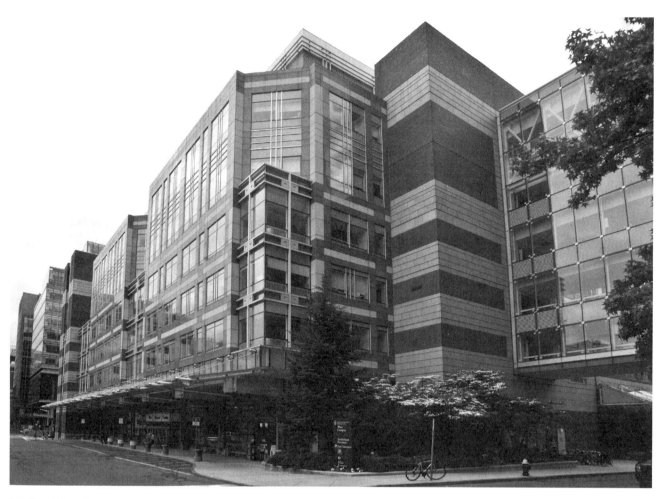

BIDMC West Campus. Bruce R. Wahl/Media Services, Beth Israel Deaconess Medical Center.

three additional orthopaedic surgeons were added to the staff: Drs. Lyle Micheli, Richard Scott, and Thomas Thornhill. Dr. Rand was collaborating with Dr. Fred Shapiro (at Boston Children's Hospital) and Albert Loskin (a HMS student) on a research project developing a tibial nonunion model in rabbits. Dr. Fink organized an elective for the fourth-year medical students on the cultural aspects of medicine and a medical exchange of doctors with Brazil. The orthopaedic case volume reported in 1993 included 167 operations in one year. Both the orthopaedic division and the plastic surgery division at Deaconess began a collaboration with the Baptist hand service in 1993.

The Board of Trustees at NEDH continued to move forward with its earlier strategy and developed:

the creation of a formal network of healthcare institutions – primary, secondary, and tertiary…what eventually emerged was Pathway Health Network…Instrumental in the creation of Pathway Health Network was the affiliation of New England Baptist Hospital…the Baptist was a specialty-referral institution with highly regarded programs in the treatment of musculoskeletal disorders and orthopedics…On July 1, 1994, New England Baptist formally joined Pathway Health Network. One of the first examples of the synergies that can be created through network collaboration was the establishment of New England Bone and Joint Institute at the Baptist, a union of the Deaconess's clinical and research programs in rheumatology and the leadership of Steve Goldring, and the

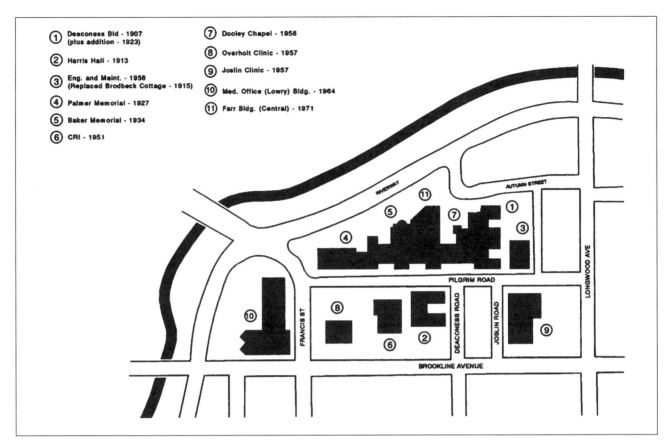

Map of NEDH, 1971. The Ruth and David Freiman Archives at Beth Israel Deaconess Medical Center.

Baptist's expertise in diagnosis and treatment of orthopedic conditions. (Brauer 1995)

By 1994, Beth Israel Hospital's financial status was precarious in the face of more intransigent insurance carriers, high debt, and restrictive governmental regulations. Providers adapted to these changes by forming larger networks, downsizing, and developing more profit-minded objectives; and there was no exception in Beth Israel's case. In 1996, Beth Israel and the NEDH merged, "a hard-won victory" (Schwartz 2009). Nevertheless, "fallout from the...merger continued for nearly a decade...Many thought the merger damaged the cultural integrity of both Beth Israel and the Deaconess. [However, each hospital] faced equally difficult choices...the Deaconess board and management feared they would be faced with absorption into the [recently formed] Partners system" (Brauer 1995).

Under the leadership of Dr. Mitchell T. Rabkin, CareGroup—the parent not-for-profit holding company—was formed in addition to the hospital merger. Dr. Rabkin became CareGroup's CEO. This additional merger had unintended consequences. The anesthesiology department left the Deaconess. At Beth Israel, anesthesiologists were salaried employees while at the Deaconess, they are independent contractors or "itinerant anesthesiologists." Subsequently, Dr. Roger Jenkins, chief of transplant surgery, moved to Lahey Clinic. CareGroup responded by dropping certain specialties and selling the real estate.

Despite these difficulties, the newly formed Beth Israel Deaconess Medical Center was strengthened. The combined orthopaedics department was led by Dr. Stephen Lipson (see chapter 55).

CHAPTER 57

BIDMC

Modernization and Preparation for the Twenty-First Century

After the Beth Israel Hospital (BIH) was opened in 1917, there were only two visiting surgeons—Drs. Albert Ehrenfried and Wyman Whittemore—who shared the sole operating room. Early in its history, Beth Israel Hospital played a key role in providing care for the increasing number of immigrants in Boston. It also became a haven of training for minority (including Jewish) medical students and physicians, who were often discriminated against by other hospitals at the time. A culture was created in which many chief residents remained on staff as visiting surgeons. **Table 57.1** lists the first five surgeon-in-chiefs of the Beth Israel Hospital, along with their years of service in this role and key accomplishments. Dr. William Silen in particular was a dedicated teacher and a highly conscientious surgeon, and although some physicians had opposed his appointment and even petitioned the board of trustees against him, he ultimately had an influential tenure.

In 1996, Beth Israel Hospital merged with the New England Deaconess Hospital to become the Beth Israel Deaconess Medical Center (BIDMC). After the merger, the financial crisis continued with declining patient volume and severe financial losses. In July of 2001, the CEO, Dr. James L. Reinertsen, was dismissed, and financial losses for the institution totalled $7.3 million for the

Table 57.1. Surgeons-in-Chief at Beth Israel Hospital, 1928–1995

Surgeon-in-Chief	Years as Surgeon-in-Chief	Key Accomplishments
Dr. Wyman Whittemore	1928–1931	First Surgeon-in-Chief Named in 1928 when hospital relocated to Brookline Avenue
Dr. Charles G. Mixter	1931–1948	Pediatric surgeon at Children's Hospital Invented "Mixter clamp" Founding member of American Board of Surgery Established residency in general surgery
Dr. Jacob Fine	1948–1966	Professor of Surgery, Harvard Medical School Noted researcher of shock
Dr. William Silen	1966–1994	Former Surgeon-in-Chief at San Francisco General Hospital Johnson & Johnson Chair of Surgery, Harvard Medical School Internationally acclaimed researcher in the physiology of the gastrointestinal tract Dean of Faculty Development and Diversity, Harvard Medical School
Dr. Mitchell P. Fink	1994–1995	Served in era of transition due to merger with New England Deaconess Hospital First Surgeon-in-Chief of Beth Israel Deaconess Medical Center

year. Following Dr. Lipson's resignation, Dr. Joseph Martin, dean of Harvard Medical School appointed Dr. Benjamin Bierbaum, an internationally known hip surgeon, as chairman of the hospital's department of orthopaedic surgery and clinical professor of orthopaedics at Harvard Medical School (HMS). Dr. Bierbaum, a professor of orthopaedics at Tufts, continued as chief of orthopaedics at the New England Baptist Hospital, a "position he has held for more than 25 years." (Schaller 2000) In the announcement of his new leadership position, Bill Schaller of the BIDMC news, stated:

> In his new role at Beth Israel Deaconess, Bierbaum will work on strengthening the orthopedic department, with an emphasis on trauma and emergency care, orthopedic oncology and specialty orthopedic surgery, including geriatrics, complications of diabetes and other musculoskeletal areas. Bierbaum's dual appointment as chairman of two orthopedic departments in the CareGroup Healthcare System, the parent organization of Beth Israel Deaconess and New England Baptist, will allow him to strategically build the Beth Israel Deaconess Department of Orthopaedics, setting a coordinated direction for efforts there and at New England Baptist... This is a wonderful opportunity to build on the strengths of two institutions which are known widely for their innovative and high quality care...this greater collaboration...will result in more efficient use of resources and will provide outstanding training opportunities that are built on strong clinical and research programs! A top priority for Bierbaum is to expand the scope of orthopaedic research at Beth Israel Deaconess and to bring clinicians and researchers together to bear on musculoskeletal disorders. In addition to selecting a new leader for the Orthopedic Biomechanical Laboratory, Bierbaum will integrate orthopedic research activities with the New England Baptist Bone and Joint Institute's Basic Science Laboratory. (Schaller 2000)

In September of 2000, BIMDC announced plans to cut many of its services in an effort to address its financial challenges, affecting thousands of patients and staff. Among the services terminated were dermatology, orthopaedics, and psychiatry. Other hospitals in BIMDC's network moved to fill the void in care by expanding their provision of these services. The decision represented a dramatic shift in approach for the hospital, from offering a broad array of comprehensive health care services to concentrating on a small number of highly profitable specialties.

At the time, the orthopaedic department at BIDMC was in disarray. No new chief had been identified after Lipson's resignation; in fact, the hospital prioritized the searches for chiefs of medicine, surgery, and anesthesia before orthopaedics. As the Harvard Combined Orthopaedic Residency Program's (HCORP's) residency director, I had repeatedly asked for a three–five-year plan, but it was never delivered. The academic mission was lost: no morbidity and mortality conferences or other orthopaedic teaching conferences were held; residents continued to be responsible for the care of indigent patients without designated responsible attendings; residents were often unsupervised in the clinics and the chief residents in the operating rooms; and the residents, especially the chief resident, had excessive night call responsibilities. Dean Joseph Martin appointed Dr. Benjamin Bierbaum as chief of the orthopaedic department in December of 2000. The apparent plan was for Dr. Bierbaum to eventually become the CareGroup chief of orthopaedics and then appoint a chief of orthopaedics at the BIDMC and another at the Baptist, following the model of Partners Orthopaedics.

Problems, however, for HCORP and BIDMC were apparent with Dr. Bierbaum's plan to move the residents from BIDMC to the Baptist for total joint and spine rotations (already satisfactory rotations at BIDMC) and to have the staff at the Baptist receive Harvard faculty appointments, which was opposed by Harvard's orthopaedic executive committee. Regarding the very successful biomechanics laboratory, the hospital leadership wanted to move the Mueller Professorship from orthopedics to medicine (Dr. Toby Hayes had relocated to the University of Oregon in 1998). The dean opposed this move. BIDMC notified the orthopaedic executive committee that they did not have the resources to recruit an assistant professor of orthopaedics, let alone a professor and chair.

In the fall of 2000, as residency program director, I became increasingly concerned about the residents' experiences at BIDMC. Through a series of written and oral evaluations of the orthopaedic services by the residents, it became increasingly clear that they were concerned about the lack of teaching, frequent cancellations of morning teaching conferences, lack of attending supervision, delays in official reading of trauma radiographs, the Level 1 trauma service coverage (except for Dr. Greg Altman, a specialty trained orthopaedic traumatologist and excellent teacher) being done by general orthopaedists (some with sports or spine specialty training) and violation of the ACGME duty hours' regulations. Most of the residents in the past had found that the PGY1 year on the surgical service excellent or superb, but recently with surgeons leaving, the surgical volume for residents had declined significantly. The only rotations they enjoyed and felt were significant surgical and educational experiences included sports medicine and total joint arthroplasty.

On October 7, 2000, the orthopaedic residents held a residents-only meeting to discuss the deterioration of some of the teaching services at BIDMC. In a memo written to the residency program director on October 10, 2000, they reaffirmed the above-listed concerns, stating:

> the number of cases performed by the BOG [Boston Orthopaedic Group] has decreased over the last year…We are concerned that the continued movement of elective orthopaedic procedures to the New England Baptist Hospital…will magnify this trend…Dr. Murphy has recently been performing more and more elective procedures (e.g. total hip arthroplasty, periacetabular osteotomy, etc.) at New England Baptist Hospital…We fear that as elective orthopaedics is moved to NEBH in the future, the experience will be completely lost to BIDMC…the PGY-4 resident is on-call for trauma every other night…PGY-5 residents now rotate through the sports service…without question, this rotation is viewed as one of the highlights of our residency program…what makes this experience unique at Harvard is the insistence by the surgeons…that the residents act as primary surgeons on their cases…Finally with regards to orthopaedic training during the BIDMC rotations, many residents have noted that the didactic schedule (e.g. morning conference, M & M conference, etc.) has become inconsistent in recent years. Indeed, a number of residents have reported that they have gone through the entire five-week rotation without having even one of the weekly morning conferences take place, due to cancellations or absence of the assigned staff member…Compromises are difficult to envision, because the history of the BIDMC is to offload service oriented work on remaining residents when vacancies or gaps in resident coverage have occurred. As the attending staff continues to expand throughout the program, and the number of residents remains fixed, the program is left with difficult decisions on how best to allocate residents. An optimal educational experience should continue to be the goal. ("The Harvard Orthopaedic Residents. Memo to Dr. James H. Herndon, October 10, 2000 [Unpublished]" 2000)

Over the objections of the program director, Dean Martin named Dr. Ben Bierbaum as clinical professor of orthopaedic surgery at HMS and supported the hospital's decision to name Bierbaum the chief of the orthopaedic department at BIDMC in December 2000, while remaining chief of the orthopaedic department at the Baptist.

Bierbaum asked Dr. Reilly to "continue to act as Vice-Chair of the Department and...appointed Greg Altman [staff trauma surgeon] to head the Musculoskeletal Unit...The Beth Israel Hospital in 1995 became a Level 1 trauma center...In 1998, the emergency department received accreditation for a Harvard Emergency Room Residency Program...[and] in July 2001, Beth Israel Deaconess Medical Center will open their new state-of-the-art Emergency Department...During the upcoming year we plan to integrate rheumatology, musculoskeletal and orthopedic surgery services to offer combined patient care and teaching for resident...[in a] Musculoskeletal Medicine Unit" (Bierbaum 2001).

In 2001, the full-time faculty included Dr. Augustus White (professor) and Drs. Gregory Altman and Robert Davis (instructors). The part-time clinical faculty included Drs. Benjamin Bierbaum and Stephen Lipson (clinical professors), Drs. Tobin Gerhart and Donald Reilly (assistant clinical professors) and Drs. Paul Glazer, Hyman Glick, Louis Meeks, William Mitchell, Jr., Stephen Murphy, Hillel Skoff, Harris Yett and Jeffrey Zilberfarb (clinical instructors).

The academic year 2001–2002 was a troublesome time for BIDMC and especially the department of orthopaedic surgery. According to Bierbaum:

> Greg Altman, MD, left early in the academic year, relocating to Pittsburgh, leaving us [BIDMC] without a trauma chief...In addition, we were dealing with a financial crisis at the hospital and the impact of the Hunter Group, which was hired to guide the hospital through its financial crises...Recruitment efforts continue, as we seek to build the department in the specialties of trauma, hand, adult reconstruction and foot and ankle surgery...At the request of the CareGroup Board of Directors [Dr. Bierbaum was also a member of the board], Donald T. Reilly, MD, PhD moved his adult reconstructive practice to the New England Baptist Hospital...Stephen J. Lipson, MD and Katherine Taft, MSN RNC moved to Harvard Vanguard Medical Associates to continue their work with patients with neck and back pain... Perhaps most exciting is our new collaboration with the New England Baptist Bone and Joint Institute Basic Science Laboratory. (Bierbaum 2003)

The only new additional staff member was Dr. Saechin Kim (clinical instructor) hired by the Boston Orthopaedic Group. No fulltime faculty were recruited within the past two years (2000–2002).

On October 3, 2001, the residency program director wrote the following letter to Dr. Bierbaum:

> In light of the significant changes that have occurred at the Beth Israel Deaconess Medical Center over the past nine months, it has become apparent that resident education and satisfaction is at an all-time low...the volume of major hip and knee replacements... has decreased dramatically, to a number that is incompatible with responsible resident training...Dr. Reilly, who ran the Joint Reconstruction Service, and did a high volume of surgical cases, has moved his practice to the Baptist... the PGY-3 resident assigned to the joint service has little, if anything, to do except cover other cases. Therefore, beginning January 1, 2002, the PGY-3 resident...will move to the...trauma position and one PGY-4 [on trauma] resident will no longer rotate through the BIDMC. Additionally, in light of Greg Altman's departure, as well as the residents' observations and complaints about their experiences on the trauma service, the PGY-2 and PGY-4/5 residents will no longer rotate through the BIDMC effective July 1, 2002. Beginning July 1, 2002, a single PGY-3 resident will remain at the BIDMC... assigned to the Sports Service for an outpatient ambulatory arthroscopy experience. He or she will not be allowed to take night call and cover

the trauma service...there is a clear consensus that the sports service rotation contributes significantly to their education and surgical training. (Herndon 2001)

In June 2002, Dr. Josef E. Fischer, the Mallinckrodt Professor of Surgery and chairman of the Department of Surgery at BIDMC, was appointed acting chairman of the department of orthopaedic surgery "and given the charge of recruiting a new department chairperson for Orthopedic Surgery" (MacDonald 2003). Harvard appointed a search committee consisting of the orthopaedic executive committee, the associate dean for faculty affairs, a professor of surgery, three professors of medicine at BIDMC, an associate professor of radiation oncology at BIDMC, the president and CEO of BIDMC, and Dr. Fischer as chair (total: 11 members). "The Search Committee met throughout the fall, winter and spring... interviewing and ranking candidates" (MacDonald 2003). In September 2003, the search committee selected Mark C. Gebhardt, MD, as orthopaedic surgeon-in-chief at BIDMC and the Frederick W. and Jane M. Ilfield Professor of Orthopaedic Surgery at Harvard Medical School.

Throughout 2002, while Dr. Fischer was serving as the acting chairman of orthopaedics, Dr. Lars C. Richardson (clinical instructor) joined the clinical part-time faculty with the practice of Drs. Meeks and Zilberfarb. Dr. Charles S. Day was also hired as the first full-time hand surgeon in the department. He was given a faculty appointment as instructor. Dr. White retired from clinical practice and focused his energies on the medical students as Master of the Holmes Society. Both Drs. Reilly and Murphy had already completed moving their clinical practices to the Baptist.

Dr. Gebhardt hired Dr. Douglas K. Ayres to head the adult reconstructive surgical service and began to actively recruit faculty in the specialty field of trauma, oncology, sports medicine, and spine surgery. At the time of his appointment as Orthopaedic Surgeon-in-Chief, Gebhardt was:

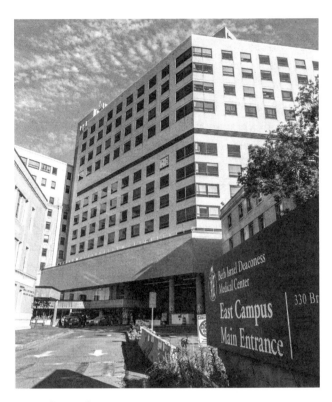

BIDMC East Campus. Kael E. Randall/Kael Randall Images.

Chair of the Core Curriculum Committee for the residency program, Chair of the Orthopaedic Residency Review Committee of ACGME...a Senior Director of the American Board of Orthopaedic Surgery and [a] member of the Board [of Directors] of the American Academy of Orthopaedic Surgeons...[He assembled] a multidisciplinary team...for the treatment of adults with bone and soft tissue tumors and metastatic carcinoma...The oncology fellowship received ACGME accreditation to include the service at the BIDMC with Children's Hospital and the MGH [3 fellows per year]. (Gebhardt 2004)

Dr. Gebhardt continued to expand the full-time faculty by adding specialists in oncology (Dr. Megan E. Anderson), sports medicine (Dr. Arun Ramappa), trauma (Dr. Ken Rodriquez as chief of orthopaedic trauma) and primary care sports medicine (Dr. Michael O'Brien). Dr. Yett also joined the full-time staff from his private practice with the

Boston Orthopaedic Group. Drs. Glick and Gerhart moved their practices to Harvard Vanguard. Gebhardt noted:

> The number of operative cases and clinic visits has more than doubled compared to last year [2004] and we are rapidly outgrowing our clinic and office space on Shapiro 2. We are planning a relocation of our academic offices next year to open up more clinic space, and we have moved arthroplasty cases to the East Campus to free up operative time on the West Campus. We now have a dedicated trauma room operating 3.5 days per week…We had the first annual Augustus A. White, MD, Spine Symposium on October 13, 2004…The Orthopaedic Biomechanics Laboratory…is active and pursing a variety of research venues…under the direction of Brian D. Snyder, MD, PhD…The Hospital is committed to providing the resources to rejuvenate this Department…and we are convinced that the BIDMC will once again be a vital part of the Harvard Combined Orthopaedic Residency Program. (Gebhardt 2005)

The HCORP had applied for an expansion of the program by two residents per year (total of 12 per year), which was approved in 2004. Because of Dr. Gebhardt's success in recruiting essential full-time faculty, residents returned to BIDMC: "two PGY-2 level residents…at BIDMC…[were] on rotations in trauma, tumor, arthroplasty, hand and sports. The addition of more residents in the program has led to an overall re-structuring…[with] an ultimate return of a total of 4 PGY-1 interns and 4 orthopaedic residents at the BIDMC." (Gebhardt 2005) The four orthopaedic residents rotated as follows: "The PGY-5 spends half of his or her time on a research elective…a PGY-2 on the arthroplasty/geriatrics service, a PGY-3 on sports and a PGY-4 on the trauma service. The reports so far indicate that the residents like the new rotations…We [also] have a vibrant conference schedule including: Weekly: Trauma Conference, Chief's Conference, Tumor Conference, and Geriatric Rounds; Monthly: Sports Medicine Journal Club, Tumor Journal Club, and Combined Sports Medicine/Radiology Conference" (Gebhardt 2006).

As of 2006, Dr. Gebhardt had continued to recruit new faculty, including "Paul Appleton, MD, (orthopaedic trauma); Navan Duggal, MD (orthopaedic foot and ankle surgery and trauma), Tamara Rozental, MD (hand and upper extremity surgery), Edward J. Vresilovic Jr., MD, PhD (spine surgery)" (Gebhardt 2006). He noted:

> We have begun construction of our new academic offices on Stoneman 10 that will include offices for an entire faculty and their administrative assistants as well as a state of the art conference room and space for resident study modules. Soon after we move into these offices in July, construction will begin on Shapiro 2 to expand the clinic space…The hospital received a nice donation to make these possible and when completed will be named the Carl J. Shapiro Department of Orthopaedics. (Gebhardt 2006)

The department is well prepared to meet the challenges of the twenty-first century with continued recruitment of orthopaedic specialists and scientists as well as its new Carl J. Shapiro Department of Orthopaedics. The new facilities add—in addition to its current research labs—modern clinic space for outpatient clinical care and needed expansion, including administrative offices and teaching conference rooms for the faculty, fellows, and residents. **Box 57.1** documents those distinguished orthopaedic division and department chiefs who served at BIH in the past as well as the department chiefs at BIDMC who continue to lead today.

Box 57.1. Orthopaedic Chiefs at BIH and BIDMC

BIH Orthopaedic Division Chiefs:
- Mark H. Rogers   1928–1941
- Armin Klein   1941–1954
- Meier G. Karp   1954–1962
- Robert Ulin (acting)   1962–1966
- Seymour Zimbler   1966–1970
- Harris S. Yett   1970–1978

BIH Orthopaedic Department Chiefs:
- Augustus A. White III   1978–1990
- Louis W. Meeks (acting) 1990–1992
- Stephen J. Lipson   1992–1997

BIDMC Orthopaedic Department Chiefs:
- Stephen J. Lipson   1997–2001
- Benjamin E. Bierbaum   2001–2002
- Josef E. Fischer (acting) 2002
- Mark C. Gebhardt   2002–

Section 8

Boston City Hospital

Refuge of sufferers! Conqueror of pain!
Healer of wounds, and woes, and misery!
Bleeding or sick, the people turn to thee,
Seeking thy touch to make them whole again!
Standing within the city's southern gate,
Stretching wide open arms to all who need;
Sleepless, thou welcom'st every race and creed,
Spring time or autumn, early hour or late.
We are they sons; each one in his own way
Gave of his best to thine abundant store,
And in thy service found, as children may,
Knowledge, strength, skill they knew not of before.
Loving, we watch thee grown from day to day,
Knowing they name is blessed evermore!

—**John Bapst Blake**. "The Municipal History of the Boston City Hospital" [One of 5 original members of the Hospital Staff]. *A History of the Boston City Hospital From its Foundation Until 1904*. Editors: D. W. Cheever, G. W. Gay, A. L. Mason, J. B. Blake. Boston Municipal Printing Office: 1906. Chapter 2, page 126.

"As I think back over this period from 1910 to 1920, I am staggered by the changes which occurred…of many men who have greatly aided our orthopaedic advance…It is good for us today to realize our indebtedness to the past."

—**Leo Mayer, MD**. "Reflections of Some Interesting Personalities in Orthopaedic Surgery During the First Quarter of the Century." *Journal of Bone and Joint Surgery*, 1955; 37:382.

CHAPTER 58

Boston City Hospital (Harvard Service)
The Beginning

A severe epidemic of cholera struck Boston in 1849. In Roxbury, on Fort Hill, the municipality organized a hospital to treat these patients—the first of whom arrived at the end of June, the last of whom was discharged in mid-November. During the intervening period, 166 of the 262 patients treated had died. At the time, the city of Boston had a population of about 13,000, and cholera claimed ~5%—around 650 people. After the epidemic, the temporary hospital for cholera was closed, but some physicians saw the necessity of a permanent municipal hospital, particularly because of how many people were turned away at or were declined admission to Massachusetts General Hospital (MGH) because of a lack of space. The growing population of the city, mostly immigrants from Ireland, overwhelmed MGH.

A memorandum to the *Boston Medical and Surgical Journal* in 1850 further illustrated the need for another hospital in Boston (**Box 58.1**). For a variety of reasons, however, the movement for a municipal hospital waned for almost a decade. Nevertheless, an endowment ($26,000) left in the will of Elisha Goodnow, a wealthy merchant, "upon condition that...it should be devoted to the erection of a hospital, situated in Wards 11 or 12...the wards of South Boston and the South End" (Cheever et al. 1906) kept the interest high amongst some physicians and the political leaders in Boston. At the time, there was a great deal of debate over the ideal location:

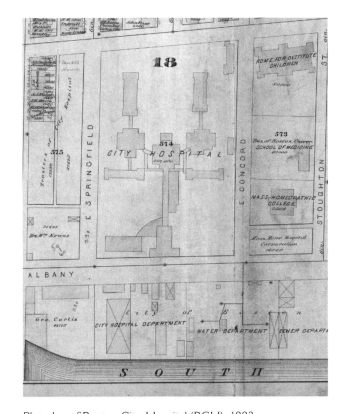

Plot plan of Boston City Hospital (BCH), 1883.
Atlas of the City of Boston: City Proper, Volume 1. Philadelphia: G. W. Bromley & Co., 1883. Norman B. Leventhal Map Center Collection, Boston Public Library.

It was thought that the only suitable sites in South Boston were "too far removed from the city proper," and after much deliberation the present site was decided...The city already was in possession of this land...Roxbury, which had many excellent sites for a hospital, was not at that time a part of the City of

293

Box 58.1. Memorandum to the Boston Medical and Surgical Journal

Proposed New Hospital in Boston

"About three years ago, an operative engaged upon the Boston Water Works, about eleven miles from the city, had his thigh fractured by the falling on a bank of frozen earth. He was removed to his boarding house, and placed in a room about fourteen square feet, where from thirty to fifty people had their meals daily…The fracture was reduced, and apparatus furnished. The patient did well… but he began to walk too soon, slipped upon the ice, and [re]fractured his limb…[It was] advised [that he be] carried to the Massachusetts General Hospital…and that his board should be paid at that institution…The patient was carried into Boston to the hospital, where they were informed that the hospital was full, and he could not be admitted. He was then brought back to his original lodging, after a journey of over twenty miles. As he was not a resident of Boston, though in the service of the city, he had no claim to admission into the House of Industry. Thus it proved that there was no place in Boston where a man, injured very seriously in the service of the city, could obtain admission…For many years, and before the hospital was enlarged, it was always stated in the cards and advertisements, that in cases of accident, patients were admitted at all hours of the day and night…long enough fully to impress the public mind that there was always provision for an extra patient, if necessity required…But if any charitable person had received the said patient into his house, subsequent to the accident, he could not be admitted unless visited by the admitting physician…If an arrangement of this kind was generally understood to exist, it would render people very cautious how they received sufferers into their houses after an accident…A hospital is wanted both for medical and surgical cases, for those who cannot be received into the Massachusetts Hospital. The latter is a private institution, not subject, I believe, in any degree to the city or State authorities; and if the trustees should determine to make it a private boarding-house for respectable invalids, or to require that none but the well-dressed be admitted, I do not know that they could be prevented. Hence the necessity for a new hospital.

"Henry B. Rogers, Esq., who had been chairman of the Committee on Internal Health, set up by the Mayor [Josiah Quincy] and Aldermen in 1849 to implement the plans of the Board of Health in combatting cholera [wrote to] John Collins Warren [and James Jackson asking] seven questions…Is an additional hospital needed? Should it be publicly or privately supported? Who would use it? Where should it be placed? etc. Warren's reply has not survived, but James Jackson, the Massachusetts General Hospital physician [replied] on January 10, 1850: 'I am satisfied that the city ought to have a hospital for this class of persons [the sick poor]! It should be located in South Boston. Possibly it might be useful to have a small hospital on the peninsula for accidents.' He advised square wards for thirty or forty patients, with a large central place. The staff should consist of one physician and one surgeon or 'at least the most two of each.' They should not be removed from office for political or religious opinions. 'These men should be well paid' he wrote, and he thought that $1,000 annually would not be too much [$28,040 in 2014]. Young men should serve as assistants, without pay, and spend two hours or so a day at the hospital. In addition to the paid apothecary, there should be two or more graduate physicians as residents, appointed annually, with full maintenance…Jackson's recommendations…followed the ward arrangement used in the Bulfinch Building…almost all of his suggestions were adopted a decade later, including the organization of the staff."

(*Boston Medical and Surgical Journal* 1850)

Boston [but] the promoters themselves had misgivings that it was not the best site…The old Roxbury canal, which carried the sewage of Roxbury to tide-water, ran through one corner of the premises, and a considerable portion of the land was salt water flats, largely of dock mud…Here we had ample space. The public domain of seventy acres could well spare one-tenth of its area for so sacred a purpose. On March 27, 1858, the City of Boston was authorized to establish a City Hospital.

(Cheever et al. 1906)

Boston City Hospital (Harvard Service)

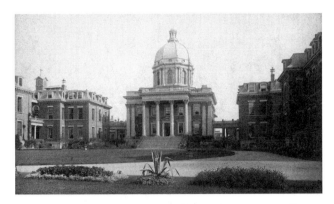

Boston City Hospital. Center building: administration. Surgery units: building on the left (north); Medical units: building on the right (south). The hospital opened in 1864. Boston City Hospital Collection, City of Boston Archives.

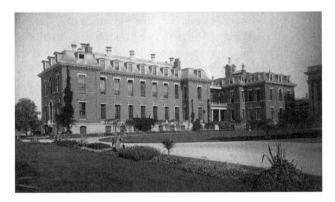

Original Pavilion I (Wards B, C, and D) and the new Surgical Building (M, N and O). Boston City Hospital Collection, City of Boston Archives.

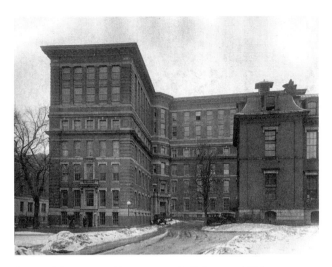

Surgical Outpatient Department Building, ca. 1904. Boston City Hospital Collection, City of Boston Archives.

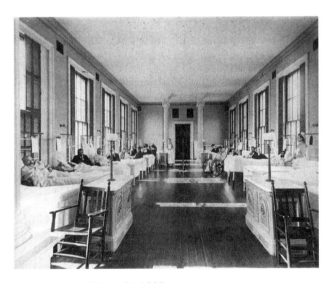

Surgical Ward (Ward B), 1895. Boston City Hospital Collection, City of Boston Archives.

The new Boston City Hospital (BCH) facilities were fashioned after those of MGH, although others later described the hospital's maze of old and existing buildings as having no plan, of developing randomly over time as the 1800s gave way to the new century—much like Boston itself. In a 1968 *New York Times* article describing BCH, Corkery notes that all of this infrastructure had been repurposed as necessary to fulfill the hospital's goal throughout its history, mainly caring for the poverty-stricken poor. Three years after authorization was approved for the hospital:

> Ground was broken for the City Hospital September 9, 1861…Four buildings constituted the original group: the Administration Building [imposing structure in the center], Pavilion I… for surgical wards A, B, C and D, Pavilion II… for medical wards E, F, G, and H and the boilerhouse…On the surgical side were accident rooms, splint rooms and accident wards. The first, second and third stories were occupied as wards. (Cheever et al. 1906)

On June 1, 1864, the BCH officially opened with 200 beds (medical, surgical, and ophthalmological). At the time, "The South…Pavilion consisted of three wards, each containing twenty-eight

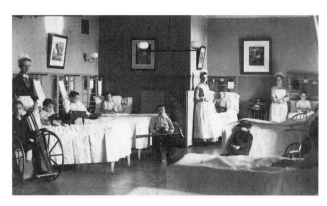

Ward O had two rooms: one large and one small. This image is of the smaller room which contained about 15 beds and was used for children (many with orthopaedic problems). The pediatric service at BCH didn't open until after 1919. Boston City Hospital Collection, City of Boston Archives.

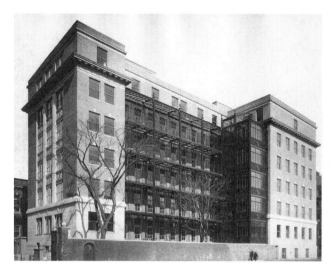

Thorndike Building, established in 1923, was the first clinical research laboratory in a municipal hospital in the US. The building housed the Harvard Medical Unit (2nd & 4th Medical Services) faculty's research labs and a clinical research ward (17 beds). Boston City Hospital Collection, City of Boston Archives.

beds [designated for medical patients]" (Cheever et al. 1906). These wards were organized by sex: "The lower and upper wards were used for males, and the centre [*sic*] wards for females" (Cheever et al. 1906). Outpatient facilities also existed in the basement. The number of hospital visits increased quickly.

"For the first days the number of patients admitted was very few, and the visiting physicians and house officers had but little work to do. Gradually, however, the public became aware that the hospital was ready to receive cases, and very soon there were no unoccupied beds…The growth of the medical department kept pace with that of the city. In 1878, the number of patients had so increased that a medical service [50 beds] was set apart" (Cheever et al. 1906).

In the beginning, BCH staff comprised 18 people—6 each of consulting physicians, visiting physicians, and visiting surgeons—all of whom had received their education at Harvard Medical School (HMS). (Four of the six surgeons would later hold faculty appointments at HMS.) The five residents selected (two in medicine, two in surgery, one in ophthalmology) would all be graduating from HMS as well just before beginning their residency. In the fall of 1864, Harvard medical students began attending teaching sessions at BCH; one of the four instructors—David W. Cheever—was a surgeon.

HARVARD MEDICAL UNIT

In addition to teaching students from HMS, the staff and house staff also taught students from Boston University School of Medicine (originally the New England Female Medical College, renamed Boston University School of Medicine in 1873) and Tufts University School of Medicine after its founding in 1893. In 1914, however, Edward Locke, then a clinical medicine instructor at Harvard, recommended a fourth service to help accommodate the number of students and allow closer instruction. In 1915, the Fourth Medical Service opened, affiliated with Harvard. Fifteen years later, operations of the Second Medical Service, comprising 112 beds, also transferred to Harvard. The fourth and second services shared the 28 beds (for men only) in Ward 2. These two services allowed staff, residents, and students to work closely together, benefitting everyone, whether

Boston City Hospital (Harvard Service)

through teaching and learning or enhanced patient care.

Another major component of the Harvard Medical Unit at the City Hospital was the Thorndike Memorial Laboratory, which had been funded through a $200,000 bequest from a George Thorndike to honor the memory of his brother, Dr. William Thorndike (no relation to Augustus Thorndike), who had been on the BCH staff as a visiting surgeon for almost 20 years in the second half of the nineteenth century. The board of trustees had appropriated another $150,000, which had been allocated for building a modern research facility at BCH. In 1921, the trustees and the HMS Dean David Edsall named Francis W. Peabody, then a physician at PBBH, as the new laboratory's director. (Peabody also became a professor of medicine at HMS.) The new laboratory opened in 1923, and it marked the first time that a tax-supported municipal hospital undertook to join with a privately endowed, university medical school in establishing a metabolic ward and a laboratory unit for clinical investigation staffed by full-time physicians. They also shared with part-time, practicing physicians the responsibilities for the care of patients, the training of the resident house-staff and the teaching of students (Finland 1964).

During the early growth of BCH around the turn of the twentieth century, Tufts University School of Medicine was in charge of two medical services: the First Medical Service (Wards L and M), the Third Medical Unit (Wards F and G), and much later a clinical research facility (1963). The BCH formalized its affiliation with Tufts in 1915 (Third Medical Service) at the time Harvard's affiliation was also started (Fourth Medical Service). Later, a Boston University Medical Unit would occupy Pavilion Three.

Because of the city's financial situation, however, in the mid-1970s, city leadership reduced the extent of BCH's affiliation with local universities. Instead of working with three schools (Harvard, Tufts, and Boston University), the city chose Boston University as the only one to retain its affiliation with the BCH. Henry Banks (affiliated with Tufts) and Thomas Quigley (with Harvard) left the hospital under predictions that it would soon cease operations because of its dire financial straits. The city pledged to keep it open, however, and thus began a long-term rehabilitation program to replace the hospital's old infrastructure and facilities with new. Approximately 20 years later, in 1996, BCH merged with Boston University Medical Center Hospital, forming the Boston Medical Center (BMC).

Surgical Services

The surgical services at BCH developed very differently from the medical services. Both Tufts (First) and Boston University (Third) had their individual surgical service, but in spite of several attempts by Harvard to form its own such service (Fifth), it was unable to ever organize a sustained

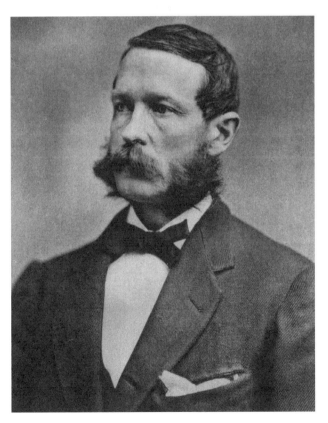

David William Cheever. Boston City Hospital Collection, City of Boston Archives.

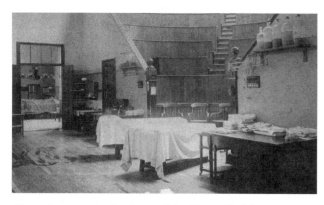

Operating room in the dome of the Centre Building. Boston City Hospital Collection, City of Boston Archives.

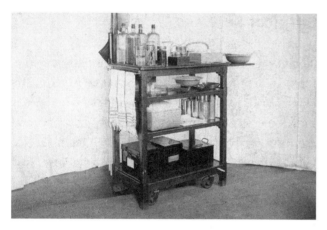

Ether tray. Ca. 1870–1880. Boston City Hospital Collection, City of Boston Archives.

Harvard Surgical Service at BCH. This was mainly because of the complexities of caring for the hospital's patients, the hospital's unclear policies, and the city of Boston's poor financial state.

One of the original six surgeons (all HMS graduates) on the staff of BCH was David W. Cheever. Cheever had studied anatomy with Oliver Wendell Holmes, and as he began teaching and demonstrating anatomy at HMS, he enhanced the process, adding brief assessments and competition among the students. He eventually began teaching residents both surgery and anatomy. In 1882, he was named a professor of surgery at HMS and began leading the Department of Surgery. During this early period of Harvard's affiliation with BCH, Cheever was the only Harvard instructor in surgery there. In 1886, however, younger surgeons—including both Edward Bradford and Robert Lovett—began being assigned to the hospital. Cheever was also an editor for both the *Boston City Hospital Reports* and the *Boston Medical and Surgical Journal*. Dr. Cheever became the hospital's first surgeon-in-chief.

Clinical Education

Eventually there were over 13 different surgeons with Harvard faculty appointments in charge of teaching surgery at BCH. Dr. Herbert L. Burrell followed Dr. Cheever. In 1907, he was named the first John Homans Professor of Surgery at HMS. Bradford (1911) described Burrell as:

> [a] man of energy and force. The chief purpose of his life was to aid in the development of the profession of surgery. As a medical student... he silently pledged his energies to the advancement of that noble art...He had little sympathy with those who made their calling chiefly an opportunity for personal vainglory, who used for personal gain their school or hospital positions. For him these positions brought with them a duty to the community and to the profession...the practice of surgery in America [during his early career] was excellent in quality, but there were marked defects in our hospital organizations which cramped the development of the average surgeon. Three months of active hospital surgical work and nine months of general practice did not offer the best chance for the training of surgeons of the greatest experience. It was his [early] endeavor to establish a continued service in the place of the short service, the universal in American hospitals, and he succeeded early in his career in arranging a continued service at the Boston Children's Hospital, although in the large civic hospital [BCH] with which he was connected all of his professional life, the establishment of a single continued service under one head was impossible. The grouping

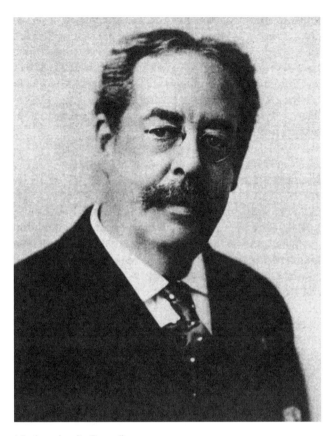

Herbert Leslie Burrell.
A History of the Boston City Hospital 1905-1964, edited by John J. Byrne. Boston: The Sheldon Press, 1964.

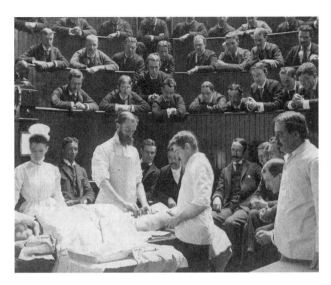

Dr. Burrell observing an operation under ether anesthesia in the dome O.R. Ca. 1880. Boston City Hospital Collection, City of Boston Archives.

of services of a selected number of surgeons, graded according to skill and seniority, and working under one leadership seemed to give an organization many advantages. It furnished a stimulus from combined efforts with a single direction continued from year to year. This system was finally adopted largely through the efforts of Dr. Burrell.

Burrell, who held many leadership positions, including secretary of the American Surgical Association, surgeon general of the Massachusetts Militia (1893), president of the Massachusetts Medical Society, and president of the American Medical Association (1907), published about 20 papers and edited one book. Most of his publications dealt with general surgical issues, but six were orthopaedic in nature and four were on surgical education.

Burrell was an innovative educator, applying the case method to teaching. This method was originally developed in the Harvard Law School. Its application was proposed by W. B. Cannon, a student at HMS, and it was used by Dr. Charles H. Frazier at the University of Pennsylvania. Bradford (1911) wrote:

> The teaching of surgery, formerly consisting of brilliant lectures by surgical leaders, or clinics where the masters of their craft displayed their skill in rare operations to a sensation-loving class, needed to be changed. The careful study of patients by small groups of students, who, under the direction of trained teachers, learn thoroughness of observation and skill of hand, presents a system of education…of high excellence, but one which needs the enrollment of earnest instructors, working less for personal advancement than from devoted interest in their profession. It was to the development of this system that Dr. Burrell gave the chief energies of his life.

Burrell envisioned the case method as a tool that would keep surgeons rooted in both

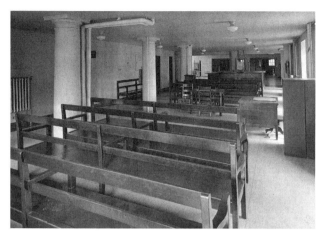

Outpatient Department waiting room. Ca. 1900–1930. Boston City Hospital Collection, City of Boston Archives.

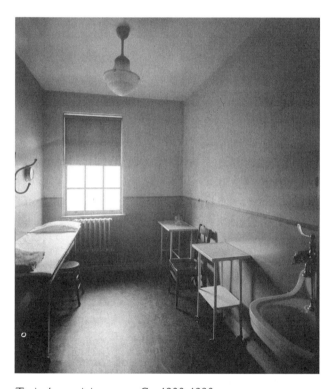

Typical examining room. Ca. 1900–1930. Boston City Hospital Collection, City of Boston Archives.

diagnostic and operative work simultaneously; at the time he felt surgeons were becoming too focused exclusively on the operative work. He wrote:

> There is a great deal of glamor about operative work; the results are brilliant, and the student is apt to deem surgery simply a question of

cleanliness and operating. In fact, surgeons of to-day do not hesitate to say that they do not make diagnoses; they simply operate. This tendency for surgeons "to work more with their hands than with their heads" is fraught with danger to the true advancement of surgery on a secure scientific basis. The "case method" system and sectional, teaching all counteract this danger and will oblige students to use their brains, not alone their hands. (Burrell 1900)

The issues of increasing specialization were also a concern of Burwell's. Bradford (1911) described these difficulties:

> Medical education twenty years ago was excellent, but the rapid growth of the sciences of medicine has made the problems of our medical schools much more difficult. When medical teaching was under the charge of the professors of a few departments, if each could attempt to make his cause the most thorough possible, an excellent school resulted, but this system brought confusion to the average student when the departments became more numerous and there was no proper sequence or proportion in the instruction given…Dr. [Burwell] worked to perfect…a grouping and arrangement of courses as would give to the student some knowledge of everything that was needed for the practitioner, and an opportunity for the more thorough study…of subjects which was most important to each individual…The subordination of the individual to the system and the perfection of the system was the creed of his endeavor.

Burrell understood this increasing specialization as inevitable and felt that curriculums must adapt accordingly. He wrote:

> Object as we may that specialization is narrowing, that it tends to destroy the ability to grasp the whole of a situation, that it has abolished the

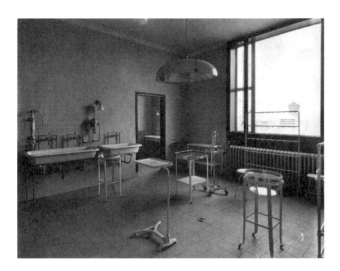

Operating room, ca. 1900–1930. Boston City Hospital Collection, City of Boston Archives.

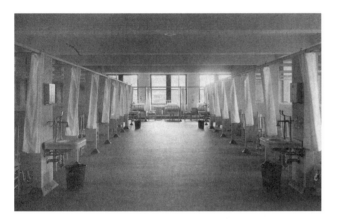

Typical ward, ca. 1920. Boston City Hospital Collection, City of Boston Archives.

well-informed general practitioner, the demand exists and it is imperative – special knowledge on special subjects founded on broad general knowledge…Elective courses…could be given by a number of instructors, not alone by the professors in the department…in order that the student should have the opportunity to obtain knowledge in a manner fitted to him… Many will insist that no specialization should exist until after the student has graduated. My answer is to this is that, "by hook or by crook," the majority of the best students who graduate…today elect that they will devote more time to one given subject than to another. This demand exists…Why not meet it and adjust our curriculum accordingly? …I believe…a minimum required curriculum [includes] the minimum number of subjects…anatomy, physiology, pathology, medicine, surgery, obstetrics and, possibly hygiene…that special knowledge should be required in such subjects as surgical pathology, therapeutics, orthopedics, genitourinary surgery, syphilis, bacteriology, medical chemistry, histology, embryology, legal medicine, ophthalmology, otology, laryngology, gynecology, neurology, military medicine, dermatology and pediatrics is open to question. If required, it should certainly be the minimum and not the maximum, as it is in many instances at present. (Burrell 1902)

Burrell met the challenges of his time in remarkable ways. Bradford described him as unique in his possession of "conspicuous power" as an organizer and administrator. Bradford (1911) wrote:

of the qualities that contribute to make the successful organizer [Burrell] had in marked degree those of being able to select the man best suited to carry out each detailed part of the work and of not interfering with his subordinates once he had placed the responsibility in their hands and was satisfied they understood the nature of it…[He] never sought to tear down what other men had reared until he was convinced that he could put something better in place.

Dr. Edward H. Nichols, another outstanding surgeon, succeeded Burrell as the surgeon in charge of clinical education in the three surgical services at BCH in 1910. Nichols had academic appointments in both surgery and surgical pathology at HMS and was head surgeon for Harvard athletics (see chapter 12). Nichols's main interest, however, was in infection after injury, e.g., osteomyelitis.

During World War I, for about one year, he was chief of the surgical service at Boston City

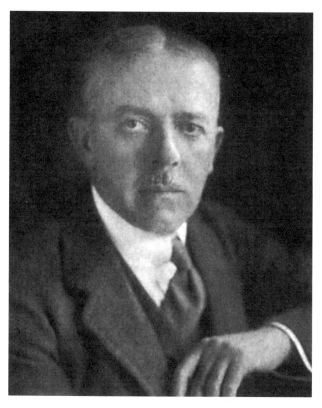

Edward H. Nichols. *A History of the Boston City Hospital 1905-1964*, edited by John J. Byrne. Boston: The Sheldon Press, 1964.

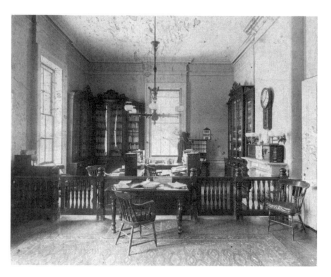

Offices of Drs. Edward Nichols and Edwin Dwight. Ca 1899–1905. Boston City Hospital Collection, City of Boston Archives.

Base Hospital No. 7 in France. After the war, he returned to BCH as Harvard's senior professor of surgery there. Although not defined as clinical clerks at the time, Harvard medical students began to regularly visit BCH. In 1915, during the reorganization of the surgical services the Fifth Surgical Service was designated Harvard's surgical service; Nichols was named chief.

By the late 1920s, Dean Edsall "initiated another attempt to found a true university service" (McDermott 1995). To do so, he appointed Dr. Edward D. Churchill to associate in surgery of:

> the Fifth Surgical Service and Director of the Laboratory of Surgical Research, which was then founded. Dr. Churchill accepted this position on a full-time basis, the first time that any surgical teacher at the Hospital was given this opportunity…However, the staff organization suffered because of occasional changes of junior men from one service to another so that there was no true continuity of service under single leadership…a serious defect in the staff organization…There was also no individual service control of appointments of interns although the appointment of the residents was the prerogative of the teaching service…the Trustees asked Dr. Churchill to draw up a plan for the development of future organization of the Fifth Surgical Service…The surgical staff blocked its adoption. As a result, Dr. Churchill…submitted his resignation [and] returned to the Massachusetts General Hospital and subsequently became its Chief Surgeon, being named to the John Homans Professorship. (McDermott 1995)

Dr. Churchill's plan had included the development of a surgical unit that would operate 24/7 (similar to the Thorndike Laboratory), but various issues at the hospital precluded this. Almost 30 years later, however, in 1954, BCH reallocated its surgical staff to accommodate just three surgical services (down from five). Because of this, many surgeons mainly interested in fractures were transferred to the hospital's Bone and Joint Service, which began handling exclusively all patients with traumatic injury to the bones and joints.

Boston City Hospital (Harvard Service)

Between 1942 and 1955, no Harvard students were assigned for surgical courses at BCH because Harvard's nominations for a chief were blocked by the staff. Harvard had a short-lived affiliation with the Second and Fifth Surgical Services, eventually "withdrawn because of seemingly irreconcilable differences about policies concerning the appointment" of the next chief (McDermott 1995). Dr. Thomas K. Richards, who had been in charge of the care of athletes at Harvard College (see chapter 12), served as chief of the Fifth Surgical Service for about nine years (1942–1951).

By 1955, BCH began the process of reestablishing multiple surgical services at City Hospital: J. Englebert Dunphy from PBBH and a professor of surgery at HMS was chosen to lead the Harvard Service; C. Gardner Child, professor of surgery at Tufts, led the Tufts Service; and John J. Byrne, professor of surgery at Boston University, led the BU Service. Byrne led the charge in coordinating the three services and creating a Surgical Advisory Board that included representatives from all surgical specialties and an Executive Committee which alternated bimonthly meetings. During Dean Berry's tenure (1949–1965), in collaboration with the trustees of the BCH and the assistance of Mayor John Hynes, Harvard had restarted its surgical department at the hospital, which also accommodated research. Earlier, in 1931, to honor the memory of Dr. George Sears, a Charles H. Tyler had left more than $1 million to provide funds for developing a surgical research lab at BCH. The hospital used that money to refurbish what was the Old Surgical Building into the Sears Surgical Laboratory.

In 1963, William McDermott Jr. left MGH to take up the position of Cheever Professor of Surgery at HMS and become the chief of the Fifth Surgical Service and director of the Sears Surgical Laboratory. During his tenure, the clinical, education, and research agendas all escalated. McDermott remained at BCH until the City of Boston allowed only Boston University School of Medicine to have an affiliation with BCH in 1974. Dr. McDermott with some of the surgical staff moved to the New England Deaconess Hospital in 1973 (see chapter 56).

Undergraduate Surgical Education

Dean Bradford supported HMS's relationship with BCH. He had been a staff surgeon there from 1886 until 1904, when he was appointed a consulting surgeon for orthopaedic surgery. Early clinical instruction at BCH during his tenure is outlined in **Box 58.2**. In 1914, Bradford was partially responsible for the surgical services moving into new and larger quarters. A second-year course in surgery was offered at the time at BCH. By 1917, the students began to express their concerns to Dean Bradford about their experiences at BCH. They were dissatisfied with the outpatient departments: not enough opportunities to see and diagnose new patients, no instructions or indications for treatment, and some students had no genitourinary experience. These criticisms had been persistent for about five years.

Except for the period 1942–1955 when no Harvard students were assigned to surgical courses at BCH, Harvard medical students had opportunities to take courses in clinical surgery each year (see chapter 9) at BCH until the affiliation with Harvard was discontinued by the City of Boston in 1974. The last course director was Dr. Quigley from the Peter Bent Brigham Hospital.

Intern and Residency Training Programs

When the hospital first opened, "there were five house officers, two medical, two surgical and an ophthalmic" (Cheever et al. 1906). The number of house officers grew to seven within five years. According to Cheever et al. (1906):

> In 1874 they were still further increased, so that each medical and surgical service had a senior and junior. In 1875 all services were given three

Box 58.2. Early Clinical Undergraduate Education at Boston City Hospital

"Teaching was begun the first autumn, in four months after opening...A small class of [Harvard] students was laboriously taught, by busy men, who, at personal sacrifice, determined to use all of their efforts to build up a clinic. At that time clinical instruction was at a low ebb. Walking the wards meant very little teaching...Dr. Cheever gave the first formal set of clinical lectures, over patients, reported for publication. It was an uphill struggle to popularize clinical teaching. Students were raw; material plenty; teachers untrained. Didactic instruction was prominent; almost exclusive...this rule of the Trustees [indicated]: 'Members of the Medical and Surgical Visiting Staff may give instruction and perform operations in the amphitheater on appointed days; and, subject to the regulations of the Trustees, may introduce patients, provided that in every case the attending physician or surgeon shall certify in writing that the patient can undergo examination and treatment without detriment; and that the superintendent and the patient consent thereto;' teaching never ceased...

"How it was in 1900 is described by Drs. Burrell and J.B Blake[,who stated:] 'It is interesting to note the increase in surgical instruction...during the last ten or fifteen years. In 1887 there was one surgical clinic and one surgical visit a week. On Fridays public operations were done by the surgeons in the amphitheater. The surgical clinic was given by the Professor of Surgery of Harvard University; large sections of the class attended the visit, and cases were shown by the surgeons. For the fourth-year class, which had recently been started, surgical visits were made on Mondays and Thursdays. The [Tuesday] clinic given by Dr. Cheever was fully attended and greatly appreciated...one of the favorite exercises of the Harvard Medical School. The ward visits gradually became less popular...finally the attendance became irregular and meagre. The amount of knowledge obtained was small...gave rise to sectional teaching in the out-patient department and small divisions of the class – ten to twenty – attended...and at present constitute one of the most valuable forms of instruction... The results of operations are shown to the students, and frequently the end result is shown them in the amphitheater...more advanced students examine the case...make their own diagnosis and prognosis, and give advice in regard to treatment...

"[Burrell and Blake further stated:] 'In the surgical clinics the students are constantly taught to explain clinical phenomena by pathological conditions, and fresh pathological material is shown whenever possible...the student attending the clinics consecutively is kept informed of the progress of the cases. When occasion arises the student goes to the autopsy. Another important step has been made in the use of clinical material to illustrate correlative didactic lectures...Another method of teaching is to have a formal consultation of a group of surgeons in the presence of the students, each surgeon expressing his views in order of seniority, the case being summed up at the end by the instructor...One of the most valuable forms of teaching is one which was carried out very carefully by Dr. Lovett in the wards of the Hospital. The students were gathered about the bed in small numbers – not over twelve – and one of the number was chosen to make a thorough examination, subject to the instructor's correction, to give the diagnosis, the differential diagnosis, the indications for treatment, the nature of the treatment and the principles of prognosis. When a student was unable to answer a question or take the next step, his fellows were invited to help him. The fourth year students have, during the last eight years, been brought more and more in contact with the patient in the ward...It will never be possible, nor is it desirable, to have students turned loose in a ward in contact with patients. They must always be under supervision, but they gain a great deal of information...by being in actual contact with patients."

(Cheever et al. 1906)

men, one of whom served six months in the Out-Patient Department, and the appointments were for eighteen months...In 1894 a clinical clerk and a dresser respectively were added to each medical and surgical service. In 1897...a man was appointed for twenty-four months, which he served in six periods of four months each. Six months of "crossed service"

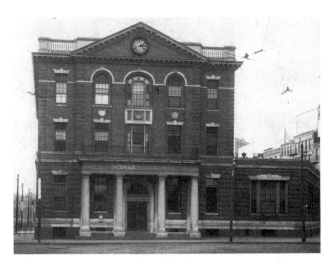

BCH Relief Station, Haymarket Square. November 5, 1905.
Public Works Department Photograph Collection, City of Boston Archives.

are provided, during which a medical man gets surgical service and vice versa. The establishment of the Relief Station [emergency room in Haymarket Square to care for industrial accident victims in the downtown area] and of the South Department (for contagious diseases) greatly extended the educational value of the Hospital for house officers, one of the four-month periods being devoted in each of these departments to surgical and medical men.

Just a few of the well-known orthopaedic surgeons who served as house officers at BCH are listed in **Box 58.3**.

Intern applicants were "subjected to a strict test of their medical knowledge" via three

Box 58.3. Some Early Orthopaedic Surgeons Who Were House Officers at BCH

- Robert Lovett (1885)
- Elliott G. Brackett (1885)
- Joel E. Goldthwait (1890)
- Robert Soutter (1902)
- Zabdiel B. Adams (1903)
- James Sever (1904)

examinations, and references were thoroughly checked for "character and general fitness" (Cheever et al. 1906). Afterward, applicants were:

> referred to special examiners, who test their ability in handling cases in the special departments for which they are candidates…a candidate must have completed at least three years of medical study and may be a doctor of medicine of equally long standing…The qualifications necessary to make a good house officer are no slight ones. He should have a broad preliminary and a thorough medical education. He must be physically strong. His morals must be good. He must have, besides theoretical knowledge, manual dexterity and aptness. He must be neat. He must have tact with patients and their friends. He must be respectful to his superiors and affable to his inferiors. He must be good tempered and patient. He must be a gentleman. (Cheever et al. 1906)

The hospital supplied sleeping facilities and meals for all house officers as well as tennis courts and a squash court, ensuring "the physical welfare of the young men" (Cheever et al. 1906). Nevertheless, "records show that at least six of them have died at their post of duty [since the opening of the hospital until 1904], mostly from diseases contracted in the Hospital" (Cheever et al. 1906). A letter dated November 28, 1939, from Dr. Irving Walker and addressed to the surgical staff, was read at a surgical staff meeting. Walker emphasized the new uniform requirements for students who were assisting during surgical procedures, reminding all that anyone not wearing the uniform would not be allowed to enter the operating rooms.

By 1920 the specialty services had begun to expand. Each service selected its own interns, and senior residents helped to oversee the junior residents, helping to perform procedures and patients consults (as approved by the visiting surgeons). When the Harvard Fifth Surgical Service came

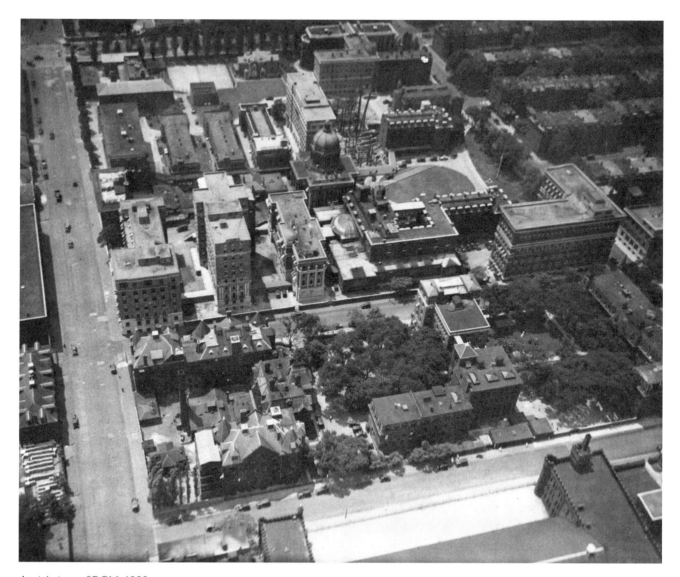

Aerial view of BCH, 1929. Aero Scenic Airviews Co., Boston, Mass. Boston Pictorial Archive, Boston Public Library/Digital Commonwealth.

into being, 18 residents received 39 months of training, rotating across clinics and all the specialty services and gaining incrementally more responsibility as they progressed. These residents were supervised by a chief resident who had completed the 39-month residency and one year as an assistant chief. By the end of World War II in the mid-1940s, the program length was five years and anywhere from 30% to 50% of these residents and interns had graduated from Harvard Medical School. A 1961 survey from the Association of American Medical Colleges ranked Harvard's Fifth Surgical Service at City Hospital as tenth nationwide (surpassed in the northeast only by the MGH program, which had been ranked fifth).

Bone and Joint Service

From the BCH's beginnings, a large portion of the surgical cases handled there were orthopaedic ones. After the hospital began operating in mid-1864, some of the first patients to be seen were treated for fractures or dislocations. During the first two decades, Dr. David W. Cheever, the hospital's first surgeon-in-chief, was the only teacher of clinical surgery. Originally a demonstrator of

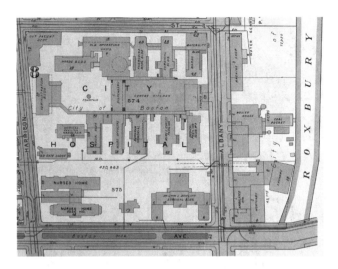

Plot plan of BCH, 1938.
Atlas of the City of Boston: Boston Proper and Back Bay. Philadelphia: G.W. Bromley & Co., 1938. Norman B. Leventhal Map Center Collection, Boston Public Library.

anatomy at Harvard Medical School, he was promoted to professor of surgery in 1882. However, it wasn't until after Dr. E. H. Bradford joined the staff in 1886 that other instructors of surgery enlarged the teaching staff. These men were all surgeons.

As specialty services with dedicated wings in the hospital began to develop around the turn of the twentieth century, orthopaedic surgery was not mentioned; only ophthalmology, gynecology, genito-urinary surgery, and later neurosurgery were noted. Throughout several surgical reorganizations the care of orthopaedic cases, the majority of which were fractures and dislocations, remained under the general surgeons and surgical house staff. And many orthopaedic cases were indeed treated during the first four decades of the hospital's operations, necessitating the development aseptic procedures:

- Dr. George Derby opens an abscess while the leg is immersed in carbolic acid (ca. 1867)
- Dr. David Cheever subperiosteally excises 9 inches of bone in a 13-year-old patient with osteomyelitis (1870)
- Dr George Day amputates a toe and applies antiseptic dressings (1878)
- Dr. Abner Post performs closed reduction under anesthesia on a 7-year-old patient with congenital hip dislocation (1884)
- Dr. Herbert Burrell uses anterior reefing of the capsule to fix a recurrent shoulder dislocation (1895)

A focus on orthopaedics began developing at the very beginning of the twentieth century. In late 1903, Edward Bradford, at the time a consulting general surgeon at BCH, volunteered to act as a consultant on orthopaedic-specific cases. Seven years later, Frederic Cotton published the now classic *Dislocations and Joint-Fractures*, and throughout the next two decades he focused his work on the treatment of fractures. It wasn't until 1928 that the VI Surgical Service (also called the Sixth Surgical Service or newly named Bone and Joint Service) was established. That January, Cotton suggested creating an "independent surgical service" (quoted in Byrne 1964). He nominated himself as chief of the service: "to be efficient I should have autocratic powers – this is a new constructive project of some difficulty. Next in line should be a Visiting Surgeon. There is one suitable man of suitable rank on our staff" (quoted in Byrne 1964). Although Cotton did not name the surgeon he recommended for the position, he may have been referring to Dr. Otto J. Hermann.

The board of trustees approved Cotton's plan four months later, officially establishing the Bone and Joint Service. The trustees named Cotton as chief, with. Drs. Otto J. Hermann and Joseph H. Shortell assisting him. The *Annual Report of the Trustees of Boston City Hospital City* (1929) notes that service began its operations in September of that same year. Dr. Joseph H. Burnett, a member of the staff also became part of the service and "junior members...Drs. Russell Sullivan and Gordon M. Morrison [staffed] the Outpatient Department. It is planned to further enhance the value of this service by adding primarily for teaching purposes, Dr. James W. Sever, Assistant Professor of Orthopedic Surgery, for Tufts Medical Classes

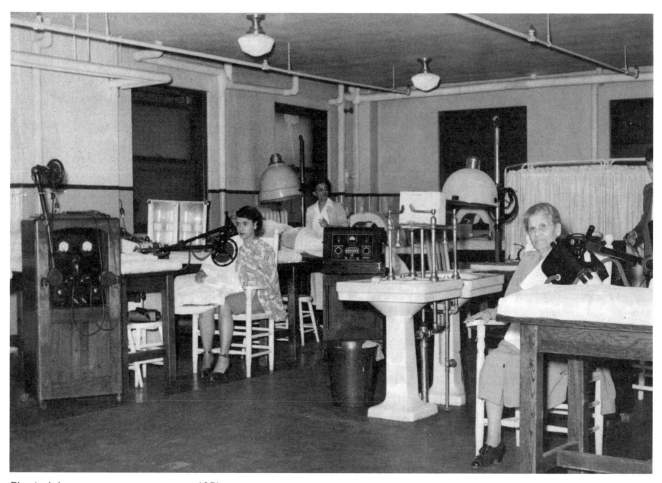

Physical therapy treatment room, ca. 1951. Boston City Hospital Collection, City of Boston Archives.

and Boston University students of medicine are expected to receive instruction on this service in the near future." **Box 58.4** includes Dr. Sever's recollections of these transformational times.

Box 58.4. Dr. James W. Sever's Recollections

"When I started doing orthopaedic surgery, The American Orthopaedic Association was in its transition stage between the brace surgeons and the surgically trained orthopaedic men; and when I was asked about that time to take over the orthopaedic surgery [teaching] at the Boston City Hospital, I was told by the surgeons that the only patients whom I could treat were those with flat feet, scoliosis, and rickets. Well, I didn't want to do that, because it didn't seem to me worth while. Dr. Brackett at that time was at the Massachusetts General Hospital and all of you knew Dr. Brackett and the wonderful work he did, not only in surgery, but also as Editor of our 'Journal' for many years."

(Sever 1955)

CHAPTER 59

Frederic J. Cotton

Orthopaedic Renaissance Man

Frederic Jay Cotton was born in Prescott, Wisconsin, on September 24, 1869, to Joseph Potter Cotton and Isabella Cole Cotton. Frederic may have developed his own extraordinary drawing skills in his father's civil engineering office, and they would serve him well in his teaching and practice as well as in his paintings and etchings. Dr. Cotton was a graduate of Rogers High School in Newport, Rhode Island, and Harvard College (class of 1890). Afterward, along with his MD degree, he earned an AM at Harvard Medical School (HMS) (class of 1894)—a form of honors degree for the most distinguished graduates in the newly developed four-year program. Some 37

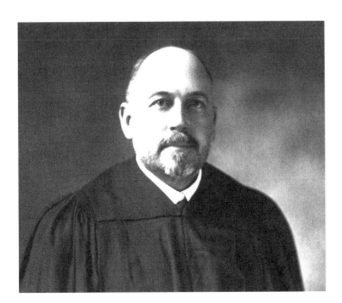

Frederic J. Cotton. Courtesy of the Archives of the American College of Surgeons.

Physician Snapshot

Frederic J. Cotton
BORN: 1869
DIED: 1938

SIGNIFICANT CONTRIBUTIONS: President of the staff and surgeon-in-chief at Boston City Hospital; established the VI Surgical Service (Bone and Joint Service) at Boston City Hospital; published the seminal text *Dislocations and Joint Fractures*; assisted Dr. Charles Scudder in the publication of *The Treatment of Fractures* by illustrating most of the drawings; collaborated with Drs. Edward Bradford and Robert Lovett on their book *Orthopedic Surgery* by completing most of the drawings; one of only two orthopaedic surgeons to give the George W. Gay Lecture (the oldest bioethics lectureship in the United States) at Harvard Medical School; influenced the medical community in the acceptance of a board certification process; identified Cotton's fracture (a unique type of ankle fracture); had several procedures named after him, including: Cotton osteotomy, Cotton advancement operation, and Burrell-Cotton operation; helped reduce the incidence and severity of infection during the Spanish American War through his efforts to improve sanitation; together with Drs. Goldthwait and Brackett organized the U.S.A. General Hospital No. 10 on Parker Hill and was surgeon-in-charge of Parker Hill Hospital; adviser to the Veterans' Bureau and the Public Health Service; assistant to the surgeon general and surgeon-in-chief at Walter Reed Hospital during WWI; founded a bacteriology laboratory at Infants Hospital; contributed to anesthesia research through the development of the Bubble Bottle Method with Dr. Walter Boothby; dedicated to the injured worker; recipient of the Warren Prize for his dissertation; accomplished artist years later when presenting a paper on osteomyelitis, Cotton would remember: "My graduation thesis was on osteomyelitis and, as I recalled it, the treatment then [1894] was a benevolent gesture. We are doing better now, but not quite well enough" (Cotton 1931). From 1893–1894, he was a surgical intern at the Massachusetts General Hospital (MGH).

EARLY TRAINING AND ORTHOPAEDIC INTERESTS

After completing his internship, Cotton spent two months in New York broadening his background by studying bacteriology. He then went to Vienna for two years, where, in addition to developing his professional skills and knowledge, he learned French and German.

Upon his return to Boston, he founded a bacteriology laboratory at Infants Hospital, and, at MGH and Boston Children's Hospitals, he pioneered new techniques in the field. Before serving as a surgeon in the Spanish-American War, Cotton demonstrated his interest in orthopaedics and orthopaedic trauma, publishing four papers. His first publication was a case report of a dislocation of the sternum with Dr. J. S. Stone, a surgeon at Boston Children's Hospital. The other three papers included "Experimental Colles Fracture" and two publications coauthored with Dr. Robert Lovett titled "Pronation of the Foot, Considered from an Anatomical Standpoint" and "Some Practical Points in the Anatomy of the Foot."

In these latter three papers, he had the support of Dr. Thomas Dwight, the Parkman Professor of Anatomy (following Dr. Oliver Wendell Holmes) and father of American forensic anthropology. In the foot-anatomy paper, Cotton noted that "material placed at our disposal by Dr. Thomas Dwight…consist[ed] of either alcoholic specimens of ligamentous dissections or relatively fresh cadavers moistened to a practically normal flexibility" (Lovett & Cotton 1898). In his experimental study of Colles fractures, Dwight provided Cotton with anatomic specimens with which Cotton studied fracture patterns in the wrist by using a mallet or a lever machine to strike the palm with the palm and fingers extended. In this paper, Cotton (1898) noted:

> The more usual cause of failure was rupture of the ligaments, especially the anterior carpal ligament in hyperextension…in some cases fracture of the carpus resulted, especially of the scaphoid [with] satisfactory results to be used in comparison there were but 10 – 7 produced by pressure and counterpressure, 3 by hyperextension…in this series all seven fractures produced [were an] actual Colles' fracture; while the three produced by hyperextension all show the reversed Barton's fracture.

These initial studies exemplify Cotton's early interest in clinical investigation. Using anatomical dissections of the foot and wrist and attempts at creating a common fracture of the wrist in cadavers, he demonstrated the pathophysiology of flat feet and the patho-mechanism of a Colles' fracture in contrast to a Barton's fracture.

THE SPANISH-AMERICAN WAR

In 1898, Dr. Cotton served in the Spanish American War as a surgeon, using his knowledge of bacteriology and civil engineering to improve sanitation, which reduced the incidence and severity of infection. He published one paper, "Malaria as seen at Montauk," in August 1898 while stationed at Camp Wikoff and a second paper of the same title published the year after. The subject of these publications was the conditions at Camp Wikoff, at Montauk Point, Long Island, where 20,000 soldiers in the Army's Fifth Corps and Roosevelt's Rough Riders had been transferred from the battlefields of Cuba.

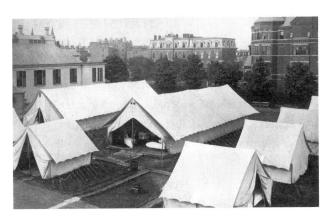

Tents set up on BCH grounds for patients during the Spanish-American War. Boston City Hospital Collection, City of Boston Archives.

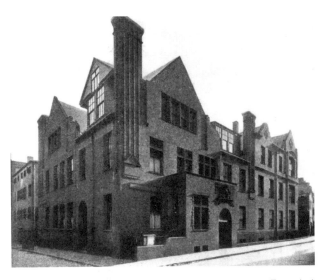

Boston Dispensary (or Boston Medical Dispensary). Founded 1796 for the care of the indigent. Merged with the New England Medical Center in 1968 to become the Tufts Medical Center. Digital Collections and Archives, Tufts University.

Between August and October 1898, these soldiers were not merely stationed at Montauk Point, they were quarantined there. Of course, they were suffering from war wounds. However, in Cuba there was not only military combat, there were swarms of mosquitoes and poor sanitation. Consequently, these soldiers sickened and died more often of infectious diseases; particularly malaria, typhoid, and yellow fever; as well as of malnutrition, than they did of their war wounds. Dr. Cotton (1898) wrote: "The above cases are from a total of about three hundred, which were under my care in the General Hospital at Camp Wikoff from the 21st of August till early in October. Of this total probably two hundred had, or had [had] malaria."

ORTHOPAEDIC CONTRIBUTIONS: 1898–1902

Upon his return from the war that same year, he was appointed a district physician at the Boston Dispensary. He also continued on staff at Boston Children's Hospital where he served for four years from 1898 to 1902. During this period, Cotton completed another experimental study in 1899 which he published in the *Journal of the Boston Medical Sciences*, "A Study of the Jerking or Trigger Knee." Cotton (1899) wrote:

> The disorder is a rare one and consists of an irregularity in the motion of extension of the knee, a sudden jerk forward at the end of the movement sharp enough to give a considerable jar and to be of much inconvenience to the patient…not associated with any disease of the joint. At the suggestion of Dr. E. H. Bradford, the writer looked up certain of these cases and attempted to explain the underlying difficulty… To Drs. Bradford and Lovett, I owe the privilege of using…older case-notes and of examining most of the patients…When extension reached 160 degrees, there was a snap and jerk and the whole lower leg was suddenly carried into full extension.

Cotton's cadaver experiments demonstrated that a loose (possible peripheral or bucket handle tear) and/or a posterior tear of the lateral meniscus could produce a "snap" or "jerk" in the knee as he extended the knee past 160 degrees. The resulting freely moving and unstable meniscus

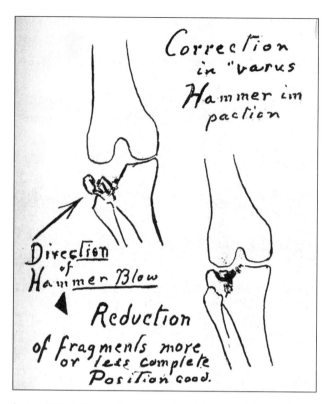

Lateral tibial plateau fracture reduced in varus followed by impaction with a hammer. Drawings by Cotton.
The Treatment of Fractures, 11th edition, by Charles L. Scudder. Philadelphia: W. B. Saunders Company, 1938. Courtesy of Charles S.K. Scudder and the Scudder Association.

created a potential block to extension. To do so, he reviewed five cases and then performed:

> a number of experiments…on dissected cadavera, the external cartilage being variously loosened, cut, mutilated, artificially thickened, etc.…no method of experiment…had any appreciable effect on the movements of the cartilages during simple flexion and extension. When the coronary attachments of the cartilage were cut away, however, leaving its end insertions intact…the range of movement of the cartilage…increased…when the knee reached an angle of 160 degrees, there was a sudden movement forward of the loosened cartilage as the tibia rotates outward [and] during the first part of extension traverses the last part of its course with a sudden jump… These experiments were repeated a number of times on different cadavers, and the abnormal movement of the loosened or cut cartilage reproduced itself almost constantly…It may be concluded, then, that the trigger knee is dependent on interference with normal extension by a damaged external semilunar cartilage… apparently always following some trauma, usually with some synovitis. (Cotton 1899)

By 1900, at 31 years old, Dr. Cotton had published a total of 11 articles, seven of which addressed orthopaedics or orthopaedic trauma. That year he published another four orthopaedic articles, but, importantly, he assisted Dr. Charles Scudder in the publication of his classic book, *The Treatment of Fractures*. Scudder wrote in his preface: "I also thank Dr. F. J. Cotton for an untiring interest in the production of most of the drawings, and in the search for fracture literature" (Scudder and Cotton 1900).

In 1901, Dr. Cotton received the Warren Prize, an award based on an original dissertation on a subject in the fields of pathologic anatomy, physiology, or surgery. It is awarded at a symposium at the MGH held every three years. The prize was founded by Dr. J. Mason Warren in honor of his father, Dr. John C. Warren. Cotton's dissertation discussed "Elbow Fractures in Children. Fractures of the Lower End of the Humerus; Lesions and end-results, and Their Bearing Upon Treatment."

BOSTON CITY HOSPITAL SURGEON-IN-CHIEF AND LATER CONTRIBUTIONS: 1902–1931

For the next 29 years (from 1902 to 1931), he treated outpatients at the Boston City Hospital—first as assistant visiting surgeon but ultimately as president of the staff and surgeon-in-chief. At Mt. Sinai Hospital (see chapter 51), which operated between 1902 and 1915, he may also have served as chief surgeon. His office was located at 520

Commonwealth Avenue in Boston. He excelled in the treatment of diseases and injuries of the bones and joints. Moreover, because traffic accident victims went to Boston City Hospital, he also became particularly experienced in treating the resulting fractures and dislocations.

Os Calcis Fractures

Dr. Cotton developed an interest in os calcis fractures early in his career. In his first of three papers published in 1908, he described (with coauthor Dr. Louis T. Wilson) the proper diagnosis and formulation of a treatment plan for crush fractures following physical examination and x-ray. He noted the fracture patterns were so complex they could not be classified. Generally speaking, Cotton said that corrections should be made by hand with the foot in plantar flexion. **Box 59.1** outlines his methods in his own words.

He published his second paper eight years later, expressing frustration that the evidence of his research had been ignored and that poor record-keeping had contributed to that status quo. He stated:

> Eight years ago I published a paper on this subject, which I have reread recently; it contains so exactly what I believe to-day that I am embarrassed. Either I was then and am now entirely wrong, or else the profession continues to be entirely wrong now, after due warning… Handicapped by poor records and the extreme difficulty in tracing the shifting artisans of big cities, I can give you no real presentation of end-results achieved, though I hope to later on.
> (Cotton 1916)

In 1921, he wrote that more than half of these patients are partially disabled and, at best, 30% or more are totally disabled. If the heel is shortened and flattened, Cotton wrote, nothing can be done. For outward deviation, he preferred to utilize the Gleich operation. His protocol further called for

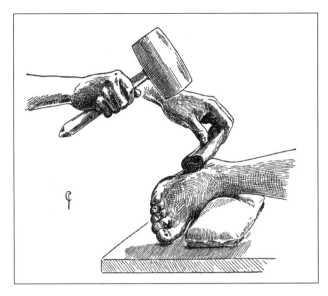

Cotton's method of treating calcaneus fractures by impaction. The foot is positioned on a sandbag, the lateral surface of the hind-foot protected by a felt pad, and the pad is struck with a mallet to reduce and impact the fracture. Drawing by Cotton. *Dislocations and Joint-Fractures* by Frederic J. Cotton. Philadelphia: W. B. Saunders Company, 1910.

the removal of bone spurs. In cases where the patient suffers a loss of lateral motion, he preferred to clear away all excess bone and forcibly manipulate the foot to clear the impediments to motion. He then detailed the appropriate schedule for cast removal and return to function: gentle motion for two weeks, then partial weight-bearing at four weeks followed by full weight-bearing at six weeks.

He reported normal function in one case and practically normal in six of nine cases he had operated upon. In 1937, Dr. C. F. Goff reported on five cases of os calcis fractures treated with a carpenter's clamp described by Yergason. In his paper, he stated: "Cotton, since 1908 has probably been responsible for the most important single contribution regarding treatment [of calcis fractures]" (Goff 1937).

Cotton's Fracture

Dr. Cotton made another of his original contributions early in his career: identifying a unique type of ankle fracture in 1908 that included a fracture of

Box 59.1. Diagnosis and Treatment of Os Calcis Fractures

"It was only after seeing a considerable number of these cases that it occurred to us to observe them…or to treat them in other than the routine way…to accept the result as inevitable…all the teachings…and all the data of the literature, warn us that we should be very careful to treat fractures of the os calcis by fixation and by putting them up in plantar flexion…to decrease the tension through the tendon Achilles, which may contribute to further displacement of the fractured heel…Such treatment of fractures of the os calcis is perfectly respectable doctrine for a date ten or fifteen years ago, but is not…what should be expected today…For our present purposes…we will consider only the type of fracture of the os calcis by crushing…We do not believe that it is possible to classify os calcis fractures according to fracture lines…All our attempts at classification have failed. There is a general similarity…The central point of the fracture…usually lies below the posterior part of the astragalus…the x-ray tells us about spurs in the sole and…the amount of vertical displacement…data must come from physical examination. Measurements we have found of no use…we have come to trust the x-ray entirely, always using the skiagraph of the other foot as a 'check'…it is practicable by clinical examination, aided by the x-ray, to determine all of the displacements which are of importance to prognosis.

"What can be done to avoid bad end-results?…proper treatment theoretically is to correct the displacement, but attempts at such correction are met with…distinct difficulties…correcting displacement…After experimenting with the Thomas wrench…and with the heavy wrench used by plumbers, we have found that none of these are more efficient…than the unaided hand…In exceptional fresh cases with great broadening, we have used the felt and mallet, striking the outer side of the bone, as a means of correcting displacement…We do not recommend it, however, as a routine. [The second difficulty is] retaining position…We have tried [tenotomy]…and found it useless and unnecessary…To maintain correction, we must pin or suture the fragments or reimpact them…Reimpaction sounds impractical. In fact, it is easy…This impaction may sometimes be accomplished by the pressure of the hands, driving the fragments in laterally. Ordinarily we have placed a firm sandbag under the inner side of the foot and then, protecting the tissues with a folded felt pad, have used a heavy mallet to reimpact the thoroughly loosened and replaced fragments in the desired position…Securing…adequate motion between os calcis and astragalus by forced pro-and supination…after treatment in…an ordinary cast…the foot is put up at about 15 to 20° of plantar flexion…usually it seems wise to secure some inversion…In a week or ten days the primary callus seems adequate to hold the connection [then] removal of the cast occasionally for massage and guarded active motion is wise. We have not allowed weight-bearing for a month…Return of full function is rather slow; probably three months will be a fair average of time…This paper is, then, a plea for more accurate study and more active treatment, a plea, in other words, for a real surgical treatment for this class of lesions."

(Cotton and Wilson 1908)

the posterior malleolus of the ankle (**Case 59.1**). Although described in his book *Dislocations and Joint-Fractures* (published in 1910), Cotton did not initially name this particular kind of ankle fracture. In 1915, he did, noting "a new fracture [which] has never been adequately described in print, and has apparently escaped the notice even of those who deal with fractures habitually" (Cotton 1915). He wrote:

Stimson records a couple of old cases belonging in this class…and Brackett, E.G., of Boston (shown March 2, 1910) and Darrach, W. of New York, have each shown plates of single cases (not published)…I have been talking about the lesion for years, until some of my house-officers at the City Hospital, wearied by long insistence, have come to refer to it as "Cotton's fracture." (Cotton 1915)

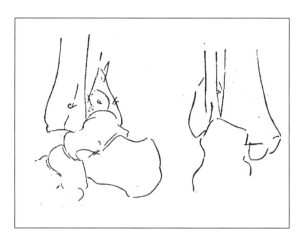

Drawing by Cotton of Cotton's fracture of the ankle, 1915.
F. J. Cotton, "A New Type of Ankle Fracture," *Journal of the American Medical Association* 1915; 64: 319.

Case 59.1. Identification of a New Type of Ankle Fracture: Cotton's Fracture

> "In 1908, [a patient], a student of the Massachusetts Institute of Technology, was brought into my office with an ankle smashed and luxated backward and outward. Obviously, this was the case I had been looking for. The fracture of the fibula and the tearing away of the internal malleolus was obvious; the foot was also luxated backward (and in this case outward as well). Reduction under light anesthesia was easy. Roentgen-ray plates taken shortly after showed a fragment broken off the posterior articular face of the tibia."
>
> (Frederic J. Cotton 1915)

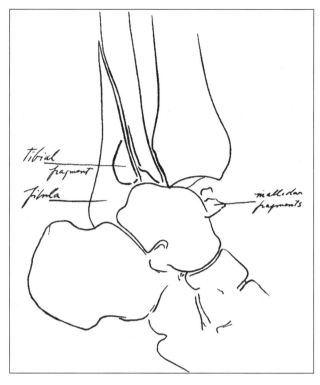

Drawing by Cotton of Cotton's fracture, 1929. F. J. Cotton, "Ankle Fractures," *New England Journal of Medicine* 1929; 201: 755.

The Cotton's fracture is a posterior dislocation of the foot that breaks a wedge-shaped fragment (posterior malleolus) off the back surface of the tibia at the joint and displaces it posteriorly or superiorly. The posterior tibial fragment is most frequently separate along with the tibio-astragaloid ligament; though associated with fracture of both malleoli, sometimes the internal malleolus and posterior tibial edge of the joint are included in one piece. The Cotton's fracture has the potential to be disabling because, if unrecognized, the ankle joint remains noncongruous with posterior subluxation or dislocation. He recalled seeing 53 cases of this type of fracture with posterior subluxation/dislocation of the ankle. He documented that the cause is a lateral and posterior twist of the foot while the weight is on the ball of the foot. Cotton (1915) noted:

> Reduction is simple if the lesion is understood. All that is called for is forward traction…in moderate plantar flexion…and then lock the reduction in maximum dorsal flexion. Hold in plaster…The after-treatment is that of Pott's fracture, save that early mobilization is absolutely essential, and no weight should be borne on the foot for at least seven or eight weeks.

Following his publication in 1915, Cotton and others referred to a fracture of the posterior malleolus with posterior subluxation/dislocation of the ankle and medial and lateral malleolar fractures as "Cotton's fracture." Almost 20 years later, in 1934, he described an operation for patients with untreated or inadequately treated Cotton's fractures, usually with a painful, crippling disability. Repair involves a reconstruction of the whole ankle by dividing the malleoli at the joint, and from the outer malleolus, opening the joint horizontally and posteriorly. Cotton and Morrison (1934) explained it was:

> an extensive reconstruction of the whole ankle, a useful operation, though formidable. The malleoli are divided at the joint level, and from the cut of the outer malleolus, the joint is opened horizontally forward. The malleolus then dragged down a bit gives access to the side of the tibia. With a large chisel (of wide curved concavity) a single cut is made horizontally across the joint, leaving a quarter cylinder concave cut...for the astragalus to set into. The next step is to loosen up the whole joint. This means extensive ligament tearing by *external* force or (not so good) instrumental leverage *within* the joint. This must be complete enough to allow the astragalus being dragged forward to a proper position. Sometimes the malleoli must be refitted. Pins or the like are not needed. Inasmuch as the cartilage of the top of the astragalus is not cut and should not be bruised, direct ankylosis does *not* occur. The results are rather better than one might reasonably expect. In the lesser cases, the remedy is less. One need only abolish the check to dorsiflexion. That means an incision on the outer side of the joint, a thin osteotome slipped in so sloped as to clear a generous wedge straight across the front of the tibia. If possible, this should be a matter of one cut, with removal of the wedge in one piece. If there has been much irritating contact, the neck of the astragalus may show overgrowth, and may be dug away, liberally. One need not fear ankylosis for there is no longer any bone contact. The only chance is of a recurrence of bony overgrowth. As a rule, the operation, very simple as it is, is well worth while.

PUBLICATION OF *DISLOCATIONS AND JOINT-FRACTURES* AND ADDITIONAL ILLUSTRATED WORKS

By 1910, Dr. Cotton had only written about 15 papers on orthopaedics and orthopaedic trauma when he published his classic textbook *Dislocations and Joint-Fractures*. Cotton dedicated the book to his father, Joseph Potter Cotton, C.E. In his introduction he wrote:

> This book was originally planned as a treatise on dislocations [but] was promptly abandoned. Dislocations...present themselves...as injuries to or near the joints...Injuries to and about joints...constitute one of the most doubtful fields of surgery, a field strewn with wrecks, – the products of mistakes and unavoidable difficulties, prolific in discontent and in resultant actions at law – actions based only too often on unavoidable uncertainty or error...It seems that the time is ripe for a summary of the subject, based on personal experience, fortified by the great mass of admirable x-ray pictures more lately produced, the data of museum specimens, and...the most recent literature... Unavoidable such a book as is here outlined must be largely personal...the book has been nearly five years in the making...For better or for worse we must study our cases of trauma, must do the best we can, and must rest on the result...so far as concerns both text and illustrations, I hold myself directly responsible. No one has even assisted in the preparation of the text. The drawings are my own; most of them were drawn for his book, and are...original; a very few were sketched from drawings in articles by others...I wish to acknowledge my great indebtedness to my colleagues of the Boston City Hospital surgical staff...Dr. William F. Whitney, Curator of the Warren Museum (Harvard Medical School), has greatly helped

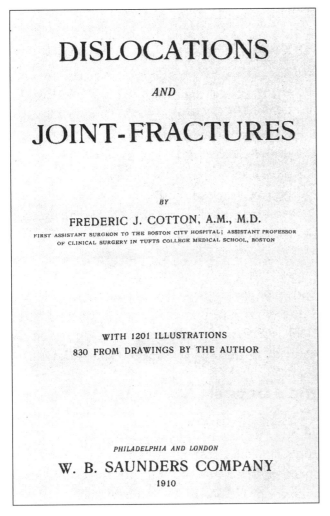

Cotton's book: *Dislocations and Joint-Fractures.* U.S. National Library of Medicine.

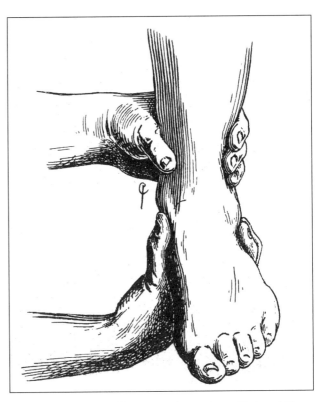

Drawing by Cotton of his test to determine ankle instability with a Pott's fracture. *Dislocations and Joint-Fractures* by Frederic J. Cotton. Philadelphia: W.B. Saunders Company, 1910.

me by placing the material of the Museum at my disposal for study. (Cotton 1910)

The book was 654 pages and contained numerous x-rays and photographs, but most illustrations were simple line drawings created by Dr. Cotton. The book was published in at least two editions. In one review of the first edition, it was stated:

In this unusual book…Cotton has reanimated one of the dullest topics in all surgery. By that work he has done a great service. Not only has he written the book himself, but he has illustrated it so that one sees visualized the victims of the injuries which he describes. The work is delightful, spirited, scholarly and original, and is not only a book of reference, but a book of casual reading…stimulating reflections, taken from the author's introductions, indicate the

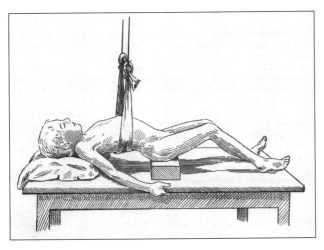

Drawing by Cotton of the use of a sling device to reduce a kyphosis allowing the application of a body cast. U.S. National Library of Medicine.

scope and nature of his work. He is an independent writer, who does his own thinking; he neither ties up to nor discards x-rays; he appreciates the work of others; he is fertile in suggestions regarding treatment; he approves of massage; he operates upon simple fractures when necessary; he gives excellent advice regarding the possibilities of actions at law; and he fills his book with vital, new and instructive pictures. Surgeons, house surgeons, and general practitioners should own and study this volume. ("Book Reviews. 'Dislocations and Joint-Fractures.'" 1910)

In a review of the second edition, Dr. Lewis S. Pilcher endorsed Dr. Cotton's emphasis on the importance of common sense and mechanical sense in fracture expertise. Pilcher (1924) wrote:

We endorse especially this statement of his, "No damage to a machinery, human or other, increases its efficiency, and in human machinery we cannot replace parts. Many breaks and dislocations do damage absolutely irreparable; many do damage entirely unrecognizable at the time…Our duty is to obtain, in the given case, the best results obtainable in this case by whatever means are at hand…No book can make a man a fracture expert…Experience, common sense, capable and trained fingers, and perhaps most important of all what you call mechanical sense, must help him out." The reviewer would like to emphasize this statement in fracture work. Common sense and mechanical sense are essential…in fracture work. It is in the degree to which this book reflects these two elements…that it is to be commended.

In this seminal book, Dr. Cotton described both a fracture type and a diagnostic test for ankle injuries that would bear his name. He explained Cotton's fracture (addressed earlier in this chapter) while not yet naming it as such, and he also detailed a simple clinical test for syndesmotic instability in a Pott's fracture. He wrote:

For accurate diagnosis it is necessary to employ the following maneuver. The ankle is grasped with one hand just above the joint, while the other hand is placed beneath the sole, with the thumb on one side of the foot, the fingers on the other below the malleoli. If the foot is grasped firmly and pushed inward and outward, the presence of an abnormal lateral mobility is easily recognized. (Cotton 1910)

In addition to illustrating both his own text and Scudder's work, he collaborated with Drs. Edward Bradford and Robert Lovett on their book *Orthopedic Surgery*, which published in 1911. Cotton completed most of their drawings.

Hip Fractures

Another major interest of Dr. Cotton was hip fractures, and he determined that an effective treatment was reduction of the fracture and subsequent impaction. He presented his technique in 1910 to the American Orthopaedic Association, publishing it in the *American Journal of Orthopedic Surgery* in 1911. This report was published 27 years before the development of the Smith-Petersen nail. He described his technique in two cases under ether anesthesia:

the leg had been dragged down, crepitus (previously absent) was readily perceived on pressure inward on the trochanter. A pad of felt was placed over the trochanter, and with the leg drawn down to its proper length and its eversion corrected, impaction was attempted. An assistant furnished counter-pressure with his hands on the opposite side of the pelvis and over the other hip. The instrument used was a large, heavy [8.5 pounds] wooden mallet. A half dozen careful blows were struck, then the result was tested; there was no tendency to reproduction of the shortening; no tendency to eversion. On test, it was obvious that the shaft of the femur now rotated not on its own axis, but on the axis of the head in acetabulum, though the sweep of rotation was less than normal, owing to the unavoidable shortening of the femoral neck. This limit was put up with a long side-splint for protection, and weight-traction was discontinued. (Cotton 1911)

Over the next 27 years, Cotton published another 11 papers on the management of hip fractures. He presented another four cases to the New England Surgical Society in 1924 and in his discussion stated: "I am not ready to talk about statistics, but I have been getting results with only an occasional failure. Prior to that you know what you get with loose fractures of the hip, and I guess everybody got the same thing" (Cotton 1925).

In 1938, the year he died, Dr. Cotton published his last paper on the treatment of hip fractures by impaction. His method included reduction of the hip, the success of which should be verified by x-ray. Cotton and Morrison (1938) wrote "the method now in use,– namely, traction in the line of the femur, hip and knee being moderately flexed; sharp adduction; knee crossed over the thigh of the sound side; sharp inward rotation of the broken limb, followed by bringing the leg down into slight abduction (20 degrees more or less) without letting up on the inward rotation…" (Cotton and Morrison 1938). They went on to say:

> When satisfactory position is attained, comes the time for converting the neutral (normal) position into valgus by impaction. The leg is abducted 20 or 30 degrees from the mid-line of the body…We use a heavy wooden mallet to impact with, the limb being protected by a single layer of heavy felt. A tightly stuffed cylindrical sandbag of four-inch thickness can be used and with this no felt is needed for protection. We have done many impactions in this way,

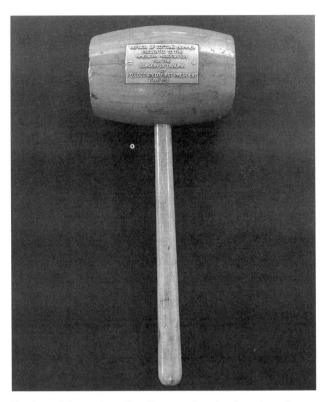

Replica of Cotton's mallet. Presented to the American Association for the Surgery of Trauma at its first meeting in 1948, by Dr. Kellogg Speed, the association's first president. It has been used by every president since to open the association's annual meeting. Courtesy of the American Association for the Surgery of Trauma.

> but we feel that the hammer gives more exact control; with this severe impaction, exactness is essential. With the hammer, the trochanter is struck and driven home. The blow is a slow swing of the heavy mallet. The direction of the blow is not in line of the neck with the old impaction procedure, but across it at an angle of roughly 45 degrees with the mid-line of the body. Since the limb is already abducted, this gives a total angle of from 70 to 75 degrees or…better stated, an angle of from 105 to 110 degrees with the shaft. The force…is applied in a line to push the neck fragment across under the head at the same time that the neck is impacted into the head. (Cotton and Morrison 1938)

He also noted, "A word of caution is necessary: It is very important that the blow be struck parallel to the table. There is a possibility of shoving the neck fragment to front or back" (Cotton and Morrison 1938). And, finally, he wrote that "Following reduction and impaction, we have nailed the fragments with Krupp nails...Then, gently, the first impaction is done with the impactor devised by Smith-Petersen, which straddles the nail and rests on bone" (Cotton & Morrison 1938). Since June 1948, in recognition of his seminal work on impaction for the treatment of hip fracture, a replica of Cotton's Hammer has been used by the American Association for the Surgery of Trauma (AAST) to open its annual meetings.

A WINDOW INTO COTTON'S THINKING ON FRACTURE MANAGEMENT

In 1911, Dr. Cotton published "Why and When to Operate on Fractures" from a talk he gave at the annual meeting of the Massachusetts Medical Society. His position that as surgical procedures on fractures have become more common, some such procedures are unnecessary. Surgery, he opined, was of course essential for certain compound fractures. Those that puncture the skin require surgery, but those that have poked beneath, but have not punctured the skin, could be managed

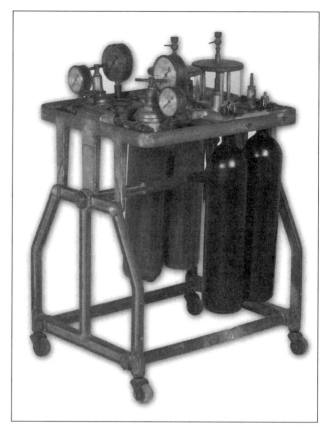

Cotton-Boothby anesthesia apparatus. Courtesy of the Wood Library-Museum of Anesthesiology, Schaumburg, IL.

Cotton's publication of a paper he presented to the Massachusetts Medical Society in which he gave a comprehensive review his method of treatment of fractures. *Boston Medical and Surgical Journal* 1911; 165: 862.

without it. The main purpose of surgery for open fractures is to prevent infections. The bone and living tissue must be cleaned, and necrotic tissue must be excised. The repair of the bone itself does not require internal fixation.

There is one exception: fracture of the patella with separation of the fragments. This injury primarily occurs occupationally to workers who depend on their mobility to continue working. The necessity to speed healing in order to allow these patients to return to work as fast as possible often requires stabilization of the fracture. Cotton wrote that the decision to perform surgery should be made based on likelihood of successful return to function but that conservative, nonsurgical management should be considered first. **Box 59.2** includes a portion of the original text he published, providing a window into his thinking on fracture management at the time.

Box 59.2. Why and When to Operate on Fractures

"I think I was one of the first in this community to do routine open operative work on fractures, eight years ago, at a time when few in Boston, except the late Drs. Porter and Burrell, used to touch any simple fracture (save the patella or olecranon), – a time when I had to get at least two seniors in consultation before I was allowed to touch a case of this sort. Since then my work has grown more radical, and my field of operative work has broadened in this class of cases as I have tested results. Within a short time a certain surgeon, not of maximum repute as to surgical judgment in other matters, has come here and declared that we should plate many fractures, if not all, and lo! what has happened? ...Not only the difficult cases are subjected to operation, but fractures of the elbow...even Colles' fractures, are subjected to surgical incision and the insertion of indiscriminate hardware...In the face of this fresh flood of enthusiasm, I feel that I am a hopeless back-number. I am not ready to say that all fractures should be operated on...I have never seen a fracture with displacement perfectly reduced without incision, but I have seen many fractures that have been so excellently handled without operation that the results have left nothing to be desired...

"I am going to present to-day what I believe...as to why and when one should operate on fractures. To begin with the most obvious problem, there is one class in which we must intervene – the compound fractures...Apart from... cases of grave crushing...compound fractures fall...into two classes...those in which the...bone...has just 'pinked' the skin, and has gone back,– and those in which the bone...has...been driven out through the skin, and often is found greatly contaminated with all sorts of dirt...It is only in the first class that we can hesitate...Everyone knows...a large proportion of these cases heal cleanly... What shall we do as a routine? ...my own answer...if... the best hospital facilities can be utilized, and if an experienced operator is at hand, I believe we are safer in opening up and radically cleansing the wound. In this class of cases I have found that my house-surgeons at the hospital... favored the 'closed' method, and justified their choice by results. My own results have been better with the open' treatment...In...the more open compound fractures – we must clean up...First of all we must clean the bone...with a brush, bite out the dirty surfaces with rongeurs, ...cut out all devitalized tissues...followed by profuse douching with normal salt solution...pack it [wound] open with gauze...My own practice is to do little [to internally stabilize the bone]...

"Are there any uncomplicated fractures which should always be treated by open reduction? I know of but one, – fracture of the patella with separation of the fragments... Most accidents occur to workingmen, laborers and artisans...With men of these types, if they are laid off for six months, they come to the end of their resources and become 'bums' of the park or of the free-lunch variety, and never become workers again. If we can halve or quarter the period of convalescence, nearly all of them will go back to work. This, to my mind, is the most cogent argument for operation in many fractures...fractures in which ordinary apparatus treatment gives poor or long-delayed results. In patella and olecranon cases incision is almost obligatory... lesions at the shoulder, fracture with luxation practically always means open operation; and all compression fractures of the os calcis are subjected to the remodeling and reimpacting process which I originated [but] are not subjects for open operation, however, save in rare instances...I believe I am correct in saying that there are almost no fractures or luxations save those above noted in which a routine primary operation is justified. In all fractures, I believe it is our duty to try non-operative first...

"I still believe we should try for the best reduction we can get, and then – within two weeks at most – get an x-ray... and decide whether we should undertake more medical treatment by readjustment under ether or by open operation to review in brief the more usual fractures and luxations...Commonest of all fractures is Colles' fracture at the wrist. When should we operate [?]...The answer is, almost never...in the worst cases, not readily held in place, the cause is a comminution not to be remedied by operation. In unrecognized cases...or in cases in which...the result is not very good, we can operate easily and successfully, but it is to be remembered...the results of operation are essentially cosmetic. The wrist will look better, but probably will not work any better, than if we let it alone. Fractures and luxations of or in the carpus are a worse problem. Many of them call for operation...if displacement [of a scaphoid fracture] or a scaphoid fracture with backward luxation of the distal row...recurs.... are we justified in operating [which] means excision of the carpus, total or partial...at least half...do eventually call for operation to get good function.

"As to fractures of the forearm...overlapping of the bone-ends will not do to leave alone...All we need here is to bring the bone-ends opposite one another, – and [secured] with plates...Fractures of the radial head and neck call for operation very often, but not as a routine. Many...do very well with…under early motion and massage…test at three to five weeks and see if motion is coming back; if not…then excise the radial head…Now as to fractures of the humerus at the elbow…Unless there is more peculiar difficulty in reducing or holding the fracture, or some injury to nerve or vessel trunks, I should not think of operating on a fresh…fracture…As to fractures of the humeral shaft, the question is different. Here we have a definite indication for interference in many cases: The humerus is a single bone, unsplinted…by a sister-bone, and displacement is often great and hardly controllable, which the chance of long-delayed union or non-union is relatively great. No quarrel is to be made with the surgeon who proposes operative interference…Personally, I do not operate often…because I think I can do things with splints [but if] splint treatment is unsatisfactory, I have had no hesitation in carrying out the open treatment. When we come to fractures of the 'surgical neck' of the humerus, or…separation of the epiphysis…Nearly always in these cases reduction without open operation is peculiarly difficult. It should be tried…If [not successful], we must cut. These fractures are hard to reduce, partly because [of interposed] soft tissues…but more particularly because the pectoral muscles adduct the lower fragment and the biceps draws it up…we must operate on a large percentage of these cases…Fractures of the anatomical neck are usually best let alone…As to pure luxation of the shoulder, there may be little leeway for judgment. In fresh luxations…practically all cases are reducible by manipulation…A certain number of cases came to us, however, usually unrecognized, at two weeks to two months after injury. These cases should be operated on…neck operations are bloody and carry much shock…Clavicle fractions do not call for operation. Clavicle luxation at the acromial joint, on the other hand, is distinctly operable…

"Next in order come hip fractures, often operated on, but in my opinion ordinarily inoperable, unless luxation is combined with the fracture. Most hip fractures are impacted…If the position is very bad (e.g. if outward rotation in extreme), we may in selected cases break up the impaction and correct the position and then reimpact…Only cases in which treatment by apparatus has been tried and has failed justify open operation…Fractures of the femoral shaft…I will only say that I believe very many of them to be operable, and think operations far too seldom done…Separation of the lower epiphysis of the femur unless easily reducible are always operated on account of the peculiar danger they present of vessel pressure and consequent gangrene of the leg…Fractures of the lower leg, responsible for much disability in very many cases, call for better treatment than they usually get [which] is usual practicable without incision, and in worse cases, those with communication, open operation is to my mind out of the question. On the other hand…any fracture so ill-reduced that the fracture surfaces are not at all in contact is too bad to let go by…these must be fixed…As to ankle fractures, the question is different: Here it is a question of reduction, not of holding the position; once reduced, these cases are easily held…Personally I have never operated on a fresh ankle fracture that was not compound. The same applies to fractures of the tarsus and foot, save for os calcis fractures, which almost uniformly call for reduction and reimpaction, but not for incision.

"This is a but rough incomplete survey…it is a plea for operative measures restricted to cases in which there is a definite reason for operating on the individual case. In general, I am inclined to fear too great an activity in fracture operating in the next few years. There are, however, two classes of fracture, by no means always to be operated on, that nevertheless deserve frequent operation because operation is often the only way to get good results, …namely fractures of the femoral shaft, and leg fractures…shortened legs, the occasional vicious deformities, the routine stiff knees, the slow unions, the common refractures [that] occur in young workingmen…also need good legs to work on…such cases…well reduced and held…today [with] 'plating' and such screw-bolt apparatus as I have repeatedly used—we can in any case can be sure of reduction and maintenance of practically perfect position and (bar sepsis) of a greatly lessened period of convalescence as well as of far better end results…

"Let me say only that I believe late operations of cases showing disability after fractures offer a field second to none in usefulness, probably even more important in the present stage of fracture treatment than open operations on fresh fractures. They are, however, incomparably more difficult than the operations on fresh cases and are successful only in proportion to the care expended in planning the operation…and to the perfection of the operative technique…Technique deserves only a word…In this work we most need – (a) A clear idea of what is to be done. (b) A clear field. (c) A minimum of cutting. (d) A minimum of handling. (e) Accurate reposition. (f) Adequate fixation, with a minimum of foreign material left in the wound."

(Cotton 1911)

CONTRIBUTIONS TO ANESTHESIA: THE BUBBLE BOTTLE METHOD

In 1911, Dr. Walter Boothby—an anesthesiologist at Boston City Hospital and on the faculty of HMS—advocated general anesthesia with Dr. Cotton, his colleague at Boston City Hospital, using nitrous oxide (and oxygen) and potentially the addition of ether. To ensure a continuous flow at the proper rate of delivery, each gas was injected through water using a "bubble bottle" or "bubble-through," method where the gases were mixed and then administered to the patient through the trachea and thence to the lungs. A bubble bottle, or bubble-through, was a glass chamber filled with water. The ether, nitrous oxide, and oxygen were mixed there. Newer anesthesia devices, developed by other clinicians, were influenced by their bubble bottle method. Over several years Cotton published eight papers about anesthesia.

INNOVATIVE EDUCATOR AND INFLUENTIAL IN THE ESTABLISHMENT OF BOARD CERTIFICATION

Dr. Cotton was a prolific researcher and published throughout his career. However, he did not confine his efforts to research, he also enjoyed teaching—particularly doctors. He was initially appointed lecturer in surgery at HMS in 1912 and then eventually promoted to the distinctive position of instructor of industrial surgery (**Box 59.3**). The specifics of his appointments vary and are unclear in the historical record, but he was "a lecturer on bone and joint surgery at Harvard Medical School and [associate in surgery at] Harvard Medical School, Courses for Graduates [and] also assistant professor of surgery at Tufts College Medical School" ("Recent Deaths. Cotton" 1938).

His lectures were effective and clear, and he taught his techniques, so they were disseminated widely and, because they were effective, they were adopted. And, of course, he did not confine his practice to academia. Hospitals all over New England sought him out for consultation. He was a consulting surgeon to many hospitals, including Faulkner Hospital, Newton Hospital, New England Hospital for Women and Children, Chelsea Memorial Hospital, Beth Israel Hospital, Cape

Box 59.3. Dr. Cotton's Appointments at HMS 1912–1914: Lecturer in Surgery

- 1814–1919: Associate in Surgery
- 1919–1920: Associate in Surgery, Graduate Courses in Medicine
- 1921–1932: Instructor in Industrial Surgery

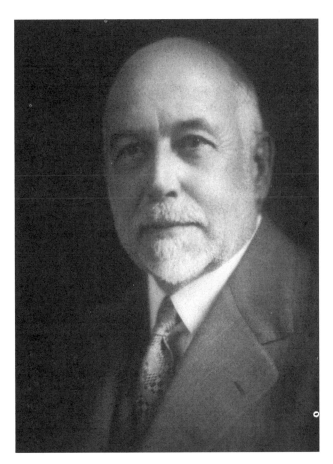

Frederic J. Cotton. Digital Collections and Archives, Tufts University.

Cod Hospital in Hyannis, the Arlington Symmes Hospital, and Malden Hospital.

Further, in order to ensure the integrity of the profession, Cotton was one of the founders of the American College of Surgeons (ACS) and one of the original 16 members of its board of regents. He was also a member of the ACS's Committee on Fractures, and:

> as a founder and member of the Board of Regents of the American College of Surgeons [a member of the Committee on Fractures for years], and of the American Board of Surgery, Dr. Cotton exerted a great amount of influence in raising the standards of surgery and of hospitals in America. (WRM 1938)

The ACS was founded in 1913 and spearheaded by gynecologist Franklin H. Martin. Martin, who also founded the journal *Surgery, Gynecology and Obstetrics* in 1905. That same year, through Martin's efforts, the ACS recruited John M. T. Finney to be president. Finney wanted to implement standards within the profession because, at the time, anyone could say they were a surgeon and there was no way to determine whether that surgeon was fit to practice. The ACS developed standards of practice around 1915 and anticipated the formation of state regulatory boards with mandatory licensure, but the ACS, like many other agencies, provided an additional credential for practice. Martin, however, encountered resistance from surgeons and institutions throughout the East Coast.

As the popularity of board certification increased in the United States (around 1922), Cotton was influential in convincing factions of the medical community to accept a board certification process for new surgeons. Cotton, along with Edward H. Bradford, dean of Harvard Medical School, put the Academy of Medicine into Martin's camp. Cotton, as a member of the board of regents, also supported the universal acceptance of these standards and most likely backed the formation of an independent certifying board (American Board of Surgery) in the early 1930s.

Dr. Cotton was also a regular attendant at numerous medical meetings: the Boston Surgical Society, the Boston Orthopedic Club (president), Boston City Hospital staff meetings, Faulkner Hospital clinical meetings, the Massachusetts Medical Society (Suffolk District), clinical congresses of the American College of Surgeons, and the Boston Society for Medical Improvement. His lectures at these meetings, which he supplemented with his famous anatomical drawings on a blackboard, were original and easy to follow, and outside the lecture hall, he willingly mentored younger doctors.

He was later chosen in 1932 to give the George W. Gay Lecture, which addressed socioeconomic and ethical issues impacting medical care. Founded in 1917, the George W. Gay Lecture is the oldest bioethics lectureship in the United States and the oldest endowed lectureship at Harvard Medical School. George W. Gay (Harvard Medical School class of 1868) donated $1,000 to Harvard Medical School for this purpose. The only other orthopaedic surgeon to receive this honor was Dr. Robert Osgood, who gave the lecture the following year in 1933. Dr. Cotton's lecture, "Medicine, Ethics and Law," covered a variety of issues: professionalism, the role of hospitals, specialty development, medico-legal issues including malpractice and physician's behavior as witnesses at trials, the need for future physician training (residencies), and ethical issues and some advice on the business aspects of medicine, i.e., billing and fee-splitting.

DEDICATION TO THE INJURED WORKER

Dr. Cotton served as a counselor of the Massachusetts Society of Examining Physicians for many years and was one of three members of a special national committee of the American Medical Association to collaborate with the American

Association for Labor Legislation to study problems of health insurance. The exact dates of his service are unclear in the historical record; however, his participation most likely began about the same time as his appointment at HMS.

Cotton had observed the results of a large number of industrial accidents, including the severity of the injury of os calcis fractures that resulted in patients being unable to return to work. The Massachusetts Workingmen's Compensation Law became effective July 1, 1912, despite previous failed attempts. Some of the provisions included:

> that the Industrial Accident Board should have a consulting surgeon upon whom should fall the duty of detail work in preparation of matters to be laid before the advisory committee [another] that insurance companies be requested to provide…specifications of services rendered by physicians…that industrial insurance companies be encouraged to allow all reputable physicians to render services in industrial accidents, provided they are willing to render such services upon a reasonable basis…that fees paid by the companies should not be less than the average minimum fee in the locality in which the service is rendered…that charges up to $50 for major operations are not excessive…that physicians appearing at hearings before the Board shall receive…compensation [and] that specialists, established and recognized by the profession as such, may receive special rates for their work, provided the case requires special skill.
>
> (Donaghue 1916)

Over a five-year period (beginning in 1916), Cotton wrote four articles published in the *Boston Medical and Surgical Journal* about workers' compensation issues: the relationship of workers' insurance to hospitals, the relationship of physicians to workers' insurance and the reasons for lack of adequate results in the management of injured workers. He noted that previously, patients were inadequately treated, resulting in unnecessary morbidity and mortality while hospitals were expected to treat patients without compensation. The new legislation permitted quality control and better results. He wrote:

> We find that our burns hang on for weeks in the out-patient department; that too many crushes and cuts go septic; that at least a third of our femur fractures never recover enough to take up their former work; that most of the os calcis cases are permanent cripples; that serious nerve involvements are common in limb injuries; that fractures of the spine are not rarely overlooked, if the cord is not damaged…Not far back, the hospital was a place for desperate illnesses and courageous surgery. Then if a man got well at all, he asked little as to weeks spent. Now, with the progress toward perfection in medicine and surgery, much that was daring and experimental has become routine [now] it has become…a question why [the patient] is not ready for work eight weeks after…an operation, instead of…six, as we have educated folks to expect…We must not only do well by the patient in the operating room, but we must study him beforehand and see him through afterward, until he is fit to get back on the job, if we care to measure up to our new standard of efficiency. Not a hospital in the country is up to this standard today…In the past the hospitals, great and small, have devoted themselves to the care and cure of the poor devil, without question of status. Now it has become a real financial factor…the insurance companies have, perhaps not unnaturally, [supported] the argument…that the hospital always did this work without pay; why not continue?…new standards are being demanded by the hospitals and their doctors, as well as by the public; that better work means better equipment, and the insurance company, which profits, should pay… We believe the insurance companies will save money by paying for more and longer care…the

amendment to the Act I [Dr. Cotton] had the honor to prepare two years ago [provides that] care continued beyond the two-week limit [is paid by] insurance companies...in many instances. (Cotton 1916)

In a second paper, Cotton summarized his thoughts about workers' accident and sickness insurance in 1916. He noted that proposed insurance regulations were passed without consulting with the medical community and that they would result in untenable financial consequences for medical professionals. He objected to authorization procedures that gave final authority to laypersons. He also noted, on the other hand:

> that some few practitioners fail in professional competency...another problem that has loomed large is the relation of hospitals to care furnished under any compensation law... some hospitals are...private...some private with provision for charity patients also. In some of these the doctor is paid in full; in some he is paid on private cases, not on ward cases...and in some instances, the older charity hospitals, the staff are not paid for any of their work at all. This variation in conditions has led to endless squabbles, and the answer is not in sight. Trustees...and...professional staff have been unable to see why arrangements conceived for the...unfortunate should be used to reduce expense accounts of commercial corporations. (Cotton 1916)

Dr. Cotton then reviewed the proposed Doten Bill and outlined the medical provisions in the third edition of the bill of the American Association for Labor Legislation (May 1916). Cotton concluded:

> Adjudication of [medical] matters by a lay board has proven unsatisfactory in the past, as one might expect. Medical matters should be in medical hands, and there should be an expert medical judgment, above that of the district supervising doctor, obviously. To sum up, I think we must accept this legislation as bound to come, sooner or later; quite likely sooner. (Cotton 1916)

In his third article Cotton stated "the war has taught us [a few things] that should help forward our civil practice...the value of organized team work which...can give...tangible results...In peace we have lost it. Worse of all, I know of no civil hospital that has clearly seized the idea or even attempted the practical solution. Nor does it seem to me likely that any general community hospital is going to do it" (Cotton 1921). He noted that quality of care was often compromised due to several barriers, including poor diagnostic protocols especially with fractures; bad surgical technique, which resulted in nerve and tendon damage; inadequate efforts to avoid infection, which resulted in sepsis; insufficient follow-up care; patient nonadherence to clinician's instructions:

> lack of after-care, or routine after-care only; lack of cooperation of the patient; lack of review of cases that are "hanging along"; lack of knowledge of what can be done-late-by proper reconstructive surgery; lack of opportunity to get such work done; lack of means of bridging over the interval between technical care and the power to do real work; lack of refitting of the handicapped to the old or to a new job...The least good average of results, I am afraid, comes from the hospitals, particularly the bigger ones, organized essentially for acute surgery, practicing more particularly abdominal surgery, large enough so that much work falls to overworked and inexperienced juniors, so large that after-care is in too many hands with no one continuously in charge of the case. (Cotton 1921)

Cotton found disparities in quality of care based on physician experts, the size or funding source of the hospitals, general hospitals or hospitals that specialize, and on patient adherence. He recommended:

> 1. Systematic review of all cases on compensation over a few weeks…
>
> 2. An arrangement by which serious cases needing expert care can be referred easily… What is needed is an institution to do this, big enough to have the services of the best experts in surgery and medicine in various branches, to have a team of skilled physiotherapy aides…adequate physical equipment, a proper record system [Dr. Cotton's proposed] a corporation called the Reconstructive Association [which] now stands ready to take cases calling for expert treatment along reconstruction lines at, practically, cost rates and give them the best treatment that can be offered…the plan is for development along lines of the army reconstruction team work… If this works out there should cease to be any excuse for many of the results (or lack of results) that some of us have seen so often in the past. (Cotton 1921)

Throughout the rest of his active career, Cotton remained dedicated to the injured worker and to the improvement of the health care system inefficiencies in their care. In 1922, he served as chairman of the Medical Advisory Committee, Industrial Accident Board. He had also served as chairman of a committee of the Suffolk District of the Massachusetts Medical Society to study the utilization of partially disabled workers in industry. As such, he made a public plea to all physicians to provide data on their patients to his committee. In a letter to the *New England Journal of Medicine*, Cotton wrote that the lack of financial return and lack of ability to assure proper follow-up care meant that surgeons avoided treating injured and disabled laborers and artisans whose injuries occurred in the course of their duties.

He was appointed by the court to participate in hearings before the state legislature on the subject of the proper care of injured workers and to "head a committee of medical men to act as medical advisers to the Board" (Cotton 1935). He involved the insurance companies. Dr. Cotton argued against the passage of House Bill 340, which would establish a single state fund for worker's compensation and exclude other insurance companies. He also treated these patients himself at the Boston City Hospital and in his private practice, developing new techniques in the process. His objective was to ensure that injured workers could get treatment by orthopaedic specialists as needed. He recorded, "for twenty years and more it has been a matter of education of insurers and employees – and the board – of slow working out of methods of cooperation of the board, the insurers and the doctors, in order to get the results" (Cotton 1935).

WORLD WAR I: MILITARY AND CIVIC CONTRIBUTIONS

In 1917, Cotton enlisted as a major in the United States Army to serve in World War I. By the summer of 1918, he was an assistant to the surgeon general and surgeon-in-chief at Walter Reed Hospital. He was an organizer with Goldthwait and Brackett and surgeon-in-charge (1919–1920) of Parker Hill Hospital (U.S.A. General Hospital No. 10), and "he was active in reconstruction work, both during and after the war" (Lund 1939). Under the Council of National Defense, Cotton was a member of the General Medical Board, and "he served on an advisory committee to the Veterans' Bureau regarding hospitalization policy along with Dr. Joel Goldthwait as chairman and Drs. C. F. Painter, W. J. Mixter and Harvey Cushing and others" (*Boston Medical and Surgical Journal* 1933). He also advised the Veterans' Bureau and the Public Health Service.

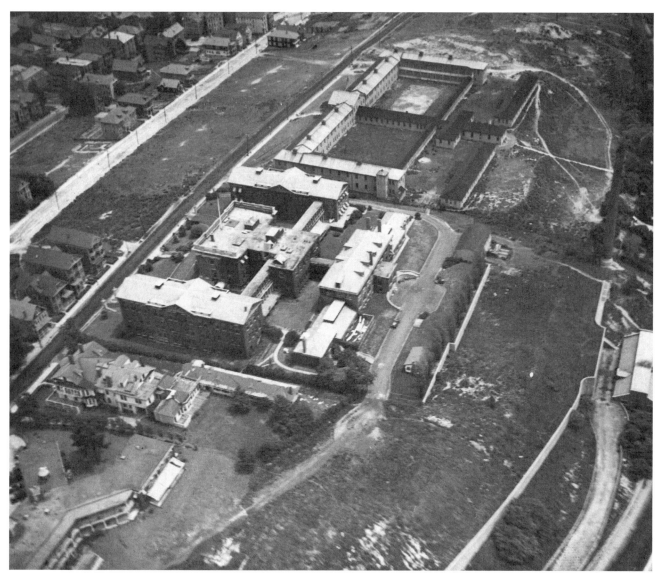

Aerial view of US General Hospital No. 10 (Parker Hill Hospital). Aereo Scenic Airviews Co., Boston, Mass. Boston Pictorial Archive, Boston Public Library/Digital Commonwealth.

ESTABLISHMENT OF THE BONE AND JOINT SERVICE (VI SURGICAL SERVICE)

On April 6, 1928, at Boston City Hospital, Cotton established the Bone and Joint Service (VI Surgical Service), which consisted of himself, a visiting surgeon, and two surgical assistants. It opened its doors five months later in September in the new surgical building. At the time, staff included Dr. Frederic Cotton, chief; Dr. Otto J. Hermann, visiting surgeon; Dr. Joseph H. Shortell, assistant visiting surgeon; and Dr. Joseph H. Burnett, junior visiting surgeon. Cotton then instituted a teaching program on the Bone and Joint Service for students at Boston University, Harvard, and Tufts and directed his staff to teach. The medical students from Boston University were under the direction of Dr. Joseph Burnett, those from Harvard were under the direction of Dr. James A. Sever, and those from Tufts were under the direction of Dr. Mark Rogers.

LEGACY

In 1931, Boston City Hospital required that Dr. Frederic J. Cotton retire because of their age restrictions, and he "resigned his position as Senior Surgeon-in-chief of the Boston City Hospital, as of July 1." ("Dr. Frederic J. Cotton Resigns" 1931) He then served as president of the hospital staff and continued as "assistant professor of surgery at Tufts" ("Recent Deaths. Cotton" 1938) and an instructor in industrial surgery at Harvard Medical School.

Dr. Cotton published more than 140 papers during his 40 years of practice; 22 papers in a single year in 1934. They covered a wide variety of topics in trauma. In addition, he gave an enormous number of local and regional lectures, presentations and discussions at Boston City Hospital and Faulkner Hospital, the Boston Orthopedic Club, the New England Roentgen Ray Society, the Springfield Academy of Medicine, the New Hampshire Medical Society, the New England Surgical Society, the American Academy of Physical Therapy, the Berkshire District Medical Society, the New England Physical Therapy Society, the Academy of Physical Medicine, the Obstetrical Society of Boston, the New England Branch of the American Urological Association, and others. His name is also on several other procedures, including:

- Cotton osteotomy: correction of flat feet by means of a medial cuneiform wedge osteotomy. The objective for the surgeon is for the patient's weight to be equally distributed between the heel and the first and fifth metatarsal heads by plantarflexing the medial column "as dictated by Cotton's concept of the foot as a tripod" (Filiatrault 2012)
- Cotton advancement operation: an advancement of the calcaneo-scaphoid ligament used rarely in flat feet
- Burrell-Cotton operation: an anterior capsule reefing with advancement of the subscapularis used to treat recurrent anterior dislocations of the shoulder

He was a member of numerous organizations throughout his career. In 1901, he was chairman of committee, Boston Medical Library. He "was also a senior member of the American Surgical Association and of the American Orthopedic Association." (WRM 1938) "He was an honorary member of the American Academy of Orthopaedic Surgeons" ("Recent Deaths. Cotton" 1938) and a member of the American Medical Association. Active his entire career in the Suffolk County District Medical Society of the Massachusetts Medical Society, he was a council member for over 12 years, served as secretary and chairman of the surgical section, chairman of the committee to study methods of re-education of disabled individuals, and served on the Committee on Public Education. In 1926, he was elected 1st Vice President of the Massachusetts General Hospital House Pupils' Alumni Association. As an active member of the Boston Chamber of Commerce, Dr. Cotton supported House Bill 1209, presented by Dr. Painter in 1924, which was a bill that would eliminate "two provisions in the present law: First, that no member of the Board of Registration in Medicine may be a member of the faculty of a medical school, and second, that no medical society shall be represented on the Board by more than three members" ("Legislative Matters. House Bill 1209" 1924).

Cotton was a well-rounded man. He was an avid fisherman, especially of trout and salmon. He was also a talented sculptor and artist, rendering excellent etchings, oil paintings, and watercolors. He brought his organizational skills to bear as charter member and president of the Physicians' Art Society of Boston. In that capacity, he organized their annual exhibits. He also helped inspire the establishment of the Massachusetts Medical Society's "hobby exhibit."

Physicians in New England began exhibiting their art in 1927, eventually forming the

Physicians' Art Society of Boston six or seven years later. Cotton was interviewed by the *Boston Globe* about the inherent artistic abilities of doctors, especially surgeons. He likened artists and surgeons to mechanics. To Cotton, the transition from medicine to art was natural because, perforce, surgical concepts had to be illustrated and photography was a new industry. Thus, surgeons had to learn to draw. Cotton remembered, "As a student at Harvard, I had a very rigorous course of training in drawing under Professor Moore. So did Mosher. When a man draws after a course like that, he knows how. Today I hardly think that I rank as an artist, but I know I'm a good draftsman…When it comes to rating artistic doctors on their art alone, I don't believe any doctor has achieved real artistic rank until he turned professional…" (Humphrey 1930). Cotton stated that as doctors reached the age of 40, they discovered that they needed a diversion. But they tended not to do abstract or modernist work, since they were influenced by the realism of their occupational lives. On the other hand, Cotton did experiment with modernism in some of his works; he noted that "*My Farm* and *Voodoo Women* are experiments in these fields" (Humphrey 1930).

A special exhibition of the Physician's Art Society of Boston's collection of paintings and sculptures was shown at the Boston Medical Library in 1934. Of the 29 artists, eight were fellows of the American College of Surgeons. Dr. Sidney C. Wiggin showed a life-size bust of Dr. Frederic Cotton that he created at that exhibition, which was praised by critics: "The portrait of 'Dr. Frederick [*sic*] J. Cotton' is fine in character and painted in a big, free way" (Philpott 1936). This was not Dr. Cotton's last gallery exhibition; he had produced a large number of original art pieces for the first exhibit of Boston physicians which was organized:

> along the lines of the New York Society… [including] 11 sculptures, 1 oil painting, 3 watercolors and 6 pen-and-ink-drawings [on] October 15 to 20, 1934, at the Boston Medical Library, as part of the American College of Surgeons Convention. [After his death a] memorial exhibit in honor of Dr. Cotton was held at the Massachusetts Medical Society Annual Meeting in 1939, at the Hotel Bradford, at which time a bust of Dr. Cotton was shown, surrounded by Dr. Cotton's many contributions of art to the Society. (Wiggin 1952)

In addition to his active involvement in many professional organizations and his major interest in art, "he also belonged to the St. Botolph Club, the Country Club, Harvard Club and R.C.R.C" ("Dr. F. J. Cotton, Surgeon, Is Dead" 1938).

On April 14, 1938, Dr. Frederic Cotton had a heart attack at his home at 239 Beacon Street. He had intended to give a lecture that day at Boston City Hospital, where he had made the hospital a premier facility for the treatment of heel fractures. His associate, Dr. Gordon M. Morrison, was summoned, but by the time he arrived, Dr. Cotton was already dead at the age of 68. He had been in failing health for three months, and, two months prior, had spent a month in the South in an attempt to recuperate. He was survived by his wife (Jane Baldwin), whom he had married in 1901, a daughter (Jean), and two grandchildren.

Dr. Cotton's funeral was held at Emmanuel Church at Newberry Street, and all staff from both Faulkner Hospital and the VI Surgical Service at Boston City Hospital were in attendance. The pallbearers were among the most prominent doctors in New England. His obituary in the *New England Journal of Medicine* read:

> Dr. Cotton endeared himself to his countless patients and associates because of his unfailing good nature and his kindly advice and generous help to those in trouble. He was always willing to lend a helping hand and to give invaluable advice to the younger generation. Of powerful build, impressive appearance and commanding personality, Dr. Cotton combined many rare

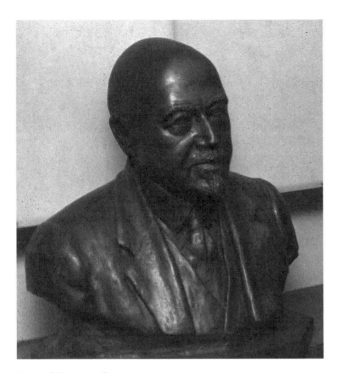

Bust of Frederic Cotton. Digital Collections and Archives, Tufts University.

qualities which resulted in making him a skillful and successful surgeon of national reputation. (WRM 1938)

His many achievements live on in the collective memory of those he influenced. Lund (1939) wrote:

> In the death of Dr. Frederic J. Cotton, the surgical profession of America lost a member of great and varied talents, industry, and ability who had greatly impressed his personality upon the surgical world, and had taken his place among the leaders of our profession…He was an enthusiastic sportsman and made regular trips to Canadian waters in successful search for trout and salmon…He had a long, active and varied career, and filled an important place in many departments of our profession. He was active in this work up to the very day of his death at his home…and so was spared a lingering illness and inactivity. He will be missed by many friends, and his loss will be felt by the entire profession.

CHAPTER 60

The Bone and Joint Service at Boston City Hospital

Other Surgeons-in-Chief

Boston City Hospital (BCH) began to treat patients for fractures or dislocations almost as soon as it officially opened its doors in the summer of 1864. However, it wasn't until 64 years later that the VI Surgical Service (also known as the Bone and Joint Service or the Sixth Surgical Service) was established in 1928. Dr. Frederic J. Cotton (see chapter 59) was named its first chief. He was assisted by Drs. Otto J. Hermann and Joseph H. Shortell.

The orthopaedic surgeons described in this chapter include those dedicated individuals who served as chief of the VI Surgical Service between 1932 and 1963. After 1963, as BCH searched for a new permanent chief of orthopaedics, various interim chiefs led the department: Dr. Arthur Thibodeau (from Tufts University), Dr. Robert Ulin (from Beth Israel Hospital), and Dr. Paul O'Brien (from Carney Hospital). The other surgeons-in-chief covered in this chapter include:

Otto J. Hermann	333
Joseph H. Shortell	338
Russell F. Sullivan	343
Gordon M. Morrison	346
Alexander P. Aitken	350

OTTO J. HERMANN

Physician Snapshot

Otto J. Hermann
BORN: 1884
DIED: 1973
SIGNIFICANT CONTRIBUTIONS: Chief of the Bone and Joint Service at Boston City Hospital 1932–1946 (during World War II); recipient of the General Leonard Wood Gold Medal for outstanding service

Otto John Hermann graduated from Harvard College in 1906 and Harvard Medical School in 1909. After an internship that he completed in 1910 at Boston City Hospital, he visited different clinics in Europe and toured in Germany. Dr. Hermann then travelled throughout the United States for six months before establishing a private practice on January 1, 1912, and joining the surgical staff of Boston City Hospital, where he practiced until he retired, specializing in the treatment of bone and joint injuries. At the time he entered practice, surgeons often had to set up their operating stations in addition to performing the actual surgery because:

> many patients insisted on being treated at home, [and] operating rooms were improvised by stripping bare all household furnishings and

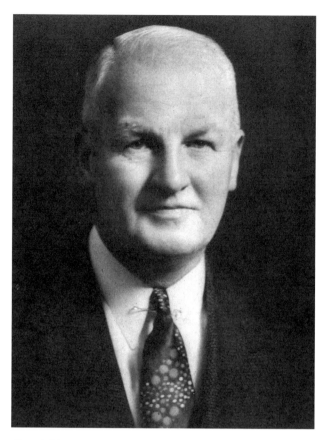

Otto J. Hermannn. Digital Collections and Archives, Tufts University.

using the kitchen table for surgery. The surgeon, accompanied by his assistant and his nurse, brought all sterile gauze, gloves, gowns and instruments. The anesthetist poured ether from a homemade cone, and the floor was protected by out-spread newspapers. All this was routine, not only for appendectomies, which were then much-dreaded operations, but for all the more challenging procedures then coming into vogue. ("Otto J. Hermann, MD, 1884–1973" 1973)

Dr. Frederic Cotton was his mentor (see chapter 59), and he appears to have introduced Dr. Hermann to organized medicine. In 1917, a committee was organized to study methods and results of reeducation of disabled individuals (World War I veterans) in the Suffolk District Medical Society. Dr. Cotton was chairman, and Dr. Hermann served on the committee along with Dr. Robert Soutter and others. Hermann was an active member of the Massachusetts Medical Society (50 years), the American Medical Association, and the American College of Surgeons.

The exact date of Dr. Hermann's faculty appointment at Harvard Medical School is unknown, but he was listed as an instructor in surgery by 1922. Two years later, Hermann moved his office from Roxbury to 520 Commonwealth Avenue in Brookline. After the VI Surgical Service (the Bone and Joint Service) at Boston City Hospital was established in 1928, Dr. Hermann and Dr. Joseph H. Shortell were named assistants on the service with Dr. Cotton as chief. Hermann had obviously expanded his clinical interest to focus on fracture treatment.

Around this time, he began to give presentations at local and regional professional society meetings and later at national meetings. Some examples included: a presentation on gangrene of the leg in a 15-month-old child at the Suffolk District Medical Society meeting held in the Cheever amphitheater at Boston City Hospital in 1927; physiotherapy and apparatus in the convalescence of os calcis fractures at a meeting of the Boston Orthopedic Club at Boston City Hospital in 1929; compound fractures at a meeting of the Massachusetts Medical Society at Boston City Hospital in 1932; frequent meetings of the clinical staff at Boston City Hospital (physiotherapy in fractures in 1932); and septic hip disease at the 1933 meeting of the New England Pediatric Society, held at Boston City Hospital.

The previous year (1932), Dr. Hermann was appointed chief of the Bone and Joint Service at Boston City Hospital, succeeding his mentor Dr. Cotton under whom he had "acquired special skills in fracture treatment" ("Otto J. Hermann, MD, 1884–1973" 1973). Two years later, he represented the Boston City Hospital as a member of the Massachusetts delegation of the New England Regional Committee on Fractures at an annual meeting of the American College of Surgeons in Boston. He also continued in a faculty role at Harvard Medical School for many years; later becoming associate in surgery while holding appointments at Tufts College Medical School. With the many political changes, including medical school affiliations, and his eventual clinical focus on fracture care, Hermann was appointed associate professor of orthopaedic and fracture surgery at Boston University Medical School in 1934 and later clinical professor of surgery at Tufts College Medical School in 1936. He was known as "a large robust, rough and ready individual, [who] presented a commanding experience. He was a fine teacher and highly competent surgeon. His influence on generations of students and residents was profound" (Banks 1999). He continued to give presentations as well, and that same year he conducted a clinic on the treatment of fractures at the Central Maine General Hospital in Lewiston, Maine.

Dr. Hermann was not a prolific writer, producing only seven publications, the majority while he was chief of the Bone and Joint Service. Two of his publications were on his special interest, os calcis fractures. The first was published in 1930 (see **Case 60.1**). In 1937, he published the results of 30 years of what he called the conservative treatment of os calcis fractures at Boston City Hospital. Of the cases reviewed by Hermann and Dr. Harold M. Childress, 152 were presented at a meeting of the fracture committee of the American College of Surgeons and published by Hermann in the *Journal of Bone and Joint Surgery*:

> The patients in the "good" class [73%] are those who, by the sixth or seventh month, had regained full functional use of the injured heel and had no pain...The "fair" division [14%] includes those patients who required seven to eighteen months to return to normalcy...the "poor" group [13%] includes those who, during the first three to four weeks of weight-bearing, had persistent pain...whom we generally did a subastragalar arthrodesis...The real advance which we have made in our conservative

> COMPOUND FRACTURE THERAPY AT THE
> BOSTON CITY HOSPITAL
>
> OTTO J. HERMANN, M.D.
> BOSTON

Title of Hermann's article in which he reviewed BCH's five-year experience treating open fractures. *Archives of Surgery* 1940; 40: 853.

> treatment of fracture of the os calcis is in the after-care. (Hermann 1937)

Seven years later, in his paper, "How to Improve the Treatment of Fractures," Dr. Charles L. Scudder wrote: "The period of aftercare or convalescence is a time of great importance. This should be regarded as a time of active treatment. One reason for Dr. Otto Hermann's successful treatment of fractures of the os calcis at the Boston City Hospital is dependent in great measure on his supervision of the minute details of the aftercare of these cases" (Scudder 1944).

Hermann performed his duties as chief "at great personal sacrifice through the strenuous years of World War II," at a time when the still relatively new service was exceptionally busy, including with large numbers of patients admitted for fracture care. During that period, it:

> included over 120 beds, at a time when almost all police-ambulance cases were brought here [Boston City Hospital] for treatment... Hermann was one of the last of the devotedly unselfish generation of doctors whose resources were derived solely from their own private practice, but who gave a major portion of their time to the wholly unpaid tasks of administering services, and personally supervising residency training programs. So successful was this work that Hermann's clinic became a major source of student teaching in the three Boston medical schools. ("Otto J. Hermann, MD, 1884–1973" 1973)

Case 60.1. Treatment of Os Calcis Fractures

"The fracture of this bone occurs most frequently in adult men whose occupation renders them liable to falls from a height of five to forty feet...and who land on the ground or other hard surfaces on their feet...a result of a direct crushing force...The results from the usual methods of treatment had been bad...ranged from permanent partial disability to absolute disability...In 1908, Dr. Frederic J. Cotton and the late Dr. Louis Wilson, both of Boston City Hospital...after five years of work adopted the following routine:

"'Ether anesthesia. Breaking up of impaction (with hands or with spindle inserted beneath the heel cord)...forced pro and supination of the foot. Re-impaction with sandbag and mallet or by manual pressure. In the after-care, a plaster of Paris cast equipped with two felt pads, one over the tendo-achilles, one over the dorsum of the foot, were used...The foot was put up at fifteen to twenty degrees plantar flexion [with] downward traction...with the hands on the dorsum of the foot, and behind, at either side of the tendo achilles...some eversion secured.

"At the end of ten days the cast was removed and massage and guarded active motion was begun. No weight bearing was allowed for a month...return of function was slow.'... It is only within recent years that several important changes have been made...in 1920...I was at work...pounding and molding one of these cases and then instead of pulling down on the heel by means of a sound inserted beneath the tendo achilles (as per F. J. Cotton) I used the regular tongs (...Edmonton Type) for traction. At this point Dr. Cotton strolled in and I...suggested leaving...the tongs...to maintain traction...[with] a Thomas splint...Tong traction was left on for two weeks and then...the regular plaster casts were applied...The use of the tongs traction was continued but only on the operating table [because of a case of skin slough].... The Thomas splint was also discarded...So by gradual steps the standardized method...evolved. I have used this method in...forty cases...the method itself:

1. Patient is turned on side opposite injury and sandbag placed under inner side of heel.
2. The tightly rolled towel is placed beneath the external malleolus and then with solid heavy blows the impaction is broken up and the piled up bone below the external malleolus is pounded down until the thumb can be easily placed in this region.
3. The heel is quickly molded....
4. With scalpel small incisions are made about 1" inch ... above the apex of the heel, the Iris tongs are driven in, locked and then lusty downward traction is made... and gives us a good arch.
5. The heel is again moulded by the fingers...If necessary, I occasionally use the mallet again.
6. Tightly folded sterile dressings are placed over the two stab wounds. ...
7. A snug roll of thick felt...is place horizontally beneath each malleolus.
8. A low plaster of Paris case is then applied with foot... inverted and in plantar flexion...
9. This cast is removed in ten days and a new one is applied...with foot at right angle.
10. A new cast is applied every ten days...up to about eight weeks. Then we apply specially contrived pads on a steel frame...pressure pads controlled by small turn buckles...followed in two weeks by a shoe that has these bars inserted in the heel with the turn buckles attached to them.
11. Massage and motion are instituted from about the eighth week.
12. Weight bearing and exercise are begun at the end of the twelfth week.

"From the third to the fifth months, the patient needs well supervised physiotherapy (baking, massage and exercise) and...cautioned against the overuse of the foot... In conclusion...I would state that the conservative construction pounding, extension, moulding method...can be used safely in all cases...In 20-25%...this method alone would not suffice; it would have to have some type of sub-astragaloid arthrodesis (preferably, that devised by Dr. Philip Wilson of the Massachusetts General Hospital) used with it...In the other 75% to 80%...[t]he method is simple and constructive...It does require meticulous care in the convalescence."

(Otto J. Hermann 1930)

Dr. Hermann had reviewed the hospital's experience with compound fractures from 1924 to 1934 and then again from 1934 to 1939. By 1940, he published the data from 1934 to 1939. During that period, the bone and joint service treated 4,491 fracture cases out of the 12,230 patients admitted to the hospital. Of the 4,491 patients admitted to the bone and joint service, 398 patients had compound fractures.

In his summary, he stated that proper treatment begins with the first responders, who should apply splints and transport patients so as to prevent further injury. Patients should receive tetanus vaccine, anti-gas-gangrene injections, and appropriate wound care so as to prevent infection. He supported both open and closed treatment depending on the type of injury and appropriate external fixation. In cases of severe infection, surgeons should evaluate the risks and benefits of early amputation given the risks of amputation while the patient is septic. He especially recommended aggressive treatment in the event that the patient develops tetanus or gas gangrene, or severe staphylococcal or streptococcal infections. The surgeon should also evaluate the necessity of bone grafting to prevent nonunion.

During the annual meeting of the American Academy of Orthopaedic Surgeons held in Boston in 1940, Dr. Hermann participated in a morning program that included Drs. Albert Brewster, Joseph Shortell, Frank Ober, and Marius Smith-Petersen, and an afternoon program of operative and dry clinics at Boston City Hospital. Other Boston hospitals that participated in the afternoon program were the Massachusetts General Hospital, Boston Children's Hospital, the Robert Breck Brigham Hospital, Carney Hospital, and the Massachusetts Memorial Hospital. In 1944, he presented a paper on fractures of the shoulder joint at the academy's annual meeting in Chicago. Dr. Smith-Petersen was president for this twelfth annual meeting of the American Academy of Orthopaedic Surgeons. Dr. Hermann presided at the Boston Orthopedic Club meeting in 1942.

Dr. Hermann held his position as chief of the Bone and Joint Service until 1946. After retirement, he remained on the courtesy staff, and in 1954 was honored by the Boston City Hospital Alumni Association with the General Leonard Wood Gold Medal for outstanding service. Major General Wood, a Medal of Honor recipient, was a graduate of Harvard Medical School and interned at Boston City Hospital in 1884.

Dr. Otto Hermann died on October 20, 1973, at the age of 89. He was survived by his widow, a daughter, four sons, six grandchildren, and one great-grandchild. He was remembered for his:

> modest nature, [and] his good works merited greater praise than he ever sought, but all his life he was beloved because of his genuine sincerity, his devoted industry, his excellent judgment, and his unfailing pleasant manners. Above all, he deserved the simple tribute that Chaucer paid the Knight in the *The Canterbury Tales*: "And ever honored for his Worthinesse." Worthiness in character was indeed one of Otto Hermann's outstanding traits. ("Otto J. Hermann, MD, 1884–1973" 1973)

JOSEPH H. SHORTELL

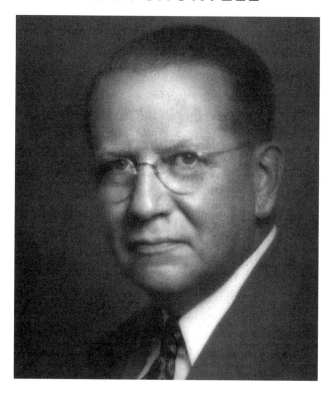

Joseph H. Shortell. Digital Collections and Archives, Tufts University.

> **Physician Snapshot**
>
> Joseph H. Shortell
> BORN: 1891
> DIED: 1951
> SIGNIFICANT CONTRIBUTIONS: Chief of the Bone and Joint Service at Boston City Hospital 1946–1950; president of the Massachusetts Society of Examining Physicians; Boston City Hospital named their newly created outpatient unit in 1952 for the treatment of fractures in his honor (the Shortell Unit)

Joseph Henry Shortell graduated from Tufts in 1911 and Harvard Medical School in 1916. He completed internships at Boston Children's Hospital and Boston City Hospital. During this period and most likely while he was an intern, he published his first paper from the surgical services of Boston City Hospital in 1917. It was a review of cases of infections of soft tissues and bones treated with bovine serum. He concluded: "Serum will control a septic process…is harmless to normal tissue…as a prophylactic agent in fresh wounds it is of value [and is] a most marked stimulant of granulations…it gives rise to no anaphylactic response" (Shortell et al. 1917).

Following his internships, he entered the American Expeditionary Forces as a medical officer (lieutenant) in 1918. Before serving in Europe with the Harvard Unit under Dr. Harvey Cushing, he received his training at Fort Oglethorpe evacuation hospital in Georgia. During both World War I and World War II, Fort Oglethorpe served as an induction and training center. It was the post for the 6th Cavalry, and, during World War I, it housed 4,000 German prisoners of war and civilian detainees.

After the war Dr. Shortell became a junior assistant surgeon at Boston Children's Hospital. He worked with others in the same category: A. H. Brewster, W. F. Cotting, and Seth M. Fitchet; along with assistant surgeons A. T. Legg, J. W. Sever, H. J. Fitzsimmons, and F. R. Ober; and associate surgeon Robert Soutter. He also was appointed to the staff at Boston City Hospital where he worked for his entire career. It was at Boston City Hospital that he began to work with Dr. Cotton and to specialize in bone and joint injuries along with Dr. Hermann.

Shortell's academic appointment at Harvard Medical School in 1924 was assistant in orthopaedic surgery, courses for graduates. His offices were located at different times on Commonwealth Avenue in the Back-Bay area, close to his home of 55 years (1937–1992) on Commonwealth Avenue near Kenmore Square. (In 1994, the MIT chapter of Alpha Chi Omega purchased his house, in which 25 members of the sorority live each semester.)

Dr. Shortell joined Dr. Cotton in his interest in fracture care and industrial accidents. In 1925, Dr. William O'Neill Sherman, who was the chief surgeon to the Carnegie Steel Corporation in Pittsburgh, spoke at the meeting of the Suffolk District Medical Society in Boston. Both Shortell and Cotton attended and commented at the end of Sherman's lecture, which was entitled "The Industrial Surgical Problem" (**Box 60.1**) Sherman

Box 60.1. "The Industrial Surgical Problem": Lecture and Discussion

At the Suffolk District Medical Society meeting, Sherman presented a brief history of trauma, especially fracture management in the United States during the rise of the industrial complex in the early 1920s. He stressed the lack of physicians' interest in fractures and the need for specialty trauma hospitals. In the discussion of Sherman's lecture, Shortell raised an important observation: graduating physicians and surgeons completing their residencies have had little or no teaching about fractures. Cotton further commented that, in New England, there are no trauma specialty hospitals because patients with fractures are commonly referred to private practitioners, who may not have experience or interest in fracture management.

In his lecture, Dr. William O'Neill Sherman stated:

"The great industrial development of the past decade, with its great technical discoveries, inventions and developments…has brought about many problems…approximately 66% of wage earners were engaged in occupations which are…hazardous. The greater value placed upon human life, the enactment of progressive humanitarian legislation, such as the Workmen's Compensation Law, has necessitated the organization of medical and surgical personnel in industry… Certain of the State Compensation Boards report that more than 50% of the applicants…must be referred for further medical or surgical reconstruction; that 17%…give a history of infection…this unsatisfactory condition in certain centers has resulted in the organization of industrial reconstruction hospitals. One would assume…that there was something… lacking in our general hospitals and personnel…Most general hospitals and surgeons take little or no interest in traumatic surgery. These cases are usually delegated to the house surgeon or junior assistant. The staff surgeon has been chiefly interested in surgery of the stomach, appendix, gall bladder and thyroid and anything in the nature of a fracture or trauma seems to be unworthy of his attention. Either the general surgeon should revive his interest in these cases or should permit others who are interested in them to treat them. The ideal plan of hospital organization is to establish wards for the traumatic and fracture cases in which a team of the general surgeon, orthopedic surgeon, physiotherapeutist or roentgenologist cooperate in the treatment of these patients. Such a plan was first organized at the Massachusetts General Hospital and is operated with great credit to that institution. Other hospitals would do well to organize along a similar plan…The recent World War gave ample evidence of our surgical unpreparedness…

"The fracture problem is not confined to industry alone, but is one for the general profession as well. There evidently is something radically wrong when 66% of the malpractice suits of the country are based upon the unsatisfactory and functional results following fractures…No open reduction for fracture should be attempted…unless the surgeon has had special training and experience, and has associated with him a trained corps of assistants…Formerly it was the practice of many surgeons to attribute their operative failures and infections to the use of catgut, or to the inferred faulty technique on the part of the operating nurse. The operator rarely considered himself as a factor, or that his own errors of technique might be the cause of the operative failure. So it is with operative fractures. It is the operator who causes the infections, chiefly through inexperience and faulty technique and improper armamentarium…Heretofore, the general practitioner and the general surgeon have not been greatly concerned in the end functional results…The real test as to function should be – 'Is the patient able to assume his former occupation and does he have sufficient function to perform his work free from pain and distress? …Maximum function can be obtained only by the elimination of infection and the correction of vicious malposition of fractures; by proper reduction and splinting…by the closed method; or…by the proper operative procedure. The tendency to discontinue treatment in the face of evident failure over many months, and the reluctance…to refer cases to a competent surgeon are frequently the cause of permanent loss of function…It is the duty of hospitals and surgeons to render to the injured, the very best that science has to offer. Hospitals and surgeons should recognize the necessity of providing better facilities for the care of traumas and fractures…the recommendation of the Fracture Committee of the American College of Surgeons, if accepted by hospitals, practitioners and surgeons…will greatly improve the end functional results and…clarify and standardize the methods of treatment…giving to the injured, better results based upon the experience and practice of…surgeons who have had extensive clinical experience in this particular field" (Sherman 1926).

Discussion

In the discussion after Dr. Sherman's presentation, Dr. Joseph Shortell stated:

"In my belief too little time is spent on this subject in the medical schools in Boston, and it is left to the student to pick up as much information as he can after his graduation...As a result...when he becomes a house officer, he is not particularly interested in cases of traumatic surgery and gives the greater part of his attention to the major abdominal cases. He is much more interested in having an appendix or hernia to do by himself than he is in treating a fractured femur or a Colles' fracture. Many of the medical students after graduation take either a medical house officership or a short mixed house officership. These men go into practice in some of the smaller cities with a very limited knowledge of traumatic surgery. They are, however, called upon to practice and are handicapped on account of that lack of training. If fractures were always treated as surgical emergencies and were reduced the same day the fracture occurred...there would be much less need of open operation. In the past there has been considerable criticism about applying circular plaster the same day the fracture occurred on account of the danger of swelling and interference with the circulation. In my experience, it has not occurred...In most cases it is not even necessary to bi-valve the plaster cast [but] extreme watchfulness should be exercised" (Shortell 1926).

Dr. Frederic Cotton followed with these remarks:

"It is a great privilege to...listen to this talk by Dr. Sherman. My first reaction was one of envy. He has solved his problem admirably but his problem is one entirely different from that which confronts us in this community...we cannot duplicate his organization and control. In this region we are dealing with scattered units and diversified control. Our cases go through the hands of private practitioners, often handicapped in...matter of convenience and technical system, not always equipped to handle the more technical cases...or else through the hospitals where the lack of continued responsibility and only too often a certain lack of interest are handicaps...these conditions have led...to the establishments of insurance clinics...not solving the problem. It is not clear how our problem here is to be solved. In the meantime, we are struggling along handicapped and less fortunate than the speaker...We are, perhaps, inclined here to do a little less operative work, and stress mechanical appliances...Dr. Sherman's handling of compound fractures...is right and the method is worthy of use, when, and only when, one can carry it out with efficient Dakinzation [to prevent infections] as he does" (Cotton 1926).

Dr. Charles L. Scudder from the fracture service at the Massachusetts General Hospital also commented:

"I will limit myself to two [points]. First: Dr. Sherman has called attention to his organized surgical unit in the Carnegie Steel Company's plant and his handling of fractures... His organization, team-work, technical operative details and results are ideal...Second: I believe that the complex situation – call it, if you please, the industrial surgical situation existing today in New England in which the following interests are involved...the laborer, the employer...the hospitals of the community, general practitioners...surgeons, the insurance companies, the accident boards or commissions...I believe that the industrial surgical situation can best be solved by the establishment of an industrial surgical center or clearing house where all interested and concerned may have the correct things done [and] could serve as an educational center of great value to the medical school. The necessity of such a center being associated...with an established hospital...with all specialists is apparent."

(Scudder 1926)

reported the use of vanadium steel for bone plates. The advantage was that they were more durable than the alternatives but were flexible enough to bend without breaking. These vanadium steel plates were fastened with vanadium steel screws, which were manufactured to fit the holes in the plates and were four times stronger than wood screws. The Fracture Committee of the American College of Surgeons had recommended the use of this device more than a decade earlier in 1914.

Shortell was active in professional organizations during his career at Boston City Hospital. For several years, he served as president of the Massachusetts Society of Examining Physicians. He was also active in the Massachusetts Medical Society and served as the secretary for the Section of Surgery and as chairman of the Committee on Rehabilitation. As a member of the Massachusetts Medical Society, he often made presentations on trauma. Active in the Boston Orthopedic Club, he also presented a paper on the fractured spine and in 1933 presented two cases of knee trauma. Occasionally, he would present a paper at the Boston City Hospital Alumni Association Meeting as well. As a fellow of the American College of Surgeons, he represented Boston on the New England Regional Committee on Fractures, along with Drs. Frederic J. Cotton, Otto J. Hermann, Mark H. Rogers, James W. Sever, Augustus Thorndike Jr., and others.

Shortell published only three papers. The first while he was probably still an intern. His next publication wasn't until 20 years later in 1937. He published a paper on accident insurance, concluding:

> The Workmen's Compensation Act in Massachusetts [July 1, 1912] appears adequate. It has been carried out by competent men, with the interest of the injured man always at heart. The matter of fees should be straightened out by the board, the Massachusetts Medical Society and the insurance companies. As regards fads in operations, I should like to give a warning against radicalism, and to express the hope that the members of society will follow conservative treatment for those injured patients. (Shortell 1937)

Nine years later, he succeeded Dr. Hermann as chief of the Bone and Joint Service in 1946. His only orthopaedic publication was coauthored with Drs. Robert Fahey and Richard Kilfoyle in 1949; a review of medical problems in a group of 100 consecutive cases, over the age of 70, with hip fractures treated on the VI Surgical Service (Bone and Joint Service) at Boston City Hospital (see **Case 60.2**). At the time of this publication, Dr. Shortell was listed as instructor in orthopaedic surgery at Harvard Medical School.

Dr. Shortell retired from his position as chief of the Bone and Joint Service in 1950. That same

Case 60.2. Medical Problems in Elderly Patients with Hip Fractures

> "[The patient], an 83-year old woman, entered the hospital on April 12, 1947, with a complaint of pain in the right hip after a fall on the night prior to admission. She also gave a history of long-standing diabetes and hypertension. The diabetes had been treated with diet alone, but she had been taking digitalis intermittently for the past year. Physical examination revealed a well developed woman in no apparent distress. The lungs showed moist rales at both bases. The heart border was enlarged to the anterior axillary line, and there was a rough, Grade III systolic murmur. The blood pressure was 190/100. There was shortening and external rotation of the right leg. The urine showed an orange Benedict reduction, and the sediment was loaded with white blood cells. Examination of the blood disclosed a hemoglobin of 65 per cent and a white-cell count of 8600. The blood sugar was 250 mg., and the nonprotein nitrogen 42 mg. per 100 cc., and the carbon dioxide combining power 49 per cent. X-ray examination showed an intertrochanteric fracture of the right femur. The right leg was placed in Russell traction, and immediate attempts to restore cardiac compensation and regulate the diabetes were instituted. The patient was given penicillin and sulfadiazine to combat the urinary-tract infection. By the 16th hospital day the diabetes was under good control, all evidence of cardiac decompensation had cleared, and the urine sediment was normal. She was then operated upon under spinal anesthesia. Smith-Petersen nail with a Thornton plate was successfully inserted. The postoperative course was smooth, and she was out of bed on the 4th postoperative day and discharged from the hospital on the 58th hospital day on crutches."
>
> (Fahey, Kilfoyle, and Shortell 1949)

THE BOSTON Medical and Surgical JOURNAL
VOLUME 194　　JANUARY 28, 1926　　NUMBER 4

ORIGINAL ARTICLES

THE INDUSTRIAL SURGICAL PROBLEM*

BY WILLIAM O'NEILL SHERMAN, M.D., F.A.C.S.

Title of William O. Sherman's article in which he advocated open reduction and internal stabilization of fractures with vanadium bone plates. *Boston Medical and Surgical Journal* 1926; 194: 139.

year, he treated major-league baseball player Ted Williams, who was also a personal friend, for a fracture in his left elbow. As a result of his expertise in the treatment of athletic injuries, the Boston Bruins retained him earlier as their physician. He had served in this capacity between 1928 and 1936. He had treated Williams 14 years later. On July 11, 1950, during the first inning of the All-Star game in Comisky Park, Williams collided with the wall in left field while catching a line drive from Ralph Kiner and sustained a comminuted fracture of his left radial head.

Dr. Ralph McCarthy, club physician, hoped but could not promise that Williams might play again before the end of the season. But the next morning, at Sancta Maria Hospital in Cambridge, Dr. Shortell found that the chipped bone from the radius impacted another bone in Williams's elbow and removed the fragment. Williams returned to play against the Yankees after only eight weeks, on September 7, 1950, after he completed his rehabilitation program. He pinched hit and walked. On September 15, he played the entire game. At the plate six times, he had three singles and three home runs for the 12–9 win. One home run traveled as far as Grand Avenue.

Dr. Joseph Shortell died on February 3, 1951, at 60 years old. In his honor, Boston City Hospital created a new outpatient unit for the treatment of fractures, the Shortell Unit, which was adjacent to the Emergency Ward. In 1951, shortly after his death, he was honored with his name on the unit. At the alumni meeting that year, the attendees toured the new Joseph H. Shortell Fracture Unit and Dr. Hermann gave a biographical sketch of Dr. Shortell before the tour. The unit officially opened on March 1, 1952.

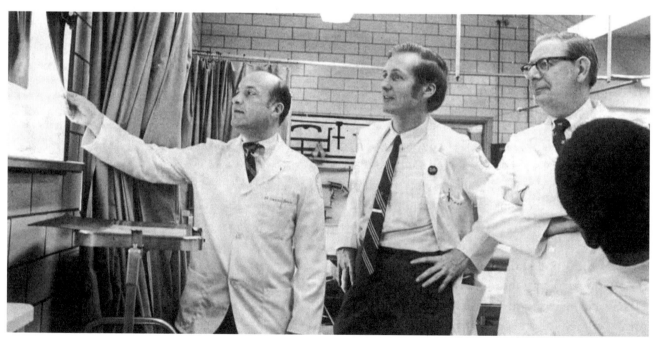

Drs. Henry H. Banks, Robert Leach, and Thomas Quigley (l–r) in the Shortell Unit of Boston City Hospital, 1970. *Scope,* November-December 1970: 15. Boston University Alumni Medical Library Archives.

RUSSELL F. SULLIVAN

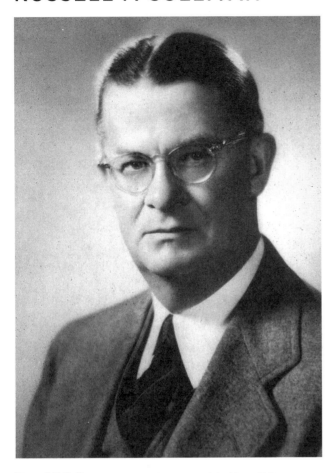

Russell F. Sullivan. Digital Collections and Archives, Tufts University.

Physician Snapshot

Russell F. Sullivan

BORN: 1893

DIED: 1966

SIGNIFICANT CONTRIBUTIONS: First board-certified orthopaedic surgeon to serve as chief of the Bone and Joint Service at Boston City Hospital (1951–1954); partnered with Dr. G. Edmund Haggert to create a combined orthopaedic residency program between the Boston City Hospital and the Lahey Clinic.

Russell F. Sullivan was born in 1893, a native to Melrose, Massachusetts. He graduated from Melrose High School and received his MD degree from Tufts University School of Medicine in 1913. After completing a residency in orthopaedic surgery at New York Orthopedic Hospital under Dr. Russell A. Hibbs, he returned to Massachusetts. He opened offices in Melrose and Malden, was a consultant on the staff at Melrose Hospital, and was appointed assistant surgeon in the orthopaedic department at Carney Hospital as well as junior visiting surgeon at Boston City Hospital. Dr. Sullivan practiced in the VI Surgical Service (the Bone and Joint Unit).

Sullivan published only four papers during his career; his most significant paper was on the treatment of vertebral tuberculosis with spine fusion, which published in the *Boston Medical and Surgical Journal* in 1924 (**Box 60.2**). At the turn of the twentieth century, spinal tuberculosis was a major problem: Sullivan reviewed related statistics at Boston Children's Hospital over an impressive 34-year period: 2,867 cases of spinal tuberculosis. He also reviewed 4,299 cases at the Hospital for the Ruptured and Crippled (HSS).

Until 1911, treatment was nonoperative: bed rest up to three years. In 1912, operative treatment was first reported by Russell Hibbs. In his paper, Sullivan reviewed the two methods of spine fusion: Hibbs & Albee. Sullivan's paper was probably most significant because he had been a resident for three years at the New York Orthopedic Hospital where Hibbs was professor. Sullivan had personally examined Hibbs's patients and analyzed the data for Hibbs' publication in 1918, in which he reviewed Hibbs' first 210 cases of Pott's disease treated by the Hibbs spine fusion method. Sullivan, in his paper, reported one case of Pott's disease he treated with a Hibbs fusion in Boston; he also summarized Hibbs' data from his 1918 publication and then reported a brief summary on a series of another 163 cases from Hibbs that Hibbs was preparing for publication. Sullivan stated that he had Hibbs' permission to use this unpublished data. An example of one of Sullivan's own later case reports (unrelated to vertebral tuberculosis) is provided in **Case 60.3**.

In 1942, Dr. Sullivan succeeded Dr. Mark H. Rogers as Professor of Orthopaedic Surgery at Tufts University School of Medicine. He remained

Box 60.2. Excerpt from Dr. Sullivan's paper "Spine Fusion in the Treatment of Vertebral Tuberculosis" (1924)

"Records from the Children's Hospital of Boston show that of the cases of joint tuberculosis admitted to the wards for treatment from 1869 to 1903, there were 2867 cases of vertebral tuberculosis and 3083 cases of all other joints combined...from 1920 to 1922...there were 422 cases of bone tuberculosis...243...of the spine. A study of consecutive cases admitted to the Ruptured and Crippled Hospital of New York City shows that there were 4299 cases of vertebral tuberculosis...The seriousness of vertebral tuberculosis is evident... 'It has been estimated that from 20% to 50% of all cases die as a result of this disease.' [Jones and Lovett] ...Until January 1911, this disease was treated by only the nonoperative method...on a Bradford Frame...Two operative methods have been devised for the treatment of Pott's Disease: 1. The Spine Fusion of Hibbs. 2. The Tibial Bone Graft of Albee. It is an interesting fact that both these operations were put into practice within a few months of each other. The first Spine Fusion was performed by Hibbs on January 9, 1911 [about a decade before Sullivan was a resident under Dr. Hibbs] ...Since all of my experience has been with the Hibbs' method, I shall not attempt to discuss the method of Albee.

"In spite of the apparent advantages of Spine Fusion, from time to time conservative orthopedists have protested against its use. Their objections have not been substantiated by a reasonable series of operative cases...at the New York Orthopedic Hospital, there has never been a death traceable in any way to operation in over 700 consecutive cases of spine fusion for this disease. I personally had the opportunity for more than three years of observing and caring for several hundred cases in the wards of this hospital, and in all that time I do not recall more than six cases that developed surgical shock. These cases yielded promptly to the usual shock treatment...The second objection is that the operation interferes with future growth of the spine... The growing centers of the vertebrae are in no way interfered with in this operation...careful measurements of the trunk and of the total height of every patient have been kept since the first Spine Fusion was performed in 1911... checked every six months, and now 12 years after...it can be definitely proved that the growth is not hindered. The third objection is that it is impossible or extremely difficult to produce solid bony fusion in young children. More than 20 children under two years of age have been successfully operated at the New York Orthopedic Hospital and...they have absolutely solid bony fusion of the operated area...

"The first official statement of results...was published by Hibbs in the *Journal of the American Medical Association*, October 26, 1918...end results in the first 210 cases. It was my privilege to have been present when these patients were examined and to have assisted in compiling the results...The next study...by Hibbs...is about to be published. It was again my privilege to have examined all these cases and to have assisted in preparing the tabulated results. Through the courtesy of Dr. Hibbs, I am quoting a few of the results in advance of the formal publication of the article. There were 163 cases considered... In the two series combined there was a total number of 373 cases examined. The total number of cases definitely cured...75%. .[with] 17% deaths...the majority...from whooping cough, broncho-pneumonia, and influenza. These results [when] compared with...Jones and Lovett's *Text Book on Orthopedic Surgery* that 20% to 50% of all cases die as a result of this disease, are most impressive... the percentage of deaths in the Hibbs' series is lower than the most optimistic estimate of cases treated by nonoperative methods...I believe that vertebral tuberculosis... is best treated by this operation."

at Boston City Hospital, with a private practice in Melrose, as a junior visiting surgeon for over 20 years. He was appointed surgeon-in-chief of the VI Surgical Service (the Bone and Joint Service) in 1951, replacing Dr. Shortell. I could find no Harvard appointment for Dr. Sullivan, but Harvard medical students rotated at Boston City Hospital only during his early service as junior visiting surgeon. No Harvard medical students were assigned to Boston City Hospital between 1942 and 1955. At the beginning of his tenure as chief, Dr. Sullivan partnered with Dr. G. Edmund Haggert,

Case 60.3. Elbow Joint Function Following an Unreduced Posterior Fracture-Dislocation

"[The patient], a 17-year-old, white male, was admitted to the Boston City Hospital October 1, 1932. He had sustained a severe injury to his right elbow when struck by a truck. He was taken to a relief station, where his arm was splinted. When admitted to this hospital a few minutes later, he was in mild shock. Examination of the posterior aspect of the right elbow showed deep ragged lacerations through which the olecranon was protruding. The forearm and hand were greatly swollen. Motions and sensations of wrist and hand were normal.

"X-rays upon admission were interpreted as showing posterior dislocation of the elbow with a fracture of the coronoid process of the ulna. The patient was treated for shock and then given the routine therapy for compound fracture. His condition while on the operating table became worse, and forcible manipulation after the first attempts at reduction had proved unsuccessful was prohibited. Although he had been given prophylactic tetanus and gas-bacillus antitoxins, on the following day he developed a definite case of gas-bacillus infection. He was critically ill for the next 2 weeks, during which time he was receiving treatment for the infection. X-rays made then showed an unreduced dislocation with the olecranon lying against the medial humeral surface about 5 cm. above the internal epicondyle.

"On October 16, or 15 days after the injury, the arm was put in traction with the elbow at a right angle. This method was not effective, and 8 days later the elbow was manipulated under the fluoroscope. This attempted reduction was not successful. The wound had filled in with granulation tissue and continued to have a moderate amount of serous drainage. The arm was then put in traction with the elbow in extension. Another manipulation was scheduled, but was not done since the patient's mother signed him out of the hospital "against advice."

"For the next 6 weeks he was treated at a private hospital, where one unsuccessful effort was made to reduce the dislocation. Skin grafts were applied to the granulating surface, and the patient was discharged home without any retentive apparatus. His elbow was completely stiff at that time, but he developed slight motion in a few weeks, and 12 months later was able to do light work in a newspaper plant. During the past 3 years he has been doing occasional heavy work. Motion at the elbow has been painless, but has not increased in range during the past 2 years. He has noticed a gradual increase of stability in the new joint and of strength in the forearm.

"On physical examination there is a marked enlargement resembling an exostosis on the medial surface of the lower humerus. The olecranon is fitted over this mass. The lower end of the humerus extends downward about 5 cm. below this point. The trochlea and capitellum are palpable beneath the skin. The ulnar nerve cannot be felt. The stability of the joint is excellent. There is about 60° to 75° of flexion. Muscle power of all the groups about the joint is about three-fourths normal. Pronation is two-thirds and supination four-fifths normal. There is no nerve disturbance."

(Sullivan and Childress 1937)

the chief of orthopaedics at the Lahey Clinic. Together they merged their two-independent hospital orthopaedic residency programs into one combined program. Dr. Haggert became the head of the residency programs. Dr. Sullivan removed the fracture service from general surgery and took charge of it in the orthopaedic department.

Following Dr. Joseph Shortell's death in 1951, for a number of years, Dr. Sullivan was the team physician for the Boston Red Sox. He was also a personal friend of Ted Williams. On March 1, 1954, Williams reported to Sarasota on the first day of spring training, accompanied by Dr. Sullivan. They had just spent several days fishing together. Within minutes of spring training, Williams attempted to catch a soft line drive by Hoot Evers, a reserve outfielder, but the ball was close to the ground and he fell. Everyone heard the sound of his collarbone breaking, but the formal diagnosis took days.

Dr. Sullivan operated on him at Sancta Maria Hospital. He wired the broken pieces together and ordered Williams to remain in the hospital for a week and then remain in Boston for two or three weeks so that he could monitor the healing process. Williams left the hospital the next day and returned to Florida within 13 days. On May 15, 1954, Williams played the greatest game of his career. The pin in his shoulder caused notable pain with use of the shoulder and he would remain in pain throughout his career, but he returned to full function.

Dr. Sullivan was certified by the American Board of Orthopaedic Surgery and was a member of the American Academy of Orthopaedic Surgeons, the American Medical Association, the New England Orthopaedic Society, and the Boston Orthopaedic Club. He was the first board certified orthopaedic surgeon who would become chief of the Bone and Joint Service at Boston City Hospital. He stepped down from his position as chief in 1954. After retiring, he was emeritus professor of orthopaedic surgery at Tufts. He died in his home in Melrose on Friday, October 28, 1966 at age 73; he was survived by his wife Thelma Cook, three daughters, and a son.

GORDON M. MORRISON

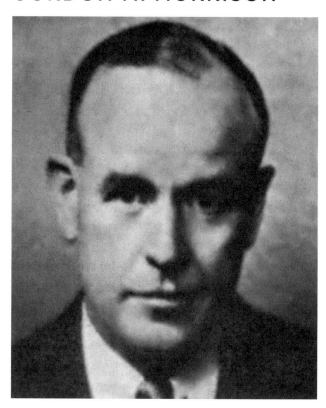

Gordon M. Morrison. Courtesy of the American Association for the Surgery of Trauma.

Physician Snapshot

Gordon M. Morrison
BORN: 1896
DIED: 1955

SIGNIFICANT CONTRIBUTIONS: Acting chief of the Bone and Joint Service at Boston City Hospital (1954); board member and president of the Board of the Massachusetts Society of Examining Physicians, i.e., Board of Medical Examiners; wartime consultant on the Medical Advisory Board and chairman of the Committee for Fracture Demonstration for the American Medical Association during World War II; president of the American Association for Surgery of Trauma

Born in 1896, Gordon Mackay Morrison served during World War I before beginning his studies at Harvard College. "He volunteered for the Royal Flying Corps and received cadet training for this uncommonly hazardous service in Canada. Only a brief [pilot] apprenticeship was allowed since the high mortality among combat pilots made the demands for replacements urgent. Morrison reached the front line in time to down one German plane before the war ended" (CHB 1956). Morrison was also an avid boxer, and "while awaiting his discharge from service, he won the heavy-weight boxing championship of the Royal Air Force" (CHB 1956). He had previously been mentored by his father, "who was noted in East Boston, both as a physician and as an amateur pugilist" (CHB 1956).

Morrison continued these athletic pursuits during his academic endeavors, and "in [his] spare time he coached football squads at Harvard, Williams, and in Iowa" (CHB 1956). He most likely did so for short periods while attending Harvard College, for one year after graduating with his AB from Harvard in 1921, and possibly intermittently or during summers while in medical school. He was listed as an assistant football coach amongst the faculty at Cornell College from 1921 until 1922. In 1926, he graduated from Tufts College Medical School. His "success [as assistant football coach] was so notable that Howard Jones, then of national prominence, asked Morrison to serve as his line coach in California. Instead, he took up a surgical internship at the Boston City Hospital where he later served, for over two decades, on the Visiting Staff" (CHB 1956).

In 1929, Dr. Morrison was appointed junior member of the surgical visiting staff in the outpatient department at Boston City Hospital, along with Dr. Russell Sullivan. The senior outpatient surgeon at the time was Dr. Joseph H. Burnett and that same year, Dr. Joseph Shortell was promoted to visiting surgeon from assistant visiting surgeon. For almost a decade, "from 1929 to 1938, Morrison was associated with Dr. Frederic J. Cotton as assistant and then as partner" (CHB 1956). Their office was at 520 Commonwealth Avenue.

Dr. Morrison published about 16 articles; the majority coauthored with Dr. Cotton. His association with Dr. Cotton "drew him exclusively into the field of bone-and-joint surgery, which became his chief interest…he conducted a very successful consulting practice, centered around Boston but occasionally reaching from Exeter, New Hampshire, to Cape Cod" (CHB 1956). **Case 60.4** illustrates an example of one of his case reports. By 1934, Morrison was assistant outpatient surgeon at Boston City Hospital and "visiting surgeon, Chelsea Memorial Hospital, junior visiting surgeon, Newton Hospital, consulting surgeon at Higgins Memorial Hospital, Wolfeboro, New Hampshire, Framingham Union Hospital and Leonard Morse Hospital, Natick" ("This Week's Issue" 1934).

He was also a trustee of the Massachusetts Memorial Hospital. I was unable to discover whether Dr. Morrison held any medical school faculty appointments.

Active in the Massachusetts Medical Society, he served on the Medical Defense Committee in the 1930s and later on the Committee on Arrangements (chairman, 1943). Along with Dr. Cotton, he was active in the American College of Surgeons, both serving on the publicity committee together, while Dr. Cotton was a member of the local executive committee of the New England Regional Committee on Fractures, and later Dr. Morrison was elected as vice-president of the Board of Governors. He was also an active member of the Boston Orthopedic Club and served on its executive council. In 1941, the New England Society of Bone and Joint Surgery was formed, and Dr. Morrison was elected secretary-treasurer and Dr. Joseph Barr was elected vice president. At its founding, they noted:

> membership is limited to those surgeons in the New England States who confined their practice to bone and joint surgery, particularly the problems of traumatic surgery. The purpose of the Society is to aid in the advancement in the methods of treatment of these conditions. The membership at present is limited to thirty-five active members. ("News Notes. The New England Society of Bone and Joint Surgery" 1941)

During World War II, "he was also wartime consultant on the Medical Advisory Board and chairman of the Committee for Fracture Demonstration for the American Medical Association. His effective work here won several national awards" (CHB 1956). The committee produced a "Primer on Fractures," a cooperative effort of the special exhibit committee on fractures and the scientific

Case 60.4. Ischaemic Paralysis from Pressure of Hematoma

"The patient, a school boy, fifteen years old, white, one hour before admission to the Boston City Hospital on January 2, 1935, at about eight o'clock in the evening, was coasting down the street on a sled. He remembered seeing the lights of a small delivery truck approaching and crashed into it, then became unconscious and awoke half an hour later in a police ambulance on the way to Boston City Hospital. He did not vomit at any time after the accident.

"Previous to the injury the patient had been in excellent health.

"Physical examination at time of admission showed a well developed and well nourished boy, conscious and rational. There was a deep transfer laceration twelve centimeters in length across the top of his scalp. The skin edges were much avulsed and bleeding profusely. There were small superficial contusions of the left thigh and right wrist.

"The left upper arm showed localized tenderness, abnormal mobility, and slight angulation deformity over the midshaft of the left humerus. There was a very tender, swollen area, about fifteen centimeters in length, extending over the medial aspect of the left upper arm. The tenderness extended completely around the arm but the swelling was chiefly over its medial aspect. The left hand was pale and cold, and the nails were cyanotic. Radial and ulnar pulses could not be felt in the left wrist. Flexion and extension of the fingers of the left hand were both very weak and the fingers could be spread hardly at all. When tested by pin pricks, there was diminished sensation over the radial distribution of the dorsum of the left hand and fingers.

"Pupils were equal and reacted to light. Knee jerks and ankle jerks were present and normal, and there was no ankle clonus or Babinski reflex.

"The patient was treated for moderate shock. Immediate x-ray showed a simple transverse fracture of the midshaft of the left humerus.

"Under ether anaesthesia, a vertical incision, about twelve centimeters in length, was made over the medial aspect of the left upper arm. A large tense area of traumatized muscle and clot was found beneath the deep fascia. The median and ulnar nerves were identified and the brachial artery was freed up for a distance of about ten centimeters. The radial and the ulnar pulses returned immediately after the brachial artery had been freed. The pressure of the hematoma caused by the fracture had evidently obliterated the lumen of the brachial artery.

"Shortly after the operation started, the pulse rate rose to 140 per minute. It was, therefore, considered inadvisable to take additional time then to plate the humerus or to attempt to inspect the radial nerve. The arm wound was closed very loosely with skin sutures only, and the arm was put up in loose traction in a Thomas arm splint. The scalp wound was cleansed and sutured at the same time.

"The patent was kept in shock position for twelve hours. His wounds healed rapidly without infection. The next morning his left hand was warm and pink with good wrist pulses. Postoperative roentgenograms showed the bone ends in good position. All sutures were removed on the eighth day after operation and the arm wound strapped with adhesive. Sensory and motor nerve lesions improved slowly.

"Eighteen days after operation, roentgenograms showed good callus formation and the arm was put up in an 'airplane' plaster cast with shoulder in right-angle abduction and elbow in right-angle flexion. After application of the cast, x-rays again showed good position of the fragments.

"Thirty-two days after injury, the patient was discharged to his home with the arm in the plaster cast.

"He was seen again six weeks after injury and the cast was removed at that time. Sensation and motion of the left hand were then almost completely normal."

(Morrison and Kennard 1935)

exhibit committee of the American Medical Association. It proved very successful, publishing six editions. He later served on the Board of the Massachusetts Society of Examining Physicians, i.e., the Board of Medical Examiners, for 10 years from 1944–1954, and "among his many professional honors were [election to] the presidency [in 1948]" (CHB 1956). His service may have been one of his "greatest contributions," and:

> few doctors realize the importance of this unrewarding, time-consuming and exasperating post, which guards the medical profession from illegitimate practices and which regulates licensure. So intense is the pressure that Board members are subjected to frequent abusive interruptions, and they often receive threats of death, sometimes even requiring State police protection. To this distasteful but essential work, Morrison gave his time persistently, fearlessly and judiciously. (CHB 1956)

At the age of 54, in 1950, Dr. Morrison became president of the American Association for Surgery of Trauma (AAST). In his presidential address, he observed that the AAST formed in 1938 to address deficiencies in the treatment of trauma. He noted that 40 to 50 percent of all patients admitted for surgery in the largest metropolitan hospitals were trauma patients, but trauma was rarely discussed at professional meetings. The AAST prescribed a training curriculum and published articles in medical journals in order to share expertise. The study of trauma improved during World War II, resulting in lower mortality, formation of bone banks, improvements in hand surgery outcomes, and treatment protocols for many categories of trauma patients. In the postwar period, AAST exerted influence in the Veterans Administration. AAST fostered improvements in anesthesia and reduction of infection by the use of antibiotics.

Dr. Morrison set out the following goals for the AAST:

- increased membership across the country
- recruitment of young surgeons to join the practice of trauma management and to conduct research
- improvement of techniques
- coordination with other specialties
- incorporation of medical ethics into training

Four years later, "in [June] 1954 he became acting chief surgeon of the Bone and Joint Service at the [Boston City] Hospital, but to the regret of all his associates, he was obliged to retire almost at once [in December], on account of a suddenly manifested heart condition" (CHB 1956). He died on December 1, 1955, at 60 years old. He was remembered as:

> universally popular [in private life]; he was a member of the Harvard Club, the Brae Burn Country Club and the Baalbeck Lodge of Masons. He was married to Alice Blodgett, who survives him with their three sons…He will be happily remembered by all who knew him for his professional skill and judgment, his frankness, his buoyance, his loyalty and his unflinching courage. (CHB 1956)

ALEXANDER P. AITKEN

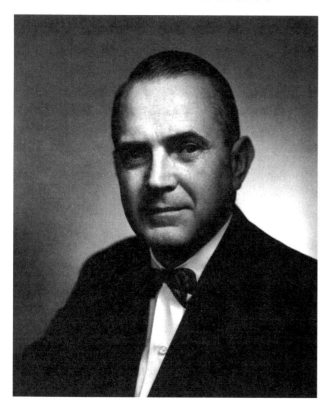

Alexander P. Aitken. U.S. National Library of Medicine/Digital Collections and Archives, Tufts University.

Physician Snapshot

Alexander P. Aitken

BORN: 1904

DIED: 1993

SIGNIFICANT CONTRIBUTIONS: Chief of the Bone and Joint Service at Boston City Hospital 1955–1963; established the first rehabilitation center for employees in the United States at Liberty Mutual and served as the center's medical director; chairman of the Subcommittee on Industrial Relations of the American College of Surgeons; chief of surgery at Brooks Hospital, Chelsea Memorial Hospital, and Winchester Hospital; in 1935 published the largest series of follow up of patients with epiphyseal injuries in the English literature, even though epiphyseal fractures have been known since the time of Hippocrates; first to type and classify epiphyseal growth injuries in 1936, 27 years before the Salter-Harris classification system

Alexander Philip Aitken was born in Barre, Vermont, on November 26, 1904. He earned his bachelor's degree at Tufts University after graduating from Boston English High School. He went on to earn his MD from Tufts University School of Medicine. He trained in surgery and orthopaedics at Boston City Hospital after successfully passing his Massachusetts Board of Registration in Medicine examination in 1928. As recorded in the list of house officers at Boston City Hospital, Dr. Aitken completed eight months of training on the surgical service during 1929. Along with one of his medical school classmates (Dr. Edward Edwards), he was:

> one of the three interns at City Hospital who have been suffering from septic poisoning, [Dr. Edwards] was removed from the danger list (December 5 [1929]). The condition of Dr. Alexander Aitken is greatly improved, and he is up and around the hospital attending to his patients. ("News of Tufts College Medical School" 1929)

That same year, he was listed as being at the Monson State Hospital in Palmer, Massachusetts, a state hospital for patients with mental health disorders, epilepsy, disabilities, or those without the financial means to obtain medical care elsewhere. I could not find any reference to house officers at Monson, but consultant physicians, including an orthopaedic surgeon, worked at the hospital. Dr. Aitken may have served as a consultant at that time. In 1931, he became a member of the Massachusetts Medical Society. By 1934, he was an assistant in surgery at Boston City Hospital, a junior surgeon at Chelsea Memorial Hospital, and instructor in surgery at Boston University School of Medicine.

Aitken made significant contributions to the specialty of orthopaedic surgery in three areas: epiphyseal injuries, end results of treatment of ruptured intervertebral discs, and rehabilitation of the injured at work. He published at least eight papers on epiphyseal injuries, contributed a chapter to Dr. Charles Scudder's book on *The Treatment of Fractures*, and published another 11 papers on ruptured discs and rehabilitation of the injured and disabled. His first two publications were in 1934, on the ankle.

Epiphyseal Injuries

His first two papers on epiphyseal injuries were published in 1935. In the first, he described the end results of 60 patients followed for two to nine years after fractures of the distal radial epiphysis; children aged four to eighteen years. This series followed for up to nine years by Dr. Aitken probably represents the largest follow up of patients with epiphyseal injuries in the English literature. This is all the more impressive because epiphyseal fractures have been known since the age of Hippocrates, especially in the late-nineteenth century. In his second paper, he added another 20 patients. He did not propose his classification system for epiphyseal fractures at the time. He concluded:

> an attempt should be made to reduce all displacements [but] repeated manipulation or osteotomy are [not] warranted...1. Displacement of the epiphysis does not persist... displacements are reduced within a year [maximum period of two to three years]. 2. Reduction is accomplished by the production of bone on the dorsum of the shaft, so that the shaft is brought up to the epiphysis. The volar portion of the shaft undergoes absorption. This loss of the volar bowing is restored within two years. 3. Temporary retardation [of growth] is commonly noticed, but is of no clinical importance. 4. Reduction occurs at any age, regardless of the proximity to the normal ossification time. 5. The one case of deformity in the series is attributed to crushing of the epiphysis, which is demonstrable by x-ray. (Aitken 1935)

The following year, Dr. Aitken published a paper on "The End Results of the Fractured Distal Tibial Epiphysis." In this paper, he classified epiphyseal injuries, for the first time, into three types:

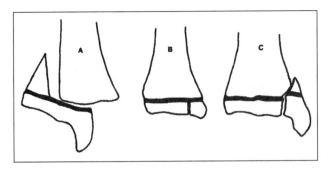

Drawing of Aitken's original three types of epiphyseal injuries from his 1936 article.
A. P. Aitken, "The End Results of the Fractured Distal Tibial Epiphysis," *Journal of Bone and Joint Surgery* 1936; 18: 685.

Type 1. The fracture line runs parallel and proximal to the cartilage plate...through the newly formed bone and emerges through the shaft...Type 2. The fracture line crosses the bony epiphysis from the joint to the cartilage plate, but there is no fracture through the plate. In about 40 per cent of the cases the plate is crushed...Type 3. The fracture line runs through the bony epiphysis, the cartilage, and the shaft. (Aitken 1936)

Probably because of his small number of cases (21 cases of distal tibial epiphyseal injuries), Dr. Aitken did not include a separate classification for a crush injury, as was done later by Drs. Robert Salter and W. Robert Harris, but he included that crush injury was part (40%) of his type 2 fractures. He reported his classification system because of the:

> great difference of opinion as to the end results of fractures of the epiphysis...In order that our conclusions may be accurate, we must have accurate statistics. A review of the literature shows that this prime requisite has been overlooked...most...authors have reported a small series of cases...to these they have...added several cases of deformity... from [other] districts. A high percentage of poor end results is thus obtained...In discussing the end results of epiphyseal fractures,

each epiphysis must be considered individually. In summarizing our work on the epiphysis to date, we are convinced that deformity is due only to crushing of the epiphysis at the time of injury or during osteotomy for correction. (Aitken 1936)

That same year, Aitken was a member of the Massachusetts group on the New England Regional Committee on Fractures of the American College of Surgeons when Dr. Joseph Shortell was chairman. He had previously become active in the American College of Surgeons with his surgical colleagues at Boston City Hospital. His clinical interest appears to have been focused only on orthopaedics and orthopaedic trauma.

Ruptured Intervertebral Discs

In his second major contribution to orthopaedics, Dr. Aitken published two papers on the end results or outcomes of patients with ruptured intervertebral discs. He coauthored his first paper with Dr. Charles H. Bradford in 1947 (see chapter 61), 13 years after the classic publication of Drs. W. Jason Mixter and Joseph Barr on rupture of the intervertebral disc. At the time, Dr. Aitken was Medical Director of the Rehabilitation Center of Liberty Mutual Insurance Company in Boston, and his position provided Aitken and Bradford with access to the company's files. Liberty Mutual had opened the first rehabilitation center for employees in the country in Boston in 1943; which was set up under Dr. Aitken.

Dr. Aitken found that the extant surgical techniques used to treat intervertebral disc ruptures led to dismal outcomes. Aitken and Bradford reviewed 170 cases of patients operated on for a symptomatic herniated disc from 1940 to 1944. They demonstrated the confusion at the time regarding the underlying pathology and the inadequacy of diagnostic techniques. For example, in one case, a procedure was performed by one neurosurgeon and two orthopaedists. The two orthopaedists disagreed about their findings, one saying there was pathology and one saying there was not. The neurosurgeon diagnosed two disc ruptures. Aitken and Bradford reviewed the diagnostic effectiveness of myelography in 102 cases and found its accuracy to be no better than chance. Out of 170 patients treated for intervertebral disc rupture with surgery, 67 patients had no disc herniation, which is significant because surgical outcomes in these patients are poor.

The authors therefore compared the outcomes in cases with disc herniation and those without. They found that symptoms did not correlate with surgical findings. For example, changes in reflexes on the involved side did not correlate with the presence or absence of a disc. In 53 percent of cases there was a herniated disc, and in 47 percent there was not. Referred pain down the leg also did not correlate and neither did sensory changes. The authors found that the pain was unrelated to anatomical changes and a proportion could be attributed to neuroses. As a result of this diagnostic unreliability, the authors recommended conservative management. They recommended bed rest of up to six weeks, heat application, massage, and traction. Only when this approach fails did the authors recommend surgery, especially since surgical outcomes are so poor. Only 20 percent of workers' compensation patients were able to return to heavy work post surgically. Some surgical failures were due to poor technique, but overall, surgery itself lead to poor outcomes, further surgeries were often necessary, and the poor outcomes did not justify the expense (25% more in the non-disc group). Slightly more than ⅓ of the operated patients remained on disability up to six years following surgery.

Five years later, Aitken published some additional observations of workers' compensation cases after lumbar spine surgery for disc disease. Dr. Aitken found defects in patient management due to poor surgical technique, ignorance about mechanics and anatomy, and a disregard of the psychological impacts of injury. He advocated for fewer surgical procedures because of poor outcomes. He opined that surgical procedures should involve a neurosurgeon and an orthopaedist, but he was emphatic that orthopaedists should not consider performing back surgery as a matter of routine and that their choice of surgery as a first-line mode of treatment minimizes the risks and overestimates the benefits of spinal fusion, laminectomy, and exploratory surgery. Spinal fusions, he maintained, should only be performed if there is instability in the back. Dr. Aitken most likely agreed with Dr. W.J. Mixter who:

> wrote to one of us (R.M.P.D.) [the patient] is of particular interest as he is the first patient in whom a ruptured intervertebral disc was recognized as such and as the cause for sciatica. Therefore, he is the man who started all the damn trouble. (Frymoyer & Donaghy 1985)

Rehabilitation and the Injured Worker

While medical director of the Rehabilitation Clinic of Liberty Mutual, Dr. Aitken published about a dozen articles on the injured worker, rehabilitation, and workers' compensation issues. He was also chairman of the Subcommittee on Industrial Relations of the American College of Surgeons, was a member of the President's Committee on Employment of the Physically Handicapped, and served on a committee chaired by Dr. Charles H. Bradford of the Massachusetts Medical Society. He wrote many insightful observations from his experience as medical director, including:

> It is clearly the physician's duty to give his very best from the minute of injury until the patient can return to work...The following statistics give some idea of our success...In the past four years 666 cases have been treated...most of these patients had multiple and serious injuries...in this age group, the earlier treatment is started, the better the result...In the average case. Six and a half months had lapsed between the date of injury and admission to the center... Despite this fact...65 per cent...have returned to gainful employment...Our experience has convinced us of the value of a combination of physical therapy and early work therapy. (Frederic J. Cotton once said, "The best way to restore a bricklayer to his job is to make him lay bricks.") (Aitken 1947)

Aitken had a holistic outlook toward treatment. He emphasized that rehabilitation must take into account the treatment of emotional disturbances. The current state of the practice at the time involved poor aftercare and did not consider the importance of proper physical therapy and psychiatric care in achieving the best functional outcomes. He most likely was referring to the entire gamut of psychiatric care, including: educating individuals on how to tolerate and live with pain, assisting patients with how to come to terms with a new disability, helping patients understand their condition (emotional response), attempting to help malingerers, and identifying secondary gains the patient may be trying to achieve.

While continuing in these endeavors, Dr. Aitken was named chief of the Bone and Joint Service at Boston City Hospital in 1955, after Dr. Gordon Morrison's unexpected death. He was also a clinical professor of orthopaedic surgery at Tufts College Medical School, as well as instructor of surgery at Boston University School of Medicine. I did not find any references that Dr. Aitken ever held an academic appointment at Harvard Medical School.

Aitken continued in his advocacy for the injured worker, actively criticizing the state of workers' compensation laws that focused on monetary compensation at the expense of patient recovery and vocational training. These laws resulted in delays in treatment and artificial limitations on length of treatment due to a treatment protocol designed by laypeople. He wrote:

Modern rehabilitation involves the total medical practice as it affects the injured. It begins with the attending physician – and even with medical school. In order for the physician to carry out his responsibilities as defined by the American College of Surgeons [adopted in 1952]. It is essential for him to recognize the total medical problem of the patient in addition to his injury, as well to his personal problems. The physician must bring to bear…all the skills and disciplines that science and society can offer, and utilize all community resources which can assist him in the accomplishments of these objectives. ("'Workmen's Compensation in the United States.' Bulletin No. 1149" 1954)

In response, the American College of Surgeons recommended a critical review of treatment protocols, financial compensation procedures, and rehabilitation protocols. ACS established as priorities diagnostic accuracy and the provision of appropriate medical care until the patient has received maximum benefit as well as which care should involve physical therapy and vocational training. Further, the ACS advocated for the requirement that a patient receive treatment until the point of maximum improvement before a determination of permanent disability is made. ACS recommended that determinations of causation, treatment course, and disability should be made by a panel of independent, salaried medical experts. Further, ACS recommended that claimants should be permitted to return to work before the patient achieves maximal improvement, especially for purposes of retraining. ACS also recommended that patients receive disability benefits and that companies be encouraged to hire disabled workers. Finally, ACS recommended that funding come from the state, from the companies themselves, or both, and that protection be extended to workers in industries that are not considered hazardous.

Dr. Aitken, in his capacity as chairperson of the ACS Subcommittee on Industrial Relations, recommended changes in workers' compensation laws. These policy changes were formulated with input from the subcommittee, the insurance industry, and government agencies. He established that the stated goals for the workers' compensation system should be to return the injured worker to gainful employment. The determination of disability, causation, treatment course, disability findings, and compensation should be overseen and mandated by trained physicians after physical examination of the injured worker. Workplace injuries must be reported to the agency promptly to begin this process. He advocated for changes in existing regulations and laws in order solve many of the problems encountered among the industrially disabled.

Continued Publications on Fracture Injuries

Aitken continued to explore his interest in fractures through his publications, and published papers on fractures involving the proximal humeral epiphysis, the distal femoral epiphysis, and the proximal tibial epiphysis. He used the same classification system he had established earlier in 1936 (which others referred to as Aitken's classification) in his 1952 paper on the distal femoral epiphysis, but in his 1956 paper on proximal tibial epiphyseal injuries, he modified his classification of type 2 injuries, writing:

> The fracture line may cross the epiphysis more or less obliquely and emerge between the bony epiphysis and the epiphyseal plate without damage to the latter; in such a case, growth disturbance will not occur. If, however, the fracture line crosses the plate and emerges between it and the diaphysis…then deformity may occur because of damage to the plate. (Aitkin & Ingersoll 1956)

Case 60.5 provides an example of one of Aitken's case reports from this time as well.

Dr. Atkins classification of epiphyseal fractures was commonly used by physicians from 1936 to 1963, and with some individuals into the 1980s. In 1963, Drs. Salter and Harris reported their classification of epiphyseal-plate injuries, which is universally used today and included five basic types. Their type II injury compares to Aitken's type 1, their type III injury compares to Aitken's type 2, and their type IV injury compares to Aitken's type 3 injury. They added a type I injury, which is a "complete separation of the epiphysis from the metaphysis without any bone fracture" (Salter & Harris 1963) and a type V injury which is a "relatively uncommon injury [which] results from a very severe crushing force applied through the epiphysis to one area of the epiphyseal plate. It occurs in joints which move in one plane only [ankle and knee]" (Salter & Harris 1963). Dr. Aitken had appreciated compression injuries with their high association of growth arrest and deformity, but he did not make a separate classification category for them as did Drs. Salter and Harris. In their article, Salter and Harris (1963) discussed classifications by previous authors:

Case 60.5. Fracture of the Proximal Tibial Epiphyseal Cartilage

"On June 8, 1949, while catching in a baseball game, [the patient], aged seventeen was standing in a semicrouched position blocking home plate when a player sliding in from third base struck the medial aspect of his right leg. He was knocked to the ground and was unable to arise because of pain in the right knee. Roentgenograms revealed a vertical fracture of the proximal tibial epiphysis in its lateral half, the fracture line emerging medially between the epiphysis and the shaft. The shaft was abducted on the epiphysis and was displaced anteriorly.

"Under pentothal anaesthesia an immediate attempt at reduction was made. The proximal tibial epiphysis could be palpated easily but slipped in all directions from under the finger like a loose body. The lateral displacement of the shaft was easily corrected but the lateral edge of the epiphysis tended to tilt upward into the joint and to become displaced proximally. Reduction consisted of manipulating the shaft in an attempt to catch and hold the elusive epiphysis. After three attempts, satisfactory reduction was obtained and a cast was applied with the knee in slight flexion. Roentgenograms made the following day showed recurrence of the anterior displacement of the shaft and proximal displacement of the epiphysis. Temporary reduction was again obtained. It was possible to reduce the fracture completely, but any motion of the leg inside the plaster or in the operator's hands caused the epiphysis to slip out of alignment. Although roentgenograms showed lateral displacement of the shaft at times on manipulation, the epiphysis itself could be seen and felt to displace in all directions. Displacement recurred after repeated attempts at reduction.

"On June 27, 1949, open reduction was performed, the cruciate ligaments and the medial meniscus were visualized and appeared to be normal. Even with direct exposure, the fragment was difficult to fix in position as it tended to displace in all planes. Firm fixation was finally obtained but there was still some persistent proximal displacement of the epiphysis. Immobilization in plaster was continued until September 13, 1949, after which it was replaced by a walking caliper brace until November 5, 1949. On November 20, 1949, an area of fluctuation developed over the fibular end of one of the bolts. Consequently one bolt and one washer were removed. Although the other washer in the fibular area was not removed, the infection cleared up promptly. The patient thereafter had no further difficulty. When seen on June 1, 1950, he had no complaints. The knee showed hyperextension of 15 degrees and a loss of flexion of 10 degrees. There was still an appreciable amount of lateral instability on abduction of the extended knee. Roentgenograms made at that time showed all the epiphyses to be closed with little evidence of residual displacement. The patient was last seen in September 1952, at which time there was full knee motion and only a slight amount of abnormal lateral mobility."

(Aitken and Ingersoll 1956)

Epiphyseal-plate injuries have been classified both generally and specifically (for a given epiphysis) by several authors. The following classification is based on the mechanism of injury and the relationship of the fracture line to the growing cells of the epiphyseal plate. The classification is also correlated with the prognosis concerning disturbance of growth.

Salter and Harris cited four articles by Aitken in their references, including his 1936 paper in which he diagrammed his classification system for the first time. They also cited an article by Dr. E. Bergenfeldt in the European literature (1933), an article by Drs. Charles O. Carothers and Andrew H. Crenshaw from the Campbell Clinic (1955), and a chapter on epiphyseal injuries by Dr. Robert Joplin in Dr. Edwin Cave's book, *Fractures and other Injuries*. Carothers and Crenshaw commented on Aitken's classification, noting his long follow up of cases (two to nine years); Dr. John Poland's classic study on epiphyseal injuries (1898); and that Dr. Joplin, in his chapter, used Dr. Aitken's classification by diagramming his three types of epiphyseal fractures. However, Drs. Harris and Salter did not fully credit Dr. Aitken or cite his name or the other authors' names whose articles they included in their limited list of previous authors of classification systems of epiphyseal injuries. But Aitken first typed and classified epiphyseal growth injuries in 1936. The Salter–Harris classification system was developed 27 years later in 1963. Because of inaccuracy of predicting growth outcomes with the Salter-Harris classification, pediatric orthopaedic surgeons continue to pursue a more accurate system of classifying epiphyseal injuries.

Legacy

Aitken had continued to maintain his private orthopaedic practice in Winchester and to work as a consultant for nine other hospitals in the Boston area while serving as chief of the Bone and Joint Service at Boston City Hospital and medical director of the rehabilitation clinic at Liberty Mutual. He stepped down from his position as chief of the Bone and Joint Service at Boston City Hospital in 1963. Subsequent chiefs included Drs. Arthur Thibodeau (Tufts), Robert Ulin (Beth Israel Hospital), and Paul O'Brien (Carney Hospital). Aitken had also simultaneously served as chief of surgery at Brooks Hospital, Chelsea Memorial Hospital, and Winchester Hospital. He was a diplomate of the American Board of Orthopaedic Surgery and a member of the American Association for Surgery of Trauma.

Little information is available about Dr. Alexander Aitken in his later years. He moved to Denver, Colorado, after retirement, where he died on February 24, 1993. He was 88. He was survived by his wife, a son, and a daughter, as well as ten grandchildren, and ten great-grandchildren.

CHAPTER 61

Boston City Hospital
Other Surgeon Scholars

After its founding in 1928, the VI Surgical Service (also known as the Bone and Joint Service or the Sixth Surgical Service) primarily treated patients with traumatic injuries, and most were cared for in the various outpatient clinics of the Shortell Unit. These clinics included a fracture clinic, the Crippled Children's Clinic (also known as the "Polio Clinic") set up by Dr. Robert Ingersoll as well as those for follow-up of patients undergoing hip procedures, procedures using Lottes nail and their outcomes, and a pediatric fracture clinic. Into the early 1960s, physicians and surgeons in these Shortell Unit clinics were seeing over 25,000 patients annually, including ~5000 fracture patients.

The VI Surgical Service provided resident education from its inception, focusing on students from Harvard, Tufts, and Boston Universities. It also began to offer an orthopaedic training program in the mid-twentieth century (see chapter 62, **Box 62.1**). However, in 1973, the City of Boston reduced the number of medical schools sending students to BCH, ending BCH's 110-year relationship with Harvard Medical School and Tufts University School of Medicine.

The orthopaedic surgeons described in this chapter are some of the Harvard surgeons who practiced on the VI Surgical Service at BCH. The surgeon scholars—Harvard's nomenclature for these clinicians—covered in this chapter include:

**Boston City Hospital:
Other Surgeon Scholars**

John D. Adams	357
George G. Bailey Jr.	360
David D. Berlin	361
Charles H. Bradford	361
Joseph H. Burnett	368
G. Kenneth Coonse	371
Robert Ingersoll	376
H. Kelvin Magill	376

JOHN D. ADAMS

Physician Snapshot

John D. Adams
BORN: Unknown
DIED: Unknown
SIGNIFICANT CONTRIBUTIONS: Orthopaedic-surgeon-in-chief at the Boston Dispensary; the first to document using a bone graft to treat scaphoid fractures

John D. Adams, a graduate of Harvard Medical School (HMS) in 1902 and associated with Boston Children's Hospital, became

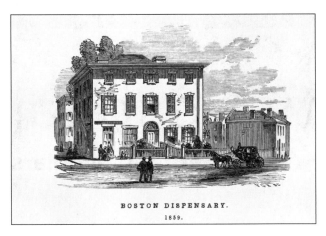

Boston Dispensary, 1859. Corner of Ash and Bennett streets, South End. Originally established in 1796 to provide medical care for the indigent. U.S. National Library of Medicine.

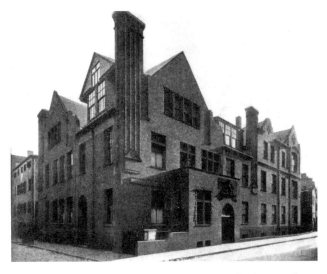

Boston Dispensary, early twentieth century. Sculpture of the Good Samaritan is above the entrance. In 1968, the dispensary merged with the New England Medical Center to become Tufts Medical Center. Digital Collections and Archives, Tufts University.

orthopaedic-surgeon-in-chief at the Boston Dispensary while in private practice with privileges at Beverly Hospital; Jordan Hospital, in Plymouth; Memorial Hospital, in Brattleboro, Vermont; and Sisters Hospital, in Waterville, Maine. His office was initially located at 43 Bay State Road, Boston, but in 1911 he moved to 261 Beacon Street.

In 1910, he reported at a meeting of the Mt. Sinai Clinical Society on his experience in treating 25 cases of back pain in laborers, which he had treated at the Boston Dispensary and in his private practice. He admitted that he offered nothing new but stated:

> there is a certain class of occupational spines which…present a functional disability, and if we have no facts to sustain an organic or bony change, we are not justified in splinting the back to the extreme detriment of its future capability…It has been the writer's experience to see far too many cases tied up in rigid apparatus, with its untoward effects, where results have been shown that they would have been far better to have supplemented a light support with counter-irritation. (Adams 1911)

Dr. Adams' interest in back pain, conditioning, and laborers' injuries continued. Under his supervision, in 1912, as head of the orthopaedic department at the Boston Dispensary, he organized a series of gymnasium classes for children (10 per session). He spoke often about back pain and conducted clinics on patients with back injuries. A decade later, in 1922, he and his associates at the dispensary led orthopaedic clinics and performed orthopaedic operations at a clinical congress of the American College of Surgeons.

That same year, at a monthly meeting of the staff of the Boston Dispensary, he gave a lecture on the meaning and value of occupational therapy. He noted: "in part, that through the introduction of occupational therapy into hospitals overseas during the war, the capacity of these hospitals was increased 50 per cent because, by it, the period of convalescence was materially reduced" (Adams 1922). He then outlined a program for a school of occupational therapy in Boston under the Massachusetts Association for Occupational Therapy. He wrote that this society "aims to make occupational therapy a part of the treatment in civilian hospitals throughout the state [including] establishment of out-patient industrial workshops in connection with the after-treatment of discharged hospital cases" (Adams 1922). Later that year, he spoke about occupational therapy at a meeting on "Rehabilitation" of the Suffolk District Medical Society. Adams (1922) stated:

> Occupational therapy is what the name implies – the idea of occupying the patient in the hospital wards in order to hasten his convalescence, restore his function, and mentally restore him to his former state of mind. It is not a diversion but a treatment applied in conjunction with the doctor…A school was organized in Boston, graduated 100 occupational therapy aids, girls, who were sent to France, who demonstrated their efficiency. The period of convalescence of the patients over there was reduced 30 percent.

At that same meeting in the discussion, Dr. James W. Sever (1922) commented that, "In regard to orthopedic surgery – the pathetic side of it is that most of the cases which require orthopedic treatment are cases we should never see, due to the fact that preliminary reconstruction surgery has not been properly carried out." Three years later, Dr. Adams was invited by the American Hospital Association to address its members at their 1925 annual meeting on the present status of occupational therapy in hospitals.

Daily clinical teaching conferences at the Boston Dispensary were started about 1928, and Adams discussed diseases of the bones and joints every Tuesday for at least 10 years. In 1929, he oversaw a clinic on arthritis at a clinical meeting of the American College of Physicians hosted by the Boston Dispensary.

The previous year—six years before Dr. Joseph Burnett's publication on scaphoid fractures—Adams wrote about a new method of treating a scaphoid fracture:

> Untreated fractures of the scaphoid almost always result in non-union…the patient [a laboring man] who needs the full strength of the wrist in movements of precision is

---

FRACTURE OF THE CARPAL SCAPHOID
A New Method of Treatment With a Report of One Case
BY JOHN D. ADAMS, M.D., F.A.C.S., AND RALPH D. LEONARD, M.D.*

Title of Adams's article in which he describes what Dr. Burnett believed was the first report on the use of a bone graft for a scaphoid fracture. *New England Journal of Medicine* 1928; 198: 401.

> incapacitated for that type of work. Such a problem stimulated us to challenge a case of non-union of eighteen months' duration to a hitherto untried method of treatment, namely, bone-graft…The usual approach was made through the dorsal incision…The fracture was transverse at the margin of the articular surface of the radial end. It was, therefore, impossible to groove the proximal fragment for a graft as it would involve the articulation with the radius. A measurement was made for the graft and a small piece removed from the tibia. A small groove was made though the cortex of the distal fragment to the length of about ½ inch… the proximal fragment was then tipped back, and a hole bored to correspond with the groove to receive the end of the graft. The graft was then cut to the proper length: the end placed in the hole in the proximal fragment and brought down into the groove. The hand was then brought into extreme adduction and flexion jamming the fragments together…[a] plaster cast [was] applied taking in the entire hand, especially the thumb…The hand was left in the cast for six weeks when passive motion was begun…He [a boxer] entered his first fight six months after the operation and won it with a knock-out with his hand. At the present writing he is free from all symptoms…The last x-ray…shows that there is bone about one-half the diameter of the scaphoid…In cases of non-union it offers a method of treatment worthy of trial…[and] fresh fractures may be treated by this method. This conclusion is based upon the

fact that a very large percentage of cases fail to unit under the present methods of treatment.
(Adams and Leonard 1928)

Dr. Burnett (1934) mentioned in his own paper on scaphoid fractures that "Dr. John Adams of Boston, so far as I know, was the first one to resort to the graft operation for these cases [painful nonunions]." See **Case 61.1** for another later example of Dr. Adams' cases.

Dr. John Adams was an assistant in orthopaedic surgery at the Harvard Medical School of Graduate Medicine and assistant demonstrator of anatomy at Tufts College Medical School. He was also a fellow of the American College of Surgeons and active in the Massachusetts Medical Society. In 1930, the Boston Dispensary merged with the Boston Floating Hospital for Children. Adams remained as orthopaedic surgeon-in-chief at the New England Medical Center.

GEORGE G. BAILEY JR.

Physician Snapshot

George G. Bailey Jr.
BORN: Unknown
DIED: 1998
SIGNIFICANT CONTRIBUTIONS: Chief of orthopaedics at Mount Auburn Hospital

Dr. George G. "Guy" Bailey Jr. graduated from Harvard in 1929 and Harvard Medical School in 1933. He was an assistant visiting surgeon on the VI (Bone and Joint) Service at Boston City Hospital. For four decades, Bailey ran a private practice, and he served as a consulting surgeon at hospitals throughout the city. He also spent more than 20 years at Mount Auburn Hospital, as both an attending surgeon and then as chief of orthopaedics (he left the latter position in 1971).

He also served as chairman of the Committee on Arrangements for the Massachusetts Medical

Case 61.1. Kineplastic Forearm Amputation

"[The patient], a 21-year-old mill hand, was referred by Dr. Harold Kurth, of Lawrence. On October 9, 1941, he caught his left hand in a carding machine. It was practically stripped of soft tissue, and all the bones of the hand sustained multiple comminuted compound fractures. It was impossible to identify the tendons, so that amputation was decided on. This consisted of an ordinary flap amputation, which left a stump measuring 20 cm. from its distal end to the tip of the acromion. The flexor and extensor muscles were fastened to the ends of the amputated radius and ulna and the fascia to give anchorage for flexion and extension. Convalescence was uneventful on the vent full and the patient returned to work in 3 weeks.

"Having heard of Kessler's kineplastic amputation, he asked me to perform one. He was instructed to exercise the stump, going through the motions of closing and opening the fingers so as to develop and train the muscles of the forearm. He was most cooperative and did this religiously.

"On March 26, 1942, the kineplastic amputation was done. Two flaps were marked out according to the Kessler technique. The dressing was not changed for 10 days. The skin grafts which were small, took well. On May 7, measurements were taken and a cast was made, pins having been left in the skin tube for the previous 2 weeks. On July 13, the prosthesis was attached.

"At the present time, the patient is working full-time. He has become proficient in manipulating his fingers and is able to pick up his dinner pail, a suitcase, and a cigarette and to hold playing cards in his hand. In other words, following the application of the prosthesis he has learned to activate the artificial fingers with the muscle motors of his forearm as though he had his own fingers. The only complication was a slight irritation of the skin at the edge of the skin tube, which was probably due to the flaps having been made a little too large."

(John D. Adams 1943)

Society. Dr. Bailey published one paper. He died on September 11, 1998, in Sanford, Maine.

DAVID D. BERLIN

> **Physician Snapshot**
>
> David D. Berlin
> BORN: Unknown
> DIED: Unknown
> SIGNIFICANT CONTRIBUTIONS: Published an article about the best position to immobilize the wrist with a scaphoid fracture

Dr. David D. Berlin was an assistant in surgery in the outpatient department at Boston City Hospital and Beth Israel Hospital. At Tufts he was an instructor in anatomy and teaching assistant in surgery. His office was located at 68 Bay State Road, Boston.

In 1929 he published an article on a controversial topic: the best position to immobilize the wrist with a scaphoid fracture. Two schools of thought existed: flexion versus extension. Encouraged by Dr. Frederic Cotton, he dissected 60 wrists. In summary he wrote:

1. The major portion of the ligamentous structure…from the dorsal carpal ligament gains insertion on the proximal two-thirds of the dorsal surface of the navicular…bone…under tension with the hand in flexion, the navicular ligamentous slip…is likewise rendered taut and pulls the proximal fragment away from the distal one.

2. The approximation of the broken fragments is distinctly favored by the tendons of the flexor carpi radialis and the flexor pollicis longus. They act together as a sling to the navicular bone on its volar surface when the hand is placed in extension.

3. The small lateral interosseous ligament in the proximal row of the carpal bones is placed under tension when the hand is flexed to either side and…displaces the fragments…to produce lateral angulation.

4. The radial collateral ligament stretching from the radial styloid to the tubercle of the navicular…favors better alignment of fragments when the hand is extended to the radial side.

5. The position of choice in the treatment of carpal navicular fractures is about 45° extension of the wrist with radial deviation, avoiding extreme or forced extension.

Little is known about Dr. Berlin's additional accomplishments and personal life.

CHARLES H. BRADFORD

> **Physician Snapshot**
>
> Charles H. Bradford
> BORN: 1904
> DIED: 2000
> SIGNIFICANT CONTRIBUTIONS: Author of *Combat Over Corregidor*, a first-hand account of a combat paratroop jump in World War II; awarded the Silver Star for bravery; historian and poet

Charles Henry Bradford, known as "Charlie" to his friends and called "Chick" by his wife, Mary Lythgoe Bradford, was born on August 2, 1904, in Milton, Massachusetts. His father was the illustrious Dr. Edward H. Bradford, professor of orthopaedic surgery at Harvard Medical School and chief of the department at Boston Children's Hospital (soon to become dean of the medical school), and his mother was Edith Fiske Bradford. He had a twin brother, Edward, as well as a sister, Elizabeth. Bradford recalled many years later to a former colleague in the US Army, whose grandfather had been a great admirer of President Teddy Roosevelt, that Roosevelt and Bradford's father were great friends, and that Roosevelt often visited his father at the family's home.

Early Training and Career

After graduating from Brown and Nichols School in Cambridge in 1921, Bradford attended Harvard College with his twin brother. In 1925, their senior year, they played football together; Charles was a defensive lineman (guard) and Edward, an offensive end, and the two alternated playing in the backfield. Charles also captained the wrestling team and threw hammer in track and field. Charles went on to attend Harvard Law School for one year after graduating magna cum laude from Harvard College; but he then enrolled in Harvard Medical School. He completed medical school in 1931 at age 27, and he interned in surgery at Boston City Hospital and fulfilled a residency in orthopaedic surgery at the University of Iowa under Professor Arthur Steindler.

Returning to Boston after completing his residency, Dr. Bradford entered private practice, joining the staffs of Boston City Hospital and many other hospitals, including Mount Auburn and Faulkner hospitals. Apparently, after just a few years in practice, Bradford wrote a strong letter on March 2, 1937, to Harvard Medical School's dean, Dr. C. Sidney Burwell. He encouraged the dean to establish a fracture teaching clinic at Boston City Hospital: "There seems to me to be such fine possibilities at the Boston City Hospital for developing a fracture clinic that I am writing you a little report on the subject…I am not urging or recommending any policy…[only] to put at your disposal information which I have gained as a resident at the City Hospital during the past year." The year was 1937. Is Dr. Bradford referring to his year as an intern at Boston City Hospital or did he take a year of residency to learn about fracture care after completing his orthopaedic residency at Iowa? I was unable to answer these questions, but from Bradford's letter, I suspect that he took a residency in fracture care at Boston City Hospital after completing his orthopaedic residency.

Dr. Bradford wrote further, making five main points: First, he advocated for fracture treatment being included as a facet of orthopaedics, rather than general surgery, especially because of its importance in training up-and-coming orthopaedic surgeons, and avoiding a limitation of their scope of knowledge. Anyone interested in specializing in bone and joint disorders today is required to take an additional residency training so as to build their specialist knowledge in trauma. Bradford then went further, suggesting that fracture care was a specialty in itself: for various reasons, surgeons must receive additional training in order to learn about the particular equipment and treatment methods required for treating fractures (closed or open treatment); the special methods necessary to avoid sepsis during surgical procedures; the ability to understand and evaluate radiographs and other imaging modalities; the particular specialized knowledge required to use tools such as pins, nails, and wires in mobilization; and the more complicated methods for using plaster of Paris. For Bradford, all of this required specialist training which general surgeons do not have. Third, Bradford pointed out the large fracture-related case volume at Boston City Hospital—up to 2,000 annually. For him, this demonstrated the need for a group or clinic that treated fractures in particular. Bradford's last two points related to financial burden and staff acceptance of a fracture clinic. He mentioned the benefits that medical schools could glean from association with a hospital-based fracture clinic, which in turn would benefit the hospital itself in terms of sharing the financial burden. Finally, he recommended that Harvard cooperate with Tufts and Boston University to fund such a clinic with the dual goals of education and research. I was unable to find any response to Dr. Bradford's letter from Dean Burwell and the Harvard Medical School.

World War II

Volunteer in England

World War II began in 1939 with the invasion of Poland by Germany. In June 1940, Dr. Bradford was one of 12 volunteers (physicians and nurses) for a medical mission to England. Robert Osgood put forth the idea to send people to help, and Dr. Philip D. Wilson, who had left the Massachusetts General Hospital five years earlier to become the chief at the Hospital for the Ruptured and Crippled in New York City, gave his wholehearted support to the project and led the contingent with which Bradford volunteered. The project was supported by the Allied Relief Fund and private donors with the purpose of helping the British care for the war injured. The volunteers were paid $200 per month (~$3,690 in 2020). The number of injured soldiers and other hospitals already established throughout the country precluded the initial plan to set up an American-run hospital with 1,000 beds. Bradford's group was sent by the British Ministry of Health to Park Prewett Hospital in Hampshire. Park Prewett normally operated as a mental hospital, but its almost 1,500 beds were reallocated during the war to house wounded soldiers.

Most of the American team stayed in the UK for a limited period because of their positions and obligations back home; Wilson stayed about four months before returning to the United States. After Dr. Wilson returned to New York, Bradford stepped into his position as head of the American team of physicians, surgeons, and nurses. Bradford witnessed the eight months of bombing of London (The Blitz), which began in September 1940 and ended in May 1941. He treated many civilians injured in these frequent German attacks. In January 1942, Bradford returned to Boston, though he was immediately commissioned as a captain in the US Army Medical Corps and entered active duty.

The 1940 annual meeting of the British Orthopaedic Association was postponed until January 3, 1941. Many distinguished guests were invited to that meeting, including Dr. Bradford. Just one month before returning to the States, Bradford invited the administrator of the American Hospital in Britain to visit Sir Henry Gauvain, an expert on tuberculosis, who led the development of an open-air designed hospital for the treatment of tuberculosis at Treolar Cripples' Hospital in Alton. I suspect that Sir Henry was known by, if not friends with, Bradford's father, Dr. Edward H. Bradford. After his visit, the administrator recalled how happy Gauvain made the patients, mostly children, when he visited the hospital

Drs. Bradford and Wilson published one paper on their experiences at the American Hospital in Britain, "Mechanical Skeletal Fixation in War Surgery." After reviewing 61 cases of external pin fixation, they concluded that it was useful in military hospitals because of its benefits in treating fractures, particularly those that are infected and those in patients with shock and on long-term bed rest, and its use as a standard method for resolving fractures of the femur. They did, however, mention the need to evaluate potential issues and hazards of the procedure.

Bradford also used the Britten hip fusion technique to treat ununited hip fractures as a salvage procedure while stationed at Park Prewett Hospital. Dr. Otto Hermann (1942) wrote:

> Dr. Charles H. Bradford, who is with the American Hospital in England, describes a hip fusion method that is being worked out by Dr. Britten, who does the equivalent of a McMurray osteotomy, slides the shaft inward and lays a wide solid piece of tibial graft above it like a roof, firmly set in the chiseled groove in the ischium just below the acetabulum. Dr. Bradford considers this type of arthrodesis to be a revolutionary development that may replace all other forms of hip fusion. I mention it because I consider it much simpler and basically sounder than the prevalent hip-fusion methods.

Battle of Corregidor

As a newly commissioned officer in the US Army Medical Corps, Bradford was assigned to the 503 Airborne Division as a surgeon, and he headed the 2nd Battalion Unit. Called "Doc Bradford" or "Charlie," the men in his unit admired the

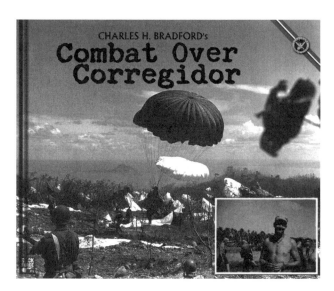

Cover of Charles Bradford's book, *Combat Over Corregidor*. Bradford is seen in the lower right inset. Courtesy of Paul F. Whitman (corregidor.org).

kindness and empathy Bradford showed the soldiers he cared for. Along with the troops, he parachuted under fire and helped to liberate the fortress at Corregidor in the Philippines (see chapter 64). Among the initial soldiers to arrive at the fortress and make contact with D company, he quickly began evaluating the company's numerous paratroopers who had been injured during fierce fighting in the night and required immediate treatment. For his bravery he was award the Silver Star.

The retaking of Corregidor in February 1945 has been described as among the most perilous of the war. One veteran who had fought with Bradford recalled, "Wherever you were, you could turn around and Charlie would be there" (quoted in "History in Sharp Focus" 2002). After that time, Bradford discussed the war very little. He did, however, write a manuscript, "Combat over Corregidor." Although he would not allow it to be published while he was living, he allowed it to be passed among the soldiers who fought with him, who read it and made copies and passed it along.

Dr. Bradford also saw action in New Guinea and later provided medical care in Cairns, Australia. While deployed, Bradford also formed close bonds with his companion soldiers. One such companion soldier, Larry Brown, recalled that they spent hours wrestling. Brown also recalled Bradford regaling him with stories of touring the United States on a motorcycle. I was unable to determine when he completed that tour.

After returning to the United States, Bradford worked in hospitals until the war ended; he was discharged in 1946. He returned to his private practice in Boston, on the staff of several hospitals, but working mainly at Boston City Hospital, Faulkner Hospital, Mount Auburn Hospital, Massachusetts Hospital School for Crippled Children, Longwood Hospital, Brooks Hospital, Parker Hill Medical Center, and New England Hospital. His office was located at 520 Commonwealth Avenue. See **Case 61.2** for an example of one of Bradford's cases.

Supporter of Civil Defense

Dr. Bradford's contributions to the literature were many: 12 articles about orthopaedic trauma, three books on history, two articles on civil defense, and 12 articles on history and opinion pieces. He also enjoyed writing poetry. A 1965 *Boston Globe* article suggested that most physicians are well-versed in not only the sciences but also the humanities, mentioning as an example the poetry Bradford wrote to engage his mind differently. Bradford had submitted two poems to the *Boston Globe*, via a letter to the editor, relating to securing the land around the Charles River as a park near the Anderson Memorial Bridge that connects Allston and Cambridge.

After the end of World War II, political and civilian unrest increased in Korea and in China. In the United States, "The Civil Defense Act of 1950…created authority for plans and preparations against the emergency of atomic war, but without unstinted public co-operation, no amount of planning can be successful" (Currier and Bradford 1951). That same year Dr. Bradford called on the medical profession to lead in the efforts to build a strong civil defense program. He described an attitude of indifference amongst physicians, stating, "The obstacle is the basic

Case 61.2. Tibial Spine Fracture

> "[The patient], a 15-year-old boy, was thrown from his bicycle and was brought to the hospital with his left knee in about 15° flexion. He was unable to extend it or to bear weight. He could flex the knee to 90°. An attempt to test the cruciate ligaments proved so painful that it was not carried out in full. X-ray films revealed elevation of the anterior spine of the tibia, together with a moderately large fragment from the upper tibial epiphysis. An attempt was made to reduce this fracture under anesthesia. Full extension could not be obtained until the operator placed his right and left thumbs on either side of the patellar tendon and pressed in deeply as he manipulated the knee toward extension. A sudden snap was then felt, giving the impression that the misplaced fragment had been reduced. Full extension could then be easily obtained, and in this position a long leg case was applied. The patient's postoperative course was uneventful. He was allowed on crutches on the 4th hospital day and was discharged on the 10th day, to be followed in the Out-Patient Department. The cast was retained for 3 weeks, after which he was allowed to walk on crutches without weight bearing. On his last visit, at the end of 3 months, he showed full, normal range of motion, and stated that he had no disability whatever. He was not limited in any way in his activity, and he had no pain."
>
> (Bradford, Adams, and Magill 1949)

belief that 'It won't ever happen to us'" (Bradford 1951). He recalled his experience in England: "The same problem confronted Britain in 1938–1939, when the possibilities of air attack were faced, and the people very wisely adapted laws that proved adequate in the crisis. They created an emergency medical service under a council and director with dictatorial powers. At the onset of the war, all doctors were subject to the orders of this service, and private practice virtually ceased" (Bradford 1951).

To emphasize the seriousness of the potential problem of an atomic bomb attack in New England, he gave the following example:

MAY 23, 1963

ANNUAL DISCOURSE

MEDICAL AIMS AND IDEALS*

CHARLES H. BRADFORD, M.D.†

BOSTON

Dr. Bradford's publication of his 1963 Annual Discourse to the Massachusetts Medical Society. *New England Journal of Medicine* 1963; 268: 1147.

It must also be remembered that the destruction of the cities will entail wholesale loss of their hospital facilities. A bomb centered over Copley Square in Boston, for instance, would certainly render ineffective the City Hospital, the New England Medical Center, the Massachusetts Memorial Hospitals, and the Peter Bent Brigham, the New England Baptist and Deaconess, the Children's, the Beth Israel, and the Massachusetts General Hospitals, as well as all the smaller hospitals in between – to say nothing of the possibility of including the Carney, St. Margaret's, St. Elizabeth's, Marine, Mount Auburn and Cambridge City hospitals, all of which lie within dangerous distance of the target area…Since this article was first prepared, it has already happened in Korea, and we hardly know on what front to expect the next assault. Although hysteria should be avoided, we must also avoid complacency or delay. "The affair cries, Haste and Speed must answer it!" (Bradford 1951)

Because of Dr. Bradford's and other leaders' efforts, "The Concord Plan" was adopted in 1951:

The Town of Concord, Massachusetts, has embarked on a training program. Spurred to

Box 61.1. Bradford's 1963 Lecture at the Massachusetts Medical Society

> "The Annual Discourse…affords a recurring opportunity for measuring the standards of our profession and for evaluating the principles on which they are based…To begin with, ours is essentially a scientific occupation, based on a scientific point of view. We deal with facts, not with faiths…let us begin by asking ourselves, what is our vision? And thereafter…What is our performance…a profession [contrasted to a trade] possesses a common purpose, under which its individual members become united and to which their private interests are subordinated…What then shall be said of medicine…I shall attempt to typify it with an illustration that I believe holds its deepest meaning. This occurred in the Philippine campaigns during the last world war, and it left a lasting impression on my mind. A messenger came running to our aid station to report that his patrol leader had been badly wounded and was being brought in by stretcher. We knew the man well, both as a fine friend and as a splendid soldier, and we hoped the wound would not prove too serious. But the runner immediately reported: 'Captain, he's hurt real bad. He's shot through the chest, and he's bled a lot, and on the stretcher, he keeps moaning, Oh, God, don't let me die; I want to live!' Before he reached the aid station, he was dead, but his words keep ringing in my thoughts for they seem to me to voice the appeal that humanity makes to the medical profession. From this incident, we can realize that here is a responsibility we share, with God. 'Don't let me die; I want to live.'
>
> "Our activities take on tremendous significance when we view them in this light. With such compelling motives, the medical profession has developed traditions of devoted service that transcend private interests and surmount social barriers, and reach to all people of all ranks, at all times. Because of this characteristic, the doctor is thrown into intimate contact with mankind as a whole, and his work becomes one of the most universal, as well as one of the most personal of all services.
>
> "This was a thought that my father recognized long ago, and described in words I have always cherished: 'The Doctor must be broadly human. He deals with the vagaries of age and the fancies of youth; the sports of boys, and the appetites of men. In his profession, he tests the aviator, rations the solder, estimates the endurance of the laborer, cares for the worried mother, and relieves the desk-ridden financier. His thought must reach to the ideals of the clergyman, and must interpret the flesh prompted dreams of the man of the world. And in this service, neither the precision of Science, nor the efficiency of business methods will suffice, for above all else, the practitioner must preserve and exercise the kindly indulgence of a considerate friend. In what academy can these lesions be taught? … As the doctor treats these tissues of mystery, he realizes how different is his profession from that of the engineer, who deals with physical forces and the physical materials, from the merchant, who exchanges commercial goods and commodities, or from the industrial laborer, who stands for long hours in the tedious production lines. The materials the doctor handles compose the very fabric of life itself; the mission he serves, the objective he seeks, and the *vision* that guides him, are best expressed in the words of the Gospel, *Give life, and give it more abundantly.*'
>
> "Here we should pause and turn from the aims and ideals of our profession to ask how far we have been able to convert our hopes into performances…it was not until about action by the outbreak of hostilities in Korea, the staff of the Emerson Hospital drew up a list of objectives, obtained the approval of the trustees, appointed a representative to act and went to work…Should a disaster occur in the Boston area today, Concord stands ready to meet the emergency with a fair chance of avoiding major confusion. (Dalrymple and MacDonald 1951)

Legacy

I was unable to find whether Dr. Bradford was on the Harvard Medical School faculty. He held an appointment of instructor in orthopaedics at Tufts College Medical School and was assistant professor of orthopaedics at Boston University School of Medicine, as a visiting physician on the

> a century ago that modern medicine began to be born. Up to that time…surgery confined itself almost entirely to dressing wounds, lancing abscesses, setting bones and amputating injured limbs. The specialties hardly existed at all, and medicine was a whole succeeded more through *Vis mediatrix naturae* – the healing force of nature – than through the physician's skills…The remarkable rapidity of their [triumphs] advance…most of their major developments have fallen within the living memories of our present senior members, or in the lives of their immediate predecessors, who taught them. They grew up in an age that is hard for us to visualize, filled as it was with 'the pestilence that walks in darkness, and the destruction that wastes at noonday.' They sat at the bedsides, and shared the sufferings and the tragedies of numberless patients who died hopelessly from complications that modern medicine could have relieved or prevented…And all this [modern surgery] is only the beginning, for medical science today is like a racket that has just left its launching pad and is approaching the edge of darkness, about to zoom off into unfathomed space…A new world of surgery awaits modern, scientific instrumentation…It even seems possible that biologic skills will learn to treat defects in the chromosome…medicine will have borrowed the role of destiny, in shaping man's future, and molding his fate…People everywhere, whether they realize it or not, live under the constant shelter and protection of the medical profession, and it becomes our obligation as doctors to make sure that adequate help is always available. We occupy both the front rank and the rear rank, the outermost and the innermost positions in the protective network of medical defense that shields the community; in this responsible position, we must never forget the lifesaving nature of our service, or the insistent duty that it imposes. If we neglect either, we cease to be physicians in the true sense of the word and become mere technicians, or merchants of health.
>
> "So much then, for our vision; so much for our performance. Of both, it may be said that they have created and thus far maintained the finest medical care ever conceived in history. Here, in America, they have produced a standard and quality of care that is nowhere excelled, and seldom equaled. Patients journey here from every continent to share its benefits, and from every nation, doctors arrive seeking its knowledge. Here, we study and adapt the brilliant contributions of foreign clinics, together with our own, and in return we render a co-ordinated type of medical practice that leads the world.
>
> "We should not close without recognizing that there is always need for further progress. What has been done well today must and will be done better tomorrow. Medicine must march *with* the times, not *against* the times, and wherever it can enlarge its service by governmental programs, it should welcome the opportunity – so long as this does not destroy the individuality and initiative and personal responsibility on which its effectiveness rests. For the future, let us hope that medicine may escape from political entrapment, that the splendid treasure house of healing will never be exposed by visionaries to the plunder of demagogues and that physicians may always continue to confront the perils of life and the challenges of death with unhindered freedom in their God-given profession."
>
> (C. H. Bradford 1963)

VI (Bone and Joint) Surgical Service at the Boston City Hospital. In 1963, he was invited to give the Annual Discourse at the annual meeting of the Massachusetts Medical Society. His lecture was titled "Medical Aims and Ideals." See **Box 61.1**.

Bradford was a long-time trustee of the Cotting School (formerly the Industrial School for Crippled Children), which was founded by his father and Augustus Thorndike. He was chairman of the board in 1967 when it was announced in the Bradford library that an open-air classroom had been replaced by a music room. It must have reminded him of his visit to Alton's Treolar Hospital to visit Sir Henry Gauvain and his open-air treatment rooms for children with tuberculosis. He was also on the board of trustees of the Massachusetts

Hospital School in Canton (recently renamed the Pappas Rehabilitation Hospital in memory of Dr. Arthur Pappas); a member of the Rotary Club and the Harvard Club; and a benefactor of the Massachusetts Historical Society, the Perkins Schools for the Blind, and Jordan Hospital in Plymouth.

In addition to his book on the Corregidor battle in World War II, Bradford published two books about the battles with the British in Boston during the Revolution. He published two papers in the Doctors Afield series in the *New England Journal of Medicine*: "Joseph Warren" and "Leonard Wood"; four papers in the Countway Happenings series: "John Jeffries, 'Astronaunt,'" "James Thatcher, MD," "John Warren," and "Resurrectionists and Spunkers"; and one unpublished manuscript, "Dorchester Heights. Prelude to Independence."

On Wednesday, May 17, 2000, Dr. Charles Bradford died of a heart attack in Jordan Hospital in Plymouth, Massachusetts. He was 95, living in Marshfield, just north of Plymouth. He was survived by his sister Elizabeth, also of Marshfield.

JOSEPH H. BURNETT

Physician Snapshot

Joseph H. Burnett
BORN: 1892
DIED: 1963
SIGNIFICANT CONTRIBUTIONS: Medical supervisor for Boston public schools; expert in secondary schools' sports injuries

Dr. Joseph Burnett had an interest in orthopaedics, especially sports injuries; his attraction to sports medicine began early in his career, when in 1919, after completing his internship, he became the medical supervisor for Boston public schools. He was later appointed junior visiting surgeon at Boston City Hospital, where he remained on staff for his entire career. Initially an assistant in anatomy at Harvard Medical School and assistant in surgery at Boston University, he was promoted to instructor in clinical surgery at Boston University School of Medicine. His office address was 520 Commonwealth Avenue, Boston.

In a Boston City Hospital Staff Clinical Meeting in 1927, Dr. Burnett reported on several cases of scaphoid fractures. (See **Case 61.3** for an example.) As a result of a discussion of his presentation by the staff at that meeting, Burnett did a follow-up study on 37 of 73 cases of scaphoid fractures treated in the clinic. When he first presented his cases, they were:

> an example of conservative therapy. At that time, it seemed desirable to approve of that treatment, rather than any other, because the results were very satisfactory. Since then the pendulum has swung in the opposite direction and it would not appear that many of the cases need an operation...these cases were grouped on the basis of good, fair and poor results... the latter two combined totaling twenty cases that were not at all satisfactory...that the cases under thirty years of age do not fare as well as those over thirty years...One of the

Case 61.3. Carpal Scaphoid Fracture

> "[The patient], chauffeur-mechanic, aged 47, fell, in August, 1929, injuring his wrist. He wore a leather splint for two months without relief. In February, 1930, he was at the hospital because of pain, weakness and inability to push. Graft operation April, 1930. In plaster case for ten weeks. Plate 1 shows the case before operation and immediately following operation: plate 2 a year later, showing presumable fibrous union, a clinically excellent result."
>
> (Joseph H. Burnett 1934)

fair results operated upon by John Adams, of the Boston Dispensary, very successfully making use of a bone graft. This is the only case… where this procedure has been performed. The other operative cases have had the usual technique of removing all of the proximal fragment, leaving a small portion of the distal [Dr. Burnett concluded]. In cases with obvious displacement, operate at once. Cases that have had little or no treatment…with a poor wrist…should be operated upon…Those cases presenting early, without displacement of fragments, should be treated conservatively, i.e., splinting for at least six to eight weeks…The cases thus treated with a poor result at the end of three months should be allowed an operation if they so desire. (Burnett 1929)

That same year, in 1929, he joined the Bone and Joint Service at Boston City Hospital. Five years later, Burnett published his last paper on scaphoid fractures. In a review of treatment of these fractures he stated:

Recent cases in good position are best treated by immobilization and rest, hoping for bony union. There is considerable difference of opinion as to just how the hand should be held… many using the cock-up position and many others using the reverse, i.e., slight volar flexion with radial flexion. Many years ago while working with Dr. Cotton and Dr. Berlin, this phase was studied at length and the conclusion arrived at that the cock-up was preferable…Dr. Berlin working on the cadaver has shown that the cock-up position gives better apposition…Immobilization regardless of how obtained should be maintained for at least six weeks, followed by baking and massage for a few weeks…The cast is applied in the cock-up position with slight radial flexion to include the palm of the hand and the base of the thumb, but does not limit the motion of the fingers…Cases with marked separation or communication of fragments should be operated on at once removing part or all of the bone. Here again… is much difference of opinion. Dr. Speed believes in removing the entire bone. Dr. Cotton believes it is better to leave in part of the distal fragment [to provide] a more stable joint. The distal fragment has a much better blood supply than the proximal…the third group of cases…represent the crippling ones that have had months of trial with the resultant pain and weakness so often seen…that have gone on to mal-union, cavity formation, bone formation along the radial styloid, to a definitely poor result…Dr. John Adams of Boston, so far as I know, was the first one to resort to the graft operation for these cases. It was thought at first that his produced bony union; but time has proved that the union is fibrous in most cases. However, clinically, this operation gives a good result in the few cases tried and should be used more extensively. The remarkable thing about it is that the patients are satisfied and feel entirely relieved from their previous symptoms. In performing this operation, I have grafted a piece of the tibia; others…use…the radius on the same arm. Some men believe in the bone peg instead of the graft. The peg operation is much easier, but…does not stabilize the parts so well as the graft. (Burnett 1934)

Burnett's early interest in sports-related orthopaedic injuries continued throughout his career—for 44 years he treated injured athletes playing football, track and hockey. Many acknowledged him as the leading expert in the field of athletic injury; he published and spoke widely of his ideas about the subject, and about preventing injury. His primary concern was for the young players, and he would not hesitate to cancel games because of poor weather. His career reached an apex when the city's English High School recognized his influence and achievements—even though he had graduated from their competitor in all sports, Boston Latin School.

In 1940, Dr. Burnett published a paper on football injuries in Boston's secondary schools. He praised the fact that Dr. Augustine Thorndike Jr. was "in complete charge of all injured players during the games and the sole judge of which of them are to continue in play. He examines these men on the field of play. What a contrast there is to the custom at one of Harvard's great rival colleges, where a trainer is sent on to the field... to judge an injured player's condition" (Burnett 1940).

Burnett reviewed the incidence and types of injuries in the Boston high schools from the 1939–40 season. Following Dr. Thorndike's example, he wrote:

> a doctor is present at all games with absolute authority as regards the continuance of injured players in the games...From this list it readily appears that injuries of a crippling or permanently disabling nature are rare...The severity of the injuries can...be...controlled by the elimination of players who have been injured during a game or who have become over fatigued. It should be the duty of the doctor at the game to see to it that all such players are promptly removed...
>
> The number of injuries sustained in organized play contrasts sharply with the number received by boys who play on the streets, in vacant lots and backyards, in parks and so forth...Judging from the records of the Boston City Hospital, the conditions created by this situation have become worse each year for the past few years. Over the week ends from late September until early December, it is customary to treat from twenty-five to thirty boys in the accident ward of the Boston City Hospital from football injuries alone...The headmaster of a Boston high school recently stated that he is constantly having absentees on Monday morning, or receiving requests from boys... to go to their doctors...or more often to hospitals, to seek relief from injuries occurred over the week end, particularly on Sundays... it is evidence that the worst injuries are to be found in unorganized groups. This type of play is unsafe...the boys play...without supervision, without officials, with no medical care... and usually without protective equipment... They play on hard ground, sometimes on pavement...subject to treatment that is against the rules, namely, clipping, piling, the illegal use of hands, holding, slugging and unnecessary roughness...It is to this unorganized group that all those interested in physical education and athletics should turn their attention in the future...Young America will play football, with or without helpful supervision, so that it is the duty of their elders to help regulate the playing of juveniles. (Burnett 1940)

> **FOOTBALL***
>
> A Review of Injuries in Boston Secondary Schools
>
> JOSEPH H. BURNETT, M.D.†
>
> BOSTON

Title of Joseph Burnett's article in which he reviewed high school football injuries in the 1939–1940 season. *New England Journal of Medicine* 1940; 223: 486.

He called on parents, teachers, coaches, playground supervisors, boys' clubs, Boy Scout leaders, athletic officials and parent–teacher associations to help in this effort. He also worked with the Savings Bank Life Insurance Company for four decades, as its medical director.

In March 1949, he was appointed the surgeon-in-chief of the Third Surgical Service at Boston City Hospital. City Hospital experienced numerous challenges that year, including difficulties with determining what medical schools it would affiliate with, issues with a service chief's retirement, and the decision by the American Medical Association's Council on Medical Education in Hospitals to decline approval of a fourth year in the hospital's surgical residency program. After this setback the trustees considered opening up affiliations with the hospital's surgical service to Harvard, Tufts, and Boston University, but it still had to grapple with the contested issue of favoring seniority in promotions. In the spring of 1951, Thomas W. Wickham, the Fourth Surgical Service's surgeon-in-chief, retired and Burnett moved into that role; Eugene O'Neil took his place as chief of the Third Surgical Service. Dr. O'Neil had established a varicose vein clinic at City Hospital and developed a peripheral vascular disease program on the Third Surgical Service. After just four years (1953–57) as a visiting orthopedic surgeon on the hospital's Bone and Joint Service, Burnett retired.

Throughout his career, he held memberships in the Massachusetts Medical Society, the American College of Surgeons, the American Medical Association, and the Belmont Masonic Lodge. Dr. Joseph Burnett retired in 1958. He died five years later, on January 24, 1963, at the age of 70. He was survived by his widow, the former Margaret Rogers.

G. KENNETH COONSE

> **Physician Snapshot**
>
> G. Kenneth Coonse
> BORN: 1897
> DIED: 1951
> SIGNIFICANT CONTRIBUTIONS: Clinical-investigator; expert in shock; chief of orthopaedics at Newton Wellesley Hospital, 1947–1951

George Kenneth "Ken" Coonse was born in 1897 of Scottish descent. He spent his early life in Seattle, Washington, where he was raised mostly by his aunt and attended public schools. His father traveled often and "his mother died shortly after his birth; he therefore had no remembrance of her" ("George Kenneth Coonse 1897–1957" 1951). He completed military service during World War I, but we have little historical record of those details. He received his bachelor's degree from Leland Stanford [Stanford] University in 1920 [and] entered Harvard Medical School in 1920, from which he graduated in 1924. He may be styled a 'self-made man,' since the expenses of his education were, for the most part, met by what he earned in outside work" ("George Kenneth Coonse 1897–1957" 1951).

Dr. Coonse then served three internships: at Boston City Hospital, Boston Children's Hospital, and the Massachusetts General Hospital (MGH). He was elected a member of the Massachusetts Medical Society in 1927. The following year, "he became assistant in orthopedic surgery at Harvard Medical School and an assistant orthopedic surgeon at Newton-Wellesley Hospital and the New England Peabody Home for Crippled Children" (Van Gorder, Dunphy, and Fried 1951). He was also on the fracture service in the outpatient department of the MGH.

In his first couple of years in practice in Boston, Coonse published two papers while at the MGH: his first was on synovectomy in chronic arthritis, which he cowrote with Dr. Nathaniel Allison (see chapter 36); his second was titled, "Treatment of Fractures of the Humerus by Mobilization and Traction," written with Howard Moore. In the paper on synovectomy, the authors reviewed 50 synovectomies completed on the orthopaedic service at MGH from 1923 to 1928. Among the 50 patients who underwent synovectomy, 33 (65%) had good outcomes, mainly pain relief and the ability to begin weight bearing. Coonse and Allison concluded that in a total synovectomy, including both menisci, helps to relieve pain more completely, especially shortly after the procedure. They did note, however, that acute arthritis resulting from gonorrhea contraindicates synovectomy.

It was at this time, while publishing his first two papers, that Dr. Coonse accepted the position of professor of orthopaedic surgery at the University of Missouri and surgeon-in-charge of the Orthopaedic Service at Missouri's University Hospital in 1929. He was also named chief surgeon, State Crippled Children's Services at the University of Missouri and consulting orthopaedic surgeon at Boone County Hospital, Columbia, Missouri. Dr. Guy L. Noyes, the dean of the University of Missouri Medical School, announced that the school would be opening numerous clinics statewide and that Coonse would be leading the process.

In his second paper on treatment of humerus fractures with mobilization and traction, published the following year, Coonse and Moore (1930) reviewed the:

> end results of more than seventy-five fractures of the humerus treated on the fracture service at the Massachusetts General Hospital, Boston, [and] one of the authors was particularly impressed with the marked limitation of both elbow and shoulder joint motion which frequently occurred. This functional limitation often handicapped the individual and prevented the resumption of normal economic and social activities for many months...We have attempted to solve the problem by utilizing standardized apparatus and recognized procedures...Thomas or Jones-Murray humerus splint to which is attached a flexible forearm piece (Pierson attachment) suspended from an overhead frame or bar...Traction is applied in the line of the humerus...traction stops are also applied to the forearm...to allow active and passive motion of the elbow joint. The humerus splint is so suspended that a moderate amount of active and passive motion of the shoulder can be maintained.

They reported their results using this new method in seven cases followed for up to 1.5 years after an average length of stay of 37 days. Coonse and Moore (1930) stated:

> The average time in which the males returned to normal economic activity was forty-one days. The average time in which the females resumed normal activities was thirty-seven days...We believe that the method described is ideal for treatment of uncomplicated fractures of the humerus[;] it prevents...joint adhesions and stiffness [and] promotes increased circulation to the injured part with consequent rapidity of callus formation and repair of the fracture [and] prevents atrophy of the muscles. Economically, there is tremendous saving to the individual...as the period of disability has been greatly shortened...The method requires careful hospital supervision.

The next year, while working with the chief technician at the University of Missouri, Coonse developed an improved, simpler, and less cumbersome apparatus for treating humerus fractures.

It was also at the University of Missouri that Coonse met an undergraduate student who was interested in medicine, Otto E. Aufranc (see chapter 40). In his autobiography, Aufranc recalled meeting Coonse and described his admiration for him. Coonse had taken Aufranc under his wing, acting as mentor and letting him help during slow times with small tasks such as changing dressings and removing stitches, and even helping patients with exercises and assisting in physical examinations. In particular, Coonse taught Aufranc to be thorough, to take time with and actively listen to patients. This early experience stuck with and benefitted Aufranc throughout his career, helping him easily cultivate great rapport with his patients.

While a student at the University of Missouri Medical School, Aufranc coauthored a paper with Dr. Coonse and Maurice Cooper (a resident), "Importance of Intrapleural Pressures and Their Measurements in Various Pathologic Conditions," describing a series of experiments they conducted on dogs. Aufranc graduated from Missouri with a bachelor of science degree both in arts and sciences and in medicine. Coonse had by then returned (in 1932) to Boston to work "as instructor in orthopaedic surgery at Harvard Medical School, orthopaedic surgeon, Newton-Wellesley Hospital, and junior visiting surgeon, Boston City Hospital Bone and Joint Service" as well as in Dr. Elliott Cutler's lab at Peter Bent Brigham Hospital (Van Gorder, Dunphy, and Fried 1951). His office was located at 370 Commonwealth Avenue. A few years later he moved his office to 270 Commonwealth Avenue.

Their relationship continued when Aufranc, at Coonse's urging, applied to Harvard Medical School and upon acceptance moved to Boston. Once in Boston, Cutler gave Aufranc a job in his laboratory at Peter Bent Brigham Hospital. In Cutler's lab, Coonse and Aufranc continued their collaboration, performing an experimental study on dogs. The resulting paper, "Traumatic and Hemorrhagic Shock, Experimental and Clinical Study," was published in the *New England Journal of Medicine*. Coonse published two more papers with Aufranc based on their research in the surgical research lab at the Peter Bent Brigham Hospital: one onintrapleural pressure effects on circulation and the other on peritoneal immunity from amniotic fluid.

During this period, Coonse simultaneously influenced the treatment of shock as a recognized

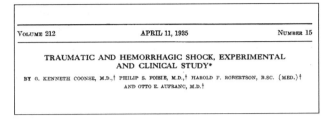

Coonse, Aufranc, and colleagues' article on shock, based on animal studies in the PBBH surgical laboratory. *New England Journal of Medicine* 1935; 212: 647.

expert at Boston City Hospital. Dr. Otto Hermann (1937) wrote, "In addition to the conventional method of shock treatment we have for the past few years treated shock by hourly intravenous injections of 50 cc. of sodium bicarbonate solution, prepared according to the formula and method advocated by Dr. Kenneth Coonse of the Boston City Hospital. If there is any shock with hemorrhage, a transfusion is given."

Coonse's personal activities included often rowing on the Charles River through the Union Boat Club. On December 1, 1939, during practice, the ice on the river cut into his outrigger, causing a leak and beginning to sink it. Coonse continued rowing toward the landing but soon had to abandon the boat; he swam to a jetty, and two teenagers who saw the accident took another boat out to retrieve him. Other than being cold and wet, Coonse was unharmed.

Despite remaining active throughout his life, in the early 1940s, "his application for service in World War II was refused after two examinations, because of high blood pressure" ("George Kenneth Coonse" 1951). He had previously served during "World War I and [was] a commissioned surgeon in the Public Health Service Reserve Corps." Coonse continued to make contributions, especially to the orthopaedic literature over the course of his career. A major original contribution was a new approach to the knee joint with a patellar turndown procedure he cowrote with Dr. John D. Adams in 1943 (see **Case 61.4**). Adams was an assistant in orthopaedic surgery at Harvard Medical School (Graduate Medicine), an instructor at Tufts, and the orthopaedic surgeon-in-chief at the Boston Dispensary. The authors described the various advantages of their contemporary procedure, which they performed on patients ranging from 18 to 70 years old. These benefits included extensive exposure (excellent for both arthrodesis and synovectomy) with little retraction required, scant trauma to the knee joint, and an incision that mostly avoids blood vessels. The approach also allows knee flexion without breaking the sutures. They also mentioned both the lack of quadriceps weakness and no functional deterioration after the procedure.

Dr. Coonse published about 18 articles and a few book chapters, and "from 1947 until his death [he] was chief of the Orthopedic Service at

Case 61.4. Patellar Turndown Procedure: A New Approach to the Knee

"[The patient], female, age 70 years. Patient stated that while outdoors on the afternoon of February 6, 1942, she slipped on the wet pavement and fell forward to the ground onto her hands and knees. In trying to get up from the sidewalk, she fell again, this time falling sharply onto her right knee, and she was unable to get up. She was assisted to her feet but her right knee was extremely painful and she was unable to move it. She was then assisted home and was brought to the hospital by the house ambulance. Patient was admitted to the ward after having been in the plaster room where a long leg cast was applied with no attempt at reduction. Closed reduction was attempted on February 9, 1942, and x-ray films showed still some displacement of fragments. On February 19, 1942, open reduction with fixation of the lateral condyle by means of two metal bolts and nuts was done. Patient was returned to the ward and the leg was suspended in balanced overhead suspension. X-ray examination on February 25, 1942, showed good position. On March 4, 1942, all sutures were taken out and the wound was clean and healed. On March 9, 1942, balanced suspension was removed and on March 13, 1942, patient was up and about on crutches with no weightbearing. Patient was discharged on March 14, 1942, on crutches with no weight bearing.

"Operative note. Under general anesthesia, with a tourniquet about the right upper thigh, the leg was prepped with 2 per cent iodine and draped with the extremity free. A 7-inch incision was made on the anterior aspect of the lower femur and knee joint in the midline. After the skin and subcutaneous tissues had been retracted, a Y-shaped incision with the stem pointed proximally was made in the quadriceps tendon. This allowed the patella to be turned down distally. The quadriceps muscle was then stripped up from the lateral condyle for about one-half its width. The fragment was opposed to the main shaft fragment and 2 bolts were inserted through drill holes to the main shaft fragment and two bolts were inserted through drill holes and nuts applied on the medial aspect. The articular cartilage in the joint was not exactly anatomical but the position was good. The wound was then sprinkled with about 3 grams of sulfanilamide crystals and the Y incision in the quadriceps tendon closed with No 1 chromic catgut continuous sutures. Several interrupted sutures were taken also. The subcutaneous tissue was closed with fine plain catgut and the skin closed with a running black silk suture. Postoperative condition was excellent. Patient returned to the ward and put in a Thomas splint with a Pearson attachment.

"On February 18, 1943, patient stated that she was able to carry on all her normal activities and had no symptoms referable to the right knee. She did not limp. Examination at this time showed that the incision was well-healed. She had complete extension. Both knees appeared symmetrical. She had flexion to about 40 degrees beyond the right ankle. No increased anteroposterior mobility and she had no appreciable increase in lateral mobility. There was a slight amount of thickening. The midpatella on the right was 14-¾ inches; upper border of patella 14-½ inches, and lower border 13 inches; midpatella on the left was 14 inches; upper border of patella 14 inches and lower border 12-½ inches. There was some creaking in both knee joints, not any more appreciable on the right than on the left."

(Coonse and Adams 1943)

Newton-Wellesley Hospital" (Van Gorder, Dunphy, and Fried 1951). He was a member of, and served actively with, various local and national professional associations (**Box 61.2**).

Box 61.2. Ken Coonse's Professional Memberships

Member
- Boston Orthopedic Club
- New England Regional (Massachusetts) Committee on Fractures of the American College of Surgeons (while Dr. Joseph H. Shortell chaired the New England chapter)
- Committee of Arrangements for Suffolk District of the Massachusetts Medical Society
- American Medical Association
- American Orthopaedic Association (1943)

Diplomate
- American Board of Orthopaedic Surgery

Fellow
- American Academy of Orthopaedic Surgeons
- American College of Surgeons (1934)

Dr. Ken Coonse died suddenly on February 15, 1951, at the age of 55. He and his wife, Hilda Gant Shepard, had two daughters. His obituary, written by an unnamed friend, was published in the *Journal of Bone and Joint Surgery*:

> It is not a difficult task for a friend who knew him intimately to eulogize Ken Coonse. Strange to say, this man was very shy and diffident and he had comparatively few intimate friends. People were attracted to him for the charm of his personality; and members of the profession recognized his ability, both as a surgeon and as a counselor. In his skill as a surgeon, he embodied the necessary qualifications of experience and judgment.

> Ben Jonson once said: "That old bald cheater, Time; beware of him." I know of no other person to whom these words can be more aptly applied than to our friend Ken. Time meant nothing to him except as the medium in which he could do the things he liked to do best. Many of his original thoughts unfortunately never came to fruition. He never allowed anything to interfere with his daily exercise, which included a three-mile run every morning with his dog, or a twelve-mile row on the river in his shell, or a game of handball at the Union Boat Club.

> A fact little known to anybody except his intimate friends was that he was a diving champion on the Pacific Coast. He defied the elements: he never wore an overcoat, undershirt or vest, rubbers or overshoes and was, in the judgment of all of us who knew him so well, the picture of health and physical fitness.

> He abhorred hypocrisy; he was sincerely honest in all his dealings, and his criticisms of individuals were always constructive. He never ventured an opinion unless he was asked for it. He could be termed a 'seeker of truth.' He was kind, modest, and gentle, ever thoughtful of the needs and desires of his friends and family. He possessed a certain quality of thoroughness, based upon a definite method and plan, and he never failed to practice the art of discretion. One of his outstanding characteristics was the charm of his humility. He accepted his failures in surgery or on controversial matters always with a smile and never with resentment.

> His life was full of things well done and presented such a wide field of activities that it is difficult to enumerate them. His great love was his farm, around which his entire life developed. He never recognized physical fatigue, and the products of his farm were generously contributed to all his friends and to the needy of the community.

> His sudden death has left avoid which will not be filled in the hearts of his friends. His

passing is a great loss to the medical profession, as his original ideas would certainly have furnished many scientific contributions in orthopaedic surgery. As a tribute to his memory, we all can say that he was a master surgeon, a wise counselor, a loyal friend, and a prince of good fellows. ("George Kenneth Coonse" 1951)

ROBERT INGERSOLL

> **Physician Snapshot**
>
> Robert Ingersoll
> BORN: Unknown
> DIED: Unknown
> SIGNIFICANT CONTRIBUTIONS: Founded the Crippled Children's Clinic (or the "Polio Clinic") at Boston City Hospital

Dr. Robert Ingersoll graduated with an MD degree in 1939 from the University of Rochester School of Medicine. He lived at 14 Bradford Street in Belmont and applied for a fellowship in the Massachusetts Medical Society (in the Middlesex South District) in 1948. Seven years later, in 1955, he founded the Crippled Children's Clinic (also known as the "Polio Clinic") to care for the numerous children affected in the then-recent polio epidemic.

In addition to working in the polio clinic, Ingersoll was an attending surgeon on the VI Surgical (Bone and Joint) Service at Boston City Hospital and on the clinical faculty at Tufts University School of Medicine. He published four papers: two on trauma, one on corrective osteotomy in Marie-Strumpell arthritis, and a paper on transfer of the peroneus longus to the anterior tibial tendon in poliomyelitis (1948–1965). In 1959, he presented a lecture on transplantation of the hand to the Massachusetts Chapter of the American Physical Therapy Association.

H. KELVIN MAGILL

> **Physician Snapshot**
>
> H. Kelvin Magill
> BORN: Unknown
> DIED: 1956
> SIGNIFICANT CONTRIBUTIONS: —

Dr. H. Kelvin Magill received both his B.A. (1931) and M.D. (1937) degrees from the University of Colorado. His appointment at Boston City Hospital was orthopaedic surgeon on the outpatient staff and assistant visiting surgeon on the fracture service. He was an instructor in orthopaedic surgery at Tufts and an associate surgeon at Newton-Wellesley Hospital. Magill was in private practice with offices located in Brookline and Winchester. Other hospital staff positions he held were at Winchester Hospital, Brooks Hospital (Brookline), and Sancta Maria Hospital in Cambridge. He authored or coauthored six papers. He died in 1956 at the age of 46.

CHAPTER 62

Pedagogical Changes
Harvard Leaves Boston City Hospital

The Bone and Joint Service (the Sixth Surgical Service) remained very active for the four decades between 1930 and 1970, mainly treating patients with traumatic injuries. Although some patients were admitted, most were seen as outpatients or in the various clinics of the Shortell Unit, e.g., the polio clinic, the special fractures clinic, etc. The service provided just 120 beds for adult patients, but there was no limit to the number of pediatric patients it could accept, mainly for fractures and other orthopaedic issues. **Table 62.1** enumerates a few of the various conditions treated and case volume of the service during 1963. That year, when Dr. Aitken left his position as chief, various interim chiefs led the service.

Table 62.1. Bone and Joint Service Case Volume during 1963

	Daily Average	Yearly Total
Inpatients (admissions)	—	1791
Outpatients	—	19,557
Shortell Unit (clinics)		25,126
Fractures	13	4698
Dislocations	1	368
Sprains	8	2952
Visits to specialized clinics	8	2744
Surgical procedures	2	757

Data from Byrne 1964.

ORTHOPAEDIC RESIDENCY PROGRAM AT BOSTON CITY HOSPITAL

The development of the orthopaedic training program at Boston City Hospital (BCH) began in the mid-twentieth century. The Sixth Surgical Service had focused on resident education since it opened in the late 1920s, and by 1964 more than 200 surgeons had been trained on the service. In his 1999 book on the history of orthopaedics at Tufts University, Dr. Henry Banks wrote that Dr. Frederick Cotton (chief of the service, 1928–31), with the help of Drs. Otto Hermann (chief, 1932–46) and Joseph Shortell (chief, 1946–1950) started to accept residents on the Bone and Joint Service as early as September 1928—the year the service opened. It remained unaffiliated with any particular medical school into the midcentury. In addition, the program was never associated with the Children's Hospital/Massachusetts General Hospital residency program, and I found no evidence that residents from the Children's Hospital/Massachusetts General Hospital program ever rotated through BCH's Bone and Joint Service.

The American Board of Orthopaedic Surgery (ABOS) was established in 1934, allowing surgeons to become board certified. Various organizations soon began applying for residencies and fellowships through the Board: In 1935, Otto Hermann received approval for a one-year residency for one resident at BCH, and R. N. Hatt received the same at Shriners Hospital for Crippled Children. In 1940, G. Edmund Haggert at the Lahey Clinic applied and was approved for a single fellow over one to three years. These residents were on duty almost daily but were paid little—just about $65 per month (~$1116 in 2014 dollars; ~$1200 in 2020 dollars). This was about the same amount I received as an *intern* at the Hospital of the University of Pennsylvania 20 years later, in 1965. Despite these initial strides in the early 1940s, however, and despite orthopaedic-related training at individual hospitals, e.g., BCH, Shriners, and the Lahey Clinic, no coordinated orthopaedic training/education program existed among these hospital programs.

A few years later, in 1946, Arthur Thibodeau created a three-year orthopaedic residency program at the West Roxbury Veterans Hospital. At that time the VA Hospital was not affiliated with any particular medical school. To be eligible for the program, residents had to have already completed a two-year residency in general surgery. They rotated among four hospitals—BCH, the VA Hospital, Massachusetts Hospital School, and Lakeville State Hospital. Residents received exposure to pediatric patients which chronic musculoskeletal conditions at the latter two locations.

In 1947, the number of board-approved residents began to increase: now two at BCH and four at the Lahey Clinic. Three years later, programs began to merge: in 1950 the orthopaedic services at BCH (led by R. Sullivan) and the Lahey Clinic (led by G. Edmund Haggert) combined to create Program 66 (as it was designated by the ABOS). Residents from both BCH and the Lahey Clinic began rotating through Shriners Hospital and the Massachusetts Hospital School in Canton (Dr. Paul Norton, of Norton brace fame, was chief there at the time) for training on pediatric conditions. The AMA listed the program in its residency directory a year later, in 1951. By 1952, the four institutions had fully coordinated to develop an orthopaedic residency program—one year at BCH, where residents saw trauma patients; one year at the Lahey Clinic, where they cared for adult patients; and one year at Shriners or the Massachusetts Hospital School, where they treated children. They also rotated through Lakeville State Hospital to gain experience in treating children with chronic conditions. The three-year program was officially called the Lahey Clinic Integrated Orthopaedic Program and led by Haggert. It accepted four residents each year, but—as in Thibodeau's program at the West Roxbury VA Hospital—only after they had completed preliminary training in surgery.

This collaboration, however, experienced issues from the start—for example, poor communication among the hospitals involved in the program and separate teaching staff at each. The chiefs at each institution met only to select residents. None of the orthopaedic surgeons from Lahey (except Leach) attended the open grand rounds at BCH. From the late-1960s, a lack of stable leadership and poor administration at BCH also caused problems: Charles Woodhouse, who became chief in 1967, dealt with many recurrent problems and was asked to resign. These issues were tempered, however, when Paul O'Brien became interim chief.

In the late-1950s, Dr. Richard Kilfoyle began a residency program at the Carney Hospital; at the time he was a member of the leadership there and at the Massachusetts Hospital School and the Lakeville Hospital (although Norton remained nominal head at Lakeville and the Massachusetts Hospital School). His program included pediatric rotations at the latter two institutions, as well as trauma and adult rotations at the New England Medical Center and BCH. (In 1990, after more than 30 years, this program was subsumed as part of the residency program at Tufts University, as a result of the field-wide trend toward building program foundations through universities.)

As more programs developed, the ABOS began dictating program requirements to help standardize them and ensure quality. In late 1969,

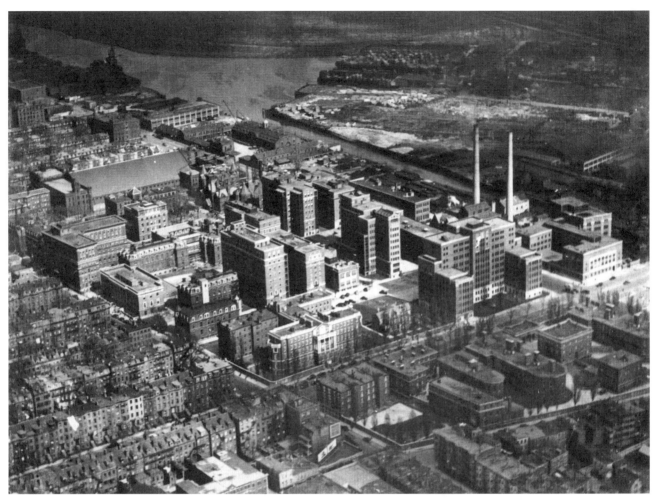

Aerial view of BCH, ca. 1960–1970. Boston City Hospital Collection, City of Boston Archives.

the ABOS required that Program 66, the Lahey Clinic/BCH program, develop an affiliation with a medical school. According to Dr. Robert Leach, who was then the chief of orthopaedic surgery at the Lahey Clinic, the ABOS proposed an affiliation with either Boston University or Tufts University as the program's parent institution. This would be a requirement of the ABOS's formal approval of the program. Leach chose Boston University; in doing so, he became a professor there, and at BCH he became the codirector of the Orthopaedic (Fracture) Service (a position he shared with Dr. Henry Banks, then just named chief of orthopaedics at Tufts University). Leach and Banks, along with Dr. Bart Quigley (a surgeon on the Harvard Surgical Service who focused on fractures and athletic injuries), created a well-respected teaching program, serving residents from various schools and hospital around the city.

The 1970s brought more upheaval to the residency scene. In 1970, the VA Hospital program became part of the larger Tufts University residency program; by that time, 55 residents had passed through a VA Hospital residency. In 1974, after five years of stability, the City of Boston determined that it had to reduce its financial commitment to BCH and thus elected to downsize the services BCH provided. To help it do so, the city's mayor, Kevin White, asked the three medical schools currently sending students there—Harvard, Tufts, and Boston Universities—to submit proposals outlining why they should retain their affiliation. The city ultimately selected Boston

Table 62.2. Clinical Courses for Harvard Students at Boston City Hospital (BCH), 1864–1974

Year	Description
1864	Clinical instruction in the surgery and ophthalmology clinics Minor surgery at the Boston Dispensary
1872	HMS published its own course catalog (separate from that of Harvard University) for three years of education No changes listed for teaching at BCH
1880	HMS increases to a four-year program Second year: surgery and clinical surgery at MGH and BCH Fourth year: clinical and operative surgery at MGH and BCH (taught at the latter by Drs. Cheever, Homans, William Thorndike, Ingalls, Fifield, and Gay)
1885	Bradford listed for the first time as a visiting surgeon (orthopaedics) at BCH; he lectured twice each week for three months First orthopaedic book recommended for students: *Human Skeleton*, by Humphreys
1886	Additional orthopaedic book added: *Joints*, by Morris
1887	Fourth year: Bradford lectures twice per week for three months
1889	Bradford now an instructor in both surgery and orthopaedics Fourth year: two lectures per week for two months
1891	Orthopaedic Surgery listed for the first time as a course for fourth-year students
1892	Third year: clinical surgery started by Bradford
1894	Third and fourth years: two lectures in clinical surgery per week for two months Second year: Clinical surgery taught by Lovett Third year: Operative surgery, with 15 practical exercises, taught by Lovett
1895	Orthopaedic Surgery listed for the first time separate from Surgery Courses for graduates now offered at BCH Courses in Clinical Surgery, Operative Surgery, and Minor Surgery offered by Lovett and other faculty at BCH
1901	Another book added for student reference: *The Treatment of Fractures*, by Scudder
1903	More books included as recommended reading: *Orthopaedic Surgery*, by Whitman *Orthopaedic Surgery*, by Bradford and Lovett *Orthopaedic Chirurgie*, by Hoffa
1904	Third and fourth years: Required orthopaedic courses on fractures, taught by Cotton Exam given for the first time New fracture course for graduates taught by Cotton

University to lead the hospital's program. This required Harvard and Tufts to find new homes for their students and residents.

Thus ended Harvard Medical School's 110-year relationship with BCH. Over that century, Harvard and Harvard Medical School had offered numerous clinical courses to their medical students who had been assigned to rotations at BCH, as described in the schools' course catalogues from 1864 until 1974. Some highlights are briefly described in **Table 62.2**, illustrating the development and expansion of orthopaedics residency training as the twentieth century progressed.

Chiefs of the Bone and Joint Service are listed in **Box 62.1**.

Box 62.1. Chiefs of the Bone and Joint Service

- Frederic J. Cotton 1928–1931
- Otto J. Hermann 1932–1946
- Joseph H. Shortell 1946–1950
- Russell F. Sullivan 1951–1954
- Gordon M. Morrison (acting) 1954–1955
- Alexander P. Aitken 1955–1963

Year	Description
1905	Fractures and dislocations courses taught by Codman (2)* Fractures course taught by Crandon (5)
1906	Fractures and dislocations courses taught by Crandon Orthopaedic Surgery at the Boston Dispensary (summer course) Only required orthopaedic course taken during the third year 15-minute exam required
1910	Books recommended to students: *The Treatment of Fractures*, by Scudder *Fractures and Dislocations*, by Stimson Summer course in orthopaedics remains at the Boston Dispensary
1916	Bone and Joint rotation started at BCH Specialty service rotations initiated at BCH Cotton becomes an associate in surgery
1928	Sever assigned to teach Harvard Medical School students at BCH
1929	Required third-year clinical exercises at Boston Children's Hospital and MGH Started required third-year clinical exercises at PBBH and BCH
1931	Clinical exercises taught by Ober and associates at Children's Hospital, MGH, PBBH, and BCH No mention of electives at BCH
1932	G. Kenneth Coonse named new instructor on faculty
1936	Third-year orthopaedic lectures (required) at Children Hospital; held daily for the first half of the year Clinical exercises (clinics) held at Children's Hospital, MGH
1938	Course in adult orthopaedics (including industrial surgery) offered at MGH, PBBG, and BCH
1942–55	Clinical experiences not offered at BCH: Harvard medical students were pulled out of BCH because of irreconcilable differences among the surgeons on the Second and Fifth Surgical Services
1953	Clinical exercises in orthopaedics resumed at BCH
1964	Required clinical exercises in orthopaedics at Children's Hospital, MGH, PBBH, Beth Israel Hospital, and BCH
1966	Introduction to Clinics (8 hours; in sections) Orthopaedic Surgery at Children's Hospital, MGH, PBBH, Beth Israel Hospital, and BCH Fractures and Related Trauma, taught by Quigley at BCH
1974	Harvard Medical School withdraws from its affiliation with BCH

(BCH, Boston City Hospital; MGH, Massachusetts General Hospital; PBBH, Peter Bent Brigham Hospital.)

*Refers to the number of times the course was offered throughout the year.

Section 9

Harvard Orthopaedists *in the* World Wars

"Those who cannot remember the past are condemned to repeat it."
—Quoted by **David LeVay**. *The History of Orthopaedics: An Account of the Study and Practice of Orthopaedics from the Earliest Times to the Modern Era*. Carnforth, Lanca, UK. The Parthenon Publishing Group, 1990:641.

"The lessons of war surgery have had to be relearned many times during the wars that have ensued. It should be remembered that in a war, many of the injuries are severe and very few are minor. Remember that delayed wound closure will not insure minor wounds and will save major wounds from the damage of infection and ischemia…in war wounds it is still necessary…to leave all wounds open and to close the wound when the danger of rapidly spreading infection has subsided."
—**Lewis N. Cozen, MD**. "Military Orthopedic Surgery." *Clinical Orthopaedics and Related Research*. 1985; 200:50.

"Sir Robert Jones calls an 'Orthopedic Conscience'…the prevention as well as the relief and cure of disability and deformity. Also, it came to mean opportunities for relief and cure where the patient himself had given up hope."
—**H. Winnett Orr**. *An Orthopedic Surgeon's Story of the Great War*. Norfolk, Nebraska, The House Publishing Co. December 1921.

CHAPTER 63

World War I
Trench Warfare

Following the assassination of Archduke Franz Ferdinand of Austria on June 28, 1914, Germany invaded Belgium and Luxembourg, then France. Britain declared war on Germany just a month later, on August 4, 1914. Throughout World War I, the approach to wound treatment would evolve significantly, as surgeons discovered that Listerian principles of chemical antisepsis, which had revolutionized surgery in the civilian setting, did not apply as well to the extensive wounds and filthy conditions that characterized a new era of trench and gas warfare. Field surgeons, trusting in the efficacy of this established approach, applied antiseptics such as camphor, formalin, carbolic acid (phenol), iodine, mercuric chloride, hydrogen peroxide, and lysol to soldiers' wounds. In many cases, they even sutured wounds after applying an antiseptic. The outcome was worse than any could have imagined. Wounded soldiers treated at the front reported to base hospitals with severely infected wounds, sepsis, tetanus, and gangrene. Among soldiers with amputation wounds that had been sutured on the field, fewer than 5% went on to heal primarily. The remainder, along with most other soldiers with wounds sutured at the front, had to have their wounds reopened to treat infection.

A breakthrough occurred in 1915 when E. T. C. Milligan published his opinion that the use of antiseptics for primary treatment of wounds was insufficient, as the infection fed on the dead tissue of the wound, grew, and spread. What was necessary, he proposed, was the aggressive excision of all foreign bodies and tissues involved in the wound—including damaged skin, fascia, and muscle—to stop the infection. Moreover, wounds should be left open to the air and allowed to drain freely, rather than be sutured and drained via inserted tubes. Milligan's proposed approach was adopted first during periods of relative calm at casualty stations and then on a broader basis at the front during the First Battle of the Somme (1916).

In adopting this approach, surgeons found that cocci rather than anaerobes (seen in gas gangrene) now populated the wounds. In addition to opening and excising wounds, surgeons also irrigated wounds with various antiseptics and eventually with hypochlorite or Dakin's solution (bleach). Combined with this irrigation, secondary suture became highly effective. Primary suture, however, quickly fell out of favor because of the poor outcomes associated with it early in World War I.

> *"Omne quod contusum est, necesse est ut putrescat, et in pus vertatur."* (Everything that is contused necessarily putrefies and is converted into pus.)
> —Hippocrates (Quoted by Serjeant-Chirgeon Richard Wiseman, attendant to Charles II, in exile in the late-seventeenth century.)

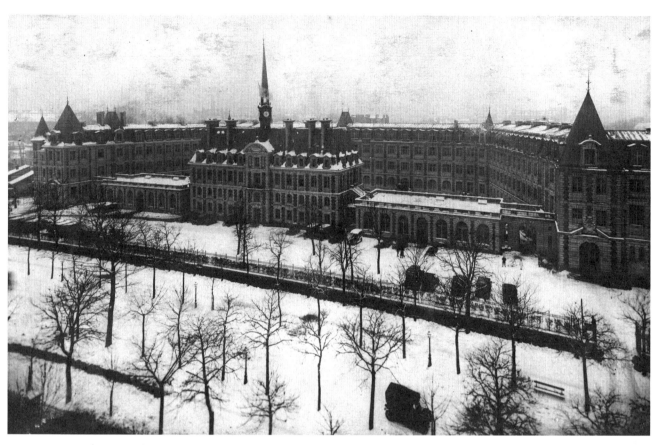

American Ambulance Hospital, Neuilly-sur-Seine, France. Located in the Lycée Pasteur secondary school on the outskirts of Paris. Courtesy of the Medical Center Archives of New York-Presbyterian/Weill Cornell Medicine.

BEGINNING OF THE GREAT WAR

After the first few months of World War I, US leaders and professionals recognized the need to aid the countries fighting Germany. The American Ambulance Field Service was the result, and "many Harvard men were among those at once pressed into the corps of workers in the [American Embassy in Paris]" (Cutler 1915). At a meeting on December 12, 1914, the president and fellows of Harvard College voted to approve "sending a contingent of surgeons from the Harvard Medical School to assume the care of the three surgical services of 150 beds each in the American Ambulance Hospital at Neuilly [France] for three months from April 1st to July 1st, 1915" ("Meeting of the President and Fellows of Harvard College" 1914).

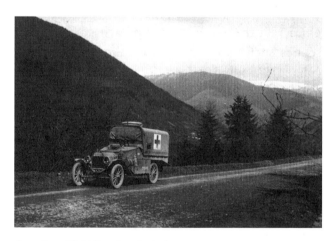

American Field Service Ambulance.
Lantern slide by Robert B. Greenough. Warren Anatomical Museum in the Francis A. Countway Library of Medicine.

Robert B. Osgood, who at the time was an assistant visiting orthopaedic surgeon at MGH, volunteered for these three months in Neuilly (see chapter 19), just outside of Paris. He was one of

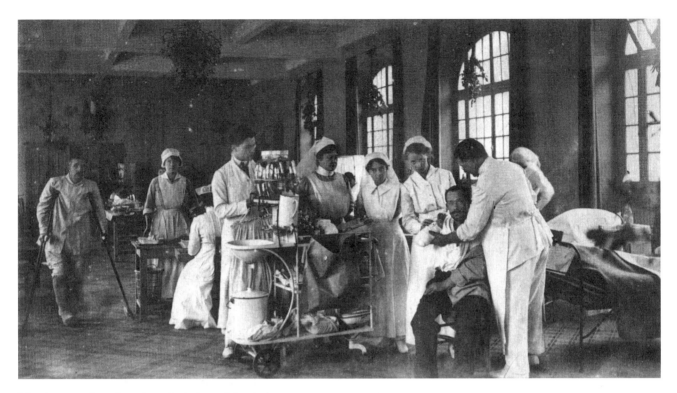

Morning rounds at American Ambulance Hospital. U.S. National Library of Medicine.

thousands of volunteers who felt a drive to contribute to the war effort in France, despite some US hostilities toward that country. Americans living in France at the time had established committees to publicize, raise funds for, and recruit for an initial volunteer ambulance service, called the American Ambulance Field Service, and this service allowed American volunteers to make a difference: 3,000 Americans volunteered to serve as drivers and hospital personnel over the course of the war, approximately 2,000 of whom were from Harvard, Cornell, and other American colleges and universities. Almost 350 of these volunteers came from Harvard alone.

In the US Army, medics and physicians, "men with medical training…[drove], looked after, and supervised" the ambulances they operated (Andrew 1920). As World War I commenced, the French ambulance service recognized the benefit of this service, whose "only role…was to get the wounded as rapidly and comfortably as possible from the battle-line to a field hospital, usually a few miles back, where they could

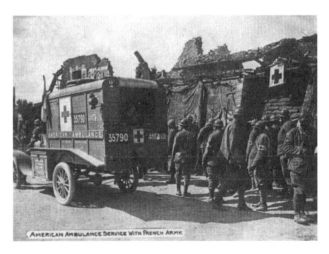

American ambulance with the French Army. National WWI Museum and Memorial, Kansas City, Missouri, USA.

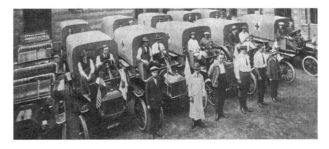

Fleet of Ford Ambulances with volunteer drivers. Boston Medical Library in the Francis A. Countway Library of Medicine.

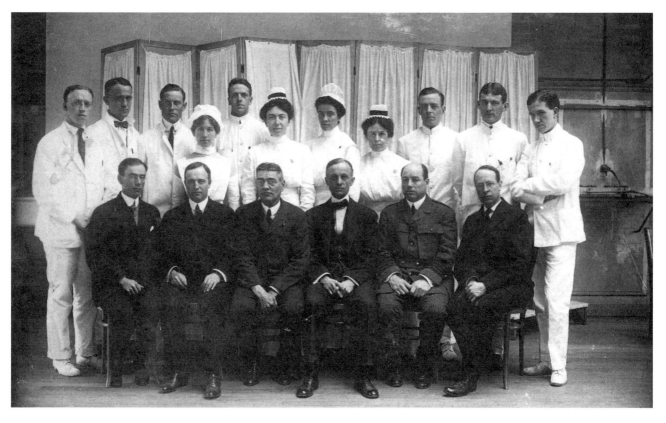

Harvard (Cushing) Unit at American Ambulance Hospital, April 1915. Dr. Cushing is seated in the middle (with bow tie). Dr. Smith-Petersen is standing at the far right. Boston Medical Library in the Francis A. Countway Library of Medicine.

receive proper treatment under advantageous conditions" (Andrew 1920). Beginning in late summer 1914, groups of 25–30 American volunteers were installed with the French army's ambulances, and their dedicated service provided "rapid transportation of the wounded…[which] rendered possible…the surgical treatment of wounded under much more favorable circumstances than in previous wars" (Andrew 1920). By the time the US Army arrived in France, 34 such groups had been working with French soldiers for almost two years, helping to ensure sanitary conditions during ambulance transports at battles like those at Ypres, Yser, and Verdun. This rapid transport of the wounded from the field to aid stations via ambulances was a key factor in reducing mortality among the wounded: "Lives saved by thousands, suffering attenuated, amputations avoided, families spared their fathers for after the war; these form only a part of the French debt toward the American Field Service" (Andrew 1920).

Even before the war began, and during its first two years, "money and hospital supplies were donated; automobiles were given and lent; men and women of all sorts offered their services… [and] a large hospital for the French wounded had been equipped and opened in the Lycée Pasteur in Neuilly…which can claim the single honor of having initiated American war relief work in France" (Andrew 1920). Housed in a converted school in a Paris suburb and boasting 170 beds, by June 1915, the hospital had expanded to 570 beds. Volunteers from Harvard came to the hospital (American Ambulance) to run the "University Service," to which 190 beds were allocated (across 18 wards) (**Box 63.1**).

The realities of World War I greatly affected the practice of surgery in the field. Immediate treatment in the field, however, had profound

Box 63.1. Initial members of the "Harvard Unit" at the Lycée Pasteur Hospital

> In mid-1915, Harvard sent a group of surgeons, residents, assistants, and nurses to staff the University Service at the Lycée Pasteur Hospital (American Ambulance) in Neuilly, France. From April through June, they provided care to soldiers wounded at the front (Cutler 1915):
>
> Dr. Robert B. Greenough, Assistant Professor of Surgery, executive officer and surgeon
> Dr. Harvey Cushing, Professor of Surgery, surgeon
> Dr. Richard P. Strong, Professor of Tropical Medicine, bacteriologist
> Dr. Robert B. Osgood, orthopaedic surgeon
> Dr. Robert H. Vose, orthopaedist
> Dr. Eben W. Fiske, orthopaedist
> Dr. Beth Vincent, assistant surgeon
> Dr. Fred A. Coller, resident surgeon
> Dr. Elliott C. Cutler, resident surgeon
> Dr. Walter M. Boothby, anesthetist
> Walter J. Dodd, radiologist
> Dr. Philip D. Wilson, house officer
> Dr. Maurius Smith-Petersen, house officer
> Dr. Lymon G. Barton Jr., house officer
> Dr. Orville F. Rogers Jr., medical assistant
> Dr. George Benet, laboratory assistant
> Edith I. Cox, operating-room nurse
> Geraldine Martin, operating-room nurse
> Helen Parks, operating-room nurse
> Marion Wilson, operating-room nurse

effects on wounded soldiers' survival, even before they arrived at the field hospitals:

> Stabilized trench warfare made prompt evacuation of the wounded practically impossible, and during major offenses, when the few roads were blocked by traffic and the wounded had only fourth priority, being superseded by men, ammunition and food, the patients reached the casualty clearing stations and evacuation hospitals in wretched condition (Mixter 1950).

One intervention that provided drastic survival advantage and outcomes was prompt and careful splinting of fractured limbs in the field before transport of the wounded soldiers. For example, about 80% of soldiers with a fractured femur died en route to evacuation hospitals during the first battle of Arras, in October 1914, when stretcher bearers did not splint injured limbs before lifting and transporting the wounded. In contrast, only about 30% of soldiers with such injuries died en route to evacuation hospitals during the second battle of Arras, in April and May 1917, when stretcher bearers *did* apply splints before transport. Specifically, Thomas splints with traction were used for femur injuries and Jones splints for arm injuries.

Soldiers did not need to have extensive wounds to be in critical condition: "It was soon evident that even the minor wounded faced almost certain death if they were operated upon as they arrived, in profound shock from exposure and starvation after hours on the battlefield" (Mixter 1950). Thus, field hospitals created "shock wards" in which to stabilize patients before they underwent a surgical procedure.

> "The five fingers that will win the war can be named men, money, munitions, food and, last but not least, health."
> —John R. McDill (*Lessons from the Enemy: How Germany Cares for Her War Disabled*. Vol. 5: *World War I Manuals*. Philadelphia: Lea and Febiger, 1918.)

In September 1915, Elliott C. Cutler wrote of the long road that soldiers wounded at the front traveled to receive treatment at a hospital:

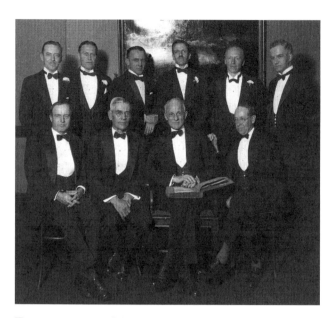

Ten-year reunion of the Harvard (Cushing) Unit of the American Hospital in Neuilly. Dr. Osgood is seated at the far right. To his left is Dr. Cushing. Dr. Smith-Petersen is standing at the far right and to his left is Dr. P. D. Wilson.

P. D. Wilson, "Robert Bayley Osgood 1873-1956," *Journal of Bone and Joint Surgery* 1957; 39: 728.

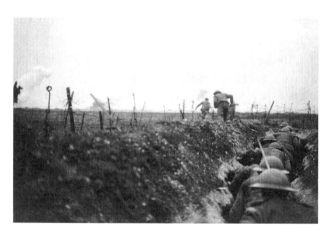

Trench warfare at the front line. John Warwick Brooke/Imperial War Museum/Wikimedia Commons.

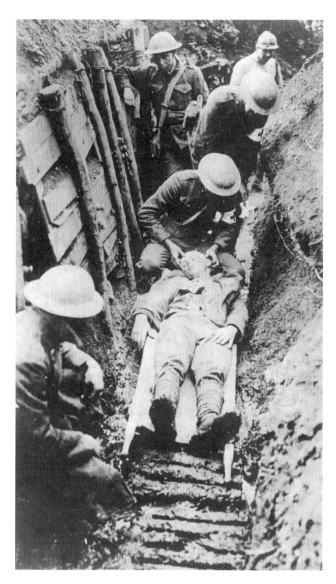

Wounded soldier receiving first aid on a stretcher in a trench on the battlefield. National WWI Museum and Memorial, Kansas City, Missouri, USA.

Under ordinary circumstances a soldier wounded in the trenches has an immediate first aid dressing applied by himself or a friend; then he walks or is carried to the poste de secours, which is the emergency dressing-station, immediately on the field of battle, generally in some sort of bomb-proof shelter; here he is observed, splints applied or an operation performed if necessity demands it, and then is at once evacuated to a first-line ambulance just beyond artillery fire; here he is again studied, his bandage changed and he may be operated on if necessary, but if his condition warrants it, he is at once evacuated to the railway and shipped south on a "sanitary train." On such trains the wounded reach Paris and the great distributing centres, and are at once divided among the local hospitals….

Cutler (1915) noted that soldiers arrived at the Lycée Pasteur hospital "within 12 to 14 hours after they have been hit…At arrival in the hospital patients were seen at once by the receiving officer [a resident], and sent...to the ward to have a bath first, or to the operating-room...The largest number of admissions to the University [Service] in any 24-hour period was 33 cases." During the initial three months of the Harvard Unit's service at the hospital, they received 295 patients, in addition to the 146 patients they were already treating. Cutler (1915) reported that "Fully 90 per cent of the wounds were badly infected," mainly because of "pieces of clothing...carried into the wounds." Among their patients' injuries were 140 fractures of the extremities, and "of all cases the compound fractures were the most serious and difficult to handle...[and in this] Osgood was an invaluable asset" (Cutler 1915). Dr. Elliot Cutler (1916) wrote of Osgood in his daily diary, noting that Osgood "is still indefatigable...[and I saw] some more of plaster-cast artistry by Dr. Osgood." Dr. Nathaniel Allison (chapter 36) replaced Dr. Osgood after three months.

While at Neuilly, Osgood (1915) described the operation of the hospital, particularly how the various members of the Harvard Unit worked together (see chapter 19): "The two residents and the three house officers [made] a careful study of the cases. Each house officer has charge of six wards of nine or ten beds each and both residents and house officers live in the hospital." He also described the extensive prevalence of "compound comminuted and infected fractures of the long bones...[which] have...needed orthopaedic treatment in the way of apparatus, to correct deformity and retain proper alignment" (Osgood 1915). Because serious problems accompany such injuries, Osgood noted that the French army was glad to have American surgeons on hand to help them. American volunteers did not stop there. Later in 1915, to provide even more assistance with the war effort, Harvard sent a second group of surgeons to Étaples—including Edward H. Nichols, an associate professor of surgery, as chief surgeon (see chapter 12)—to work with the British Expeditionary Forces.

Osgood (1915) also mentioned two types of injury occurring often as a consequence of nerve

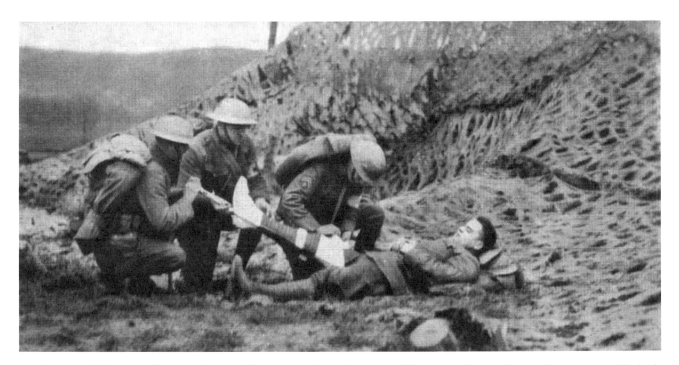

Application of a Thomas splint for a fractured femur on the front line. In the 1950 Annual Oration for the Massachusetts Medical Society, Dr. John W. O'Meara cited "splint 'em where they lie" as "a slogan of World War I." National WWI Museum and Memorial, Kansas City, Missouri, USA.

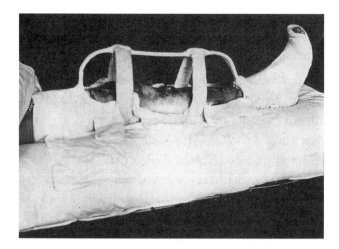

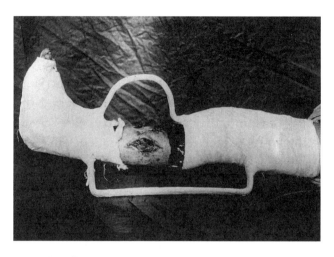

Examples of severe extremity open fractures treated in casts with outriggers to allow for wound care. Lantern slides by Robert B. Greenough. Warren Anatomical Museum in the Francis A. Countway Library of Medicine.

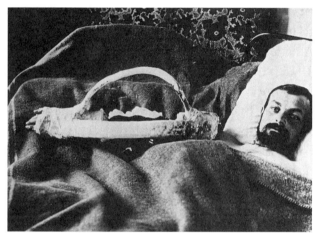

lesions and presenting as local paralysis: "wrist drop from injury to the musculo-spiral nerve, and…foot drop due either to a spinal cord injury or to a lesion of the external popliteal nerve. Mr. Robert Jones has also emphasized in cases of paralysis…the importance of preventing overstretching of the paralyzed muscles by allowing the malposition to be maintained…[The] apparatus [i.e., sprints and braces] may be not only retentive, but corrective as well…The apparatus work in the Ambulance is already of such a high grade that I fear we may have simply brought coals to Newcastle." It was essential for treatment, in Osgood's view, for an orthopaedic patient to be kept in the hospital, where splints and braces could be applied and discharge could be planned to the appropriate facility, such as a convalescent home, where rehabilitation could be continued in a medical setting.

He helped to establish this process during his time in Neuilly.

In 1916, the year after his return from France, Osgood summarized his experiences at the American Ambulance Field Hospital in an article published in the *Boston Medical and Surgical Journal*. He named three elements that were necessary for orthopaedic treatment of wounded soldiers in a field hospital:

1. A person interested in orthopaedic surgery, and in those mechanical principles which have to do with the fixation of inflamed joints and broken bones, and also with the restoration of function in stiffened joints and the obtaining of proper final alignment in fractures. 2. Proper materials with which the work may be done [see **Box 63.2**]…3. Given interest and materials, one must have time and assistants to use them. We have been several orthopaedic surgeons… "doing their bit" and doing it splendidly, but unable to do the kind of work which their training best fitted them to do and which in our opinion in this war is second in importance to none, because their time was fully occupied either with administrative matters or

Box 63.2. Equipment Necessary for Orthopaedic Work in a Field Hospital

According to Robert Osgood (1916), physicians required various equipment to be able to care for patients with orthopaedic injuries:

- "Dry, fine-ground plaster of Paris and a medium meshed, starch-sized crinoline
- "Simple shop and tools, a good vise, file, cold chisel, metal saw…drill, hammer and tweezers…screws and tap, flat iron…very thin stove pipe iron or sheet zinc…one may make almost any form of metal base
- "A fracture table of some sort will be found of the greatest convenience; one may almost say a necessity
- "Various appliances, such as the steel bars of Goldthwait…for the application of plaster jackets…"

the routine surgery necessary on account of the septic nature of nearly all of the wounds or because they must do it alone.

Osgood praised the Harvard Unit for such work at the American Ambulance (Hospital) in Neuilly. In his view, the group's "foresighted organization" allowed them to achieve "all these necessary conditions [and] the most ready help of the house surgeon and nurses [who were] constantly available" (Osgood 1916).

THE UNITED STATES ENTERS WORLD WAR I

In the United States, before World War I, with improvements in anesthesia, equipment, and operative technique, surgeons were increasingly drawn to performing surgical procedures that were elective and involved working inside of body cavities. This type of surgery was lucrative, convenient to schedule, and stimulating. Although this trend was advantageous to surgeons in many ways, it also resulted in many surgeons shunning treatment of fractures and other trauma-related surgery. Moreover, as insurance companies and industrial commissions began to establish policies governing the care of trauma-related injuries, the profitability of performing trauma-related orthopaedic surgery decreased and the paperwork it required increased. Therefore, the sudden and massive need for trauma care that emerged with the onset of World War I ran counter to the professional focus and desires of many American surgeons of the time.

Some surgeons, however, recognized the importance of embracing trauma surgery and the important role surgeons could play in caring for those injured in the war. In early 1916, Dr. Elliott G. Brackett (see chapter 35) presented to the Central States Orthopedic Club in Ohio, describing the efforts of Sir Robert Jones, a major general in the British Royal Army Medical Corps and the director of military orthopedics for Great Britain and Ireland: "[Jones] was undertaking the establishment [of orthopaedic centers] in each of the British Military Hospitals…There were neither trained surgeons nor surgeons to train… [to staff] these proposed centers" (Orr 1921). Brackett urged the American surgeons present to volunteer, and some, including Dr. H. Winnett Orr, were willing to answer the call. Throughout 1916, however, no such organized volunteer efforts materialized. But "when America entered the war…in the following April (1917), the call came in direct from…the British Commission that came over immediately upon our entrance into the war…[bringing] a request from Sir Robert Jones for twenty orthopedic surgeons to be sent to Great Britain" (Orr 1921) (see chapter 19).

A 1917 editorial in the *American Journal of Orthopedic Surgery*, in addition to acknowledging that Britain needed the help of orthopaedic surgeons from the United States, argued for segregating orthopaedic patients from other surgical patients (those with abdominal or urologic injuries, eye injuries, etc.):

Such surgeons [orthopaedic] can find their place of service only in hospitals set aside for the treatment of bone, muscle and tendon…the great importance of the segregation of the wounded will be appreciated by any surgeon who will make a study of the wounded now being returned to their homes. Let America learn by the failure of the past. Britain invites her to profit by the imperfections of her organization. France proffers her dearly bought experience to the student of medical organization. ("Editorial" 1917)

Orthopaedic surgeons from the United States had been practicing a specialty that was recognized as such as early as 1887, when the American Orthopaedic Association had been established. On the contrary, by 1914, when World War I began and Britain declared war, orthopaedics was not a special area of practice distinct from other surgical specialties in Britain, and orthopaedic specialists were rare. Jones created two prototypical military orthopaedic hospitals—first at Alder Hey in Liverpool, followed shortly thereafter at Shepherd's Bush in West London (which had 1,200 beds available for patients with orthopaedic conditions and injuries). When he demonstrated the success of these programs in treating and rehabilitating soldiers with orthopaedic injuries, he was "able to convince the War Office of the need of specialization and for the segregation of patients with back and extremity wounds in orthopedic hospitals…" (Orr 1921). Few orthopaedists had been trained or were ready to practice at all, while the number of orthopedic hospitals was only increasing, and he was "was acutely aware of both the need for orthopaedists…and how few had been trained and were available in Britain" (Orr 1921). In the end, orthopaedics became an official specialty in only Britain in 1918, the year when both the war ended and the British Orthopaedic Association was founded.)

PERSONNEL AND TRAINING

In 1916, the American Orthopaedic Association (AOA) and the Orthopaedic Section of the American Medical Association (AMA) organized their orthopaedic committees on preparedness, both chaired by Joel E. Goldthwait, in anticipation of the potential need for orthopaedic surgeons in the War in Europe (see chapter 33). In addition to Goldthwait, the AOA committee comprised Dr. A. Mackenzie Forbes, Dr. W. G. Erving, Dr. Nathaniel Allison, and Dr. M. S. Henderson; the AMA committee included Osgood, Dr. E. W. Ryerson, Dr. Russell A. Hibbs, and Dr. Eben W. Fiske who were: "Charged to consider and determine what would be needed in the form of orthopaedic surgeons, hospitals, and supplies to treat the wounded should America become involved in the conflict" (Green and DeLee 2017). The AOA committee shared its findings with members at the annual meeting in Pittsburgh, Pennsylvania, in May 1917:

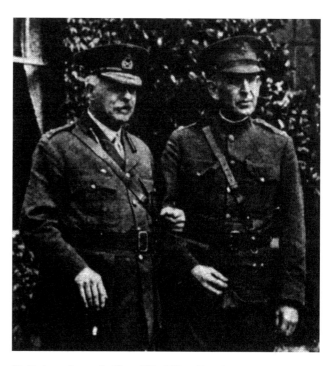

Sir Robert Jones (left) and Dr. Elliott Brackett. MGH HCORP Archives.

At this meeting it was voted that the association should offer the services of its members to the Government in any way most acceptable, and suggested that aid in orthopedic methods of examination, treatment, and instruction of conditions affecting the soldier in training, would be a practicable activity. On July 2, 1917, the resolutions passed…were presented to the Surgeon General…and the suggestions…were accepted by him. He requested that the committee prepare a brief of directions for distribution to surgeons in camps to serve as a basis of instruction and examination in matters of orthopedic interest. This brief comprised instruction in regard to the foot and footwear, and to the affections of joints, spine, etc., and was intended to serve as a guide for the standardization of orthopedic work in military usage. (Weed 1927)

Medical Corps Colonel Elliott G. Brackett (see chapter 35), a reserve officer working for the surgeon general, "was detailed to take charge of the part of the work that included orthopedic surgery and physical reconstruction" (Weed 1927). Reports from Europe indicated that injured soldiers would require extensive orthopaedic care, and that in the case of the United States joining the war, the country should prepare "on a large scale for the care of our soldiers when they should be returned to this country" (Weed 1927). An orthopaedic advisory council organized by the surgeon general's office and comprising former leaders of the AOA and the orthopaedic section of the AMA, surveyed orthopaedic surgeons nationwide "for the purposes of obtaining data on their qualifications and their availability for service" (Weed 1927). This council had seven overarching goals:

To provide for the care of future orthopedic cases in France by the establishment of hospitals especially equipped and supplied with the special personnel; to provide for the demand for a large increase of available surgeons who could aid in carrying on this increased work, both in France and in the United States; to provide hospital facilities for orthopedic reconstruction of disabled soldiers returning to the United States; and at the same time to provide the means for the industrial reeducation of these same men, to fit them for return to civil life…to provide a large corps of specially trained masseurs to treat the joint and muscle conditions and deformities…to arrange for the necessary hospital equipment overseas, and to develop plans for orthopedic reconstruction in the United States. (Weed 1927)

All of this planning proved prescient: on April 6, 1917, the United States declared war on Germany. By that time, orthopaedic surgery was still a relatively fledgling specialty in the US compared with other specialties such as obstetrics, gynecology, and ophthalmology. It claimed only about 100 orthopaedic surgeons, most of whom practiced in large cities such as New York, Philadelphia, Boston, Chicago, St. Louis, Pittsburgh, Baltimore, and Minneapolis. Furthermore, at the time the specialty focused mainly on pediatric patients with chronic and congenital conditions.

> Orthopedic surgery may be said to have come into its own…the specialty of a principle and not of a portion of anatomy [and has] vindicated itself at least on a conspicuous scale.
> —Robert B. Osgood, MD ("The Orthopedic Centres of Great Britain and Their American Medical Officers," *Journal of Orthopedic Surgery*, 1918;10:140.)

In light of this fact, the orthopaedic advisory council's survey highlighted a concern. Even after "enrolling…the available trained orthopedic surgeons" to supplement the "original personnel of the division of military orthopedic surgery" (Weed 1927), it became evident that their numbers would be inadequate: "It was clear that the source of this supply must be found among the younger general surgeons and…many young practitioners who had…acceptable training along surgical lines…Early in September, 1917, arrangements were made with the postgraduate department of Harvard University [see chapter 16] and with the New York Post Graduate Medical School and Hospital to establish a course of instruction, and a definite syllabus…was prepared with the advice of the orthopedic advisory council" (Weed 1927) (see the addendum following this chapter, "Military Orthopedic Surgery").

In October 1917, the Office of the Surgeon General published a notice from Brackett, by then the director of the Department of Military Orthopedic Surgery, describing this course: "For those members of the Medical Officers' Reserve Corps, or those intending to apply for commission, who have had only a general surgical training and who desire to be assigned to the Orthopedic Service of the Army, a course of intensive instruction in the fundamentals of orthopedic surgery…has been arranged. This course is of about six weeks' duration, and will be given at various universities" ("War Notes" 1917). The goal was to maintain "a definite continuity of orthopedic treatment as soon as a man is injured…the lesson that we have learned from England's mistake, not to make a radical change in the treatment, but to establish the principles of orthopedic treatment close to the firing line and to continue until the man is discharged" ("War Notes" 1917). That autumn, the military opened an orthopedic service at the Walter Reed General Hospital in Washington, DC, "and the use of the wards and clinical material was offered…with the [aforementioned] proposed course…as part of the Army Medical School" (Weed 1927). Other Army facilities such as Camp Greenleaf, Fort Oglethorpe, Georgia, also offered courses. (It was at Fort Oglethorpe where Dr. J. H. Shortell [see chapter 60] trained before joining the Harvard Unit in France led by Dr. Cushing.)

The main concern about the lack of organized care of the wounded in Europe during the early

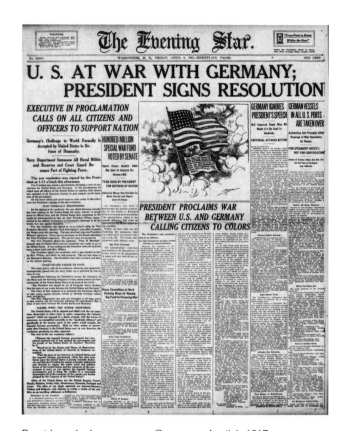

President declares war on Germany, April 6, 1917. *Evening Star*, April 6, 1917: 1. Library of Congress.

years of the war led to another significant decision by the surgeon general—this one related to rehabilitation of soldiers upon their return home. In late-August 1917, the Office of the Surgeon General had asked Brackett and Goldthwait, both physicians at Boston Children's Hospital and MGH in addition to their war-related efforts, to formulate a curriculum. Also at Children's Hospital, Dr. Robert Lovett [see chapter 16] and Janet Merrill, then the director of the Department of Physical Therapeutics, developed programs intended to train reconstruction aides, beginning in 1918. Between 1921 and 1929, reconstruction aides and postgraduates were trained at the Harvard Graduate Medical School. Dr. Arthur T. Legg (see chapter 18), Dr. James Warren Sever (see chapter 17), and Merrill taught the introductory graduate course through 1945. By 1930, however, Boston boasted two medical schools—Harvard Medical School (courses 441 and 442) and the Boston School

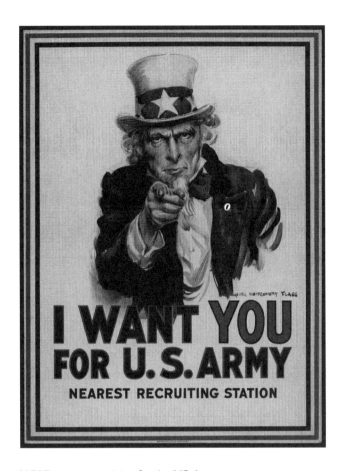

WWI poster recruiting for the US Army. Library of Congress.

of Physical Education—that met the educational requirements of the AMA in physical therapy; only nine other schools throughout the country did the same.

Whereas practicing surgeons and physicians were called on to attend these new courses on wartime orthopaedics and rehabilitation, "the war… disrupted undergraduate and postgraduate medical education in this country" (Ober 1943), just as it had disrupted medical students' education in Europe. This caused three significant problems for the medical profession at home:

> first, because…the armed [forces] have called into service all physically fit medical students who are limited to one year of hospital training which practically nullifies the pools from which doctors are obtained who wish to go into special fields; second, physically fit physicians who are the ones that go in for postgraduate courses have been called to active duty; and third, the teaching school faculties have been so depleted that there are scarcely enough teachers to maintain the teaching of the undergraduate, especially under the speeding up of the whole medical program. (Ober 1943)

Frank Ober (see chapter 20), writing in 1943 in relation to World War II, highlighted the steps needed to keep the medical professional salient in wartime, particularly in relation to medical education. These steps had been learned during the First World War almost 30 years earlier:

> It is vitally necessary then if we are to keep our standing in the medical world that preparations be started now to organize a program of graduate education which will meet the demands that must surely come when the war is over. It should be our duty to supply adequate additional educational advantages for all those young doctors who have had a one-year internship, and also for all those older doctors who wish to improve their education before returning to their practices. There will be thousands of both, and schools and hospitals will be expected to help fill the deficiencies in their education. Many will desire more hospital experience…It is up to us…orthopaedic surgeons, to do our part in promulgating plans for the future of graduate medical education… (Ober 1943)

Ober (1943) ended with optimism that these decades of wartime experience would help later generations: "Let us hope that our successors have learned from us all we have to give."

GOLDTHWAIT LEADS VOLUNTEERS

In an effort to help the allied forces, the orthopaedic leadership in the United States and the surgeon

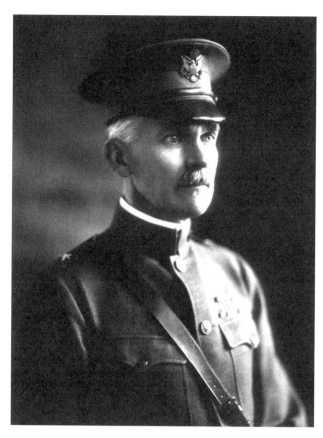

General Joel Goldthwait. U.S. National Library of Medicine.

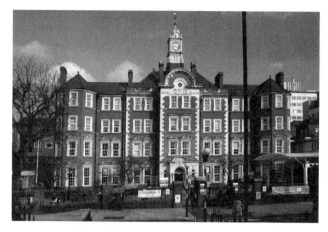

Special Surgical Hospital (now known as Hammersmith Hospital), Shepherd's Bush, London. Petr Brož/Wikimedia Commons.

general, in collaboration with Sir Robert Jones (who requested 20 orthopaedic surgeons from the US), introduced some orthopedic surgeons to the injured soldiers in England under direction of the recently experienced surgeons and orthopaedic surgeons in the United Kingdom. Joel Goldthwait stepped up to lead these American surgeons: he "immediately accepted a commission as Major and set about the organization of the first Goldthwait unit...organized at once from volunteers by telegraph" (Orr 1921). Goldthwait's unit comprised 21 surgeons, including Orr. The group traveled to Liverpool, arriving May 28, 1917, where they were met by Jones, who lived there and provided them with their "first accurate ideas of the British scheme for the care of the war wounded" (Orr 1921). They met Osgood there also. They stayed for two days, during which Jones described the need and his plans for orthopaedic surgeons in England.

They then went to London (Shepherd's Bush) and began learning from Goldthwait "the treatment of war wounds and fractures, and methods in war hospitals" (Orr 1921). Over 10 days they learned about:

> the administrative, surgical and training methods by which the British wounded were rehabilitated after their physical injuries in France. At this time, it was already more than two and one-half years since the beginning of the war… [and] we had our eyes opened to the very serious character of the war wounds. It was almost beyond belief to see how very extensive was the physical damage done. The infections were appalling. Large open wounds involving bones and joints were bathed in pus. In those who had survived, there were some fearful evidences of the destructive power of gas gangrene… we saw a few amputations done and a few patients recently amputated who gave us some impression as to what the loss of limb as well as the loss of life for America, was going to be. (Orr 1921)

During their time at Shepherd's Bush, Goldthwait and his unit focused on six main areas of interest:

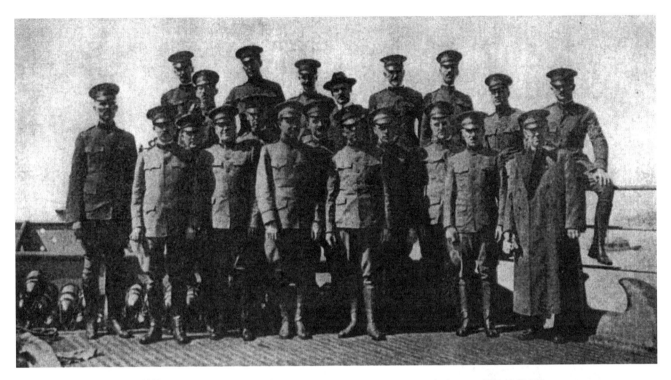

First Goldthwait Unit, WWI. C. Parker, "Correspondence," *American Journal of Orthopedic Surgery* 1917; s2-15: 791.

1. Methods of immobilization for compound infected bone and joint injuries.
2. The cleaning up of infected wounds involving bones and joints.
3. The correction of late deformities after war wounds of bone, joints and soft parts.
4. The repair of peripheral nerve injuries.
5. Postoperative splinting by the method of Hugh Owen Thomas and Sir Robert Jones.
6. Rehabilitation of war cripples by vocational training. (Orr 1921)

The team saw a great many difficult cases during their time at Shepherd's Bush. But despite the horrendous injuries and the often-overwhelming number of wounded soldiers to care for, the British service was "effective." Orr (1921) described one patient who:

> had gone to France for the first time on Thursday. His company went into action about noon on Friday. He was hit in the leg by late Friday afternoon, and he was back on a hospital train in Great Britain on Saturday morning. I…saw him in bed in a Base Hospital the same evening. Moreover, he had on a good splint, a good dressing and had antitetanic serum during the first few hours that he was hurt. How the British did this for their hundreds of thousands was what the Americans had come to learn.

CURATIVE WORKSHOPS

King Manuel II of Portugal, then living in exile in the UK, supported Portugal entering the war and made himself available to the Allies. Although disappointed when he was assigned a post in the British Red Cross, he was very active visiting hospitals and wounded soldiers in hospitals on the front, and he participated frequently in fund drives and conferences. He was responsible for the creation of the orthopaedic department with its curative workshops at Shepherd's Bush Hospital,

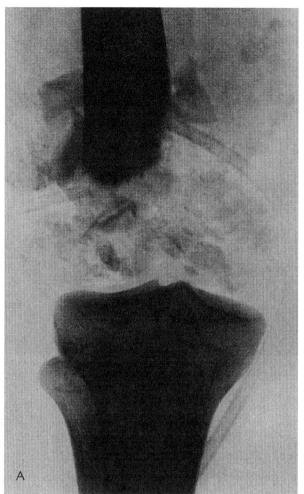
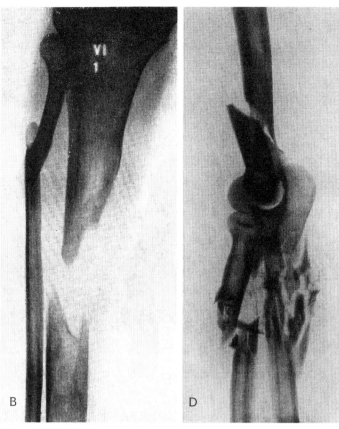
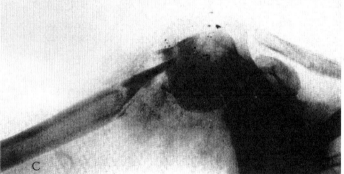

Examples of severe open-bone fractures. Major issues confronting the treating surgeons included infection, malalignment, shortening, stiffness, and major limitation of useful function of the injured extremity.

The Medical Department of the U.S. Army in the World War, Volume XI: Surgery, under the direction of Maj. Gen. M. W. Ireland. Washington, DC: Government Printing Office, 1927.

supporting their function until 1925. Orr (1921) recalled the effects of these efforts:

> All of the problems...had been solved to a considerable extent at the time we arrived... With money largely collected by King Manuel (formerly of Portugal), excellent curative workshops had been built and five or six hundred men were working daily. The shops served three purposes:

1. They gave occupations to a number of men whose recovery was hastened by the mere performance of certain arm and leg movements.

2. Other men were learning new trades adapted to their changed physical conditions.

3. The shops produced a large amount of splints, carpenter work, mattresses, brooms, brushes, etc.

At the request of Robert Osgood, a friend of King Manuel and then the assistant director of military orthopedics in the United States, in 1918 King Manuel wrote an article "on the organization and results obtained in the curative workshops which have been established in the Orthopaedic Centers in the United Kingdom." He described his invited visits in 1915 to the British war hospitals in Rouen (Roi Albert I Anglo-Belgian Hospital) and Paris (Grand Palais), and his subsequent belief that the same type of care provided there should be provided in England. He noted, "At that time there was only one military orthopedic hospital in this country [England], viz., at Alder Hey Hospital, in Liverpool…in March 1916, it was decided to establish a big Orthopedic Center in London" (King Manuel of Portugal 1918)—what became Shepherd's Bush Military Hospital, now known as Hammersmith Hospital. In Shepherd's Bush, Jones was able to add a larger orthopaedic inpatient service for the wounded. Alder Hey was the first hospital where Jones had begun an orthopaedic service.

King Manuel elaborated on his deliberations about the importance of rehabilitation with Sir Robert Jones and Major Walter Hill (then the registrar of Shepherd's Bush Hospital) during the first half of 1916. King Manuel was mainly interested in avoiding idleness among wounded soldiers being treated at the hospital. The three men:

> considered the great advantage of having workshops established at that Hospital…We had… to consider that an orthopaedic hospital… [was] different from a general hospital, as the majority of men are not in bed. Our first object, therefore, was to give occupation to the men; secondly to choose such occupations as would be useful for that injury; and, thirdly, to find occupations which would have a beneficial psychological effect on the men. After discussions, many difficulties and worries, it was decided to establish the first curative workshops at Shepherd's Bush. (King Manuel of Portugal 1918)

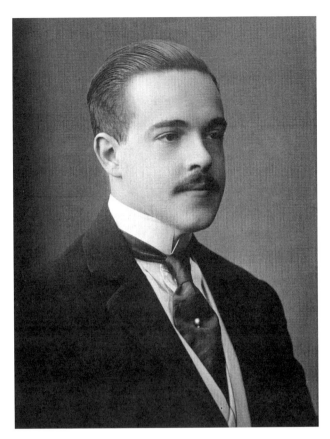

King Manuel of Portugal, ca. 1915–1920. Library of Congress.

These workshops began on October 1, 1916, at Shepherd's Bush Hospital, with "the expense of equipping them being borne by the…British Red Cross Society and Order of St. John of Jerusalem in England" (King Manuel of Portugal 1918). The men's participation was voluntary. They could practice various trades (**Box 63.3**), and soldiers usually were assigned one they had been working in before the war. The popularity of the workshops spread throughout the United Kingdom, and by 1918, public fundraising efforts had enabled the curative workshops to be established in 11 urban centers through Britain—for example, Bristol and Liverpool in England; Aberdeen and Glasgow in Scotland; and Dublin in Ireland.

With an overall goal to keep the soldiers busy during their time at the orthopaedic hospitals, these workshops had a twofold purpose: "Being a military organization, the first duty of

Box 63.3. Trades Practiced in British Curative Workshops

> Splint making
> Boot and shoe making (principally surgical boot work)
> Carpentry
> Tailoring
> General engineering
> Fret working
> Painting
> Commercial photography
> Electrical work
> Plumbing
> Ironworking
> Cigarette making
> Printing
> Sign writing
> Net making
> Basket weaving
> Leather embossing
> Wood carving
>
> (King Manuel of Portugal 1918)

the orthopedic centers is to try to get men fit as soon as possible to go back [to fight, whereas] disabled men…at the completion of their treatment, will be discharged from the army and go back to their civil life…[Second,] with the curative workshops we have tried to build a bridge between the military and the civil life" (King Manuel of Portugal 1918). King Manuel and the other men who developed these workshops "have tried to take as our basis and ideal the old Latin rule of '*Mens sana in corpore sano*' ['a sound mind in a sound body']…a guiding principle in all our work" (King Manuel of Portugal 1918).

The workshops "had the added benefit of cutting down on discipline and morale problems in the hospitals" (Green and DeLee 2017). King Manuel (1918) also described the clinical and "practical results" of the curative workshops:

> [I]n many cases the manual curative treatment has helped wonderfully the recovery of the injured limbs. We see men who have been idle for months, start working, gain interest in their work, and begin again the active life they formerly led, while still undergoing treatment… We have no doubt, from the military point of view, that the curative workshops have been a great help…the men were getting fit more quickly as a result of the classes of treatment received in the workshops, i.e., the direct and the indirect. For men who have been in the hospital for a long time; the psychological treatment has an importance at least as great as the direct treatment of the injured limb in the shops.

Goldthwait and his unit of orthopaedic surgeons saw these workshops at work. After their time at Shepherd's Bush, the unit attended to patients at the Star and Garter Hospital, also in London, which had been "established and rapidly enlarged for the care of men hopelessly crippled because of spinal cord injuries" (King Manuel of Portugal 1918). King Manuel (1918) recalled "One poor chap [who] was doing quite well making and selling flies to fishermen." The group then moved on to the hospital at Roehampton, where they recognized "an atmosphere of hope" (King Manuel of Portugal 1918). At the time, "With two thousand men minus arms and legs, almost everyone was busy. Mr. Muirhead Little [son of Dr. William John Little of Little's disease] in charge… is doing excellent work…stumps were being improved surgically, deformities…corrected, [and] temporary and artificial limbs were being put on" (King Manuel of Portugal 1918). Not only were the surgeons and other personnel at the hospital busy: "best of all, the vocational schools were really working. From the motor repair training

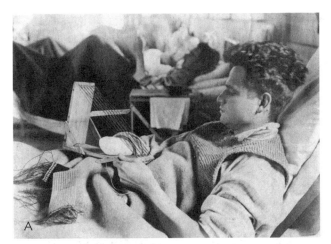
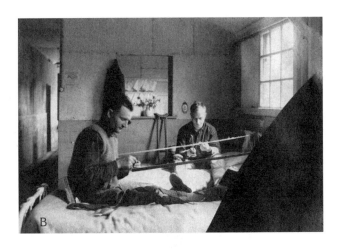

Examples of Curative Workshops. A and B: National WWI Museum and Memorial, Kansas City, Missouri, USA. C: Courtesy of Picture Parlour Antique Prints.

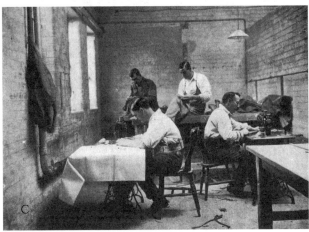

schools alone, about fifty…men were…graduated for work as expert motor mechanics or drivers… We found that the British had achieved wonders in their preparation for and care of the wounded" (King Manuel of Portugal 1918).

The Americans (Goldthwait and Osgood) appreciated the British curative workshops: "It is a great comfort and encouragement to have seen this scheme approved by great authorities, such as Major Joel Goldthwait and Major R. B. Osgood" (King Manuel of Portugal 1918). Likely at the two men's urging, the American Army intended to begin a similar project. In fact, Goldthwait's second unit included three technically trained nonphysicians, who were recruited from the Sanitary Corps to develop and direct curative workshops in each orthopaedic hospital overseas. Elliott Brackett (1917) described the direction the US Army would take these workshops: "Since…

the development of the so-called Curative Work Shop is a natural part of the general orthopedic equipment, and since the reeducation and training for industry is a natural development of this…a special advisory committee…the Active Vocational Board has been appointed…All affairs relating to military orthopedic surgery will pass through this department, and when bearing the signature of any of the three Directors may be regarded as official and representing the policy" of the newly created Department for Military Orthopedics. King Manuel (1918) noted that "it [is] a great pleasure to know that the scheme of curative workshops is being followed in the orthopedic hospitals of the United States."

In a 1918 report to the US surgeon general, Osgood described the benefits of the curative workshops implemented at American orthopaedic hospitals and the benefits they have for soldiers:

> Very little in the way of vocational training for our men is being planned in France, but with the present attitude of the Expeditionary Staff toward helping the man once over on the other side…something in the way of occupational and curative work must be established…Everyone who comes in contact with the severely

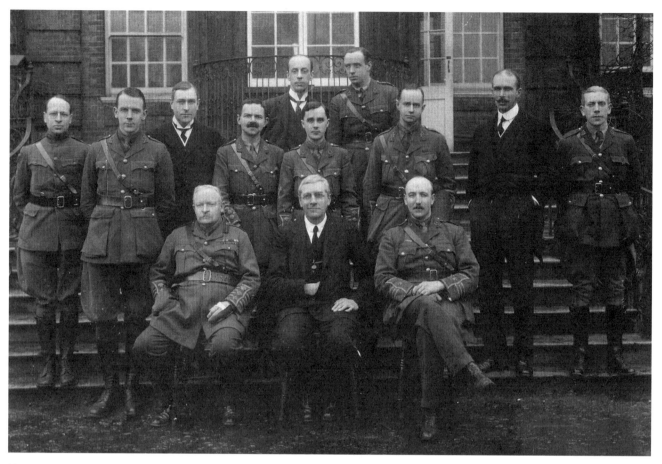

First meeting of the newly formed British Orthopaedic Association, Roehampton, February 1918. Dr. Osgood is standing at the far left. James Koepfler/Boston Children's Hospital Archives.

wounded soldier, who has been through hardships and suffered and has emerged in a more or less crippled condition, recognizes the importance of beginning, as soon as possible, to combat the idea of crippledom and to awaken and foster a spirit of future usefulness. If at this stage the soldier can be given something to do with his hands and to occupy his mind as well, and he can come in contact with a stimulating personality who is not a soldier…he gains comparatively quickly the conception of a possible wage-earning capacity and a return to a useful place in the body politic…There were being established, just as I was leaving [February 1918], convalescent camps, in which much of the military discipline of the training battalions was being instituted…under medical supervision.

THE US JOINS THE FIGHT

The 21 orthopaedic surgeons in Goldthwait's first unit were soon assigned for duty in hospitals in nine cities throughout the United Kingdom: Oxford, Leads, London, Liverpool, Aberdeen, Glasgow, Belfast, Edinburgh, and Cardiff (**Box 63.4**). They had been appointed to a six-month period of service. Soon after their arrival, however, Goldthwait returned to the Office of the Surgeon General's in Washington, DC, where he spent July and August "with Col. E. G. Brackett, Director of Orthopedic Surgery in the United States…developing plans for the American orthopedic surgeon in the United States, [including] plans for the American orthopedic activities in France and… recruiting the second Goldthwait unit for service overseas" (Rauer, n.d.).

Box 63.4. The American Experience on the Front Lines

> "In the summer of 1917, among the first Americans to enter into World War I was CPT Stanhope Bayne-Jones [physician]. Reporting for duty at the 69th Field Ambulance in war-torn Belgium he began what he would later describe as 'a great job – and rather lively.' For the next twenty days, Bayne-Jones was under fire at an advanced dressing station where he worked continuously among the wounded and dying of the British Expeditionary Force (BEF). He also contended with the continual danger of shell fire and poison gas. Recognizing the hazards he faced, Bayne-Jones later remarked, 'I have not been as scared as I thought I would be,' although 'the war is horrible beyond imagination.' Working with his British counterpart, he performed his duties under all the circumstances that came to characterize life in the World War I front lines. Additional duties, outside treating the wounded, consumed much of Bayne-Jones' time, mainly preventative medicine measures that later became the focus of many American medical officers. He had to supervise sanitation, check personnel for venereal disease, and conduct sick call. Bayne-Jones was responsible for both keeping his men healthy and returning them to good health after sickness, disease, or wounds from combat. Bayne-Jones' experiences are typical of what many American physicians would see during their World War I service with BEF."
>
> (Rauer, n.d.)

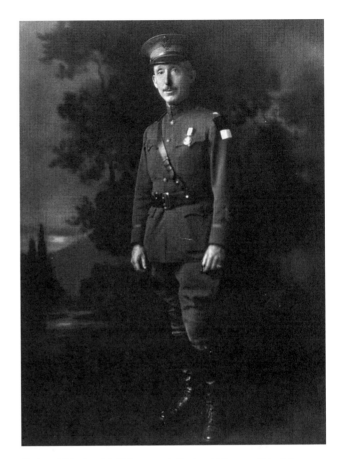

Colonel Nathaniel Allison. U.S. National Library of Medicine.

During Goldthwait's hiatus, he visited with Colonel Brackett. As a result of their discussions and some promising statistics, the surgeon general decided to organize a Department for Military Orthopedics: "[A] very large percentage of casualties…require special orthopedic…treatment (from 30–40%) and the large percentage of these cases…can be restored to military usefulness (from 70–75%)…[Thus] the Surgeon General…[created] an organization to care for these cases…designated 'The Department for Military Orthopedics,' and will have to do with the work that is required both at home and abroad" (Brackett 1917). Brackett himself, then a major in the US Medical Reserve Corps, became the new department's director; Major David Silver became assistant director. (After the war, Silver became a professor of orthopaedic surgery at the University of Pittsburgh.) Goldthwait was appointed as the director of military orthopaedics for the expeditionary forces and reported to Brackett. Osgood, who at the time was stationed at Base Hospital No. 5, and Nathaniel Allison, a captain stationed at Base Hospital No. 21—both in France—were assigned to be Goldthwait's assistant directors.

Brackett (1917) detailed Osgood's and Allison's roles in their new positions: "Major Osgood will be temporarily assigned to Col. Robert Jones, the Director of Military Orthopedics for the British Forces, for the study of details of organization and methods of treatment, and Capt. Allison will be temporarily assigned to similar study with the French and Italian forces." Bracket also named an advisory orthopedic board, which included Dr. Robert W. Lovett of Boston; Dr. Albert H. Freiberg of Cincinnati; Dr. G. Gwilym Davis of Philadelphia, Dr. F. H. Albee of New York, and Dr. John L. Porter of Chicago; these men were tasked with helping the directors of the new Department of Military Orthopaedics.

During his two months in the States, in July 1917, Goldthwait—who had brought back with him fresh insights into the casualties resulting from the war in Europe—wrote an editorial in the *American Journal of Orthopedic Surgery* describing his thoughts on the role of the orthopaedic surgeon during the war:

> There are two kinds of service in which the orthopedic surgeon finds a definite place. The first is in connection with the work of the "base" hospital, which is located comparatively near the actual conflict, and to which the men are sent as soon as the first dressings are applied at the field hospital or first-aid station. These hospitals are naturally under the direction of general surgeons and the orthopedist's position is that of assistant, the cases in which special mechanical problems exist being turned over to him for care…The second form of service that is open to the orthopedic surgeon in time of war is that which would be rendered in hospitals to which patients would be sent from the base hospitals, and kept as long as necessary, not only for the purely surgical treatment, but for such reeducation along occupational lines as is indicated, so that when discharged there will be the least possible physical handicap, with the greatest amount of industrial fitness. Such hospitals are designated by the Army and the Red Cross as general hospitals for orthopedic…purposes. They should be located in or near large cities…[and] the staff… made up of men skilled in orthopedic surgery.

Goldthwait (1917) went on to describe "a type of this form of cooperation and organization" embodied by an orthopaedic unit at the Robert B. Brigham Hospital and the City Hospital in Boston. The unit was staffed by two services: the first with Brackett as surgeon-in-chief and Lloyd T. Brown (see chapter 46) and M. S. Danforth as surgeons; the second with Charles F. Painter as chief (see chapter 45) and Mark H. Rogers (see chapter 53) and Loring T. Swaim (see chapter 45) as surgeons.

In summer 1917, and into that autumn, while the new Department of Military Orthopaedics found its footing and Goldthwait recruited members to his second unit of volunteers, the directors and advisory council members debated the role of the American volunteers:

> in the war and as to the future of the Orthopedic Service. Original plans had been that we should remain on duty with the British only a few months; and that American orthopedic participation in the war would require our services in France or perhaps even our return to the United States by November. However, it had become clear that there was no particular need for most of us in France and that our greatest field of usefulness for the present, lay with the British. Consequently, most of the members of both the first and second Goldthwait units remained or were now assigned for duty with the British. (Orr 1921)

Upon his promotion to lieutenant colonel in early November, Goldthwait and Osgood, his first assistant, began making:

> More definite plans for the conduct of the Orthopedic Services in France…It was, however, some months before Col. Goldthwait's original ideas had much effect upon the organization and operation of the hospital service in France…The British had got so far behind in the care of their amputated men that they

were compelled to send them home from the hospitals as soon as their primary wounds had healed. The intention was to bring the men back to the limb fitting centers...as rapidly as possible...Neither the hospitals nor the artificial limb factories...were able to keep pace with this demand. In 1918 there were said to be about 10,000 men waiting at home. (Orr 1921)

Orr, in his 1921 book about his experience in the war, described the issues for injured British soldiers that resulted from such delays or breaks in treatment:

Our experience with these men showed how important it is to make the treatment continuous from the time of the original operation. Of 500 patients who returned to Whitchurch...more than 300 required either reconstruction or surgical treatment, or both, before their limbs could be put on. Many of the men had discharging sinuses from osteomyelitis or from foreign bodies in the stump, that had not been removed. Others had contracture deformity, flexion of the thigh, flexion of the knee, adduction of the arm, etc., so severe that an artificial extremity could not be put on in a position to be worn. All of these things had to be corrected.

In November 1917, "Goldthwait arrived in London with the second orthopedic group" (Orr 1921), which was composed of 45 officers—including 12 nurses, the orthopaedic surgeon George W. Van Gorder (see chapter 40) and two other physicians from Boston, Drs. Frank W. Marvin and James B. Montgomery. This group would begin their service in England, where they would "work under our own American officers who have been at the British orthopedic service for the past four or five months" (Rauer, n.d.), and they would eventually staff the American war hospitals in France, once they were made ready.

With the coming of winter and the specter of more fighting on the Western Front come spring, British leadership recognized the need to get men back to the fight or clear out the hospitals. In December in Liverpool, Jones led "a conference of all surgeons on duty in the British Military Orthopaedic Centers" to discuss the problems and determine what was to be done:

The British hospitals of all kinds...were filled...Many sick and wounded were arriving in the British Isles daily...[and] an investigation...revealed the fact that patients were being detained in hospital longer than necessary...the result both of failure to provide prompt treatment upon arrival at hospital and efficient treatment afterwards...It was soon found that a considerable number of cases could be returned to usefulness much more promptly by transfer from general to orthopedic hospitals. This was true particularly of those patients who had been months in the hospital with foot drop, contraction of the hip or knee or some other disabling deformity that could be corrected surgically or by mechanical apparatus. It was also found that many men were delayed in hospitals because of failure to systemically re-examine patients; consequently, they were not promptly discharged when ready. It is not commonly appreciated how much unnecessary disability there is because of failure to inspect frequently patients of this class. (Orr 1921)

Jones and the assistant directors of medical services decided to make their rounds "of British hospitals during the winter" and had "the authority to examine...every patient who had been in the hospital more than sixty days. They were to discharge all such patients at their discretion" (Orr 1921). These visits led to the Ministry of Pensions requiring hospitals "to furnish more satisfactory written reports...It was found that the patient's record...of many hospitals had been very seriously neglected" (Orr 1921). The American volunteers, however, had been using "card index systems which had been in operation for nearly six

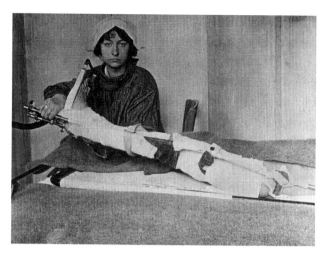

Patient with a fractured femur being treated in traction with a Thomas splint. Lantern slide by Robert B. Greenough. Warren Anatomical Museum in the Francis A. Countway Library of Medicine.

months supplied us promptly with most of the information which was called for" (Orr 1921) (an example is shown in **Case 63.1**). Although well-intentioned, this requirement placed additional burden on hospital staff to complete all the necessary documentation.

During their visits, Jones and his team realized that treatment of femur fractures was "far from as good as [it] should have been" (Orr 1921). Approximately 60 percent of soldiers who had a fractured femur as a result of a gunshot wound died during the first year of the war, although by the third year of the war this number was drastically reduced—to 12 percent—as a result of emergent splinting in the field. "Now, however...there was found to be a large amount of shortening and deformity in the femur and leg...due largely if not entirely to failure to maintain continuity of treatment as good as the first splinting. Somewhere between the advanced dressing station, and the base hospital the treatment broke down and the patients were recovering with serious deformity and...permanent disability" (Orr 1921). The British War Office instituted changes to the treatment of femur fractures to try and avoid these residual problems: "The principal factors in this change were the

Case 63.1. Example from the Americans' Card Index System for Tracking Patient Records

> **Patient Record (Index Card):**
>
> Name – Litchfield, A.
>
> Rank, Pte. Regt., No 14336.
>
> Unit 1st Coldstream Guards.
>
> Age, 24.
>
> Ward, M.1.
>
> Admitted, 28-3-17.
>
> Diagnosis (in detail G.S.W.L. leg. Back.
>
> Fracture. R. Leg. (No. IX. 4).
>
> X-ray No. 2534. 2930
>
> Time in previous Hospitals. Six months.
>
> Discharged from W.M.W.H. _____
>
> To _____
>
> **Reverse Side**
>
> History: Wounded Sept. 15th, 1916 in France. Bullet went through a point above patella and came out inner side of knee joint. Knee joint stiff, foot in position of varus. Short 2 ¼ inches. Skiagram shows fracture of lower end of femur. 19-4-17. Operation. Inner sinus enlarged. Sequestrum removed. Full drainage established. Previous treatment. Drainage, dressings, etc.
>
> Treatment here. 19-4-17. Inner sinus enlarged. Sequestrum removed. Bone scraped. Full drainage established. 18-7-17. Not yet healed. Sinus 3-inch. Hot fomentations. 3-9-17.
>
> Examination Board: No attempts at extension. Through and through drainage. Sequestrotomy. Arthrodesis of second toe and tenotomy by Major Smith 22-9-17. Operation of femur, also Sequestrotomy. 19-11-17. Wounds healing satisfactorily. Latest X-ray shows signs of bony union in good position. Shortening 1 ½ inches. Thomas splint with extension. 1-12-17. Erysipelas. To Ely Isolation Hospital. 24-12-17. Readmitted from Ely Hospital. 5-1-18. To get up. To have caliper splint and S.W.C. (Soldiers Wounded Convalescent). Boots.
>
> (Example quoted from Orr 1921)

more general efficient use of the Thomas splint; the employment of traction by ice tongs and certain other measures that came to be insisted upon in the orthopedic and other hospitals" (Orr 1921).

Worries about "the spring offensive on the Western front...started by the Germans," proved well founded, and "the British sustained some very serious punishment. From February until May the British wounded were brought across the channel in thousands," and the American volunteers and the British personnel in the war hospitals were "hardly able to meet the tremendous surgical and hospital problems" (Orr 1921). "Just when things were getting to their worst," however, "the Americans entered the fray and by their inspiring early victories gave us...definite hope that the new forces from America would be able to turn the tide against Germany" (Orr 1921).

In autumn 1918, a British publication "[defined] the scope of orthopedic surgery in the British hospitals...[and] specified that all bone, joint, peripheral nerve and soft parts injuries with existing or impending deformity should be classified as orthopedic and referred to orthopedic centers or consulting orthopedic surgeons for treatment or advice" (Orr 1921). "The Americans on duty with the British were thoroughly impressed with the importance of the prevention and early correction of deformity" that Jones had identified during his tour of British hospitals, and "Col. Goldthwait succeeded in early 1918 of having a similar circular issued from headquarters of the American Expeditionary Force in France" (Orr 1921). Part of this American publication, Circular No. 11, is set in **Box 63.5**.

By the time the United States officially joined the war, American volunteers had been a huge boon to British hospitals. Frank E. Weed shared Jones's depiction of orthopaedics in Britain and how British hospitals had benefitted from America's surgeon-volunteers. Weed was a physician and transportation officer (hospital trains and ambulances) in charge of moving the war injured the first six months of 1919 from Europe to the United States. Jones's words in **Box 63.6** illustrate how those surgeon's efforts made all the difference to British soldiers with orthopaedic injuries.

As the fighting went on and America became entrenched in the war, some of the orthopaedic surgeons in both of Goldthwait's units were eventually sent to American hospitals in France. Dr. H. Winnett Orr (1921) wrote about his experiences with both neglected injured soldiers and apathetic medical officers at Base Hospital No. 9 at Chateauroux:

> One found here as elsewhere a considerable number of wards in which, either because of lack of knowledge, lack of interest or lack of industry on the part of the ward surgeons, there were uncorrected, unsplinted, and otherwise more or less neglected patients. This neglect showed itself in a few principal ways. There was shortening and deformity of some fractures, especially of the compound fractures. There were also many patients with shoulders, elbows, wrists, knees and ankles...healing after compound injuries in bad position. One of the most striking illustrations of this was to be found in the upper arm and elbow injuries... patients...returning from the front in...hinged ring Thomas splints...with the whole arm straight and the hand pronated...[—]a good splint for transportation...[but] a bad treatment splint...because the straight stiff arm is a useless arm...One found in the Army hospitals a considerable number of surgeons who were never able to adjust themselves to the problem of splinting a compound fracture...I was extremely anxious to apply here...the methods of Sir Robert Jones...to my genuine sorrow, however, I found neither in Base Hospital No. 9 nor elsewhere a receptive attitude in this matter...Those who had little or no experience whatever...were apparently even less willing to learn...

Box 63.5. Circular No. 11

France, March 3, 1918

The following instructions are issued for the guidance of all Medical Officers:

1. Injuries to the bones and joints, as well as of the muscles and tendons adjacent to these structures, represent a large percentage of the casualties of both the Training and the Combat Periods of an Army.

2. To restore useful function to these injured structures is one of the purposes of the Medical Organization of the Army. The problems involved in this have to do not only with the cleansing and healing of the wounds, but also with the restoration of motion in the joint or strength to the part. This latter part naturally follows the first, but it is essential that the first part be carried out with reference to that which is to follow. Unless this second part of the treatment, the restoration of strength and motion, is carried out much of the first part is purposeless.

3. To insure to the man not only the proper treatment for this type of injury, but the proper supervision until he is as fully restored as possible, necessitates some form of radical control that makes it impossible for a man to be overlooked in inevitable transfers, from service to service, or hospital to hospital.

4. Since as much of the ultimate result in these conditions depends upon orthopaedic measures after the first treatment of the wounds has been carried out, the following will govern:—The Director of Orthopaedic Surgery is responsible for the treatment of the injuries or diseases of the bones or joints, exclusive of the head and face.

   He will be held responsible for the treatment of injuries or diseases of the ligaments, tendons or muscles that are involved in the joint function, of the extremities.

   Officers attached to other Divisions may operate upon and treat such conditions, but the Division of Orthopaedic Surgery, through its Director, will be held responsible for the character of the treatment and for the final results.

   It is expected that the direction and supervision of the treatment here indicated will be carried out, in so far as is possible, in co-operation with the Director of the Division of General Surgery.

5. To carry out the instructions of this circular, the Director of the Division of Orthopaedic Surgery will arrange so that representatives of his Division will see all cases of the nature described, to determine whether or not their management is proceeding satisfactorily so as to obtain the best possible results.

   These representatives will report to the Commanding Officers of the hospitals in which such patients are being treated and their services as consultants will be freely utilized; any recommendation made by them as to change of treatment, transfer to some other professional service, or hospital will ordinarily, if the military situation permits, receive favorable consideration.

6. It is not the intention of this order to interfere with the routine work of hospitals, but to insure to the soldier proper supervision during the time of his treatment and the period of his convalescence.

By command of General Pershing:
  APPROVED: A.E. Bradley
J.G. Harbord,   Brig. Gen. N.A.
Chief of Staff.   Chief Surgeon.

ORTHOPAEDIC SURGERY ACCEPTED AS A SPECIALTY

Although orthopaedic surgery had established itself as a specialty in the late 1800s, until America's entry into World War I, the US Army had not recognized it as such. Soon after Goldthwait's first unit arrived in England, he reported to Gorgas that 1,000 of the 1,350 soldiers who had received orthopaedic care at Shepherd's Bush Hospital were able to return to duty and the remainder were released in a state of functional fitness, both orthopaedically and vocationally. In this way, he illustrated how orthopaedic surgery was contributing significantly to the war effort. Despite this, it was only after Congress had voted to enter the war that Surgeon General William C. Gorgas created the Division of Orthopedic Surgery as a distinct and separate entity. In the end, the war and the demand it created for orthopaedic surgeons both elevated and empowered the specialty.

> "The war has done more to bring Orthopaedic Surgery into its true inheritance than would have been accomplished by other agencies in many years, if indeed anything else would ever have brought about such complete emancipation of our specialty."
> —Herbert P. H. Galloway, MD (AOA President's Address, "Readjustment to Changing Conditions," *Journal of Orthopaedic Surgery* 1919; 1(7):39.)

Leaders within the newly formed Division of Orthopedic Surgery were ambitious and farsighted regarding the role of orthopaedic surgeons contributing to the war effort. They viewed orthopaedic care as integral, not peripheral, to the medical care that wounded soldiers required. Building on the already generous scope of practice that Surgeon General Gorgas had granted them, which included establishing specialized hospitals and acquiring equipment as needed, division leaders sought constantly to expand their purview in order to afford the wounded with the most comprehensive and effective orthopaedic care possible. For instance, Brackett, then the director of military orthopedics, insisted that the goal of the military orthopaedic surgeon should not be merely to save the soldier's life or help him regain strength enough to be shipped home, but to rehabilitate him to the point that he could return to active duty or engage productively in industrial work.

Goldthwait, too, shared this bold, holistic vision of military orthopaedic practice. Beyond providing the wounded with sufficient hospital beds, of which he had more than 30,000 constructed on his arrival in France, he developed a more effective method for triaging them. This process featured a chain of stations for orthopaedic care that extended along evacuation routes from the front to the north shores of France, from whence soldiers would eventually depart for home. An orthopaedic surgeon and two orderlies staffed each station, splinting or re-splinting injured limbs with Thomas (for legs) or Jones (for arms) splints. Goldthwait was particularly concerned with preventing shortening and/or angular deformities as well as preventing or treating joint contractures—which he knew, if left unattended, could result in deformities that would require more extensive treatment later.

This expansion of orthopaedic practice offended some general surgeons in the Division of General Surgery, such as Charles W. Mayo and William W. Keen, who viewed it as an encroachment on their turf and saw no need for an independent division of orthopaedic surgery. In a letter to Mayo, however, Goldthwait adroitly addressed his counterpart's concern by describing what he saw as the necessary and mutually beneficial division of labor between orthopaedic and general surgeons. Orthopaedic operations, he posited, could be performed by any type of surgeon with a certain level of skill, whereas the true focus of the orthopaedic surgeon was on the rehabilitative care of the patient following surgery, which required knowledge of specialized exercises and equipment and which could last for months.

In the summer of 1918, the Office of the Surgeon General was reorganized. The Section of Orthopaedic Surgery was led by Colonel E. G. Brackett, chief of the section, and Lieutenant-Colonel David Silver, assistant chief; consultants to camp inspectors and general and base hospitals included Lieutenant-Colonel Osgood and Major Zabdiel B. Adams (see chapter 40). The surgeon general appointed a committee in December 1918 to determine which medical conditions should fall within the orthopaedic section's ambit, and the committee identified five main categories:

1. All cases of amputation
2. Deformities of extremities due to or associated with contractures of muscles, ligaments and tendons

Box 63.6. American Surgeons Save British Lives

Sir Robert Jones, in charge of the orthopaedic efforts in Britain's Army, described the overwhelming shortages of surgeons and physicians Britain experienced as their qualified medical men went to the front:

"The Great War made so extensive and sudden a demand upon medical overseas service that we were faced with a serious shortage of young medical men at home. This shortage became more and more acute as time passed, and was experienced in every department of surgery. Were it not for the great ability and vision of our Director General (Sir Alfred Keogh) events would have proved much more tragic than they did. As it was, fractures and wounds which had been carefully treated abroad lacked an adequate continuity in their treatment on arrival here – for, owing to the character of our struggle and the sudden and ever growing demand for beds, a fear naturally rose that a stasis would seriously dislocate military operations. Under such conditions a choice of evils favored the rapid emptying of our beds. In the same spirit that the soldiers sacrificed their lives, a further sacrifice was demanded of our wounded. In 1916 we were ordered to start an orthopedic hospital for military cases in Liverpool, but at that time so short of hospitals were we all over the country that only 250 beds could be afforded to the so-called chronic or orthopedic cases. At that time, it was not fully realized that an ideal orthopedic hospital was primarily intended to prevent the occurrence of disability and deformity, which in so large a proportion of cases were the results of hurried evacuation and inefficient treatment. The wards were immediately filled with a ghastly array of derelicts. In spite of the fact that we were seriously handicapped for want of staff, the experiment proved so successful that I was practically given a free hand to increase our beds in Liverpool and start similar establishments in other centers. In a few months we had increased our bed accommodation from 250 to nearly 20,000. By degrees the orthopedic hospital was found in London, Leeds, Edinburgh, Aberdeen, Glasgow, Newcastle, Manchester, Bristol, Newport, Cardiff, Dublin, Belfast, and other towns. Instead of dealing merely with cases which result from want of continuity in treatment, and which were hopelessly crippled, we received many directly from abroad. This was the opportunity which was needed in order to stem the tide of deformity. Our aim in forming an orthopaedic center was to procure:

1. A staff of surgeons who had had previous experience of the principles and practice of orthopedic surgery, operative, manipulative, and educational.

2. Men who though not specializing in orthopedic surgery were interested in it, and only needed experience to fit them to take charge of wards as new centers were formed.

3. Still younger men, who were ultimately to go abroad where a training in the elements of orthopedic work would be to their great advantage.

4. The center would further consist of a series of auxiliary departments, each under an expert in the particular methods of treatment under his direction, such as

3. Derangement and disabilities of joints; including articular fractures
4. Deformities and disabilities of the feet
5. Cases requiring tendon transplantation... (Osgood 1919)

Whether a patient should be treated by a general surgeon or an orthopaedic surgeon depended on which coexisting condition was more severe. The chiefs of surgery were evenhanded in making these determinations. Their main goal was "to place the surgeon best qualified to care for the case or group of cases in charge of these patients without regard to the specialty to which he belonged. The main difficulty of the Chief of the Orthopedic Section has been to find for both overseas and America enough orthopedic surgeons who were well qualified to deal with the acute and chronic surgical problems as well as to supervise

> departments for electricity massage, muscle-reeducation, hydrology, and gymnastic drill.
>
> "Every center contained on its staff, in addition to specialists, a well-known surgeon, a neurologist, and a physician and consultations were of weekly occurrence in which every member participated.
>
> "A great feature of these centers was the curative workshops. They acted directly and indirectly on the welfare and recovery of the patient – directly as a curative agent when the work done gave exercise to the disabled limb, the work being employed as an agent in restoring coordinate movements; indirectly in the psychological effect produced by the stimulus of work. King Manuel, representing the British Red Cross and St. John of Jerusalem, was our tower of strength in this department.
>
> "Before the development of these hospitals was in any way complete we were hard pressed to the point of despair for the want of young orthopedic surgeons. It was anathema to keep any young surgeon in the country. The authorities on this were adamant. Their views were, that as it had become necessary for surgeons with families to go abroad, no excuse could hold good for the retention in this country of young men, no matter how expert. Could not the older men be trained to do orthopedic work, we were asked. At last permission was given that we could retain 12 young surgeons, and we were promised that under no circumstances would they be sent abroad. This was a great gain; but 12 men could not do justice to so vast a problem as that which confronted us, and the work was sorely handicapped."
>
> Jones then elaborated on the hugely valuable work done by American surgeons in England during the war:
>
> "It was at this moment that your great nation came to our assistance. Sir John Goodwin placed before the American authorities a statement of our difficulties, and they promised us help. I shall never forget the thrill of joy I experienced when there arrived in Liverpool five young orthopedic surgeons placed at our disposal by the American Government for the period of the war. They were an extraordinarily fine body of men, keen, enthusiastic, and well trained. These units were distributed amongst the various centers and were given charge of wards. It is impossible to speak too highly of their loyalty, discipline, and devotion to duty. There sprang up immediately a bond of fraternity between them and their English colleagues, and the relationship was maintained throughout. The American Government wisely decided that their young surgeons on their way to the war area should spend a few weeks in the English orthopedic centers in order to gain experience. This arrangement was of distinct benefit to both nations. We often had over a hundred American surgeons working in the country at one time.
>
> "I should like to pay a tribute of gratitude to America for the splendid service rendered by these young men. They came in to us in our extremity; they filled a gap which seriously threatened to sterilize our reconstructive efforts, and they filled it with distinction and success" (quoted in Weed 1927).

that detailed and often tedious special treatment… [for] the return of the greatest amount of function in the shortest possible time" (Osgood 1919).

Wounded men were treated on the front in various facilities and hospitals (**Figure 63.1**). These facilities were mainly of three types: a field ambulance, a casualty clearing station, and a general hospital (specialty hospitals, which included orthopaedic hospitals, were located both at or near the front and off the battlefield near base hospitals). In a 1919 article about "Medical Work in the British Armies in France," published in the *Transactions of the American Clinical and Climatological Association*, George Cheever Shattuck described these three arenas of treatment:

> A field ambulance was attached to every fighting division in the field…[Its] functions…were to collect the wounded from the regimental aid posts and when necessary from the field, to put on dressings and splints, stop hemorrhage, and evacuate cases with the least possible delay to the casualty clearing stations in the rear, where most of the operating was done…
>
> A clearing station can ordinarily accommodate five hundred cases and has facilities for expansion to 1,000. Every army at the front had a number of these units…[and] they moved with it when necessary, but moves were not frequent during the period of trench warfare….

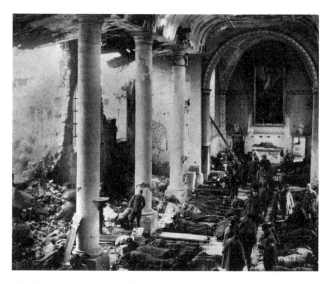

Field hospital in a partially destroyed church.
National WWI Museum and Memorial, Kansas City, Missouri, USA.

Fig. 63.1 General Scheme of British Hospitals.
G. S. Cheever, "Medical Evacuation. British Armies in France," *Transactions of the American Clinical and Climatological Association* 1919; 35: 140.

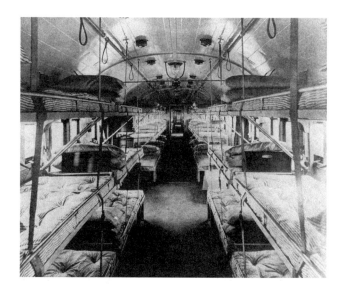

Interior of a typical US Army Hospital Train.
The Army Medical Department 1917–1941 by Mary C. Gillett. Washington, DC: Center of Military History, United States Army, 2009.

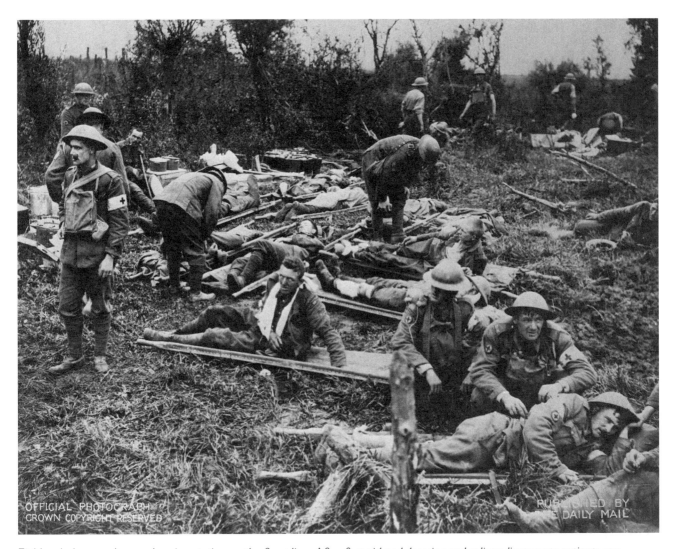

Field ambulance: advance dressing station on the front line. After first aid and dressing and splint adjustments patients are transferred to the casualty clearing station (CCS). Wellcome Collection.

The large hospitals to which the clearing stations evacuated their sick and wounded were called "general hospitals." These were on the coast, some in towns where they occupied permanent buildings, and others in open country where huts and tents were erected… Patients came to them by ambulance car from the hospital train. The principle avenues for evacuation were the "convalescent camps" in France and the "hospital ships" for England.

The capacity of most of the "general hospitals" was increased several times during the war and finally reached 2,400 comprising about 1,400 permanent beds and roughly 1,000 stretchers or bed sacks.

Shattuck (1919) went on to characterize in detail the operation of the 22nd general hospital, which was staffed by American physicians, surgeons, and nurses, many of whom were from Harvard:

All the administrative officers [initially] were British…[I]t had two divisions, a surgical and medical…[and was staffed by] thirty-two officers…Two wards of 60 beds each with from 10 to 20 new patients a day was found to be more than a new man could handle efficiently…, whereas the same man a few months later could learn to handle twice that number of stretcher cases…

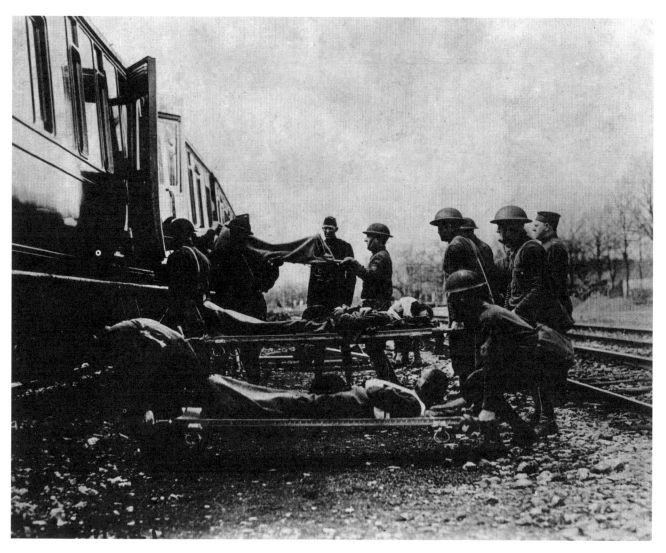

Wounded soldiers being loaded onto a hospital train. *The Army Medical Department 1917-1941* by Mary C. Gillett. Washington, DC: Center of Military History, United States Army, 2009.

In 1917 and 1918, the number of officers on duty…was at times below the authorized establishment…

Because a "wounded man passes through five or six hands before reaching a base hospital and he usually receives a different kind of treatment at each station" (McDill 1918), standardization of care was a necessity. Splints were one main element of care that lent itself to such standardization, particularly by "[limiting] their number to a certain few patterns" (Osgood 1918). Osgood (1918) noted, "This seemed of great importance since…many medical officers had been unfamiliar in civil life with the most efficient types of military splints, and many…had given little attention to fractures." The American Expeditionary Forces' chief surgeon, General Alfred E. Bradley, named six men to a "splint board": Osgood, Alexander Lambert, Joseph A. Blake (all with the rank of major), William S. Baer, Nathaniel Allison (both with the rank of captain), and the board's chairman, Colonel William L. Keller. "This board agreed on a standardization of splints, limited the number for use on the front to seven, and…wrote a manual" that was completed and approved in October 1917. A total of 25,000 copies of the manual were "distributed…to all medical offices

World War I

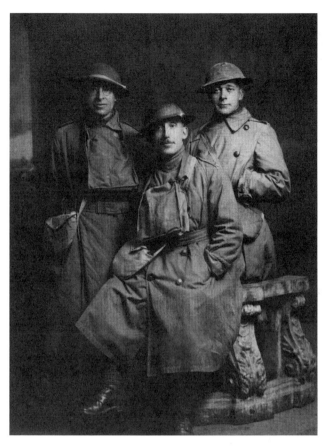

Dr. Osgood (left) and Dr. Allison (center) in uniform.
National WWI Museum and Memorial, Kansas City, Missouri, USA.

abroad" (Osgood 1918). Allison, who was also part of the Division of Orthopaedic Surgery, oversaw the combat divisions and field hospitals and taught officers and stretcher-bearers the proper techniques for applying splints. British soldiers set a two-minute record "for applying a Thomas leg splint…and the recognized time which all stretcher-bearers are expected to better is six minutes. The wounded men with fractures are [now] coming back in splendid shape to the evacuation hospitals" (Osgood 1918).

At the request of the surgeon general, Osgood also described the organization of medical care in the American Expeditionary Forces. First, he shared details about the days before combat began: "Casual surgical and medical cases…occur in small numbers. They are sent to the base hospital…." To the surprise of physicians and military leaders, however, the work required of those serving in the division of orthopedic surgery was "much larger than was anticipated"—not because of war injuries, but because in many regiments between 15 and 20 men were unfit for combat because of back conditions, poor footwear, or foot strain. They had been quickly drafted and were not fit enough to sustain intensive training. This caused issues for the men's morale and put strain on the physicians providing care: they were unfit for duty but had no surgical or medical issues, and the physicians sent them back on duty. After a few days, they would be back at the base hospitals. This was a blow to their morale, because "they themselves knew they were not 'quitters,' [but] they were being considered so…[and] useless to the Army" (Osgood 1918). James Bevens, a colonel in the 26th Division, proposed a way to make these soldiers "fit for combat": training by line officers "under medical supervision of orthopedic medical officers. The experiment…proved successful beyond any anticipation. After three months…something like 80 per cent of the men…returned to combat duty after an average gradual training of about six weeks… [and] 90 per cent could be made fit for work in some capacity in the Army" (Osgood 1918).

In his report, Osgood (1918) went on to describe the process of delivering care once combat started: "When the division goes into action… the most acute attention is being focused on getting the cases back to the evacuation hospitals in the best possible condition…in the shortest possible time. Practically no surgery, except the stopping of hemorrhage, the halting of a case in shock and an occasional abdominal or chest emergency is done in the field hospital [field ambulance]." Each combat unit had a specialist in each of three areas: genitourinary, psychiatry, and orthopedic surgery.

Osgood (1918) expanded on the care provided once soldiers have been removed to evacuation hospitals:

> The surgery is almost wholly that of emergency surgery and must be entirely in the hands of

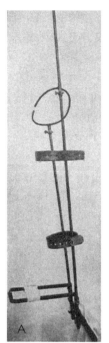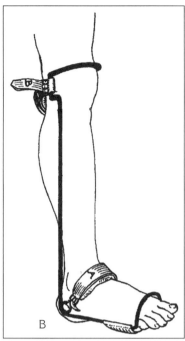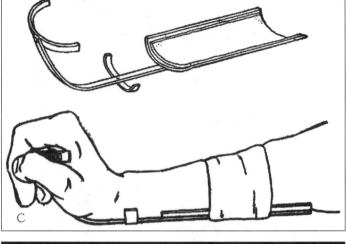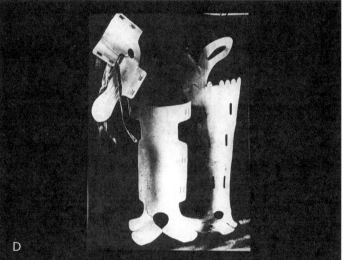

Example of standardized splints used in WWI. A): Thomas splint made of Shelby tubing. B): Line drawing of a wire splint for a drop-foot deformity. C): Line drawing of a wire splint for a wrist-drop deformity. D): First aid splints of thin sheet aluminum or zinc. They were packed flat and bent to shape when used.

A and B: R. B. Osgood, "Orthopaedic Work in a War Hospital," *Boston Medical and Surgical Journal* 1916; 174: 109. C: R. B. Osgood, "The Transport Splints of the American Army," *Journal of the American Medical Association* 1981; 71: 737. D: Lantern slide by Robert B. Greenough. Warren Anatomical Museum in the Francis A. Countway Library of Medicine.

the general surgeons...the different specialists being asked to come in for consultation as they are desired.

When the cases can safely be removed from the evacuation hospitals, they go back either to the base hospitals of the advanced zone, the special hospitals of the advanced zone, or sometimes directly to the base hospitals of the intermediate and base zones. The special cases of bone and joint injury are segregated as far as possible and sent to the special bone and joint hospitals. One is already established in the advanced zone and several others in the intermediate and base zones. In the advanced zone these are known as bone and joint hospitals...their senior medical officer [is] either a general surgeon skilled in bone and joint conditions or an orthopedic surgeon qualified to deal with fractures...

Osgood (1918) gave particular attention to the treatment of soldiers requiring amputation:

From the base hospitals in the advanced zone, cases of amputation are sent to a special center and segregated. There the early treatment for weight-bearing is begun. At Base Hospital No. 9 such a center is already established under the direction of Capt. Philip Wilson [see chapter 40], a man of large surgical experience and fine training in the artificial limb problem through a long service in the Red Cross Bureau of Mutilés

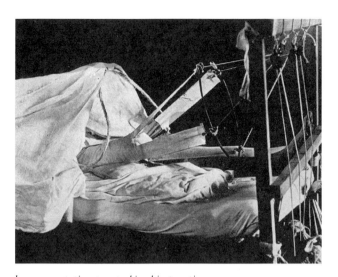

Leg amputation treated in skin traction.
The Medical Department of the U.S. Army in the World War, Volume XI: Surgery, under the direction of Maj. Gen. M.W. Ireland. Washington, DC: Government Printing Office, 1927.

[in Paris]. Here the cases are fitted to pilons and to temporary limbs with the same joint mechanism as the permanent limbs and a consecutive training without waste of time is begun, to be continued on this side [back in the United States], where a more permanent and finished limb will be applied. By the time the stumps are ready for their final most perfect mechanism the men should be ready for wage-earning also.

He recognized the economic importance of appropriately treating amputations and did not hesitate to share this in his report:

An enormous loss of time and labor to a nation is suffered when large numbers of cases wait much longer than the condition of their stumps requires for the fitting of the artificial limbs. In one of the belligerent countries, there are probably…10,000 men waiting for more than six months longer than necessary for the fitting of the limbs. When one realizes that this represents, in actual time lost to the nation, the entire labor of a man for 5,000 years, one begins to see the importance of the economic waste. (Osgood 1918)

Finally, Osgood (1918) explained how soldiers with bone and joint injuries were handled under:

the Division of Orthopedic Surgery, to whom the long-standing cases originally come in the special orthopedic hospitals. It does not mean that the orthopedic surgeons have entire charge or care of these cases. Perhaps they have been more accustomed than general surgeons to determine whether the greatest amount of function…has been gained…It seemed fair… to ask their consultation as to methods of treatment most likely to bring about the best possible result. The "check-up"…is the important thing…in…the various base hospitals…and consulting with the various surgical and orthopedic men stationed in these hospitals. It was apparent that all cases were being handled extremely well, and we may hope…that our burden of preventable cripples will be lightened. We should like to emphasize again the general atmosphere of team play…among the professional divisions…No one wishes to be considered, over there [in the US], a specialist, except in so far as his previous training has made it possible for him to render one type of service better than another.

AMERICAN BASE HOSPITALS: HARVARD UNITS

Each of the first six American base hospitals that took over six British general hospitals in France in the spring of 1917 "was organized under a director, and on each, with one exception, was an orthopedic surgeon…The director of the Harvard unit was Maj. Harvey Cushing, and Capt. Frank Ober [see chapter 20] was orthopedic surgeon" (Osgood 1919). Allison, who had graduated from Harvard and would eventually return there as a professor of orthopaedic surgery, worked as an orthopedic surgeon with the Washington University unit and had two assistants.

Because the military needed to mobilize quickly and on short notice upon the United States' official entry into the war, plans for the May 1917 construction of a demonstration hospital on the Boston Common fell by the wayside. Various units of Harvard surgeons, physicians, nurses, and other personnel based at hospitals throughout the Boston area formed for deployment. The American Expeditionary Forces created 78 base hospitals in total, six of which were lent to the British Expeditionary Forces for a year, to provide the British with much-needed personnel; of those six, Base Hospital No. 5 remained with the British Expeditionary Forces for the rest of the war. According to Harvey Cushing, these six hospitals treated more wounded soldiers than the other 72 base hospitals combined. **Table 63.1** describes three of the Boston-derived base hospitals; these hospitals are described in details in what follows.

Base Hospital No. 5

In late May 1917, Cushing and the team of Base Hospital No. 5 "arrived at Camiers and took charge of No. 11 General Hospital adjoining the Harvard Surgical Unit at No. 22," whose chief then was Dr. E. H. Nichols. The medical officers at Base Hospital No. 5, the "Harvard Unit," were all affiliated with Harvard and came from various hospitals across Boston:

- Major Harvey Cushing, director (from PBBH)
- Lieutenant Walter B. Cannon, director of the laboratory section (from HMS)
- Captain Horace Binney, a genitourinary surgeon and chief of the surgical service (from Boston City Hospital)
- Captain Elliott C. Cutler (from HMS, MGH, and PBBH)
- Major Roger I. Lee, chief of the medical service (from MGH)
- Lieutenant Frank R. Ober, the unit's orthopedist (from HMS, Boston Children's Hospital) (see chapter 20)
- Major Robert B. Osgood (MGH) (**Box 63.7**)

American Medical Corps personnel like Osgood became integrated into every aspect of the British Expeditionary Forces throughout the theatre of war, sometimes working with more than five British organizations. They fulfilled "capacities…intended to take advantage of their knowledge, skills and expertise…once the floodgates of U.S. Army Medical Corps had been opened in May 1917, they entered nearly every aspect of service within the British forces in Europe…" (Rauer, n.d.).

In the first month, the hospital treated more than 3,000 patients. On August 1, 1917, just as the Third Battle of Ypres began, 964 patients were admitted and "[by] war's end, over 45,000 British and American…patients had been treated at Base Hospital No. 5" ("Formation of the Base Hospitals," n.d.). In **Box 63.8**, Cushing describes the urgency and frightening circumstances those as Base Hospital No. 5 faced during its two years of service in France.

The American medical staff new to the base hospitals required training at the front and so, in

Table 63.1. Three Main Boston-derived Base Hospitals

Base Hospital No.	Boston Hospital	Director	Location During War
5	Peter Bent Brigham	Harvey Cushing	Camiers and Boulogne, France
6	Massachusetts General	Frederick A. Washburn	Talence, France
7	Boston City	John Joseph Dowling	Joué-le-Tours, France

Box 63.7. Robert Osgood's Posts Throughout His Tour of Duty

> Osgood was a surgical instructor at Harvard Medical School and was commissioned on May 5, 1917, when he began his work with the Harvard Unit. He subsequently held various important posts throughout the war: He was appointed chief of surgery on September 14, 1917, and after a year was sent to the orthopedic section of the American Expeditionary Forces. On February 14, 1918, he began a post at "the War Office, London, as Assistant Director of Military Orthopedic Surgery, A.E.F. February 14, 1918, [he was] transferred to France as Orthopedic Consultant, Headquarters Medical and Surgical Consultants, Neufchâteau" (Cushing 1919). Six weeks later he was transferred again to assume his post at the office of the chief surgeon in Tours. Osgood was later "on duty in the Surgeon-General's office, Washington, as Orthopedic Consultant. [He was] promoted to Lieutenant Colonel July 29, 1918" (Cushing 1919). Osgood published nine articles while on active duty, including the well-known "Manual of Splints and Appliances for the Medical Corps of the United States Army" in November 1917 with Nathaniel Allison, William S. Baer, Joseph A. Blake, William L. Keller, and Alexander Lambert.

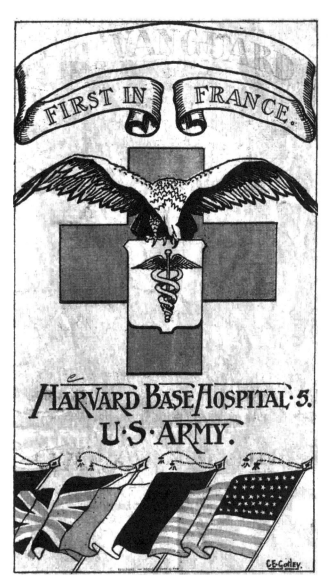

Cover of Base Hospital No. 5's monthly newsletter *The Vanguard: First in France*, May 1918. Boston Medical Library in the Francis A. Countway Library of Medicine.

summer 1917, US personnel became "part of the rotation of supplemental personnel to the CCSs [Casualty Clearing Stations], teams of surgeons and operating room nurses" (Rauer, n.d.). By June, all six American Base Hospitals, including Base Hospital No. 5:

> underwent a period of familiarization and training…it was recognized that these American medical personnel should gain some first-hand front-line experience…to understand the complexities of the medical situations they would face. Beginning in July and lasting through December 1917 the original…surgical teams…quickly found themselves in CCSs [Casualty Clearing Stations] that were a few miles behind the front lines on the Western Front. Here medical officers attended to the routine tasks of dressing wounds, and…operated on the wounded to stabilize each man for the next stage of the evacuation process… The teams improved their surgical techniques through experience and no group of surgeons burned out from constant work at a CCS…
> (Rauer, n.d.)

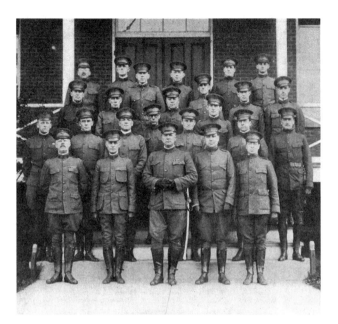

Officers of US Army Base Hospital No. 5 in Fort Totten (Queens, NY) on May 10, 1917, just before sailing to France. Dr. Ober is at the far left in the back row and Dr. Osgood is in the front row on the far right. Dr. Cushing is second from the left in the first row. *The Story of U.S. Army Base Hospital No. 5* by Harvey Cushing. Cambridge: The University Press, 1919.

Box 63.9 includes a 1917 letter to the editor of the *American Journal of Orthopedic Surgery*, in which Osgood wrote about some of his experiences at US Army Base Hospital No. 5. The hospital became fully staffed, but there were some administrative and procedural differences between the British and the American militaries, and with regard to certain policies, for example, whether soldiers were required to or prohibited from bringing their firearms into the base hospital. Nonetheless, the US and British medical staff worked well together and with the supplies they had:

> Once the American hospitals began their transition into General Hospitals it became very apparent that they were understaffed. Base Hospital No. 5 absorbed forty American enlisted men, fifteen nurses and a few more physicians…Eventually all six of the American base hospitals acquired the necessary

Box 63.8. Base Hospital No. 5: The First 2 Years

> "It was the first [unit] to suffer casualties at the hands of the enemy…Five members of the Harvard contingent [of the American Ambulance in 1915], Drs. Boothby, Cutler, Cushing, Osgood and Strong, subsequently enrolled themselves as members of the organization which came to be Base Hospital No. 5…No. 11 General…was the most northerly of the whole series of hospitals, very near the station at Dannes and flanked on the north by a large Portland cement works…[and] a large ammunition dump not far beyond…The Casualty Clearing Stations in forward areas were of course continually subjected to nocturnal bombing raids…But the Base so far had been exempt until on the night of September 4, 1917, without warning…a Gotha [twin-engine bomber] swept over the Camiers area and dropped a succession of seven bombs, five of them being direct hits in Base Hospital No. 5's compound. Twenty-two bed patients…were…seriously rewounded [numerous staff were wounded and four were killed]…
>
> "Although the move had been anticipated since June 1 [1917], it was with mixed feelings when orders from a clear sky were received on October 31 for the Unit to proceed forthwith to Boulogne and take over No. 13 General…The Transfer was made on short notice, and November 1 found the first installment of US in charge of the Casino…the hospital was the nearest of all general hospitals…to the Boulogne station and to the landing stage of the Channel packets, one of its functions was a place of temporary detention for slightly sick and wounded…whole convoys of cases destined to England might be deposited at the Casino if they reached Boulogne too late for the boat, or if, as not infrequently happened, the winter storms rendered the Channel unfit for crossing or necessitated extra sweeping to assume freedom from floating mines" (Cushing 1919).

staff for their new responsibilities. The Americans quickly established routines and began to treat the patients that arrived. Col. Harvey Cushing, at General Hospital No. 11 described

Box 63.9. Osgood's Letter to the Editor of the American Journal of Orthopedic Surgery

"On the surgical side at No. 11 we have an eye ward, a dental ward, a ward for head cases, two wards for orthopedic cases [and] twelve general surgical wards…it is necessary to send many cases back to England sooner than one would wish…Thus far no objection has been raised to our keeping important cases until it was possible to transport them without danger of jeopardizing the end-result, and, in badly septic comminuted thigh and joint fractures, this means many weeks – nine or ten at the least….We have a large ward kept full of cases of joint lesions without external wounds, backs strained by the weight of earth in which the soldier is often buried by a shell explosion, an occasionally unrecognized vertebral compression fracture, a common sacro-iliac or lumbo-sacral sprain, a deep hematoma, a rupture of the spinal ligaments. One of the ways in which the Army keeps its more or less inactive men in good condition is by insisting on football practice…when played by men unaccustomed to the game and on a somewhat irregular ground, [it] is the source of many sprained ankles, torn and dislocated semilunar cartilages, ruptured lateral and crucial ligaments – a veritable El Dorado of the very lesions which make it possible to practice orthopedic surgery in civil life…We are still being governed in cases of gunshot wounds of joints by the same principles which an earlier French experience had laid down…If a foreign body has perforated a joint and its tract appears to be reasonably clean, the joint is immobilized and carefully watched…At most, an aspiration is done and…bacteriology determined…In the case of a penetrating wound with the foreign body still present…in the joint…or imbedded in the articular ends of the bones…[It] should be removed…the joint is washed out for at least ten minutes with a weak bichloride or sterile normal saline or perhaps even the antiseptic solution devised by Dakin….a soft catheter tube inserted into…the joint, the joint cavity is tightly closed…and the external wound only partially sutured or not at all…

"The compound fractures make up the largest number of lesions, and complicated as they all are by sepsis, call for the most efficient methods of fixation, which must…provide adequate room for copious dressings and treatment by the Carrel technique…At the primary operation…tissues damaged beyond repair are removed…[but] never to remove even seemingly completely separated fragments of bone….excisions of joints and…bone fragments…the results of these procedures…are often deplorable…plaster-of-Paris dressings with wide openings bridged by loops of metal or plaster offer the most perfect fixation and greatest comfort to the patient…Thomas and Jones splints…are admirably adaptable, easy to make, capable of quick application, can be supplied in large quantities to the first stations, and allow…comfortable transportation…There is every indication…for the adoption of these unit types of splints by the American War Department" (Osgood 1917).

the transition thus: "Beginning to take over…We are effectively swallowed up in the British Army Machine, and already Base Hospital No. 5 has completely lost its identity…Our young officers have taken hold valiantly, and the wards, with the nurse's help, are already improved in appearance…It seems small when compared to the 70,000-bed capacity of this district." Working in the British General Hospitals saw some administrative friction as differences between the British and American regulations became apparent…American procedures directed patients should keep their entire "kits" with them. Unfortunately for the British this meant that the American soldiers would keep weapons in hospitals…British regulations prohibited soldiers entering medical facilities with weapons, holding that it violated the Geneva Convention…

By August 1917 the American-run General Hospitals were a fully functioning part of the British military medical establishment…A British inspection noted the Harvard unit [Base Hospital No. 5] had shown "much

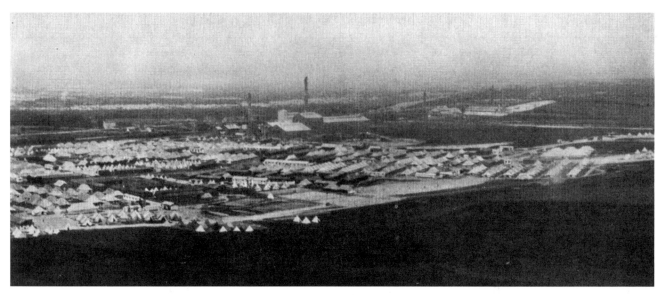

Aerial view of the northern part of the group of five hospitals in Camiers, including General Hospital No. 11 on the left. Sand dunes and the sea are in the background. *The Story of U.S. Army Base Hospital No. 5* by Harvey Cushing. Cambridge: The University Press, 1919.

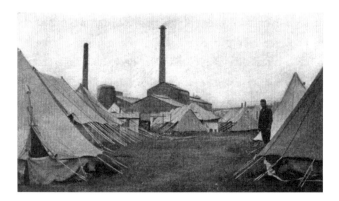

Although initially planned for a temporary period, the tents of Base Hospital No. 5 remained for about five months before the unit moved to Boulogne. *The Story of U.S. Army Base Hospital No. 5* by Harvey Cushing. Cambridge: The University Press, 1919.

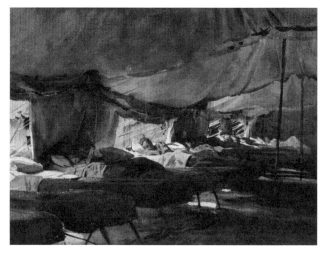

"The Interior of a Hospital Tent" by John Singer Sargent, 1918. Imperial War Museum/Wikimedia Commons.

improvement" in adapting the Casino building and surroundings to hospital purposes…The relations with the British and Colonials continue excellent, and the supplies furnished by the British are fairly satisfactory… (Rauer, n.d.)

Being on the front was a frightening and stressful experience. All personnel in Base Hospital No. 5 were traumatized by the sheer number of devastating injuries and high mortality rate, as well as the incessant German bombardment.

Some physicians lost their lives while trying to save patients because they left the dugouts to retrieve and treat wounded soldiers: "The CCSs were subject to aerial bombardments in addition to the other hazards of forward duty…[one physician] described his thoughts on his time at CCS No. 61. 'The horrible wounds, the suffering, the high mortality, tended to depress one and this was added to at night by the disturbing visits of the Hun planes'" (Rauer, n.d.).

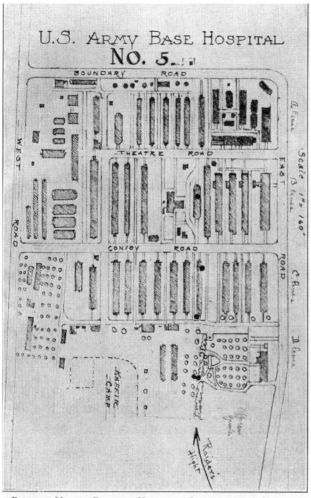

PLAN OF NO. 11 GENERAL HOSPITAL, CAMIERS. THE HEAVY BLACK DOTS IN LINE OF ARROW SHOWING WHERE BOMBS WERE DROPPED

Plan of General Hospital No. 11, Camiers. Black dots are the locations where the bombs struck the hospital.
The Story of U.S. Army Base Hospital No. 5 by Harvey Cushing. Cambridge: The University Press, 1919.

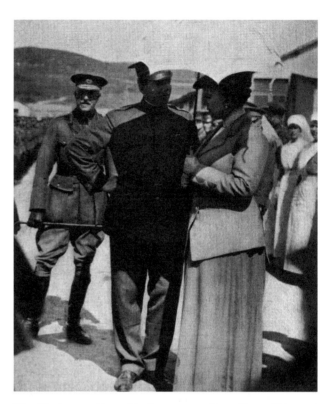

The Queen speaking with the commanding officer of General Hospital No. 11.
The Story of U.S. Army Base Hospital No. 5 by Harvey Cushing. Cambridge: The University Press, 1919.

In total, ~1,650 US physicians worked with the British Expeditionary Forces (B.E.F.). Of those, "37 lost their lives either while serving with the B.E.F. or as an immediate result. Twenty-five stemmed from front line combat service…In contrast, the A.E.F. had 28 physicians killed in action and 24 who died of wounds…first lieutenants (21 in A.E.F., 12 in B.E.F.)…captains (five in the A.E.F., three in the B.E.F.)….while two majors were killed with the A.E.F." (Rauer, n.d.). Some of the American medical officers had went further, past the CCSs, and into the thick of the fighting:

at the front lines, under fire from the Germans…in harm's way…It was here that physicians were in the greatest danger of injury and death. Often, they would leave the semi-protection of their dugouts…to treat an injured soldier…a young medical officer [recalled]… "When shells began to fall, Stan lay in the mud while the ground leaped like the surface of a pond under rain. The mud was also thick inside the captured German bunker where he received the wounded; the flies on the walls swarmed over one another, while all about and overhead the earth was beaten by huge steel flails as the bombardment moved ahead of a German Counterattack…when the firing quieted enough to let the stretcher-bearers out, he triaged the wounded. As many as twelve men were needed to manage a single litter over the mucky, cratered ground. Not all the wounded could be moved, and the hard rule of triage was

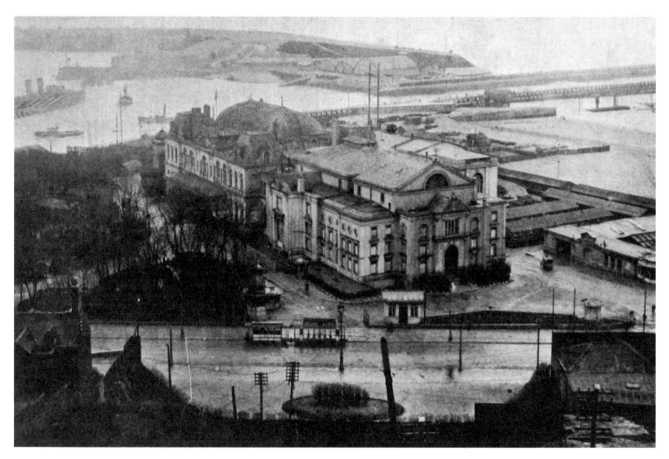

Casino Boulogne-sur-Mer—site for the US Army Base Hospital No. 5 (General Hospital No. 13)—on the coast of Normandy, France. The large breakwater is seen in the upper right. *The Story of U.S. Army Base Hospital No. 5* by Harvey Cushing. Cambridge: The University Press, 1919.

to save those who might survive and let the others die. At that unearthly hour, Stan had to play God and decide who went and who did not…" (Rauer, n.d.)

> "The orthopedic surgeon of the future can neither adequately represent our specialty, nor meet creditably the demands which will be made upon him unless he be conscious of possessing wide general surgeon training and experience."
> —Herbert P. H. Galloway, MD (AOA President's Address, "Readjustment to Changing Conditions," *Journal of Orthopaedic Surgery*, 1919; 1(7):39.)

By the end of December 1918, Base Hospital No. 5 was reduced to two surgical wards that remained active. Personnel at Base Hospital No. 5 had treated ~48,000 patients in their 20 months on site. The officers and men were transferred to Camp Devens, Massachusetts, to be demobilized. By early January 1919, "all other replacements [from Mobile Unit No. 6 in Argonne], numbering in the vicinity of seventy, were also returned to the American Expeditionary Forces. Late in January, the hospital was emptied of patients and the hospital was officially closed on February 1, 1919" (Hatch 1919).

World War I

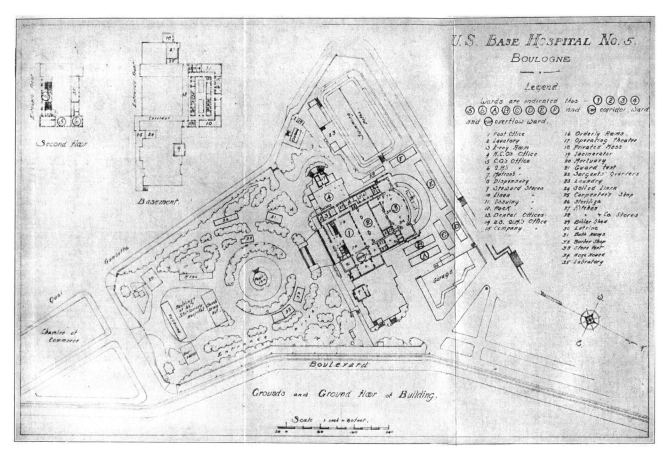

Map of the grounds and the ground floor of the Boulogne Casino. *The Story of U.S. Army Base Hospital No. 5* by Harvey Cushing. Cambridge: The University Press, 1919.

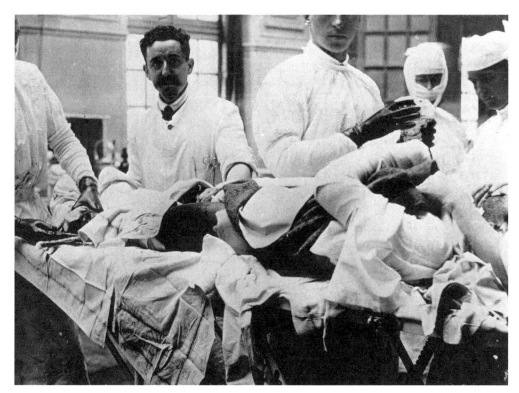

Operating room (Base Hospital No. 5) with injured soldier and medical staff.

Lantern slide by Robert B. Greenough. Warren Anatomical Museum in the Francis A. Countway Library of Medicine.

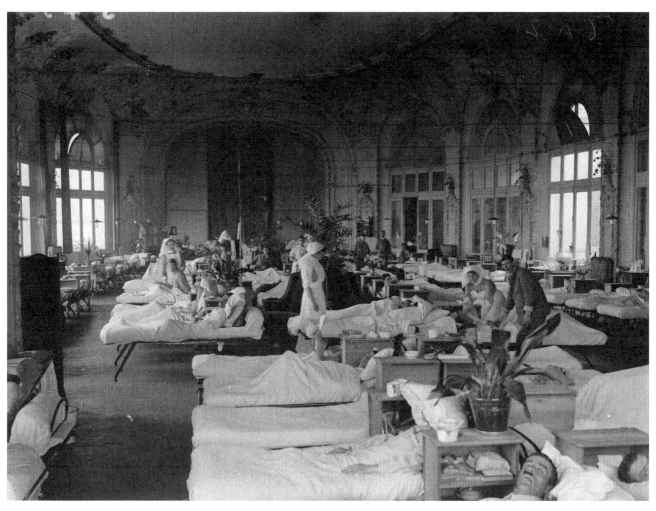
Patient ward in the Boulogne Casino. ©Imperial War Museum (Q 29162).

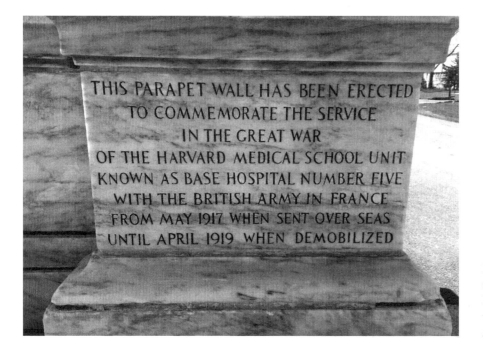
Parapet wall commemorating the service of Harvard's unit, Base Hospital No. 5 in WWI. Located at the entrance to HMS on Longwood Avenue. Photo by the author.

World War I

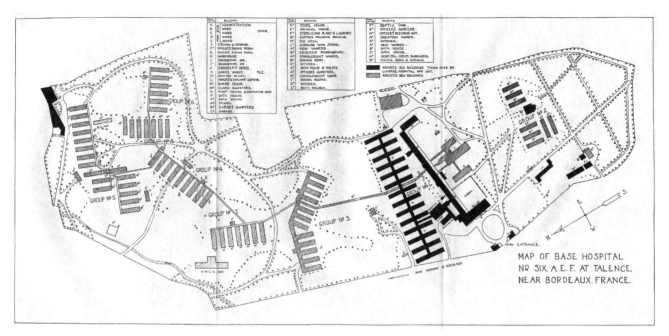

Map of US Army Base Hospital No. 6, Talence, France (on the outskirts of Bordeaux), 1917–1918. *The History of U.S. Army Base Hospital No. 6 and its Part in the American Expeditionary Forces, 1917-1918*, edited by George Clymer. Boston: Massachusetts General Hospital, 1924.

Base Hospital No. 6

More than a year before the war began, Dr. Frederic A. Washburn, who would become the commander of Base Hospital No. 6, wrote to Surgeon General Gorgas to discuss creating civilian hospital units for army service. General Gorgas agreed to a plan of organizing reserve hospital units in hospitals in the United States. Examples of such hospitals included the Massachusetts General Hospital and the Johns Hopkins Hospital. The MGH trustees consented to the creation of such a reserve unit at MGH on March 17, 1916: "That Dr. Washburn be authorized to accept the position of Director, and to organize at the Massachusetts General Hospital a mobile unit to be ready for service for the Army in case of war…Base Hospital No. 6 was thus early authorized…to organize and pledge its officers and nurses under the Red Cross and to arrange for equipment" (Washburn 1939).

In a history of Base Hospital No. 6, Warren L. Babcock (1924) describes the well-trained and well-prepared MGH hospital unit:

Few hospital units left the States as well equipped in professional personnel as did the Massachusetts General Hospital…Base Hospital No. 6 maintained throughout its entire history the high ideals and unswerving loyalty of purpose that were characteristic of the original unit. The leavening influence of the highly

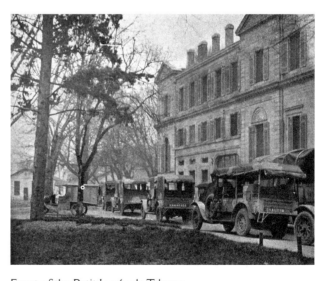

Front of the Petit Lycée de Talence.

The History of U.S. Army Base Hospital No. 6 and its Part in the American Expeditionary Forces, 1917-1918, edited by George Clymer. Boston: Massachusetts General Hospital, 1924.

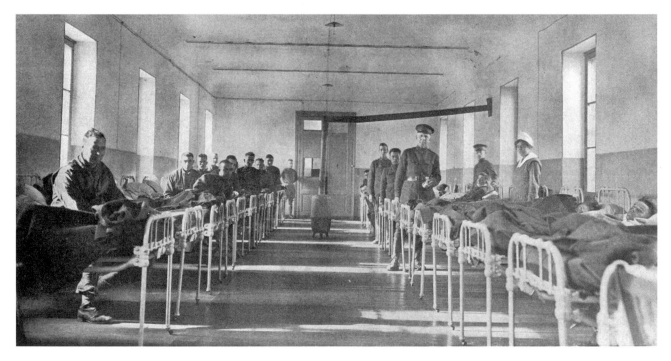

Ward in the Lycée building. *The History of U.S. Army Base Hospital No. 6 and its Part in the American Expeditionary Forces, 1917-1918*, edited by George Clymer. Boston: Massachusetts General Hospital, 1924.

trained professional groups was constantly apparent…The first Commanding Officer [Colonel Washburn] was a hospital administrator of well-known ability. He brought to his work a training and military experience acquired as a volunteer officer in the Spanish-American War. Base Hospital No. 6 was the only one of the early phase hospitals commanded from the start by a civilian medical reserve officer.

Training and preparation began immediately. The preparation by Washburn and the reserve team at MGH:

showed its value. Men were soon enlisted. The necessary officers for organization were mustered into the service in May…The enlisted men and certain officers went to Fort Strong, on Long Island in Boston Harbor, for training…Surgery [was headed] by Lieutenant Colonel Lincoln Davis…Base Hospital No. 6 was but one of the many hospitals thus organized. When they became going concerns in France and England they gave the American soldier a high-grade hospitalization that he had never had in previous wars. These hospitals were the backbone of the Medical Department in the American Expeditionary Forces… (Washburn 1939)

A little more than a year after its establishment, as the US entered the war in April 1917, Base Hospital No. 6 became "one of the first units in America to respond to the call of the Allies for medical assistance was established early in Bordeaux…[and] at once became the marker and pattern for other similar units that were stationed later in this region which formed one of the largest centers of hospital activities of the American Forces in France" (Shaw 1924). Washburn (1939) went on to write:

when the Base Hospital unit sailed from New York on the *Aurania*, July 9, 1917, it was a real military organization, uniformed and disciplined. It carried with it equipment for a

World War I

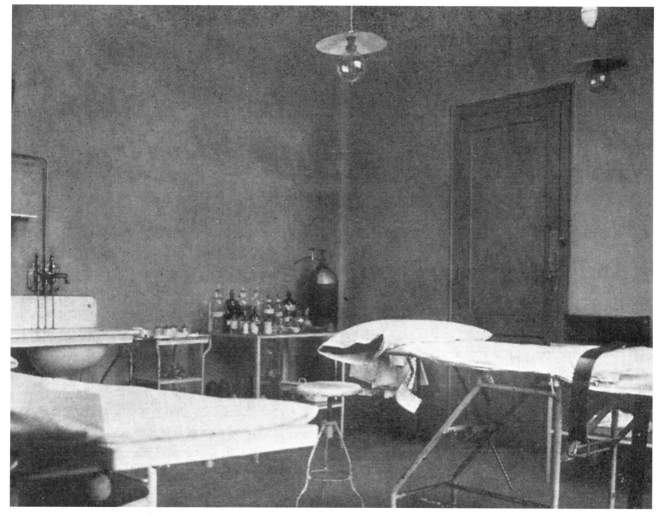

Operating Room in Base Hospital No. 6. *The History of U.S. Army Base Hospital No. 6 and its Part in the American Expeditionary Forces, 1917-1918*, edited by George Clymer. Boston: Massachusetts General Hospital, 1924.

500-bed hospital...[but] when in full activity [the hospital] had 4300 patients at one time... The unit landed at Liverpool, crossed England to Southampton, thence to Le Havre, then to Bordeaux, and finally to Talence, a suburb of Bordeaux.

Just a few months after delivering the MGH team to France, the RMS *Aurania* (the second of three of that name, built in 1916) was attacked by a German submarine and sunk by torpedoes. No one survived.

In 1924, Paul Dudley White quaintly described the beginnings of Base Hospital No. 6: "In the little town of Talence on the outskirts of

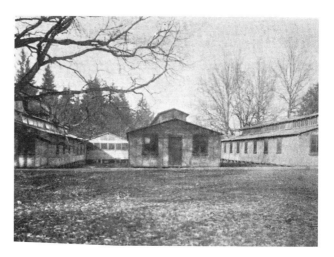

Surgical & Orthopaedic Wards, Base Hospital No. 6.
The History of U.S. Army Base Hospital No. 6 and its Part in the American Expeditionary Forces, 1917-1918, edited by George Clymer. Boston: Massachusetts General Hospital, 1924.

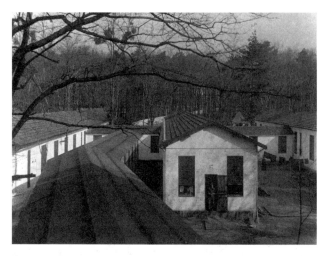

Corridor from receiving to the new hospital (Base Hospital No. 6), April 1918. National Archives and Records Administration/Wikimedia Commons.

Bordeaux there lived for a year and a half, during the World War, a group of pioneers of the Medical Corps of the American Expeditionary Force." In Talence, the French had converted the Petit Lycée de Talence, a school, into a hospital (Hôpital Complémentaire No. 25) at the beginning of the War: "On this French site of approximately sixty-seven acres, ensconced in a grove of sturdy oaks, was the nucleus for the development of one of the largest single base hospitals in the A.E.F." (Babcock 1924). According to Washburn (1939), the MGH unit:

> was the first American organization to enter Bordeaux and was one of the first to be established in what was later known as Base Section No. 2…the French [however] were rather reluctant to give up their hospital…[and] wanted to share it with the Americans…Finally on the first of September…the Médecin-Chief of the French Hôpital…turned over the buildings to Major Washburn for use by the American Base Hospital…On August 21, 1917, about ten days before the hospital was officially turned over…the first American patient was admitted to U.S. Base Hospital No. 6, A.E.F.

American soldiers slowly made their way into southeastern France and the Bordeaux region. From its opening until the American forces pulled out of Europe in January 1919, ~25,000 patients would be admitted to the hospital:

> By the time of the armistice, one year later, Base Section No. 2 and Bordeaux in particular were swarming with American soldiers… The first patients were admitted to the hospital on August 21, 1917. On October 1, 1917, there were 160 patients in the hospital and 200 beds. On the last day of the year, there were 325 patients and 500 beds. The diseases for which they were admitted at that time were mostly acute infections: measles, scarlet fever, mumps, and lobar pneumonia…During the three months of October, November and December, 1917, 231 surgical operations were performed… Various opportunities during the fall were given to members of the personnel…for two weeks' stay to the British first…to observe the methods of the French and British in the war zone…
> (White 1924)

As more wounded soldiers arrived, they were moved into larger wards in Group 3, designated as the orthopaedic service. By 1918, more and more nurses were enlisted to dress these wounds because of the sheer number of casualties. As the injured arrived, hospital personnel reviewed their medical history, usually to be found in envelopes around their necks, and sent them through the process of having their dressings changed, receiving x-rays, having splints and other apparatus administered, and receiving further treatment. On April 25, 1918, Colonel Washburn was "upon recommendation of General Bradley, then Chief Surgeon of the American Expeditionary Forces… detached from command of Base Hospital No. 6 at Talence and sent to England to have charge of the hospitalization of American troops there" in Base Section No. 3—which composed Great Britain, Ireland, and the Murman Coast in the far

World War I

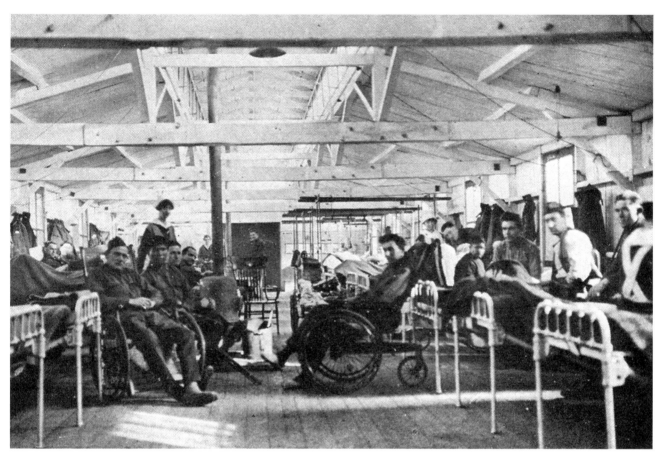

Surgical ward in the new American hospital, Base Hospital No. 6. *The History of U.S. Army Base Hospital No. 6 and its Part in the American Expeditionary Forces, 1917–1918*, edited by George Clymer. Boston: Massachusetts General Hospital, 1924.

northwest of Russia (Washburn 1939). He was replaced by Lt. Colonel Warren L. Babcock, who was former superintendent of Grace Hospital in Detroit.

Colonel Washburn had started construction at Base Hospital No. 6 through a joint effort of both the American Corps of Engineers and the French Military Engineering Service. Progress was slow, however. Throughout the summer of 1918, multiple buildings were constructed, mainly of wood, connected by long corridors because of the deep mud present during the rainy season. Under Babcock's leadership, construction expanded from a goal of 2,200 beds to over 4,000 beds. The hospital had only about 1,000 beds when the Americans initially arrived. Captain Z. B. Adams (see chapter 40) had obtained essential equipment—Balkan frames, Thomas splints, weights, pulleys, and other items—and organized the orthopedic service itself (Marble 1924).

Adams directed the orthopaedic service at Base Hospital No. 6. In fall 2017, Osgood, Goldthwait, and Mosher had previously visited Base Hospital No. 6 on a Red Cross–sponsored inspection tour of US hospitals. On October 26, 1917, Nathanial Allison, then a captain in the St. Louis Unit, also toured the hospital. At the time, the few severely injured orthopaedic patients were housed in the small orthopaedic wards (6, 7, and 8), all under the care of Captain Adams. At the end of Allison's visit, Adams had left with him to visit Tours and Lyons to study orthopaedic and reconstruction work. During this period, orthopaedic cases were managed first by Captain Henry Marble and then "were for a while under the care of Lieutenant…George A. Leland,

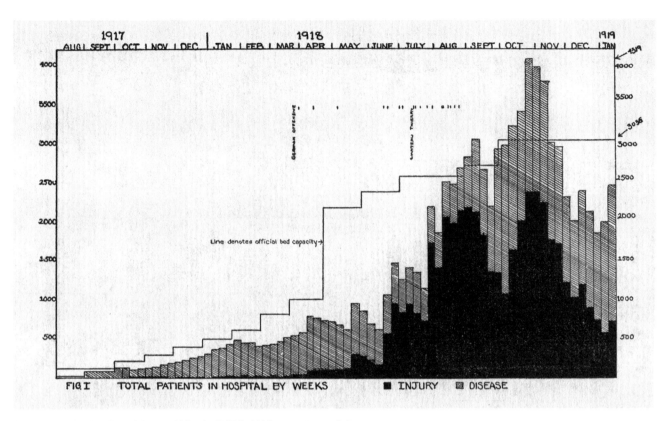

Patients treated at Base Hospital No. 6, 1917 & 1918—injuries and diseases. *The History of U.S. Army Base Hospital No. 6 and its Part in the American Expeditionary Forces, 1917-1918*, edited by George Clymer. Boston: Massachusetts General Hospital, 1924.

Jr., and later under the care of Capt. Henry G. Turner, of Unit O, who had had an intensive short orthopedic course before sailing overseas." (Marble 1924). Captain Marble (see chapter 40) wrote:

> When the more serious cases began to arrive in the hospital…it was decided at once that it was necessary to have more adequate accommodations for these cases. They were then moved to a set of wards in Group 3, and placed under my [Capt. Marble; see chapter 40] care. These were wooden buildings beginning with Ward 24, and extending to Ward 31. They had been built by Colonel Washburn and were of the monitor type of building, of ample width, moderate height, and although designed to hold thirty patients, it soon became necessary to put forty, and later in the war as many as fifty in each ward…

> As the summer of 1918 wore on, these wards became filled with bone and joint cases, and it was at this time that orders were issued designating them as the Orthopedic Department, with the writer [Capt. Marble] as head of the service. All the appliances which had been prepared by Captain Adams were now put in use, and here in this small group of wards could be found between three and four hundred cases of bone injury. There was a nurse in charge of each ward, and under her were orderlies. In view of the large amount of work it became necessary for the nurses to do practically all the dressings, and the load they were called upon to bear was tremendous, mainly because of the scarcity of medical officers. In some wards there were as many as fourteen or fifteen compound fractures of the femur, all in Balkan frames with weights, pulleys and splints, and with septic wounds to dress. (Marble 1924)

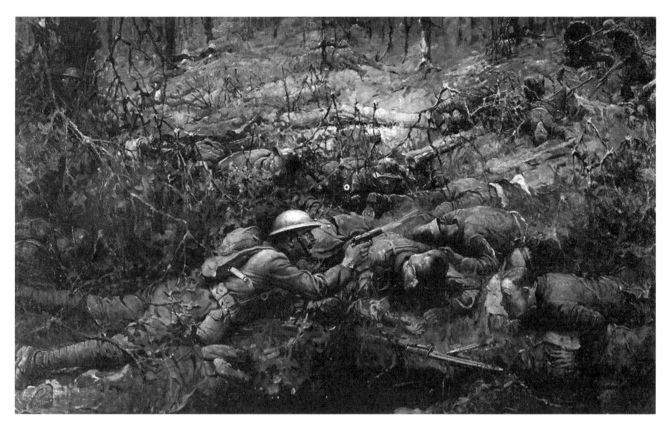

"Sergeant Alvin C. York." Painting by Frank E. Schoonover. Sgt. York received the Medal of Honor for leading an attack on 35 machine gun nests in the Battle of the Argonne Forest (Meuse-Argonne Offensive) on October 8, 1918. He killed 25 enemy soldiers and captured 132 prisoners, which helped lead to the eventual surrender of Germany. Marshall Ferdinand Foch, Commander-in-Chief of the Allied Armies, stated it was "the greatest thing accomplished by any private soldier of all the Armies of Europe." Wikimedia Commons.

The providers at Base Hospital No. 6 developed a patient flow process that allowed smooth triage and treatment of the wounded patients that arrived from the field:

> Patients usually arrived direct from a field hospital or from a hospital in the advanced field zone. They came on hospital trains, and were transported from the trains in ambulances to the hospital receiving room. Here they were sorted by the Receiving Officer, and the bone and joint injuries were assigned to the Orthopedic Service. Usually when patients arrived in the wards all dressings were taken down, and records of the case, which usually came in a small envelope around the patient's neck, read and studied. The dressings were reapplied, and the patients were sent at once to the x-ray department for pictures. The splints were readjusted and the patients generally suspended in Balkan frames. The usual routine was to treat the open wounds by the Carrel-Dakin method, and the subsequent dressings were as a rule carried on by the nurse in charge of the ward. The splinting and care of the Balkan frames and the other apparatus on the patient was detailed to the men of the hospital corps. In many of these cases major surgical operations had to be done, cleaning up infected areas, removing shell fragments, and loose pieces of bone. Following these operations, the aftercare consisted of reestablishing the Carrel-Dakin routine and the resplinting of the members. The wounds being healed, and the alignment of the fractures being

satisfactory, the patients were then loaded into litters and sent directly to the United States.
(Marble 1924)

The huge number of wounded soldiers requiring orthopaedic care necessitated help from elsewhere. Many of those who were assigned to provide assistance were not medically trained but were invaluable. As 1918 progressed, reconstruction and occupational aides joined to provide much-needed additional help (**Box 63.10**). Being responsible for the care of this great number of patients, it was necessary to obtain help from various hospital corpsmen, and during this strenuous period there were assigned to the orthopedic service several, who although not medically trained, aided in caring for the wounded. These men became quite expert in the care of fractures, and equally expert in the making and application of fracture appliances. With these diligent young soldiers, it was possible to keep this large group of patients moving along smoothly.

Throughout the latter half of 1918, the office of the Disability Board was a busy place. Its personnel saw thousands of cases. Major Brenzier was at that time supervising the orthopaedic service, and Captain Marble, originally assigned as the unit's registrar, was working as an orthopaedist. Casualties continued to flood in throughout the summer and early autumn of 1918 (see **Table 63.2**). The peak occurred in October and early November 1918 because of the Argonne offensive, and patients with influenza began to join the orthopaedic cases.

Table 63.2. Patient Census at Base Hospital No. 6, Summer/Early Autumn 1918

Month	No. of Beds	Admissions	Total No. of Inpatients	Surgical Operations
July	2600	3115	2332	325
August	2600	3165	2971	673
September	2750	2330	2996	590
October	3000	4378	4235	582

Box 63.10. Reconstruction and Occupational Aides

> "During the latter part of the summer, two groups of Reconstruction Aides were attached to our organization. The first group [14 physical therapists] had to do with massage and physiotherapy. They massaged the wounded limbs, gave the soldiers exercises, and by these means started the injured members back to normal function. The work was hard and the hours were long, but they were interested in the work and the results were most gratifying.
>
> "The second group were the Occupational Aides [13 occupational therapists]. Their work was the establishing of bedside occupations, and in a small way vocational training. Some of the wards were literally bee-hives of industry, and the wounded men who had been lying in bed, some of them for months without occupation, or any way of filling in the long hours, now had work to do. They made toys, baskets, and paintings. Distinctly the whole tone of the ward was changed, and these idle hours became most profitable" (Marble 1924).

The November armistice resulted in the gradual drop in casualties: "On the 12th of November 1918, there were 4,319 patients in the hospital… the largest in the hospital at any time. After the armistice on the eleventh, patients decreased in number very rapidly, so that by December 4, there were but 2,400 cases in the hospital…By December 31 it had dropped to 1,500…" (White 1924). Base Hospital No. 6 did not officially close until midnight on January 14, 1919, however. Despite the end of the fighting, "[there] was little celebration of the armistice at Base Hospital No. 6 until several weeks after, simply because everyone was so rushed with work that there was no time…The work grew much lighter…[and by] the first of January [1919]…all were restless, and anxious to get away, counting the days from that time on until relieved from duty" (White 1924).

Just after the new year began, leadership of Base Hospital No. 6 received instructions from the chief surgeon of the American Expeditionary Forces to release the hospital—all equipment and property—to US Base Hospital No. 208 and its commanding officer. Immediately afterward, the chief surgeon ordered Warren L. Babcock, the commanding officer, to oversee transport of remaining wounded soldiers back to the United States. "The month of February was largely taken up with preparations to return. Every one packed, said farewell to French friends, and asked daily for news of sailing orders" (White 1924). The nurses and medical officers of Base Hospital No. 6 boarded the steamship *Abangarez* and sailed to the United States: "At New York orders were received for transportation to Camp Devens; there in March 1919, the members of Base Hospital No. 6 were mustered out of service, after nearly two years of active duty as part of the A.E.F." (White 1924). Base Hospital No. 6 officially demobilized on April 1, 1919.

During the approximate one and one-half years (July 1, 1917–January 14, 1919) that the hospital functioned during the war, a total of 24,122 patients (averaging 1304 per month) were treated. There were 434 deaths (1.9%). Gunshot wounds numbered 6,751; 1,966 patients had been gassed; 1,352 patients had pneumonia; and 1,045 patients with fractures were treated. The highest mortality rate was pneumonia (21%); fracture deaths were 0.8%, deaths from gunshot wounds were 0.6%; and deaths from being gassed were 0.4%.

Base Hospital No. 7

The third Base Hospital from Boston, affiliated with Harvard Medical School and staffed primarily

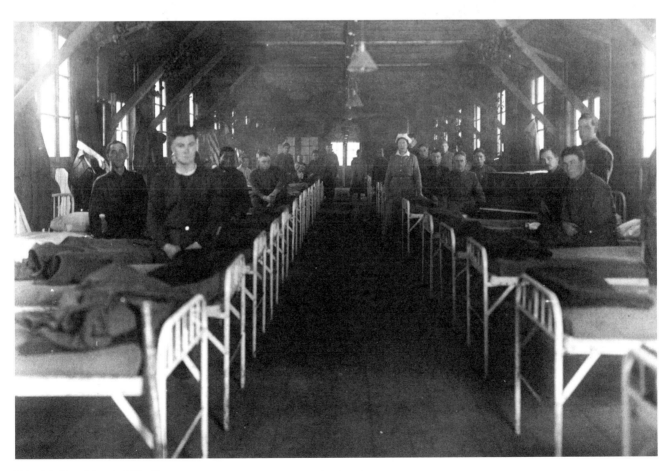

Ward 6, Base Hospital No. 7. National Archives and Records Administration.

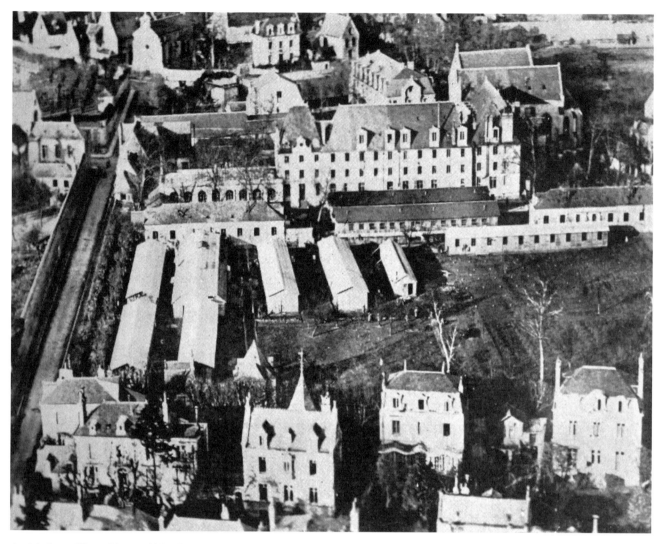

Aerial view of Base Hospital No. 7, Joué-lès-Tours (largest suburb of Tours).
The Medical Department of the U.S. Army in the World War, Volume II: Administration American Expeditionary Forces, under the direction of Maj. Gen. M.W. Ireland. Washington, DC: Government Printing Office, 1927.

from Boston City Hospital, was Base Hospital No. 7. It had begun to organize before the United States entered the war on April 6, 1917. That year, Dr. John J. Dowling, who was the superintendent of Boston City Hospital, was named commanding officer of the unit. Emma Nichols, who was superintendent of nurses, recruited, with the help of Dr. Edward H. Nichols (see chapter 12), 35 physicians, 100 nurses, and 200 enlisted men to serve in the unit. The recruits underwent training in providing wartime medical care at Camp Devens. At Étaples in 1915, Nichols had previously been engaged with the British Expeditionary Forces,

first Harvard Unit. He "was commissioned an honorary lieutenant colonel in the British army during the World War and took over the Harvard Unit" ("Obituary. Resolutions on the Death of Edward Hall Nichols" 1922). Two years later at Base Hospital No. 7, Nichols, a major in the US Army, was chief of surgery. Other Harvard faculty from Boston City Hospital who served with Nichols included Drs. Robert C. Cochran and Somers Fraser, both assistants in surgery, and Dr. Halsey B. Loder, an orthopaedic surgeon.

The officers and enlisted personnel of the unit assigned to Base Hospital No. 7 arrived in Brest,

France, in July of 1918, having sailed from the US on the infamous ocean liner *Leviathan*, which a few months later would be the site of a major outbreak of the Spanish Flu among American troops en route to France. The unit camped under tents in a mud field at Brest for two weeks, although Major David D. Scannell and Captains Cochran and Fraser, along with a small team, went ahead to Tours to assist at Camp Hospital 27. The bulk of the unit arrived at their designated base hospital in Joué' les Tours on July 28. The town was just 3 miles from Tours, which was a central supply hub for the US Army. The hospital had 2,800 beds and was prepared to receive patients. The first group of wounded—600 men, many in poor condition and many from the 26th Massachusetts Division—arrived in early August from Château-Thierry.

In early October, Captain Cochran and a surgical team were ordered to the Argonne to serve at Evacuation Hospital No. 110. They remained there until the Armistice, arriving back at Base Camp No. 7 on November 20. Throughout the course of the unit's seven-month deployment in Joue-les-tours, they treated 8,000 patients and had remarkably few deaths, but did lose three nurses—all from Boston City Hospital—one due to spinal meningitis, one to pneumonia, and one to influenza. Early in 1919, the unit received orders to return to the US. However, many volunteered to stay to serve at other hospitals and to aid with reconstruction. Before returning home, several received promotions from the Office of the Surgeon General: Major Nichols to lieutenant colonel and Captain Fraser to major. Nichols, "the surgeon in charge of Base Hospital No. 7…was cited by General Pershing for exceptionally meritorious and conspicuous service at Base Hospital No. 7, Joué-les-tours, France" ("Obituary. Resolutions on the Death of Edward Hall Nichols" 1922). Members of the unit who were returning home departed St. Nazairre on March 8, 1919, and were discharged a month later at Camp Devans.

RECONSTRUCTION HOSPITALS IN THE UNITED STATES

Well before the end of World War I, the US Medical Department began planning to build military reconstruction hospitals in the US to provide care for the anticipated hundreds of thousands of wounded American soldiers returning home. Department officials estimated that four such hospitals would be required, and it became the focus of orthopaedic surgeons at home to properly equip and staff them.

Six months after the United States entered the war, Major Elliott Brackett, director of the Division of Orthopaedic Surgery in the Office of the Surgeon General, spoke to the American Public Health Association about rehabilitation of returning injured soldiers: "Usually the soldiers who have come back from war disabled and diseased, have been cared for only by the emergency… they…created. The Surgeon-General, however… has anticipated that and has taken steps toward the control and caring for these men who…are coming back…after our part of the war begins" (Brackett 1918). In a 1917 editorial to the *American Journal of Orthopedic Surgery*, C. L. Furbush, a major in the American Medical Corps, relayed the surgeon general's "request to readers to send to the Surgeon-General short life histories of any partially handicapped persons who have been successful. Names of the handicapped are not at all necessary" (**Box 63.11**).

In a paper presented in October 1917 to the American Public Health Association and published in that association's official journal in 1918, Brackett described the duty of the government to care for returning injured soldiers:

> These men…taken into the Army…are wards of the Government…Therefore it is the duty and privilege of the Department of the Army to care for these men until they are put back into civil life as nearly restored physically and

Box 63.11. Major C. L. Furbush's Editorial in the *American Journal of Orthopedic Surgery* (1917)

> Dear Sir [Editor]:
>
> The Surgeon-General directs me to invite your attention to the following:
>
> He is arranging for special treatment for wounded, including special efforts for functional restoration of damaged parts and vocational re-education for those who, from the nature of their illness or injury, are unable to follow their previous occupation.
>
> It will be a very great help if he can know just what those who are suffering from chronic illnesses or who are partially disabled, as a result of injuries, are now doing in the United States. As example: one having lost the right hand may still be a successful carpenter or a market gardener; one having lost both the lower extremities may be successful in some line; one with chronic heart disease may have found a suitable occupation. The collection of these experiences should be of remarkable assistance as showing what the various types can do.
>
> The Surgeon-General very earnestly requests that the medical society of which you are secretary aid in this matter by getting through its members and the various local agencies, a list of the partially disabled in your county who are successfully following a trade or occupation. The information desired in reference to each case is as follows:
>
> Character of disability, medical or surgical.
>
> At what is the patient employed and how successful is he?
>
> In what way did he learn or enter his occupation after his injury or illness?
>
> The names of the disabled are not necessary.
>
> If any man who has been successful after an injury or illness desires to write a short autobiography, stating his experiences, the same might be exceedingly useful in this work, in preparing a booklet to be distributed to the men at the proper time.

industrially, as possible...to be kept under the control and under the guidance of the Army until all of this is accomplished...Therefore... special hospitals already have been ordered and are under way, so that these men who are injured shall promptly have the care of those specially trained physicians and surgeons in order to avoid the disabilities that come and have come always in wars from delay...When the disabled arrive in this country, there will be special hospitals to be known as Reconstruction Hospitals.

> "The war gave us a marvelous opportunity to learn some about accident-injury-reconstruction— orthopaedic surgery. The war hospitals were an enormous laboratory for surgery. Many experiments were tried. The careful students learned much. Those who saw a great deal and worked hard arrived at certain conclusions."
> —H. Winnett Orr (*An Orthopedic Surgeon's Story of the Great War*, 1921:13. Norfolk, Neb: The Huse Publishing Co.)

Such hospitals had already been functioning in the United Kingdom with the assistance of the American orthopaedic surgeons in the two so-called Goldthwait units. At the request of Goldthwait, Captain Carleton R. Metcalf, M.D.R.C., United States Army, wrote an article for American orthopaedic surgeons about the work of the United States orthopaedic unit in Belfast, Ireland:

There have been established ten orthopaedic or reconstruction hospitals: four in England at London, Liverpool, Leeds and Bristol; three in Scotland at Aberdeen, Glasgow and Edinburgh; two in Ireland at Belfast and Dublin; and one in Wales at Cardiff. The group provides nearly five thousand beds, all under the general supervision of Colonel Sir Robert Jones...Many come from base hospitals, some from command depots...

while a few are ex-soldiers...discharged from the Army, and drawing a pension. After they have been reconstructed...are retired to civil life, an effort...made...to provide them with suitable employment. They may then continue to visit an orthopedic hospital as outpatients... Perhaps a third of the patients leaving hospital are fit for further military duty...returned to these units or to a command depot [with treatment facilities]. A man may...stay at a command depot not more than three or four months. (Metcalf 1917)

Metcalf described in depth how the successful British system of reconstruction hospitals (**Box 63.12**) could, if appropriately modified, work in the United States:

So adopted, the United States will have its hospital units, each with workshops and other subsidiary departments, a group of surgeons trained in the proper technique and treatment...[military orthopedics is different from civil orthopaedics] the treatment of a peripheral nerve that has been cut or otherwise injured... [is more common]...Fractures have been largely absorbed into the orthopaedic group. Many are malunited, with overriding, angular deformity or errors of rotation. For ununited fractures, we are leaning more and more to bone grafts; after gunshot wounds, metal plates have proved generally inefficient. "Latent sepsis" is so common that one is advised to delay grafting for at least six months after a septic wound has healed... Foot deformities are common...many men were admitted whose feet were not adapted to the vicissitudes of a soldier's life. Defects have been accentuated by marching, by frostbite or that disease known as trench-foot...A chapter, too, might be written on the proper position for fixation after joint injuries. Many men come to us with elbows fixed in extension, with shoulders in adduction, with a foot in varus. Initial fixation in malposition is often

Box 63.12. Metcalf's (1917) Description of the Organization of British Reconstruction Hospitals

For orthopedic patients we have:

1. Four wards containing fifty beds each. A fifth ward contains limbless patients...
2. An electro-therapeutic department conducted by trained women...electrical treatment or massage... for muscle atrophy, injuries of peripheral nerves, stiff joints and the like...
3. An excellent x-ray plant
4. A plaster room...the American invasion has increased the number of plaster splints, jackets and casts
5. A gymnasium
6. A photographic room and
7. Curative workshops. Here the patients are to be given tasks carpentering, tailoring, boat-making, leather-working. The workshops are mainly curative...not...necessarily to teach a man a trade... on a doctor's prescription, he is put at work with certain tools...which will bring into action the joint or muscle that needs exercise...

the cause. Another interesting group of cases is classified as "functional." A patient will hold his foot or hand in a distorted, unnatural spasm; or will complain that he is unable to move an arm, despite the fact that sensation is normal and that muscles react intelligently to a Faradic current. Some of these patients are doubtless malingerers...others have an indefinite nerve lesion; still others a hysteria, to be relieved by psychotherapy...

The United States Orthopedic Unit has been distributed...among the several orthopedic hospitals. Personally, I am looking after some fifty or sixty beds, collecting data for two or three papers and reading the English books on this particular phase of war surgery. For those who expect to undertake reconstruction work...I can recommend: 1. Jones' Notes on Military Orthopedics...2. Jones' Injuries to Joints...3. Bristow's Treatment of Joint and Muscle Injuries...4. Stewart and Evans' Nerve Injuries and Their Treatment... [Metcalf recalled meeting Sir William Osler in London]...two of us were accosted on the street by a strange gentleman, who...recognized our uniforms. He exclaimed: "Hello, boys, I'm glad to see you. I'm Sir William Osler. Who are you?"...We were delighted to see him, chatted for a few minutes and he left us with this Parthian shot: "Remember that I have a first-class hotel at Oxford. If you get lonesome run down and put up with me." Hasn't changed much, has he? (Metcalf 1917)

Published in 1917, Jones's *Notes on Military Orthopaedics* was dedicated to King Manuel II of Portugal, "In recognition of his sympathy, co-operation and enthusiasm in the promotion of Orthopaedic Centres for disabled soldiers..." (Jones 1917). Jones (1917) wrote in the preface:

"Curative workshops" started in each centre owe their existence and success to the initiative and inspiring enthusiasm of King Manuel, who has acted as representative of the British Red Cross Society. These workshops have already proved to be of very real value, and are the latest but not least important advance in the orthopaedic treatment of wounded men suffering from physical disabilities of their limbs...when the preliminary stages of operative and surgical treatment are over, there is a steady gradation through massage and exercise to productive work, which is commenced as soon as the man can really begin to use his limb at all. If his former trade or employment is a suitable one, he is put to use tools he understands, otherwise some occupation suitable for his disability, and curative in its character, is found for him...Those of us who have any imagination cannot fail to realize the difference

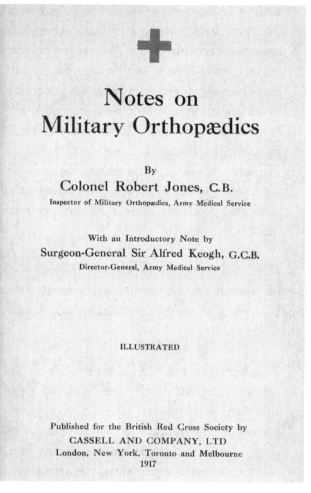

Title page of Sir Robert Jones's book, *Notes on Military Orthopaedics*. London: Cassell and Company, Ltd., 1917. Wellcome Library.

in atmosphere and morale in hospitals where the patients have nothing to do but smoke, play cards, or be entertained, from that found in those where for part of the day they have regular, useful and productive work. Massage and exercise is no longer a mere routine: it all fits in and leads up to the idea of fitness – fitness to work and earn a living and serve the State in an economic sense, even if not to return...and fight once more in the ranks of the Army.

In July 1917, the *American Journal of Orthopedic Surgery* published an editorial and three articles on the importance of rehabilitation and specialty hospitals in treating wounded disabled soldiers and returning them to gainful employment after their discharge:

> The first of these is the introduction written by Col. Robert Jones, to his small book just published, *Notes on Military Orthopaedics*… The second is an address read at the American Orthopedic Association meeting at Pittsburgh, June 1917, by W.E. Gallie of Toronto, and shows what the Canadians are doing. Dr. Gallie is in charge of one of the reconstruction hospitals established at Toronto. The third is the report of the Committee on Preparedness, appointed a year ago by the American Orthopedic Association, and the Orthopaedic Section of the American Medical Association, and this report indicates what we must do, and what already has been accomplished…
>
> This work of the extended care of the wounded soldiers has been done in England under the name of 'general hospitals for orthopedic cases,' but lately there has come to the forefront a new name, which seems to be much more comprehensive…the word "reconstruction" to take the place of "orthopedic." We feel it carries a more definite meaning and has a broader use, and we like it. It brings out the idea that there is much more to be done than just the surgical or orthopedic work…It is impossible to predict just how much work will be sent back to us, because no one knows how long this war will last…the Government is laying its plans for at least three years of war…It would be folly not to profit by the experience of the other countries [especially England]…Now are we ready, or will be ready in this year to really care for 10,000? We would be swamped at the present time, and…must get ready… now…It is not humane to allow these men to be discharged without a proper chance to be so "reconstructed" that they are capable of being useful citizens…This is "reconstruction," and it includes more than good surgical or orthopedic work, — it includes educational and industrial work as well…done on a big plan. This is the work for the men with orthopedic training; the call is sure to come and we must be ready to meet it. ("Editorial. Reconstruction" 1917)

Goldthwait, as chairman, in his 1917 report of the committee on preparedness of the American Orthopaedic Association (identical to his report of a similar committee that he chaired in the orthopaedic section of the American Medical Association), wrote about the two roles of the orthopaedic surgeon during wartime:

> The first is in connection with the work of the "base" hospital, which is located…near the actual conflict…These hospitals are…under the direction of general surgeons, and the orthopedist's position is that of assistant, the cases in which special mechanical problems exist being turned over to him for care…The second form of service…open to the orthopedic surgeon in time of war is…in hospitals to which patients would be sent from the base hospitals…kept as long as necessary…for the purely surgical treatment…[and] for…reeducation along occupational lines as is indicated, so that when discharged there will be the least possible physical handicap…Such hospitals are designated… as general hospitals for orthopedic…purposes. They should be located in or near large cities… [ensuring] the greatest case in officering and equipment. The staff would naturally be made up of men skilled in orthopedic surgery…No hospital…should be established with less than 200 beds…The hospitals can be built…[or] a still better plan…is to use some already existing institution…work…taken over entirely by the Government, or for the Government to pay… the existing management for the care of the patient on a per diem basis.

He went on to describe such a hospital that had been organized between the City of Boston and Robert B. Brigham Hospital:

As a type of this form of coöperation and organization, a hospital unit has been worked out in Boston with the Robert B. Brigham Hospital and the City of Boston. The hospital, which is designed for the chronic case, many of whom are crippled, is equipped…with the usual operating rooms, x-ray outfit, laboratory facilities, etc., but has a fully equipped hydrotherapeutic plant and an organized industrial department for occupational training. Adjoining the hospital is a park belonging to the City of Boston, and this is so laid out that tent or shack wards can be erected…that would accommodate about five hundred patients. On the land of the hospital proper, additional space for one or two hundred patients is available if needed. The service, heating and power plant of the hospital is adequate…In this way is the shortest possible time and with the least expense to the government, efficient care of five or six hundred men is available.

The organization of the staff for this Orthopedic Hospital has been worked out in the light of the experience abroad…[with] one chief of service…would be responsible for 250 patients. The assignments are as follows: First Service – Surgeon-in-Chief, E.S. Brackett; surgeons, L.T. Brown [see chapter 46], M.S. Danforth…Second Service – Surgeon-in-Chief, C.F. Painter [see chapter 45]; surgeons, M.H. Rogers [see chapter 53], L.T. Swai[m] [see chapter 45]. In charge of the physical therapy, including – muscular reeducation…Miss Marguerite Sanderson and Miss Marjorie Bouvé, of the Boston School of Physical Education. (Goldthwait 1917)

In the United States, the military reconstruction hospitals would feature gyms set up to provide orthopaedic rehabilitation via exercise, electrotherapy, and hydrotherapy. They would also offer settings for occupational rehabilitation, such as workshops and simulated workplaces, resembling departments already established at Massachusetts General Hospital and the Shepherd's Bush Military Hospital. The shift from caring for children with disabilities to caring for wounded soldiers that many orthopaedic surgeons faced would prove to be easier than might have been expected, as so many of the soldiers were 18-year-olds (the Selective Service Act, which permitted the draft, having just been passed in July of 1917). The surgeons who were caring for these young men were motivated by the goal of rehabilitating them so that they could become productive citizens and workers. Dr. Frederic Cotton and other orthopaedic surgeons were leaders at the time in the development of worker's compensation regulations, and in 1921, Congress created the Veterans' Bureau, which combined all veterans' programs. The bureau absorbed the veterans' hospitals of the Public Health Service and initiated a bold plan for building additional hospitals to meet the need of veterans of World War I.

Reconstruction Base Hospital No. 1

In 1917, Elliott Brackett and Cotton "came before the council of the Massachusetts Medical Society with a reconstruction program which we, with Dr. Goldthwait, had worked out, based on our knowledge of the problem [war injuries] and of the excellent work that had been done by French, British, and Canadians to cope with the problem as it has come to them. This was the first public appearance of the 'reconstruction' idea in America" (Cotton 1919). In June of that year, only two months after the United States entered the war, plans were in place for the first reconstruction hospital in the United States:

Reconstruction Base Hospital No. 1, for the United States War Department is to be built here in Boston on Parker Hill, on the site of the Old Parker Hill Reservoir, now graded to level, next to the Robert B. Brigham Hospital. Its object is the "reconstruction" of the crippled soldiers, likely to return to us not long hence. This work is special work, not adapted to the

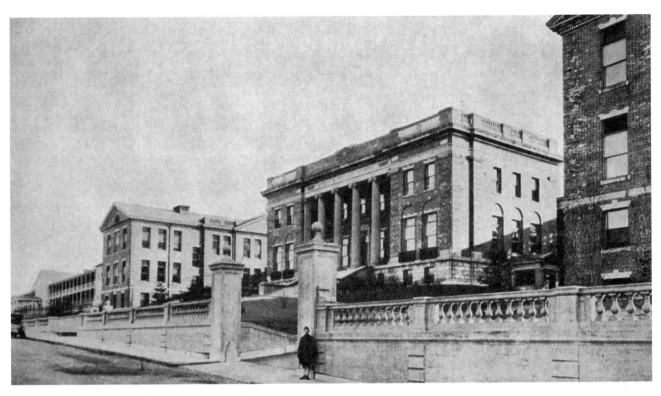

Front of General Hospital No. 10 (Reconstruction Base Hospital No. 1), Boston.
The Medical Department of the U.S. Army in the World War, Volume V: Military Hospitals in the United States, under the direction of Maj. Gen. M.W. Ireland. Washington, DC: Government Printing Office, 1927.

general base hospitals at the front or here. It means the reconstruction, by operation, by apparatus, by education – reeducation – of those who came back with fractures ununited or ill-united, with stiff joints, with nerve palsies from injury or shock – of those who need plastic operations to remedy contractures or defects, or need appliances to supplant a missing limb, and the necessary education in their use. (Cotton 1917)

The Brigham Hospital provided resources. Robert Breck Brigham Hospital, which adjoined the rehabilitative hospital, furnished light and heat, and a kitchen, laundry, chemical laboratory, x-ray plant, and other necessities. Funding was sought from the community, as the War Department provided no funding; partial funding was indeed secured. and vocational education became an important element of the treatment there. Cotton wrote:

Most of these men, if discharged early, would be permanent cripples – a burden on the community…This Boston hospital for reconstruction…has been accepted and endorsed by the War Department. Thanks primarily to the efforts of Dr. Joel Goldthwait…Mayor Curley has had the Parker Hill Reservoir levelled off (it had long been planned to make this a park)…and the Robert Brigham Hospital, next door, able to share something from its wonderful central plant, As to professional, a unit of eleven men has been gathered…the Brigham Hospital is ready, the site is nearly ready…In the meantime the community must help… [as] the War Department has no funds…[for] the erection of our buildings…We want – for now – four wards of temporary type, of twenty-four beds each. Each will cost about $4000 to build and fit out…The plans are all ready not only for this group of buildings…but for eventual expansion to five hundred beds when this shall have

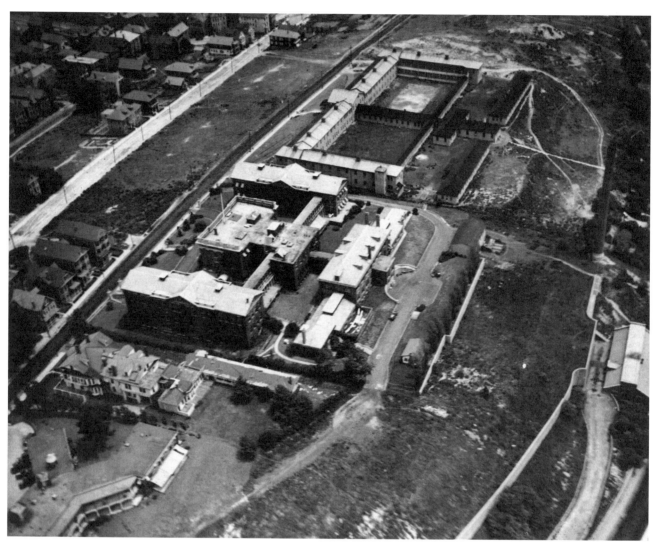

Aerial view of General Hospital No. 10 (Reconstruction Base Hospital No. 1.) Parker Hill, Boston. Aereo Scenic Airviews, Boston, Mass. Boston Pictorial Archive, Boston Public Library/Digital Commonwealth.

become a War Department hospital. We have money enough for one ward already…all that lies between us and…completion of the small hospital…is money. (Cotton 1917)

The main goal was to rehabilitate the whole patient—not just to fix bodies, but to allow their ability to function and work after discharge, or to return to service: "It will be observed that the work goes entirely beyond the purely surgical repair that will be a portion of it, and extends to the final disposal of the patient…Probably one of the most interesting problems to be undertaken will be the vocational education…It will be a new feature in hospital work, but it is of the utmost importance from the standpoint of the patients" ("Editorial. The Scope of a Reconstruction Hospital" 1917). Such rehabilitation was one unexpected outcome of these hospitals: "One of the surprises of this war has been the success of both the Allies and Central Powers in rendering again serviceable thousands of men who would have become derelicts under the old régime" (Cotton 1917).

Many injured soldiers were amputees, and functional ability was an even larger issue for those missing limbs. If amputees were discharged too early, they could become permanently disabled. Surprisingly, many of the injured soldiers

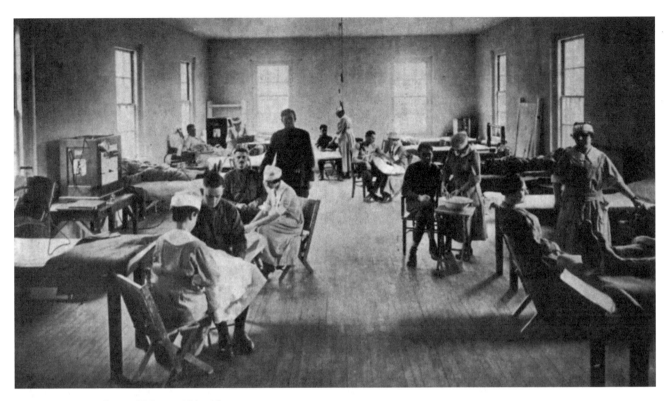

Physiotherapy at General Hospital No. 10. Courtesy of CardCow.com.

were able to be returned to service as a result of the rehabilitative success at the hospital. Brackett (1918) wrote:

> Attention to the mechanical features of treatment includes in many cases the fitting of artificial limbs. Too little thought and time has been given in the past by the medical profession to this most important subject, not only to the proper selection of the substitutes, but also to the fitting and training in their use, and to the early preparation of the stump for their reception. As much time and personal attention should be given by the surgeon to this important subject as to that of splints and apparatus for acute joint affections. This subject is now beginning to have the proper realization of its importance by the prominence of its demands.

The Benevolent Order of Elks offered to fund the reconstructive hospital (Reconstruction Base Hospital No. 1) on Parker Hill, just near the Robert Breck Brigham Hospital. Surgeon General Gorgas accepted their offer on behalf of the US government. The Elks paid approximately $300,000 to finance the Elks' Reconstruction Hospital, which was built in 1918. It was a crucial member of US General Hospital No. 10—comprising the Elks Hospital (Reconstruction Base Hospital No. 1), the Robert Breck Brigham Hospital, the West Roxbury plant (Boston City Hospital—leased by the government for one dollar per year); and the Massachusetts Women's Hospital (to be used for nurses quarters)—and was designated as a treatment hospital, "furnished with heat and light and operating facilities by the adjoining Robert B. Brigham Hospital, through tunnel connections" (Cotton 1919). Although somewhat small, the Elks hospital provided:

> accommodation for over three hundred patients, [and had] a fully equipped building for electrotherapy, hydrotherapy, and mechanotherapeutic work, a shop building 150 feet by

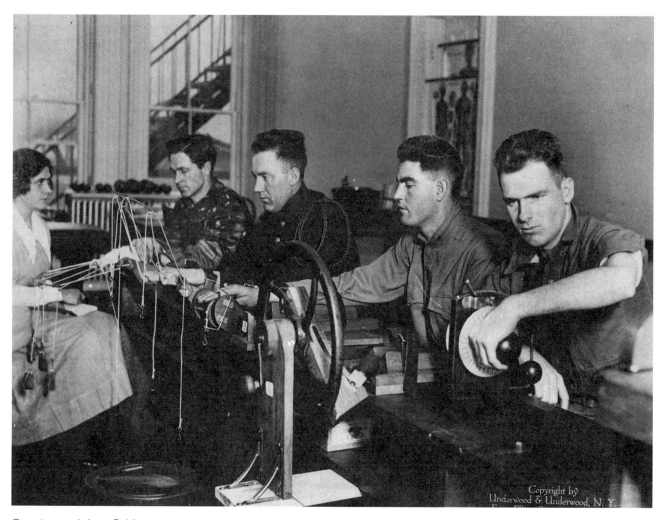
Curative workshop. Soldiers using various devices with their hands. National WWI Museum and Memorial, Kansas City, Missouri, USA.

22 for curative work and for the surgical appliance shop, and a barracks building. The whole block of building is 300 by 150 feet, with 45,000 feet of floor space. The equipment…is army equipment, save for the excellent outfitting of the shops, which the Red Cross did, and for the furnishing of a ward by the people of the town of Belmont. After the erection of the Elks' Hospital, it became evident that the need was greater than had been foreseen. It was too small.

Then the trustees of the Robert B. Brigham Hospital…entered into an agreement with the Government by which they turned over their hospital for war use, taking care of the patients of their charity elsewhere. At the same time Mayor Peters, for the City of Boston, offered the West Department of the City Hospital in West Roxbury, for the use of the Government during the war period. This is an elaborately modernized hospital plant of two hundred and fifty beds, fully equipped, prepared by the City for a contagious hospital, but not yet used. It is six miles away from Parker Hill, but so well equipped as to be suitable for a half independent unit. It was accepted and is in use. Besides all this, the Massachusetts Women's Hospital (the old Charity Club) was offered and was leased for nurses' quarters. (Cotton 1919)

Colonel Joseph Taylor Clarke became commander of US General Hospital No. 10,

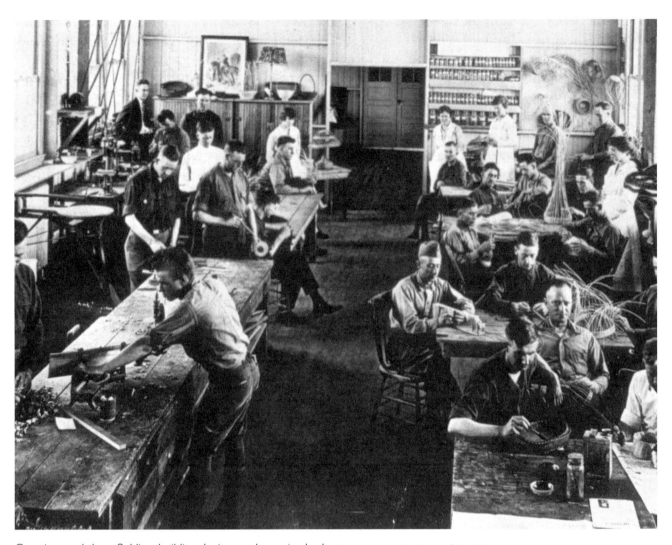
Curative workshop. Soldiers building devices and weaving baskets. U.S. National Library of Medicine.

overseeing the orthopaedic, physiotherapeutic, and educational work being done:

> It looks as if the work were to be predominantly orthopedic…calling for high grade work of specially trained men and for the very best operating conditions…first rate shop work, including the making and fitting of artificial limbs…The physiotherapy department…looks strong and the plans are laid for a great deal of work by the doctors and the excellent staff of trained women aides. Rather unusually extensive use of electrical treatment is contemplated, and of hydrotherapy. The educational department amply staffed from Washington…is already busy. The plan of work is in no large essential different from what is projected elsewhere – what has been done…at Walter Reed Hospital in Washington and three or four other places… In the past, our civil work of this sort has been poor, not so much because we did not know as because we were not in shape to coordinate our special workers and special means of care. Here, today, we have an institution, particularly favoring the working out of such coordination. (Cotton 1919)

In a 1919 article, Cotton (see chapter 59) reviewed the concept of reconstruction hospitals, both military and civilian.

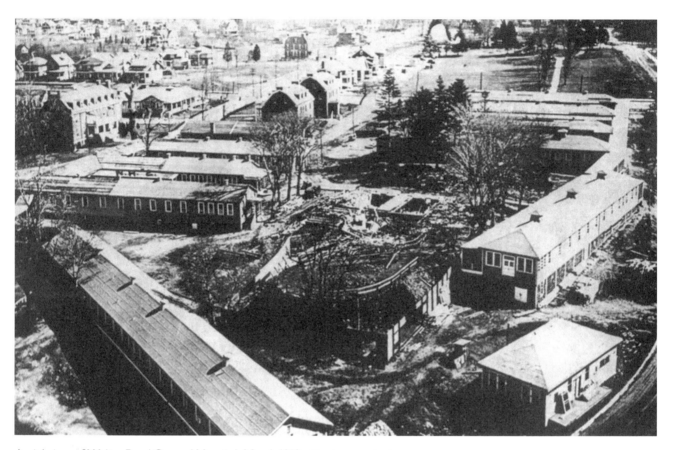

Aerial view of Walter Reed General Hospital, March 1919. *The Army Medical Department 1917-1941* by Mary C. Gillett. Washington, DC: Center of Military History, United States Army, 2009.

The reconstruction movement, like the movement for hospital efficiency, [Ernest A.] Codman's drive for the end-result system, the standardization movement of the A.C.S. [American College of Surgeons], means that we need better work, completer work, than we have been doing in our hospitals, and it means that the special problems of the wounded – the potential cripples of war – has jarred us into action. A few have long known that only by shifting our point of view to the results end, and coordinating surgical and allied staffs to reach that end…can real results be achieved…That the war hospitals in this country…as they have shown, results in the way of functional restoration beyond all experience of us old hands in civil hospitals, is a marvel…Let us not make the mistake of considering the work done in the war a military matter only…save for the Carrel-Dakin treatment the discoveries have been almost negligible…New institutions had to be reared…free from hampering traditions, and in a couple of years it has been possible to go farther than in a decade of peace…

Cotton (1919) went on to describe his wish to use US General Hospital No. 10, of which he had been chief of staff, as a model for civilian hospitals moving forward:

This is the plan I want to see put into civil practice here and elsewhere…I want to see…the reclaiming of our great army of cripples and past cripples in the community, whether they have fought in France or got hurt in a factory or on the street…What I want to do today is to ask how…we can secure for our civil work the advantages of a war hospital and get something like the war results, as we have not done in the past in civil life. It is possible to teach old dogs some tricks, but old institutions, never, and I believe our problem is to erect new institutions or better yet, take over those now doing army work in reconstruction [after the war].

Moreover, with a premonition of this problem, No. 10 has largely been staffed by Massachusetts doctors, nurses and aides, – they are available. Let us hope that Massachusetts may lead again…In this community we are not likely to lack for alleged scientific work, – what we need most is the human "repair shop."

ORTHOPAEDIC SERVICES IN US HOSPITALS

As described earlier, conditions falling within the scope of the orthopaedic surgery service included amputations, deformities of extremity caused by soft tissue contractures, injuries to bones, joints and feet, and those requiring tendon transplantation. The biggest hurdle was to find enough properly trained orthopaedists to staff these services. The services overseas required supervision so as to prevent cases from becoming more serious as they entered the orthopaedic service, and orthopaedists in the surgical services needed the skills to return these patients to the highest possible level of function as quickly as possible. Robert Osgood (1919) emphasized the importance of maintaining vigilance in continuing appropriate care for wounded soldiers upon their return to the US:

> the cases returning to America presenting bone, joint, and muscle lesions as the result of battle wounds, have shown very conclusively the result of treatment oversees…in the early years of the war…[a] very high percentage of deformities which might have been prevented was truly alarming…There has been a constant danger that, manned as our base hospitals have been until recently with medical officers without experience with our overseas forces, these deformities would develop in America in the course of the healing of wounds…the great value of the system of supervision overseas has been clearly demonstrated and the need of constant watchfulness at home has been emphasized.

During the first year of the United States' involvement in the war, the military established the following types of hospitals with orthopaedic services in the United States: general hospitals (23), embarkation hospitals (2), debarkation hospitals (9), and base hospitals (17). Of the approximately 23 orthopaedic services at general hospitals, two—Walter Reed and Letterman General Hospitals—housed major amputation services, although several others accepted amputation cases, and some had neurosurgical services. At Walter Reed, the amputation:

> service began to assume important proportions in June 1918, as the first overseas wounded began to return. Major T.M. Foley…the Chief of Service [Orthopaedic Surgery] for several weeks…was succeeded by Major Albert H. Freiberg as Chief [CH/MGH resident]… Over 800 cases of amputation have been in the wards of the Walter Reed Hospital at one time. Since it was the first amputation center to receive large number of cases, it has been here that the plan of provisional limbs, conceived by Lt. Colonel Silver [an HMS graduate], in charge of the amputation work, has been worked out. Colonel Silver has acted as consultant to the Walter Reed Hospital in connection with amputation work…
>
> After the armistice, Major Freiberg was relieved of duty at his own desire…The service these days numbered over 1200 patients… nearly all cases of osteomyelitis, and…many of the bone and joint cases requiring surgical attention, were divided…to the orthopedic section and some to the general surgical

section...the orthopedic staff...numbers 19... Colonel Allison and Major [Murray S.] Danforth [an assistant orthopedic surgeon in the outpatient department of MGH], have been assigned to the Walter Reed on the orthopedic service. Major Philip Wilson has been given full charge of the amputation section [he was still serving by April 1919]. (Osgood 1919)

Various orthopaedic surgeons from the Harvard community also served in other general hospitals: Lt. John Dane (chapter 23) at the USA General Hospital No. 2, Fort McHenry, Maryland; Major Henry C. Marble (chapter 40) and Lt. Armin Klein (chapter 53) at USA General Hospital No. 3, Colonia, New Jersey; and Major Frederic J. Cotton (chapter 59) at USA General Hospital No. 10, Boston. At No. 10, Cotton:

originally exempted to orthopaedic surgery, has been chief of the surgical service since the opening of the hospital. He was released to general surgery while acting as chief of the surgical service in the Walter Reed Hospital. His long interest and wide experience in bone and joint conditions fit him especially for this post, since a very large proportion of the surgical cases sent to No. 10 are operative in type...in addition... the Government has taken over the buildings of the parental home in West Roxbury, which furnish convalescent beds for 400 more cases. USA General Hospital No. 10 is designated as a neuro-surgical centre and an amputation centre. There was on April 1st [1919] 674 overseas cases in Boston. (Osgood 1919)

The principal embarkation hospitals were in the ports of Hoboken, New Jersey, and Newport News, Virginia. At least nine debarkation hospitals existed, including Hoboken and Newport News:

When the cases first began to be transported [back to the US], there was a good deal of difficulty experienced because of the failure of surgeons...to realize the importance of maintaining fixation until the patients landed. The soldier would often request to have the splints removed and their condition not being acute, the surgeons would frequently comply with these requests and in many instances unnecessary shortening and preventable deformities occurred. This difficulty was also experienced in the debarkation hospitals...Orthopedic surgeons, were on this account, sent to the ports of debarkation and a more careful supervision of splinting was instituted, both before the cases were removed from the transports and while under treatment of the debarkation hospitals... [Now] the cases arrive at the general or base hospitals as a rule well splinted. (Osgood 1919)

After debarkation, soldiers would be transferred to an onshore base hospital; more than 17 of them provided orthopaedic services. In Massachusetts there was a base hospital at Camp Devens. Captain Henry J. Fitzsimmons (Boston Children's Hospital; see chapter 23) was the chief orthopaedic surgeon there with a staff of six other orthopaedic surgeons. At Camp Taylor, Kentucky, Major Ernest A. Codman (MGH; see chapter 34) became chief of the surgical service; according to Osgood (1919), "Codman's interest in bone and joint cases and his wide experience in bone and joint surgery are a great asset to the service." Captain E. B. Mumford was appointed orthopaedic surgeon (he had spent 12 months in the orthopaedic division's service). At Camp Taylor, "[a] very close liaison is being worked out between the orthopedic convalescent cases in which joint function must be increased and the reconstruction activities. Careful records are taken of the weekly progress in joint motion. The work assigned is specially planned for the restoration of function" (Osgood 1919). At Fort Riley, Kansas, toward the end of August 1918, Major Mark Rogers, from MGH, became chief of the orthopaedic service (see chapter 53); he "developed a most useful service in connection with the large number of overseas cases which began to be sent home" (Osgood 1919). Rogers was later discharged at Fort Riley.

At the end of his article on a survey of orthopaedic services in US hospitals, Osgood (1919) praised the work of orthopaedic surgeons and those who worked with them:

> Little has been said of the devoted and unspectacular work of the orthopaedic medical officers assigned to camp work. Their original careful examinations of the draft cases and their important services on discharge boards may seem to have passed unnoticed, but this is not so. It has been generally recognized as necessary and important by the Division Surgeons. If, in the treatment of the wounded soldiers, the attention of the surgeons has been directed to the importance of combining conservation of function with the treatment of the wound itself, a service to surgery as well as to the soldiers may have been rendered.

WORLD WAR I CHANGED ORTHOPAEDICS FOREVER

Before World War I, general surgeons cared for patients with fractures, and orthopaedics began to be a specialty in its own right, moving away from treating solely skeletal deformities—mainly in children—with nonoperative means. As a result of their service in the war, orthopaedic surgeons began to gain respect within the medical community, and many continued their training and practice in orthopaedic surgery after returning home:

> Many of the surgeons assigned to the Division of Orthopaedic Surgery in World War I had little, if any, exposure to bone and joint surgery at the time that they were sent to Europe. They learned under the few senior orthopaedic surgeons [many from Boston] and by treating wounded men…many sought additional

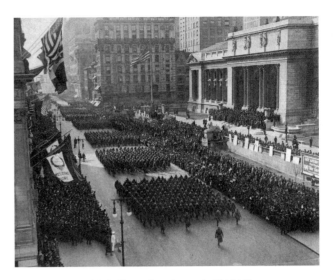

Parade in New York City after the end of WWI. National Archives and Records Administration/Wikimedia Commons.

> training and became full-time orthopaedists upon their return to civilian life. Two marvelous examples…are Ralph K. Ghormley [see chapter 40] and J. Albert Key. Both went to France with the Johns Hopkins Unit before they had graduated from medical school…enlisted as corpsmen; after performing with distinction, they were graduated from medical school "in absentia," promoted to lieutenants, and assigned to the Division of Orthopaedic Surgery… (Green and DeLee 2017)

This expanded role allowed orthopaedists to gradually take over the treatment of patients with fractures and, eventually, nerve injuries, and to focus on the prevention of amputation and contractures:

> Not only were most fractures treated by general surgeons, but injuries of the peripheral nerves virtually had been ignored. The massive number of troops with extremity injuries resulted in the realization that nerve injuries [needed to be treated: repaired and splinted]… at some point during the war, it was mandated that all peripheral nerve injuries be sent to the orthopaedic centers for care.

> In most previous conflicts [and in civilian life]…the standard treatment for an open fracture was amputation, lest the patient die of infection…in the first year of the Great War, patients with open femoral fractures had an 80% mortality rate…Because most…surgeons had little orthopaedic experience, failure [to properly immobilize or splint fractures preventing shortening, angulation and malrotation]…resulted in a myriad of malunions, nonunions, [shortening], contractures and joint deformities…Antibiotics would not become available until World War II, so osteomyelitis was rampant… (Green and DeLee 2017)

Surgeons at the frontlines "were taught maximum salvage of limbs, [open circular amputation techniques], prevention of contractures was emphasized, and early mobilization with temporary appliances was encouraged" (Green and DeLee 2017). Their reputation was enhanced because they significantly reduced the number of deaths from femur fractures—from an earlier 80 percent mortality rate—and, through their treatment of casualties in the field, reduced the numbers of amputations, infection, and cases of permanent disability.

Rehabilitation became a priority in the orthopaedic service as well, so that orthopaedic casualties could be returned to as much function as possible. To that end, rehabilitative hospitals were established so that patients could receive physical therapy:

> Restoration of function and return to useful employment are now well-established orthopaedic principles, but these were new concepts in 1917.…credited primarily to the influence of Sir Robert Jones [and Cotton, Goldthwait, Osgood, Wilson, and others in the US], emphasis was given to rehabilitation…[Jones] thought "that no soldier should be discharged from the Army until everything is done to make him a healthy and efficient citizen, and when the war is ended, he should not be discharged until he is declared to be fit…to enable him to take an honorable part in life." (Green and DeLee 2017)

In all, British military hospitals had increased about 12-fold throughout World War I, and that "large number meant there were specialized facilities for all medical fields" (Rauer, n.d.). Throughout the war, "some 583 surgeons served with the Orthopaedic Division of the AEF. Among these were a generation of future leaders" in orthopaedic surgery (Green and DeLee 2017), with 13 going on to become president of the American Orthopaedic Association and 6, president of the American Academy of Orthopaedic Surgeons.

> "The most frightful war in all history has happily terminated long before the most optimistic of us thought possible one short year ago; and with the lifting of the cloud of dread and uncertainly which rested upon civilized humanity for four dreadful years, we once more realized how true it is that "there is a Divinity which shapes our ends, rough hew them how we will."
> —Herbert P. H. Galloway, MD (AOA President's Address. "Readjustment to Changing Conditions" [1919]. *Journal of Orthopaedic Surgery*, 1919; 1[7]: 395.)

ADDENDUM

The following is the text of a 1917 Harvard Medical School course pamphlet, courtesy of the Countway Medical Library, reproduced here in its entirety.

MILITARY ORTHOPEDIC SURGERY

Duration of the course – 6 weeks

33 hours per week to every man

Approximately 190 hours of instruction in the course.

126 hours. General Instruction

74 hours. Special Instruction

Hospital facilities

    Harvard Medical School
        Anatomical Building
        Warren Museum
        Library and Lecture Rooms
    Children's Hospital
        Orthopedic Department
        Amphitheatre
        Wards
        Out Patient Department
        Appliance Shop
    Massachusetts General Hospital
        Orthopedic Wards
        Out Patient Department
    Boston City Hospital
        Surgical Wards
        Out Patient Department
    Peter Bent Brigham Hospital
        Surgical Service
    State Hospital School, Canton
    Libraries of the Harvard Medical School and
    Children's Hospital,
    Boston Medical Library

INSTRUCTORS

Maj. Robert E. Lovett	Dr. John Homans
Capt. M. H. Rogers	Dr. David Cheever
Lieut. R. J. Cook	Dr. John E. Fish
Lieut. Edward King	Dr. William F. Whitney
Dr. Robert Soutter	Dr. E. W. Taylor
Dr. A. Ehrenfried	Dr. C. A. Porter
Dr. H. J. FitzSimmons	Dr. C. L. Scudder
Dr. A. T. Legg	Dr. G. W. Holmes
Dr. J. W. Sever	Dr. Lloyd Brown

Dr. Channing Simmons

Demonstration in application of plaster paris bandage. Opportunity afforded for application of plaster by students in the Out Patient Department and post operative cases – 4 periods.

Muscle function and physiology with clinical study of selected cases – 10 periods.

Operations as selected and studied cases – 8 periods.

Joints – their phenomena and anatomy – 3 periods.

Operations on the cadaver performed by students under instruction including: Tendon Transplant, Tonotomy, Osteotomy, Astragulectomy, Fasciotomy and Nerve Suture, – 5 periods.

Demonstration and study of selected cases. – Cases in the ward being assigned and presented by the student before the class — 5 periods.

Conference and quiz. – discussion of course, short written examination reviewing completed work – 4 periods.

Bone pathology – 3 periods.

Visit to State Hospital School, Canton, Massachusetts. – Industrial Rehabilitation – 2 periods

Clinics at Peter Bent Brigham Hospital. – selected cases demonstrated on the Wards and Amphitheatre. – apparatus and X-Ray. Demonstration and discussion – 3 periods.

Clinic at Boston City Hospital – selected Ward cases. Bedside teaching. X-Ray interpretation. Out Patient Department – fresh fracture clinic with treatment by students. Application of splints and fixation apparatus – 4 periods.

Warren Anatomical Museum. – Exhibition of selected specimens of pathological bones. Demonstration and instruction – 3 periods.

X-Ray Interpretation. Plates and lanters [sic] slides demonstrated by students. – Quiz – 4 periods.

Bone Tuberculosis. Character, distribution, diagnosis, treatment in detail – X-Rays – 1 period.

Muscle Testing. Spring balance muscle test. Muscle Training – 2 periods.

Non union in fractures with treatment, bone grafts, etc. – 1 period.

Osteomyelitis. Types and differential diagnosis – 3 periods.

Osteotomies for bony deformities – 1 period.

Deformities of neck and spine – 1 period.

Fractures of spine – 1 period.

Examination.

INSTRUCTION AT MASSACHUSETTS GENERAL HOSPITAL

Theory of nerve diagnosis. Demonstration, dissection. Reaction of degeneration and use of electricity – 2 hours.

Fractures in joints – 2 hours.

Peripheral nerve surgery – 2 hours.

X-Ray diagnosis – 3 hours.

Posture – 1 hours.

Osteomyelitis – 1 hours.

Clinical work in Out Patient Department under instruction – 17 hours.

Demonstration of selected cases – 8 hours

ASSIGNMENT OF HOURS

	Hours
Plaster of Paris	
Demonstrations	8
Fracture in application	12
Anatomy – Muscle function	15
Joints	5
Joints – Physiology & Pathology	3
Apparatus	12
Bone Pathology	3

The foregoing subject should be taken up first as fundamental.

The others follow without special recommendation as to order

Shop work	8
Muscle function and training	5
Operation to illustrate principles	20
Artificial limbs	2
Vocational training	2
Physical therapy	8
X-ray interpretation	6
Operative surgery on cadaver	12
Principles of tendon surgery	3
Camp accidents and their treatment	10
Conferences and examinations	6
Nerve Dissection	12
Foot	12
Back	10
Joints (pathology, diagnosis & treatment	16
Collateral reading	—

SYLLABUS OF TOPICS

Plaster Of Paris

Schedule

<u>Materials</u>, varieties, names, special uses, cement

<u>Bandage</u> material, varieties, names, special uses

<u>Bandage</u> preparation, tearing, washing, etc. rolling, use of machines

<u>Bandage</u>, keeping of, tin, etc. commercial bandages.

<u>Bandage</u> application, water warm, use of salt, use of glue, paper wrapping

<u>Skin</u> protection, flannel, wadding, stockinet

<u>Drying</u> of plaster bandages, do not cover with bed clothes, X-rays through them, allow
    24-48 hours. Avoid finger dents, and reverses of bandages.

<u>Signs</u> of danger, odor-dermatitis, localized pain, swelling, obstruction of circulation

<u>Reinforcement</u> by plaster rope, iron strips, wire, wire gauze, wood

<u>Windows</u> to allow inspection, dressing, relief of pressure, how to make them

Bracketted [sic] plasters, mode of application

<u>Removal</u> of plaster bandages. Removable plasters

<u>Plaster sheets</u> for posterior leg splints, etc.

Plaster Bandages (regional)

Spine for Tuberculosis of the spine in hyperextension as standard

(1) suspension from head, head and arms, head-piece, Sayre, Calot method (sheets) bandage method.

(2) frame

On face webbing, apron, how to obtain hyperextension by lowering hammock.

On back in hamock [sic], Goldthwait, Brackett or Silver rods emergency, between

    tables on hammock by suspended loop.

    Inclusion of head Calot's technique, other techniques. Rope head plaster for torticollis, or fracture of cervical spine. Use, for cervical lesions or dorsal above 9th dorsal vertebra.

    Inclusion of hip

Shoulder On the Hawley table
    In the sitting position
    Off the end of the table
    Practically always in ABDUCTED position
    Combination with the airplane splint

Elbow Most often in acute flexion
    Complete extension in olecranon fracture

Forearm and Hand

Seldom used as permanent dressing except when complicated with lesions higher up. Position midway between pronation and supinations, wrist in dorsiflexion.

Hip and Pelvis

    Hawley table, use of
    Sacral or pelvic supporst [sic]
    Improvisation by automobile jack
    Position: Fracture of hip
          Marked abduction, midrotation of thigh, flexion not to exceed 10 Degrees

Long spine; down to the toes, up to nipple, foot at right ankle, indications for

    Short spine; firm grip of the femoral condyles, cut away in front and behind to permit flexion of the knees.

Knee: Complete immobilization requires inclusion of pelvis.

    Unless dressing extend[s] at least to the groin, fixation will be unsatisfactory. Patella must be carefully padded.

Foot and ankle:

    Always at right angle to leg, except for special reason, such as paralytic calcaneus.

Removable Dressings

    Plaster of Paris

        (a) by cutting circular plaster dressing

        (b) plaster splints, reinforced or not with other materials.

Method Demonstrations, 8 hours, followed by

    Application to patients by instructor assisted by students, 12 hours.

Time 20 hours in all.

FUNCTIONAL ANATOMY OF MUSCLES AND MUSCLE TRAINING.

The function of muscles and muscular groups in connection with their nerve supply – Intended (1) to enable students to make a diagnosis of nerve injury from muscular involvement (2) to teach the principles of careful muscular examination (3) to throw light on the theory of tendon transplantation (4) to enable correct and sound operating in tendon transfer.

    Instruction on wet specimens of muscular dissections at anatomical laboratory, demonstration preceded by quiz.

    Demonstration at Hospital of muscular examination of patients with infantile paralysis.

    Muscular training and its use, muscle balance, muscle contractions.

    Effect of stretching muscles.

    Demonstration of muscle training exercises on cases of poliomyelitis and other similar conditions.

JOINT ANATOMY

A review of

Anatomy, structure, function, structural weakness and strength and vulnerability of the six important joints, hip, knee, ankle, shoulder, elbow, and wrist.

Method

Anatomical laboratory

Cadaver, wet specimens, diagrams, models.

Time

Five hours.

Comment

It was thought especially important that full demonstration of the anatomy of the knee be given and some comment on the other joints, particularly shoulder and foot.

JOINTS

Physiology, General Characteristics, Reaction to Trauma, and Infection

Schedule

General Phenomena

Structure Joints consist of bone, cartilage, ligaments, synovial membrane, muscles.

Synovial membrane most important to study – endethelial [sic] layer on fibrous base – synovial fluid, use of, composition, secretion increased by use.

Reaction of joints to trauma, toxin and infections – process in synovial membrane swelling, increased secretion, hyperaemia, pain, tenderness, perhaps restricted motion.

Muscular atrophy from disuse and reflex – avoidance by avoiding disuse, Importance as after effect

Normal muscles necessary for normal joint

Muscle spasm: significance in acute joint affections

Progress of synovial reaction:

(a) Recovery, absorption of fluid, restoration to normal, restoration of complete function;

(b) Chronic process with continuance of acute phenomena

(c) Suppuration with pus formation, perhaps with cartilage destruction

(d) Chronic process with adhesions and perhaps fibrillation of cartilage.

Ankylosis as end result from formation of cicatrix.

Partial or total, fibrous or bony (latter always total)

Ankylosis always represents lesion to joint.

Fixation as cause of ankylosis – ankylophobia

General control of ankylosis is control of acute process and

Limitation of its extent.

Measures to control acute process.

Method

General statement followed by clinical demonstration of cases illustrating different types and stages.

Time

Three hours.

APPARATUS

Principles of use of orthopedic apparatus and indications.

Material – iron, steel, aluminum, wood, wire, celluloid, leather, pasteboard, plaster of Paris, etc. – character of each

Improvised apparatus – no especial rule.

Military Splints:

Description and definition of use, measurements, material, covering, practical drill in measurement for such splints as specified in the manual.

Method of Instruction:

Exhibition of splints, explanation of use and construction, rules for measurement and fitting, personal drill in taking tracings and fitting all apparatus, which is ready for trial, under supervision of instructor. Patients in wards and outpatient department shown in apparatus, students criticize fit and usefulness of apparatus. Special drill in measurement and fitting of military splints.

Definite quizzes on latter subject.

Stock civil splints: — typical forms in general use (for plaster apparatus see that section) made from tracings of limbs, or casts.

   Hip: Thomas hip splint – single, double.
           Taylor traction.
           Perineal crutch

   Knee: Traction jointed knee splint for traction
           Splint to limit knee motion
           Thomas caliper splint
           (Thomas knee splint – see military splints)

   Ankle: Foot plates to correct inversion and pronation
           Uprights on shoe to correct inversion or eversion deformity (Jones, Injuries to Joints, fig. 21)
           Uprights fastened to plate
           Type of Taylor varus or valgus splint.

   Spine: Taylor back brace without and with head support
           Tempered steel uprights
           Leather or canvas corset or belt

   Neck: Thomas collar
           Goldthwait wire collar

Time:
   Twelve hours.

CLINICAL AND MICROSCOPIC PATHOLOGY OF BONE:

Osteomyelitis, tuberculosis, syphilis, bone growth and repair.

Bone-grafts

New growths

Time:
   Three hours.

SHOP WORK

Schedule
   Rudimentary demonstration of routine methods used in an apparatus shop by workman, at first under an instructor, later to students (in sections) on the following topics: -- braizing, welding, soldering, tempering, shaping and bending to tracing or casts, shortening and lengthening, covering, repairing, rivetting, sewing and shpaing [sic] leather covers, and general routine shop work of this sort.

Time:
   Eight hours.

Comment
   This part of the course seems most useful to the students and is intended to teach them what to tell a blacksmith about how he shall change, repair, or construct apparatus for use in emergencies.

OPERATIONS TO ILLUSTRATE PRINCIPLES

Operation to be shown must be in a measure dependant [sic] upon available cases. These would be:

Tendon operations –

Osteotomy, correction of ankylosis by manipulation, correction of deformity by manipulation and fasciotomy, astragalectomy, arthredesis [sic], bone grafting, arthrotomy, (for drainage and exploration) osteomyelitis, excision of nerve, sutures and lengthening.

Time
   The time allotted is twenty hours.

Comment
   There is a great demand to see operating and the course could be made largely operative. We have felt that fundamentals were more important and that one or two operations as types were sufficient for an experienced man to see.

ARTIFICIAL LIMBS

Leg:
   Early care of stump: protection of remaining foot in cases of amputation of one leg; crutch paralysis and types of crutches used to avoid it; method of testing for contracture of stump.

   Temporary artificial legs; advantages methods of construction of cheap types.

   Permanent artificial legs; difficulties in fitting and in use; construction.

Arms
    No effective substitute: artificial hands practically of esthetic value only; in actual work some form of mechanical hook only mechanism of value. Demonstration of cases and artificial limbs.

Time
    Two hours.

VOCATIONAL TRAINING

Talk on principles of vocational training, illustrated by examples and instances drawn from Cripples School, with exhibition of patients. Visit to shops.

Method as above

Time
    Two hours.

Comment
    This seems more practical than a purely theoretical talk.

PHYSICAL THERAPY

Theory of massage.

Nucleous therapy -theory of an applied to war surgery
    Curative workshops
    Apparatus for muscle training and joint mobilization.

Heat and Light
    Hydrotherapy – Electricity with especial reference to diagnosis and prognosis. Its therapeutic use as a means of muscular exercise. Dangers of overuse. Joint mobilization – need of care in manual attempts. Dangers of manipulation under anesthetic.

Time
    Eight hours.

X-ray Interpretation
    In addition to instruction in this subject allotted under special headings by demonstration.

Time
    Six hours.

OPERATIVE STUDY ON CADAVER

    Students operating as far as possible
    Tendon-lengthening and shortening and transplanting joints.
    Incision for operative approach
    Incisions for drainage

Bones
    Bone transplantation
    Osteotomies, — excisions

Time
    Twelve hours.

TENDON OPERATIONS

Schedule

    (a) for muscle injury   (b) for nerve injury

    Transplantation based on anatomical plan. Two dangers (1) insufficient correction (2) over-correction. Balance must be studied. Tendons may be transplanted into. (a) other tendons (b) extended by silk if necessary and inserted into bone or periosteum. Technique – importance of asepsis – after treatment – preliminary treatment, which should consist of avoiance [sic] of stretching and removal of existing deformity.

Tendon fixation
    Tenedosis [sic] – fastening of tendon of paralysed [sic] muscle to bone to act as suspensory ligament.
        Tenotomy and plastic tension lengthening
        Tendon shortening

Method and Time
    Talk on principles and technique, three hours
    Tendon Operations inculded [sic] in operative time

CAMP ACCIDENTS AND THEIR TREATMENT

If it can be arranged an instructor with the class should visit a camp by arrangement and see with the surgeon in charge cases of routine orthopedic accidents in consultation. It would seem as if such an exercise would make the men more valuable as camp assistants.

    Time
        Ten hours.

CONFERENCES AND EXAMINATIONS

The best use of conferences has seemed to be in getting from the men criticisms of the course, a statement of their requirements and short-comings with some discussion of topics already considered. It is recommended that weekly tests be given, perhaps in connection with the conferences, preferably oral in character. At the close of the course a written examination should be given the the [sic] marks furnished to the Surgeon General's Office.

Time
  Six hours.

NERVE ANATOMY

Men in sections an anatomical Laboratory
Dissection by each squad of the important nerves and plexuses on one side of the body on the cadaver, with quizzes.

Time
  Twelve hours to a man in sections.

Method
  Dissections followed by demonstration.

FOOT PROPHYLAXIS

Shoes – care of the feet
Affections of the foot
  Examination
Sprains
  Deformities resulting from injuries
  Static deformities and disabilities.
Time
  8 hours.
Back
  Anatomy of spin [sic] and X-ray interpretation physiology
  Examination
  Various back lesions
    Strain and trauma
    Fracture and dislocation
  Traumatic Spondylitis (Kimmel) Tuberculosis, arthritis, static deformities.

Time
  Ten hours.
Treatment:
  Conservation
  Operation

JOINTS

Pathology – diagnosis – treatment
Hip
  Examination and X-ray Interpretation
  Motions
  Deformity – actual and practical shortening line of deformity
  Limitation of motions – bony ankylosis – fibrous ankylosis – muscular spasm.
Lesion
  Synovitis and Arthritis
  Trauma and Fractur [sic] and Dislocations
Treatment
  Prevalent deformity
  Protection and Fixation
  Prevention   (use of plastic braces
                (Balkan frame
                (Traction
Corrections   (Traction)
              (Plaster of Paris
              (Manipulation
              (Operative   (Arthrodesis
                            (Osteotome [sic]
Operations
  Methods of Approach
  After-Care
  Excision
  Artheotomy [sic]
Knee
  Examination and X-ray
  Lesion
  Traumatic strain
  Rupture on int. sat. leg
  Fractures into joint
  Semilunar dislocation

Injury to crucial ligaments
Tuberculosis
Synovitis and arthritis   (infections
                                     (hypertrophic

Treatment
   Fixation
   Protective   (Splints
                    (Bandages
                    (Strapping
   Fracture
   Operation methods of approach
   After-care
   Upper extremity
       shoulder, elbow, and wrist
       see general scheme for other joints

<u>Time</u>
   Twelve hours.

<u>Collateral Reading</u>

A list of text books should be prepared to supplement the official manual.

This should consist of
   (a) text books
   (b) reference to important monographs and periodical literature.

CHAPTER 64

World War II
Mobile Warfare

The evolution of orthopaedics and fracture care at the turn of the twentieth century and following World War I set the stage for care during World War II. In the United States in the early years—the late 1880s through the early 1900s—many in the field of medicine disregarded orthopaedic surgeons, referring to them as "strap and buckle" surgeons despite their renowned skills as surgeons and impressive outcomes in working with patients with disabilities. Robert Jones, a Welsh surgeon practicing in Liverpool, UK, was the most well-known orthopaedist, but despite his achievements even he was called simply a "bonesetter." This too was despite the fact that the American Orthopaedic Association (AOA) and the Orthopaedic Section of the American Medical Association (AMA) existed well before World War I.

At the time, some orthopaedic surgeons insisted that those in their specialty should be more involved in managing patients with trauma, and, as early as 1891, Dr. Virgil P. Gibney (the first president of the AOA) believed that, in the future, orthopaedic surgeons would be treating fractures and malunions. Nevertheless, before World War I, many surgeons had little training in or experience with trauma, particularly to the extremities. Dr. Leo Mayer wrote, "It is only fair to conclude that orthopaedic surgery at the turn of the century did not demand surgical skill and knowledge as a prerequisite. The change in emphasis from mechanics to surgery has been one of the noteworthy advances of our specialty" (1955).

Dr. Abel Phelps, the eighth president of the AOA (1899), had agreed with Dr. Gibney: "It is my earnest conviction that within a very few years fractures and dislocations will be treated by the orthopaedic surgeons" (quoted in Cave 1961). After the discovery of x-rays, the management of fractures began to change from surgeons to orthopaedic surgeons, and within the first decade of the twentieth century, a fundamental shift in fracture care from general to orthopaedic surgeons was underway. Mayer continued, "Let no one gain the impression that this transition was easy and peaceful. Inevitably it precipitated a clash with the general surgeon, who disputed the new surgical claims of the young specialty" (1955). In his 1894 AOA Presidential Address, Phelps had stated, "The orthopaedist was always at war with the general surgeon...There never was a time when they could lie peacefully together in the same bed, excepting 'like the lion and the lamb – one inside the other, and the poor *orthopede* was always inside'" (Mayer 1955).

However, the opportunities afforded by World War I not only dramatically improved the reputation of the specialty but aided it in establishing standards of practice that promoted its development in the decades to come. Their work on the front lines—where the orthopaedic surgeon had to learn quickly to effectively treat traumatic injuries to the extremities—grew their knowledge and their clinical abilities. With more than 65% of the injuries treated orthopaedic in nature and nearly two-thirds of all casualties in the war resulting from orthopaedic conditions, the critical need for specialists in orthopaedic care was never greater.

Toward the end of the World War I, Massachusetts General Hospital (MGH) developed a unique approach to fracture care: a cooperative effort of the orthopaedic surgeons and the general surgeons. In 1917, Dr. Charles Scudder, with the support Dr. Robert Osgood, founded the Fracture Clinic at MGH, which—according Dr. Carter Rowe—was likely the first "in the world" (Rowe 1996). It was an outgrowth of the "fracture squad" originally started by Scudder, and within two years it "became an independent unit under the guidance" of orthopaedic surgery and general surgery (Rowe 1996). During this period, "Dr. Daniel F. Jones, Chief of Surgery, and Dr. Nathaniel Allison, Chief of Orthopaedics, shared responsibilities" (Rowe 1996). In his 1917 AOA presidential address, Dr. John L. Porter said, "I believe a new era has begun for our specialty through the impetus given by war. The old conception of orthopaedic surgery is undergoing transformation rapidly" (Cave 1961).

The burgeoning of the field of orthopaedics following World War I, as noted by Sir Harry Platt, manifested perhaps most significantly in the emergence of fracture services, rehabilitation services, and, in bigger hospitals, orthopaedic departments. Almost 600 military officers had spent time serving in the army's orthopaedic division. Moreover, collaboration between British and American orthopaedists in developing the standards of practice during World War I resulted in the establishment of similar standards of orthopaedic practice in the two countries in subsequent years. Smith (2015) noted, "More than any single advance, World War I illustrated the profound difference that existed between a knowledgeable and skilled…orthopaedic surgeon and even a well-trained general surgeon when it came to management of complex extremity wounds involving fractures. It also sent a message to the orthopaedic community – we needed to further study fracture management."

In particular, it spurred the development of many techniques to address one of the greatest challenges to a surgeon: treatment of compound fractures with associated osteomyelitis. These techniques included timely reduction of the fracture, proper immobilization, rest, drainage, debridement, the packing of dressings into wounds, internal and external skeletal fixation, plaster casting, and sulfonamide drugs. About a year after the war ended, H. P. H. Galloway wrote that it "has done more to bring orthopaedic surgery into its true inheritance than would have been accomplished by any other agencies in many years" (Cave 1961).

In addition to the impetus provided by World War I, the rapid increase in the number of compound fractures resulting from automobile, farm, and factory-related accidents spurred interest in fracture management in the United States. Because laypeople and general practitioners provided emergency care for 95% of such cases, a key role of orthopaedic surgeons at the time was to provide accurate information on fracture treatment to this broad audience. Unfortunately, in many cases, poor initial management of fractures by caregivers ignorant of proper techniques led to secondary trauma in patients and complicated the work of orthopaedic specialists who followed up with them.

The Fracture Clinic at the MGH continued to grow, and it held its first fracture course on October 16, 1928, eleven years after it had opened its doors. That first course—about two weeks in duration—was widely attended by "134 doctors from three states" (Rowe 1996). The clinic continued to be led by both a general and an orthopaedic surgeon. Despite the experience with trauma that surgeons obtained during World War I, it did not immediately translate into clinical practice in orthopaedics. It would be another 20 years—with the onset of World War II—that orthopaedics would definitively break with general surgery to focus more explicitly on trauma.

World War II

> **Author Recollections**
>
> While a surgical resident from 1965 until 1967, I remember at the Hospital of the University of Pennsylvania that fracture call was still divided between the general surgeons and the orthopaedic surgeons, each service alternating weekly on the fracture service.

WORLD WAR II BEGINS

After World War I ended, there was a worldwide recession followed by the Great Depression, which began on Black Tuesday in 1929. The United States still had not recovered from the war. Germany, Italy, and Japan were unhappy with their political and economic status. Declaring the need for more living space ("Lebensraum"), Adolf Hitler began to ignore the provisions of the Treaty of Versailles. He built the Luftwaffe in the 1930s, which was prohibited by the treaty; actions that were ignored by the West. Then on September 1, 1939, he invaded Poland. Afterward, both France and the United Kingdom declared war on Germany.

The United States began to feel "the effects of the war socially and economically" at this point (Faxon 1959), as supply chains for and exportation of food and other necessities were disrupted. At the time, America had adopted an isolationist policy, although President Franklin D. Roosevelt

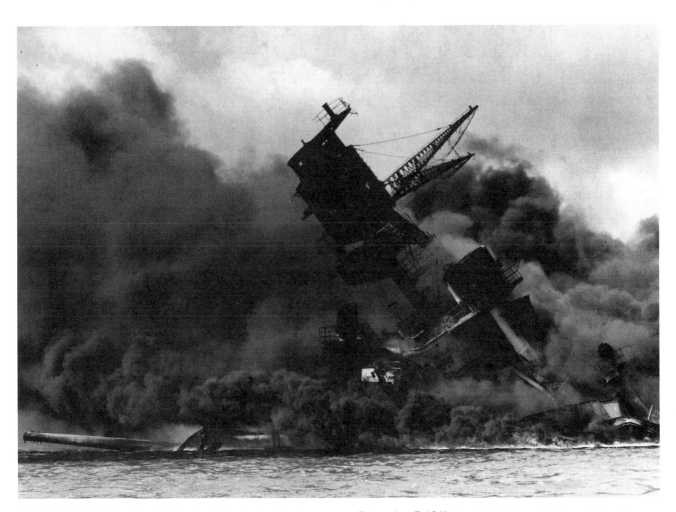

Battleship USS *Arizona* bombed in Pearl Harbor by the Japanese on December 7, 1941. Franklin D. Roosevelt Library, National Archives and Records Administration/Wikimedia Commons.

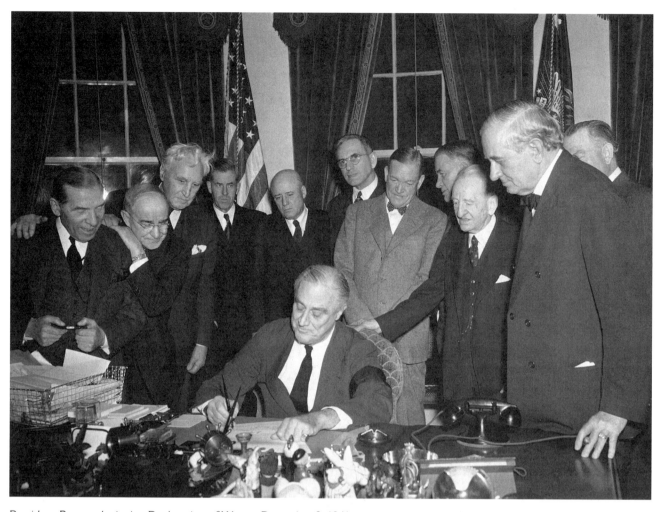

President Roosevelt signing Declaration of War on December 8, 1941. Associated Press.

spoke publicly about the dangers of the leaders in Germany, Italy, and Japan, and he supported England via arms sales. The majority of Americans were opposed to entering any war, however, even after Germany invaded France and waged the Battle of Britain. But after the bombing of Pearl Harbor on December 7, 1941, the United States Congress declared war on Japan the next day.

Orthopaedics as a specialty had continued to advance in the intervening years between the wars. Although orthopaedists disagreed over certain matters, it was a healthy disagreement based on a common foundation of knowledge and goals. Spencer's comments on scientific research in general seem especially pertinent to the practice of orthopaedics during this time:

The efforts of numerous independent seekers carrying out their research in different directions constitute a better agency for finding the true method than any that could be devised. Each of them struck by some new thought which probably contains more or less of basis in facts – each of them zealous on behalf of his plan, fertile in expedients to test its correctness, and untiring in his efforts to make known its success – each of them merciless in his criticism of the rest – there cannot fail, by composition of forces, to be a gradual approximation of all toward the right course. Whatever portion of the method any one of them has discovered must, by the constant exhibition of its results, force itself into adoption; whatever wrong practices he has joined with it must, by repeated experiment and failure, be exploded. And, by this aggregation of truths and elimination of errors, there must eventually be developed a correct and complete body of doctrine. Of the three phases through which human opinion passes—the unanimity of the ignorant, the disagreement of the inquiring and the unanimity of the wise – it is manfest [sic] that the second is the parent of the third. (Spencer 1861)

By the time the US entered World War II, orthopaedic surgeons were far better prepared to meet the challenges of caring for wounded soldiers than they had been a generation earlier. Orthopaedics now claimed over 700 certified specialists, who were unified by a well-established set of treatment principles that guided their practice.

IMPACT ON US HOSPITALS AND TRAINING PROGRAMS

Disturbance from the war extended to hospitals, too. MGH experienced such disruption through a loss of staff—physicians and surgeons joined the armed forces and other personnel "left the Hospital to work in war industries, attracted by the higher wages" (Faxon 1959). One example was that of the nursing school at MGH. Enrollment of men declined rapidly in 1943, from an average number of 30 to only eight. Women, too, were more attracted to the Cadet Nursing Corps training program. The war delayed the building of the new Vincent Memorial Hospital and changed priorities of research by the Office of Scientific Research and Development to focus on fitness, war injuries, and other issues related to the war.

During World War II, training programs were greatly affected with both a decline in staff and house officers in orthopaedics. In order to have an adequate number of physicians in the army and navy, all medical school graduates were required to enter the medical corps after a 12-month internship; which later was reduced to nine months. House officers were ordered to be reduced by 15%. At MGH, this meant a reduction from 321 house officers to 230. At Boston Children's Hospital in 1942, Dr. Frank R. Ober (see chapter 20) noted that:

the Army regulations do not permit more than one year of internship following graduation from medical school. This means that there has been a good deal of disruption of the house staff service so it is about fifty percent of normal…In meeting our needs [orthopaedics at BCH and MGH], it has been necessary to suspend temporarily the preliminary eight months training in the Department of Pathology…Our visiting staff has always been small in number and barely covered the several services of this Department so that even a depletion of two staff members plus the loss of house staff throws a heavy burden on those who are left. Several of our staff also take care of the orthopedic patients and orthopedic teaching at the Peter Bent Brigham Hospital. (Ober 1942)

In addition, Thomas Parran Jr., surgeon general at the time, mandated that all medical schools be reduced from four years to three. Thus, these newly minted doctors had little clinical experience before being thrust into the responsibility of caring for large numbers of severely injured soldiers. In order to improve this deficiency and to allow more physicians to remain caring for patients in the inadequately staffed teaching hospitals in the United States, the surgeon general activated the so-called "9-9-9 rule." This mandate allowed one-third of the house officers to remain in their training program an additional nine months; one-half of the second group could then remain an additional nine months. Thus, a small number of house officers could complete a total of 27 months in their training program before being called to active military duty.

In 1944—one year before the war ended—Dr. Ober discussed the challenges that Boston Children's Hospital had faced. They had continued to serve similar numbers of orthopaedic patients with significantly reduced staff. He wrote in his annual report:

> The bed capacity has not been cut down but it was found necessary to change the Out-Patient Clinic from six days a week to three, and operations are scheduled three days a week alternating with Out-Patient days. This was done because there were not enough members on the Visiting Staff to do the necessary work and furnish proper care to all the orthopaedic patients coming to the hospital. This has proven to be a very satisfactory arrangement…The House Officer Service has been difficult the past year owing to military requirements. We have had to make substitutes for vacancies several times, but have had help from the Surgical Service, which allows some of their interns to serve part of their time on the Orthopedic Service…The Visiting Staff has been under considerable pressure the past year but this was relieved to a great extent by having the operating and Out-Patient Clinics work on alternate days. (Ober 1944)

Many hospitals in the United States were left severely short-handed during the war, but they were innovative in adapting to the necessary circumstances of the times. These vacancies were quickly filled, however, after the war ended and training programs were able to resume in full. By 1945, Ober wrote that:

> the Orthopedic Department of the Hospital [Boston Children's Hospital] has had a very busy year in all its various divisions. The depleted House Staff became augmented quite rapidly after peace was declared, and there was no dearth of applications for appointments to fill vacancies. It has been decided to change the setup of house officers by appointing assistant residents. There will be a return of the combined House and Residence Service [stopped during the war] with the Orthopedic Department of the Massachusetts General Hospital in 1946, thus resuming the training of these men in both adult and children's orthopedic conditions. This method furnishes a well-rounded program in the education of those who are going to specialize in Orthopedic Surgery. Related to the training program, it should be noted that the recently expanded clinical and orthopedic teaching facilities at the Peter Bent Brigham are coordinated with the teaching activates of the Children's Hospital… [the house officer] service was run on a short-handed bases…When peace was declared it became possible to secure men from the armed services to fill the gaps so that before the year was finished, this Service was going on in a most satisfactory manner…The Visiting Staff remained unchanged throughout the year. It will have its full complement restored in 1946. (Ober 1945)

INTRODUCTION OF PORTABLE SURGICAL HOSPITALS

World War II introduced the quick mobilization of troops and the extensive use of blitzkrieg and heavy artillery, which had their own consequences for extracting wounded soldiers. MacFarlane (1942) wrote, "When we went to war in September 1939, many of us thought in terms of 1918 [but] two decades between wars is a tragic interval." Even with air ambulances, it was difficult to transport injured soldiers to the field hospitals. Mixter (1950) discussed this change from trench warfare to mobile warfare: "Stabilized trench warfare [during World War I] made prompt evacuation of the wounded practically impossible…patients reached casualty clearing stations and evacuation hospitals in wretched condition." Suddenly surgeons were presented with a new dilemma: they had to take themselves, their team, and all necessary equipment to the wounded. For this, they needed "vehicles which can move as quickly as the armored divisions which [they serve]" (MacFarlane 1942). These mobile teams became known as portable surgical hospitals, the precursors of the Mobile Army Surgical Hospital (MASH) units later deployed in the Korean War.

> "I would remind you again how large and various was the experience of the battlefield, and how fertile the blood of warriors in the rearing of good surgeons."
> —Hieronymus Brunschwig, lived circa 1450–1512
> (Quoted by Thomas C. Allbutt in LeVay 1990, 641.)

IMPACT ON WOUND MANAGEMENT

Walter Lippman, a Harvard alum and a journalist and political commentator who won two Pulitzer Prizes, paraphrasing the German philosopher George Wilhelm Friedrich Hegel, stated, "the lesson of history is that the lesson of history is never learned." For Michael DeBakey, Lippmann's words resonate with regard to applying the experiences of war to the field of surgery. He believed that surgeons in World War II forgot the lessons hard-learned during World War I—use of antiseptics to sterilize wounds failed, primarily closed wounds became septic, the need for sufficient debridement—and that being cognizant of previous knowledge of military surgery could have saved limbs and lives during World War II and in general surgical practice. In **Box 64.1**, MacFarlane describes this impact on wound care at the time, and in **Case 64.1**, he contrasts wound care performed for a patient during World War I and for one during World War II. Bristow (1943) agreed with DeBakey, noting:

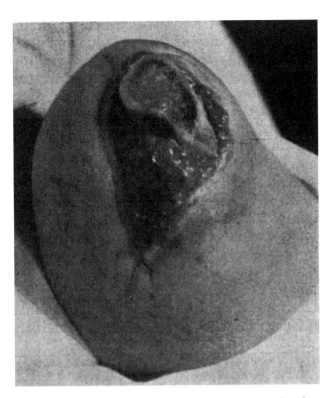

Guillotine amputation with bone exposed—two months after procedure with retraction of soft tissues. An open circular amputation and use of skin traction avoids this major problem. U.S. National Library of Medicine.

Box 64.1. MacFarlane's Notes on Wound Care

> "A large number of wounds have been operated on in the forward area. The recognized débridement was carried out in as many early cases as possible. The wounds were saucerized, dusted with sulphanilamide, and packed lightly with vaselin [sic] gauze. All these cases did extremely well. Some wounds had been sutured, but, with the exception of very few cases, were badly septic on arrival at the base…Operation entails enlargement of skin wounds and incision of the deep fascia."
> (MacFarlane 1942)

To recapitulate, the same old mistakes, which we learned to avoid during the Great War, have given the most trouble. We must remind ourselves that wounds must be left open and not sutured, that amputation flaps must not be closed, that plugging of wounds must be avoided, that vaseline [sic] gauze should be used

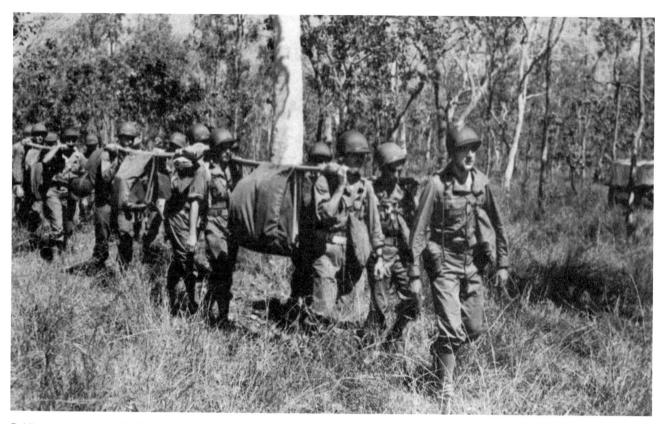

Soldiers carrying supplies/equipment for a portable hospital (MASH Unit). U.S. National Library of Medicine.

as a covering not as a plug, and that skin must not be sacrificed unnecessarily in performing a wound toilet.

During World War II, two components of wound management emerged that began to counter the stigma associated with military surgery: standardization according to solid principles of practice and phased wound management. Surgeons were directed to leave wounds open after they'd been cleaned and debrided, to refrain from suturing limbs after amputation, and to use a split or bivalve cast for soldiers who would be transported elsewhere—all important aspects that had barely been understood during World War I. Based on the work of Edward Churchill (from MGH) in the early period of the war, surgeons also followed three phases of surgical management, which, they found, could be applied to all wounds: "initial wound surgery, a function of advanced hospitals…reparative surgery, a responsibility of general hospitals in the Zone of Communications…and reconstructive surgery, a function of general hospitals in the Zone of the Interior" (DeBakey 1947).

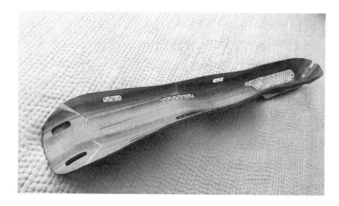

Eames molded plywood leg splint. Designed by Charles and Ray Eames who were contracted by the US Navy in 1943 to design a lightweight splint to replace the heavier metal Thomas splint used by the Army. It was molded to the lower extremity, flaring out at the proximal end to fit against the buttocks and tapering distally to fit the lower leg and foot. More than 150,000 Eames splints were made between 1943 and 1945. Photo by the author, from his personal collection.

> "Infection in war wounds has always been the *bête noire* of military surgeons."
> —Lewis N. Cozen, MD ("Military Orthopedic Surgery," Clinical Orthopaedics and Related Research, 1985; 200:50.)

Case 64.1. Wounds in War: Changes from WWI to WWII

> In March 1942, Dr. Colonel J. A. MacFarlane saw a patient who had previously been wounded in the Great War in 1918. He wrote:
>
> "The patient, an Englishman, was wounded by a shell fragment in the right buttock [1918]. The bone was not involved. Roentgenograms revealed no evidence of old injury or of infection. There was no indication of a sciatic-nerve lesion. The wound, therefore, involved only the soft tissues of the buttock, including the glutei. The patient reached a casualty clearing station some twelve hours after injury, and was operated upon. He was subsequently transferred to a large hospital in France, where he remained for six months. One or two drainage operations were performed during that interval. Dressings were changed three times a day, and the wound was 'syringed.' Following the discharge from the hospital he attended an out-patient department for another six months. A very good result was obtained, and the patient is now a corporal in the Provost Corps in the Canadian Army.
>
> "It is interesting to contrast this case with that of a patient injured in the great air raid on Coventry [November 14, 1940] who suffered a bomb wound in exactly that same area and approximately of the same degree.
>
> "The patient's wound was explored, foreign bodies were removed, and a thorough debridement was carried out. He was then put in a plaster spica. He was in the hospital two months, during which time he had in all three changes of plaster and dressing. At the end of the third month he was able to return to his work in the factory."

ADVANCEMENT OF SURGICAL SPECIALTIES AND ORTHOPAEDICS

By March 1942, four months after the United States entered World War II, Major General James Magee, Surgeon General of the US Army, had added a professional consultants division in his office. Magee appointed "a civilian specialist to advise him concerning surgery and the surgical specialties...At the same time, consultants in major specialties and subspecialties were appointed to overseas hospitals and units" (DeBakey 1947). The civilian specialist focused on selecting experienced and dedicated consultants to oversee the various theaters of operation and so avoided many of the problems the army faced in getting its surgeons where they were needed during World War I; they were chosen "with the utmost care, on the basis of training, ability, accomplishments and professional eminence" (DeBakey 1947). At the time, "the chief consultant for the Mediterranean Theater was Colonel Edward D. Churchill [MGH] and the chief consultant for the European Theater was Brigadier General Elliott C. Cutler [PBBH]" (DeBakey 1947).

Despite his great responsibilities and his isolation from other leadership, e.g., the president's chief of staff and the secretary of war (who along with others at higher levels seemed to view the medical department in terms of only the amounts of rations and ammunition they used), the office of the army surgeon general led the medical department well and achieved smooth and proficient functioning of his consultants, specialists, and medical officers and staff. Surgeon General Norman T. Kirk (**Box 64.2**), who served after Magee, made significant improvements in the care of the wounded, and he was responsible for the expansion of the medical corps from 1,200 to 47,000 physicians who cared for approximately 599,724 wounded soldiers. Another major improvement developed by General Kirk was the establishment of specialty centers, centers where soldiers with similar injuries would be hospitalized in units specifically designed for their care under specialists in the field. The most commonly known example is the nerve and hand centers in the US, authorized under the leadership of Dr. Sterling Burwell; others included spinal cord injury, amputations, eye injuries, and others: "appropriate specialists to the points at which they could be most useful and by the concentration of patients with special types of injuries in centers equipped and staffed for their care… Under his leadership…[the] medical profession [was] fully committed to the principle of specialization" (DeBakey 1947). Two major changes had also occurred in civilian medical practice supporting this strong move toward specialization, accreditation of specialty residency programs and certification of specialists.

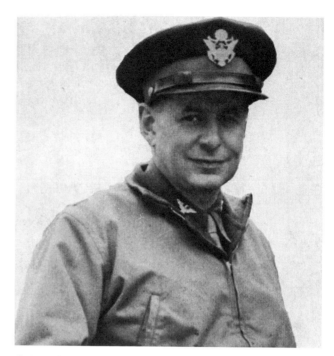

Colonel Edward D. Churchill. C.D. Wright, "Historical Perspectives of the American Association for Thoracic Surgery: Edward D. Churchill 1895–1972," *The Journal of Thoracic and Cardiovascular Surgery* 2011; 143: 2

Box 64.2. Major General Norman T. Kirk: US Army Surgeon General 1943–1947

> Major General Norman T. Kirk was an orthopaedic surgeon and a career army officer. After graduating from the University of Maryland Medical School in 1910, he was a house officer at the University Hospital in Baltimore. While stationed on the surgical service, "at Walter Reed in 1919, he transferred his practice from general surgery to bone and joint surgery. He was credited with treating at least one-third of the major amputations incurred in World War I…[and] was acknowledged as one of the leading experts in the United States on amputation" ("Norman T. Kirk" 2009).
>
> After the first world war, he studied at both MGH and the Johns Hopkins University Hospital. I was unable to find how long and what he studied at MGH, but I think he may have spent his time with the new fracture service, a combined service with general surgery and orthopaedic surgery (Charles L. Scudder and Robert B. Osgood) or with Dr. Philip D. Wilson, also an expert on amputations.

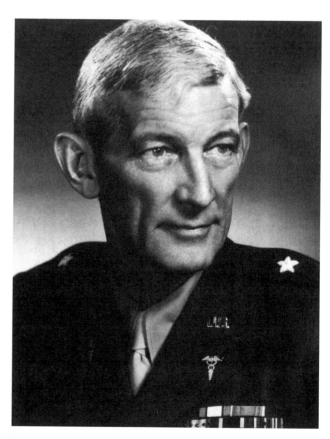

Brigadier General Elliott C. Cutler. U.S. National Library of Medicine.

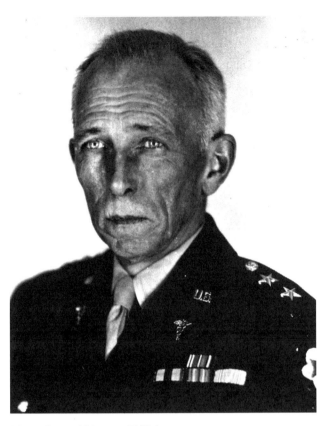

Major General Norman T. Kirk. U.S. National Library of Medicine.

ORTHOPAEDICS AS A SPECIALTY

Two publications appeared at the initial threat of another world war: *The Division of Orthopaedic Surgery in the A.E.F.*, published in 1941 by Dr. Joel Goldthwait, and *Medical War Manual No. 4 Military Orthopaedic Surgery*, published in 1942, written by a subcommittee on orthopaedic surgery of the Committee on Surgery of the Division of Medical Sciences of the National Research Council. Dr. Goldthwait stated in his introduction that his purpose for writing the book was to pass on knowledge gained during the Great War that might prove useful to surgeons in the event of a second global conflict, which event he viewed as likely. The latter publication was edited by orthopaedic surgeons who were recognized as authorities in their specialty. They attempted to prepare orthopaedic surgeons who had not served during World War I for the management of the severe war wounds they would treat for the first time in their careers. The subcommittee was chaired by George E. Bennett and members included: LeRoy C. Abbott, William Darrach, J. Albert Key, Guy W. Leadbetter, Frank R. Ober, Harold R. Conn, Robert H. Kennedy, Frederick C. Kidner, Paul B. Magnuson, M.H. Smith-Petersen, and Philip D. Wilson.

Medical War Manual No. 4, however, was largely useless to orthopaedic surgeons providing primary care of wounded soldiers on the front because it took the perspective of civilian practice and focused mainly on techniques for reconstruction, which were only appropriate for those working in base hospitals. It often omitted or covered in only a cursory manner the information that would have been most helpful, that is, the emergent treatment of joint and bone injuries. This critical information stayed hidden within historical accounts of the First World War and inaccessible to the surgeons facing casualties in the new war, and so American surgeons were forced to learn again by trial and error.

> "The lesson of history is never learned... The lesson will need to be relearned all over again, as it has with each war."
> —Trueta 1959

Nevertheless, one of the largest surgical subspecialties established during World War II was orthopaedics, and "surgical teams sent to the forward areas were staffed by orthopaedic surgeons as the supply would allow. Wounds of the extremities made up 70 per cent of the case load of evacuation hospitals" (Cave 1961). Of particular note, the open circular approach to amputation was identified as more effective than the guillotine approach, as the latter resulted in insufficient soft tissue to provide bone coverage, and thus required follow-up surgery to correct. An adaptation of the circular technique continues to be used today.

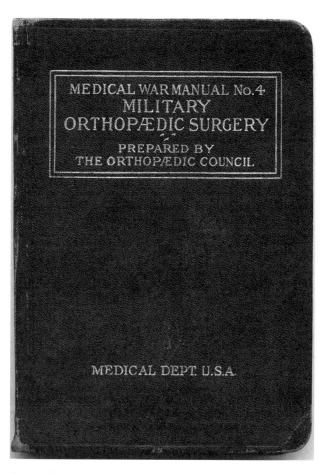

Cover, *Medical War Manual No. 4: Military Orthopaedic Surgery*. Philadelphia and New York: Lea & Febiger, 1918.

AMERICA BASE HOSPITALS

After World War I, pursuant to the National Defense Act of 1920, the US War Department decided to close down their base hospitals but retain the ability to reactivate them should they be needed in the future. Among these was "Base Hospital No. 6 [which] was included as a unit of the Organized Reserves…[and] existed as a 'paper unit' and no more…There existed no facilities at all for unit training…Inadequate funds and lack of personnel in the Regular Army…precluded institution of a training program" (Faxon 1959). As World War II began and Germany and its allies began invading Europe—Poland, Denmark and Norway, France—the War Department began considering such reactivation. In 1940, the army surgeon general wrote the director of MGH about staffing old Base Hospital No. 6, which was to be reinstated as the 6th General Hospital and would again be affiliated with MGH. The hospital trustees approved the request.

By 1942, the 5th General Hospital and the 105th General Hospital (Harvard University's two reserve hospitals) were each activated as well. As **Table 64.1** shows, station hospitals and general hospitals were fifth and sixth out of six levels of medical care provided to wounded US soldiers in terms of distance from the battlefield in Europe. Members of the MGH staff included:

- 123 active staff
- 176 residents and interns
- 158 nurses
- 175 employees
- 11 additional unidentified members

6th General Hospital

When the old Base Hospital No. 6 reopened as the 6th General Hospital, MGH—at the surgeon general's request—assigned medical officers and nurses and chose a unit director. The hospital selected Colonel Thomas R. Goethals, one of its surgeons in obstetrics and gynecology, for approval by the surgeon general. The War Department would select the high-level officers in charge—commanding, executive, supply, and administration officers—and all enlisted soldiers who would serve with the unit.

Personnel and Training

The 6th General Hospital became active at Camp Blanding in May 1942. During the eight months following activation, personnel of the 6th General Hospital underwent basic military and medical training (similar to content in mission training plans 8-1 and 8-10) at the Camp Blanding Station Hospital. This included enlisted members and nurses, along with the schools of motor transport and chemical warfare (certain officers). Ahead of that time, and from "the time the United States entered the war, in December, 1941 [until] the date of activation…all the authorized nurses had been enrolled as well as fifty-eight of the required seventy-one officers…[However] fourteen of the officers and fifteen of the nurses who had been originally enrolled [were transferred to other organizations]…" (Faxon 1959).

Professionals and officers of the unit taught courses on medical theory and practice. These instructors included 41 officers, 17 of whom were surgeons, including Lt. Colonel Marshall K. Bartlett, MC (a member of the Back Bay practice of Drs. Horatio Rogers and Richard Miller). According to Faxon (1959):

> All personnel of all services and departments were given thorough basic and advanced military training, including semiweekly road marches…Morale was kept at a high level despite the minor frustrations experienced by some in their adjustment to military life, and by the natural tension caused by the uncertainty as to when orders for alert status might be received…The Service Chiefs [included] Lieutenant Colonel [Horatio] Rogers, Chief of Surgery. (Faxon 1959)

Camp Kilmer and Deployment to North Africa

The 6th General Hospital went on alert in mid-December 1942, cancelled leaves, and began to pack up and mobilize. Finally receiving orders on January 20, 1943, the unit travelled via train from the Camp Blanding Station Hospital to Camp Kilmer, where it staged until February 7, engaging in further training and readiness drills. By that date, it was:

> temporarily designated as Task Force 5995-DD and broken down into six groups for overseas shipment, entrained for the New York Port of Embarkation, where in the late afternoon it was embarked on six ships of the convoy [50 ships carrying over 50,000 people] then

Table 64.1. Levels of Medical Care Provided by the US Army in Terms of Distance from the Battlefield

Level of Care	Distance from Frontline	Type of Care Rendered
Frontline	—	Each soldier has first aid packet Contains 6 gm. of sulfanilamide Already received tetanus vaccination
Litter Bearer's Section	—	Compound fractures splinted
Battalion Aid Station	300–800 yards	Hemorrhage controlled Morphine & sulfa given Splints adjusted & blankets given
Collection Station	1000–2000 yards	Continued medical care Patients prepared for evacuation by ambulance
Hospital or Clearing Station	4–5 miles; beyond rifle range	Patients in shock or needing wound care admitted Patients slightly wounded are treated and returned to their unit Others are transferred by ambulance
Surgical or Field Hospital	4–5 miles	Full surgical facilities for emergency operative procedures
Evacuation Hospital or Area Station	10–20 miles	Established on a railhead Additional wound debridement Shock wards Patients admitted for more than a few days
General Hospital	>50 miles	Continued care, including specialty care

(Adapted from N. T. Kirk 1941.)

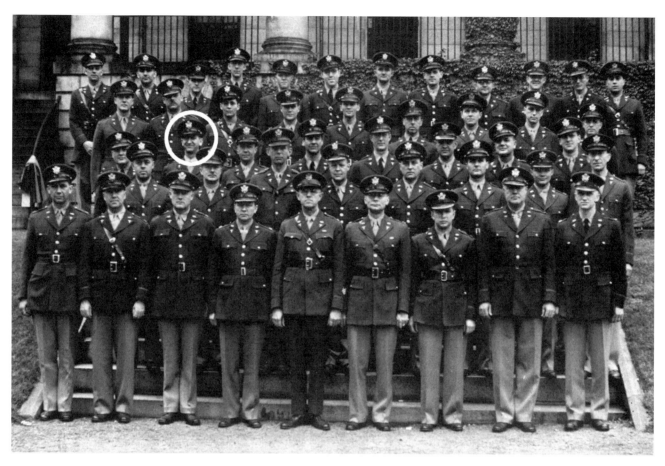

Medical Staff of the 6th General Hospital. Dr. Aufranc is second from the left in the third row. Massachusetts General Hospital, Archives and Special Collections

preparing to sail. In the darkness of the early morning hours of February 8, the convoy pulled out from its docks in New York Harbor. Even at this time the hospital had no inkling of its destination. The two most likely guesses were that it was destined for Great Britain or North Africa…[they] gradually swung to the belief that they were headed for the Straits of Gibraltar…There was the grandeur of this [enormous] convoy…moving across the ocean in a constantly changing zigzag pattern, shepherded by destroyers, battleships, and cruisers…the medical contingent was only a small part of the troops on board…About twenty-four hours before a landfall was made it was announced that the envoy…was destined in part for Casablanca, French Morocco, and in part to another North African port, on the Mediterranean…

Several detachments of the 6th were landed in Casablanca on February 19, in the dark and rain…a tour of duty began in that Moroccan city which was destined to last for not quite fifteen months. (Faxon 1959)

On arriving in Casablanca, detachments of the 6th General Hospital stayed in a massive, trash-strewn warehouse across the street from the hospital itself. It was cold and raining, and their quarters lacked water, toilets, and lights. Soon, the enlisted men were moved to a bivouac area in a nearby park, where they lived in pyramidal tents, and the officers were assigned quarters in hotels, the Boy's School (L'École des Garçons), and in private dwellings.

The 78 men of the Surgical Service settled in and within three days had set up an operating room to handle emergencies. They organized the hospital across three locations:

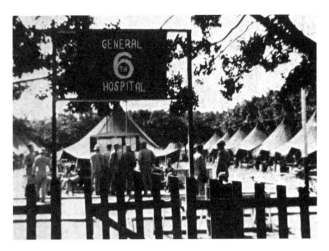

Signpost indicating location of the hospital in Casablanca, French Morocco, February 1943. The hospital's official stay in Casablanca lasted from February 27, 1943 to May 14, 1944. *The Story of the Sixth General Hospital*, ca. 1946. Massachusetts General Hospital, Archives and Special Collections.

> The largest of these included the buildings of a girls' school, the Collège de Jeunes Filles, Mers Sultan. Across the street…was a large warehouse, La Marocaine des Bois…which was to be used for ambulant sick and injured. Some three hundred yards away was a smaller school, L'École de Garçons, Mers Sultan…for installation of the Neuropsychiatric Service. Preliminary inspection of these premises indicated that they were more than adequate to contain 1,000 beds. (Faxon 1959)

Upon opening, the hospital had 78 beds, and it received its first patient on February 27. The

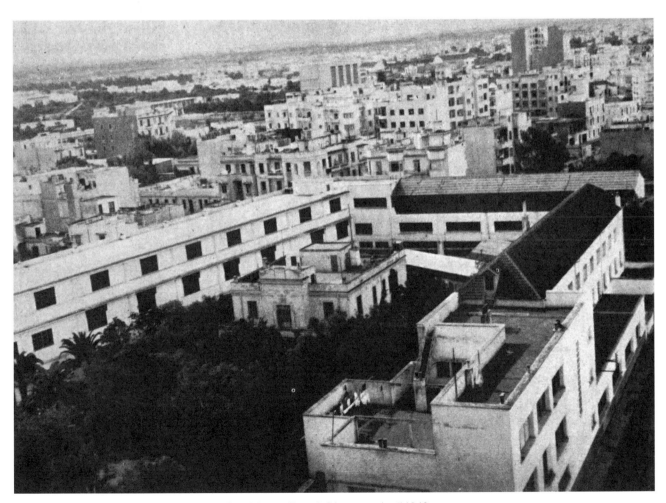

Aerial view of the 6th General Hospital in Casablanca, French Morocco, April 1943. *The Story of the Sixth General Hospital*, ca. 1946. Massachusetts General Hospital, Archives and Special Collections.

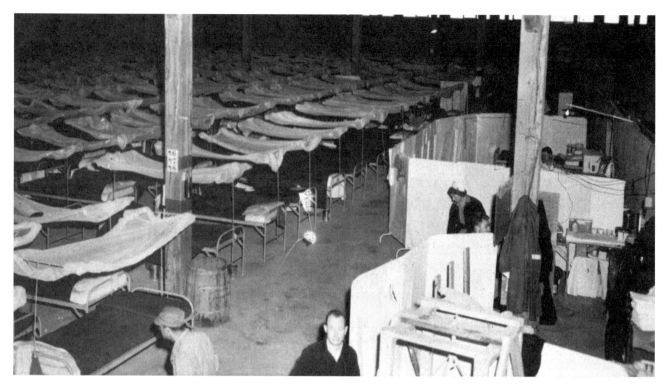

One of the wards in the 6th General Hospital. U.S. National Library of Medicine.

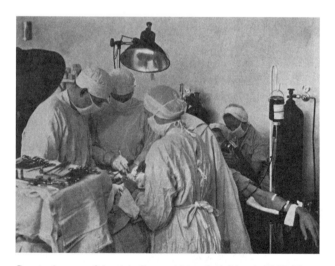

Surgical team of the 6th General Hospital, March 1943. The unit's first surgical ward opened on March 6, 1943.

The Story of the Sixth General Hospital, ca. 1946. Massachusetts General Hospital, Archives and Special Collections.

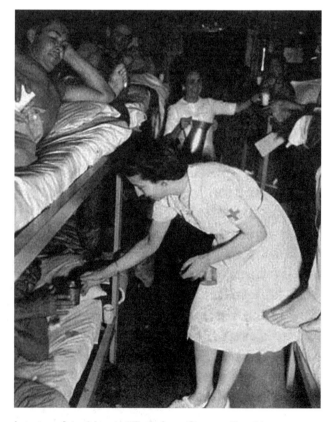

Interior of the Hospital Train from Oran to Casablanca.

The Medical Department: Medical Service in the Mediterranean and Minor Theaters by Charles M. Wiltse. Washington, DC: Center of Military History, United States Army, 1987.

surgeons there could only perform emergency surgery because the operating rooms were not yet ready for use; any elective surgeries were handled at two nearby evacuation hospitals until mid-April. (see **Box 64.3**) By mid-June, the hospital had 1,263 beds available—its maximal capacity throughout the war. Both General Patton (minor

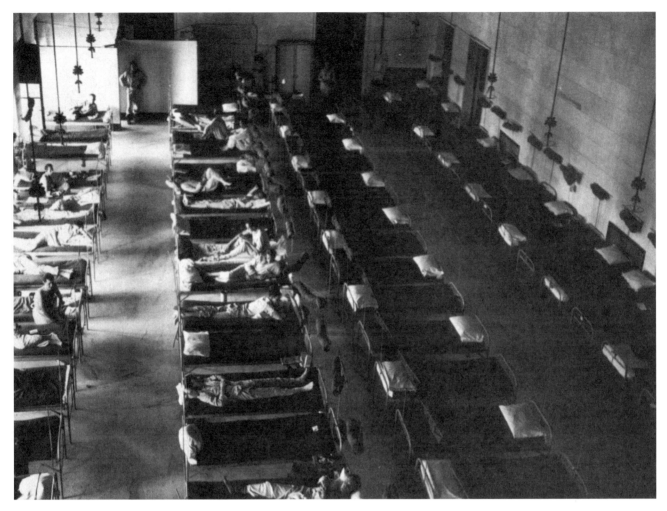

Hospital ward in Naples, 1944. U.S. National Library of Medicine.

facial procedure) and Winston Churchill (chest problem) were treated at the 6th General Hospital.

With the end of combat operations in North Africa in May 1943, planning began for the eventual relocation of the 6th General Hospital. However:

> although combat operations in North Africa came to an end in May 1943, it was twelve months later before the 6th General Hospital closed station at Casablanca, and by this time it had received and treated over 18,000 sick and injured patients. A surprisingly high percentage (over 22 per cent) of admissions were neuropsychiatric patients…from local units or evacuated from combat zone…the warehouse… now under the title of "the Moroccan Building"

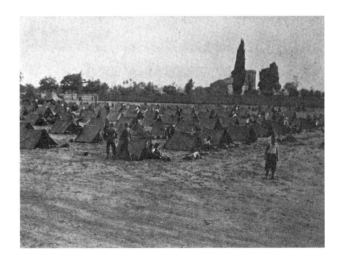

Enlisted men's bivouac and staging area in Maddaloni, Italy, June 3, 1944. Maddaloni (in the province of Casserta) contained a rail station and is located 19 miles north of Naples and 120 miles south of Rome.

The Story of the Sixth General Hospital, ca. 1946. Massachusetts General Hospital, Archives and Special Collections.

Box 64.3. The First Two Months at the 6th General Hospital

"For approximately the first two months…the 6th General Hospital received patients from local units in addition to those evacuated from the combat zone and from hospitals located in the Mediterranean Base Station…Thirty-five airplane convoys were admitted during March and April, each delivering from one to eighty patients. The first Hospital Train convoy from Oran was admitted…on March 1… from May 1943 on, the majority of evacuated patients were received by Hospital Trains. A plan for sorting patients was quickly perfected. When a train was expected, two teams of officers would drive to Fez, board the train there, and… working from each end, would meet in the middle before the train arrived at Casablanca. Each patient would have a card attached, assigning him to a specific bed in a specific ward. Three hundred patients were transferred from one train to their beds within an hour…the 6th General… [also became] a port-of debarkation hospital."

(Faxon 1959)

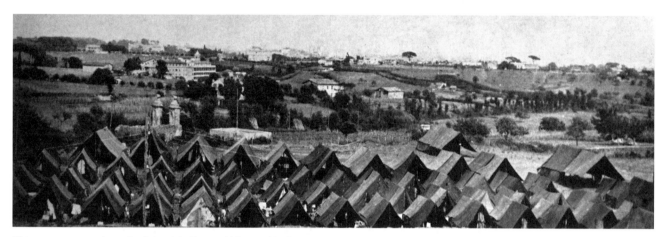

Temporary camp (tents) of the 6th General Hospital before moving into the "Insituto Buon Pastore" in Rome, Italy. *The Story of the Sixth General Hospital*, ca. 1946. Massachusetts General Hospital, Archives and Special Collections.

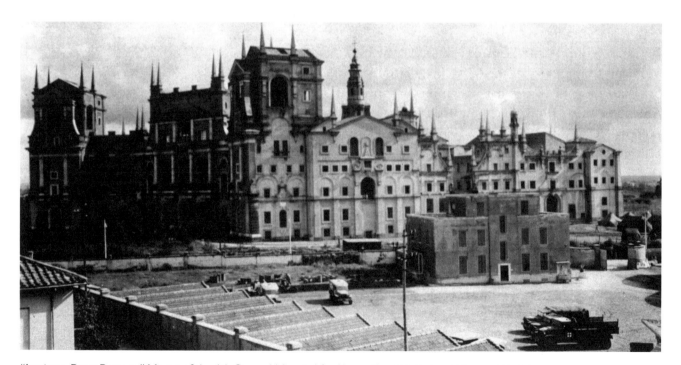

"Instituto Buon Pastore." Home of the 6th General Hospital for 11 months. U.S. National Library of Medicine.

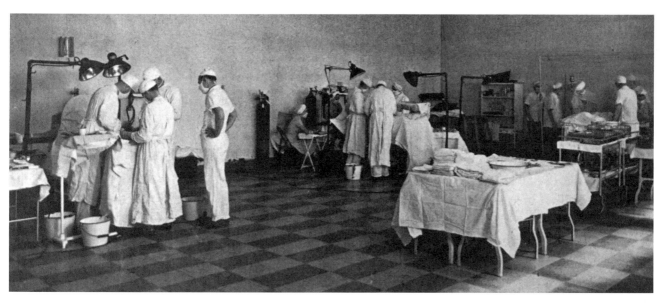

Operating room in the 6th General Hospital in Bologna, Italy. *The Story of the Sixth General Hospital*, ca. 1946. Massachusetts General Hospital, Archives and Special Collections.

contained eight wards for ambulance patients, one in the rear of the boys' school taken over by the Neuropsychiatric Service, and one in the detachment area… (Faxon 1959)

Finally, in early 1944, the unit received orders to move to the Peninsular Base Station in Italy. With assistance from nearly 60 Italian prisoners of war, who arrived in two groups on February 10 and March 27, unit personnel packed up and readied for departure. The unit closed its Casablanca station on May 24, staged in Oron, Algeria.

Peninsular Base Station and Deployment to Italy

After closing the Casablanca station, they then departed North Africa on May 31 aboard the US Army Hospital Ship *Shamrock*, arriving in Naples on June 3: "On landing at Naples…plans had been made to place practically all the officers of the Professional Division of the Hospital, as well as all nurses…on detached service at various hospitals already at station…only the…officers of Hospital Headquarters…went into camp near the town of Maddaloni, same ten kilometers from Caserta…"

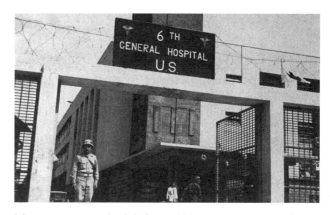

Main entrance to the 6th General Hospital in Bologna, Italy. *The Story of the Sixth General Hospital*, ca. 1946. Massachusetts General Hospital, Archives and Special Collections.

(Faxon 1959). After two weeks of personnel serving detached in various hospitals in Naples or camping, the unit once again mobilized and, from June 17 to 19, traveled to Rome. Their next hospital station was located across the Tiber River, in hilly countryside. Originally built with American funds as a home for troubled girls, the Institute of the Good Shephard (Instituto Buon Pastore) had most recently served as a hospital for the Italians and Germans, the latter having abandoned many supplies in their haste to depart. With four levels plus a basement, the hospital could house 2,423 beds.

The Peninsular Base Station (PBS), which comprised hospitals in Naples (15,000 beds), Rome (6,000 beds), and north of Rome (4,000 beds), was responsible for a total of 28,900 beds (which also included other hospitals in the Caserta region and Mostra Fairgrounds in Bagnoli). Impressively, the PBS admitted 281,823 patients in the space of less than 10 months (from October 14, 1943, to August 31, 1944), 213,624 of whom returned to duty after release from care. About half of all admissions were combat-related.

The 6th General Hospital ended operations in Rome on December 22, 1944. **Box 64.4** details those who held command afterward. Despite officially ending operations, most personnel were requested to serve at other hospitals in the PBS, and one detachment served from January 17 to May 1, 1945, on a hospital train (No. 42-A1, "Kelley's Comet"). According to Faxon:

> The name was applied facetiously by the train crew because after we received an urgent appeal to assume the operation of the train at Leghorn, we did not move from the siding for a period of six weeks. In fact, our anticipation of a busy schedule, shuttling patients from the front back to Rome and Naples never materialized, for during our whole assignment, we did not carry patients for more than thirty-six hours… (Faxon 1959)

Bologna, Italy was liberated by April 21, 1945, and command chose the city "for the third and final overseas installation of the 6th General Hospital" (Faxon 1959). The hospital opened its doors with 1,500 beds at the new location on May 9, "exactly one week after hostilities had ceased in Italy following the German surrender" at the University of Bologna (Faxon 1959). Despite the large number of beds available, "the greatest number occupied at any one time was 1412, on June 19. During the months of May, June, and July 2733 patients were admitted" (Faxon 1959) . Of these patients, most were prisoners of war. The Bologna site closed to patients on July 24, 1945, but for about a month it continued "to serve as a boarding house for troops en route to 'recreational detached service' in Switzerland" (Faxon 1959).

Orthopaedic Section of the 6th General Hospital

Major Henry H. Faxon, a general surgeon, served as chief of the orthopaedic section of the 6th General Hospital. He was supported by two ward officers, Captain Otto E. Aufranc (see chapter 40) and Captain Oscar S. Staples (see chapter 40). Dr. Aufranc, who had been an orthopaedic surgeon at the MGH, entered the war as a captain serving in the 6th General Hospital in Casablanca and later served in Naples, Rome, Leghorn, Florence, Pisa, Pistolia, and Bologna before returning to practice at MGH. He was eventually promoted to major and received the bronze star. Aufranc relates his experience at the 6th General Hospital in **Box 64.5**.

Closing of the 6th General Hospital

The 6th General Hospital officially closed on August 10, 1945. In Casablanca, the hospital had treated 18,052 patients; in Rome, 8,171 patients;

Box 64.4. Leadership After Ending Operations in Rome

> "On March 19, 1945 Colonel Goethals was relieved from assignment to the 6th General Hospital and transferred to the command of the Lovell General Hospital at Ayer, Massachusetts. Lieutenant Colonel Marshall K. Bartlett succeeded to temporary command of the 6th, he in turn being succeeded for short periods by Lieutenant Colonel Steward Hamilton and Lieutenant Colonel Edward Bland until May 5, shortly after transfer of the Hospital to its new location, when Colonel W.C.H. Prosser assumed command…."
>
> (Faxon 1959)

Box 64.5. Captain Otto E. Aufranc's Experience at the 6th General Hospital

"When I went into the war, I was given the rank of Captain and was assigned to the 6th General Hospital. I was the only trained orthopedic surgeon in the unit but because I only had the rank of Captain, I could not become the Chief of the service…Although my training made me eligible for the rank of Major or Lieutenant Colonel, I would not get the appointment at that time [having not taken his Board exam]. The chief surgeon in the Mediterranean Theater made the 6th General Hospital the training center for orthopedic surgeons. I had surgeons rotating through my section who had no training at all in orthopedics and most had only one month of preparation.

"We all had a lot of work to do in Casablanca where I was stationed for 14 months. There was a Naval hospital there without an orthopedic surgeon so every Friday night I went over and worked on their cases. One patient was a Norwegian seaman who had been afloat on a raft for three weeks. He had a fractured femur that was three inches short with a piece of the femur sticking out below the knee…[which] was sequestrating. I elected to excise the dead bone, debride the wound and pull the distal fragment down and put the spike of the proximal femur into the condyle of the femur by bending the knee and then impacting by straightening the leg. The bone healed by primary intention and the function was very satisfactory. This seaman walked out of the hospital and came over to our hospital to give me his cane on his way home.

"I was moved to Naples right after it fell to the Allies and was assigned an eighty-patient hospital tent of freshly injured soldiers the day I arrived. The next twelve hours I spent evaluating these people, getting blood into them and operating on those who needed it immediately. We were short of trained anesthetists so I rounded up supplies and enough pentothal and taught my nurse to give pentothal anesthesia…Then I moved up to Anzio and into Rome where we stayed eight months. Later on, we moved to Leghorn, Florence, Pisa, Pistolia and Bologna. By this time the war had ended.

"My work in Bologna was over very quickly now that the war was over. We had captured a German hospital with over two hundred German soldiers as patients. Most of them had orthopedic problems and they looked like the people from Dachau. They were skeletous, and their wounds had not been debrided. One boy had been injured in Libya two years before and all that had been done for him was dressing changes…He [hospital administrator] sent to a POW camp and rounded up healthy German POW's and brought them in as blood donors. I transfused every one of the patients, some getting three or four transfusions. They began to eat and thrive and we began to debride their wounds and straighten their fractures. There were over a hundred fractured femurs in that group, all in terrible shape and all with infected wounds. As our soldiers captured the German hospital in Bologna one of the German Lieutenants was shot by one of our men. The bullet broke his femur above the knee…I debrided his wound right away and closed it. I put a drain in for 24 hours and the wound healed without any problem and without an infection. Word spread very rapidly that we had taken good care of their lieutenant. Every morning when I came in he called his men to attention. There was not a word spoken while I made rounds in those days. I felt very embarrassed about this, so I told him one day to let the men be at ease while I made rounds. After that, we had a very good relationship. When they were to be shipped back to Germany, they wrote a letter of gratitude. It was a very moving experience.

"When I returned from Leghorn, I waited for about a month for transportation back to the United States. I had been booked to go to Japan, but when the bomb was dropped, this was cancelled. It was now 1946 and I was 37 years of age. I had spent three and a half years in the Army and learned a lot. I don't believe that army experience is valuable unless you've had good training before you get there…Those who had a full surgical training benefitted most from the war experience. Those whose surgical training was only the war experience developed a rather false sense of their ability. Although their trauma experiences would be helpful in civilian practice, the many finer points of surgical technique would have to be developed. The young and healthy soldier could recover from the most brutal injury, the civilian is not always so healthy.

> "During the war, I had a machine shop make me some instruments. I had a portable clothes rack...[that] I would move...over a stretcher or operating table, put a couple of pulleys on it and hang a bucket of water down at the end. If I was debriding a femur or an arm, I would put a Kirschner wire in for traction using the water as a variable weight and the portable clothes hanger as an overhead frame...
>
> "I was promoted to Major while in Rome and was made the Chief of the Orthopedic Service. Our return to the U.S. was in a Liberty ship of the World War I vintage. That old concrete hull tossed, rolled and pitched for eighteen miserable sea sick days. We landed in Hampton Roads, Virginia where we were treated to much needed clean clothes, good food, and a phone call to the family. In March 1947, I was finally mustered out of the Army with the rank of Lieutenant Colonel. One tries to forget the war: The constant fatigue, the fears, the filth, the brutality – the inhumanity of man toward man – all the things that finally resulted in what is called 'victory' – where no one wins only one side has lost more...When I returned from the war, I was welcome by family, friends and doctors. Dr. Smith-Petersen assured me that I was still in practice with him and I resumed my appointment at the M.G.H.... [but] there were few beds available in the hospital. The doctors who had not gone to war had been extremely busy and the hospitals were full. I joined the staff at the Newton-Wellesley Hospital where I operated on weekends and holidays. I was gradually able to resume full practice at the M.G.H."
>
> (quoted in Butler and Dickson 1995)

and in Bologna, 2,743 patients. Disease accounted for 55%, injuries for 17%, and 25% battle causalities. Only 0.2% (64) died. Approximately 3% of those treated were prisoners of war. The supreme allied commander of the Mediterranean theater of operations awarded an official commendation to the 6th General Hospital and to the MGH Board of Trustees in September 1945 (**Box 64.6**).

5th General Hospital

The 5th General Hospital, whose physicians (46) and nurses (44) were from the Harvard University Unit, was activated on January 3, 1942, at Fort Bragg, Fayetteville, North Carolina. Major Edwin F. Cave, Major Augustus Thorndike Jr., and Captain Thomas B. Quigley were officers in the 5th General Hospital.

Personnel and Training

Hospital personnel arrived via train at Fort Dix in Wrightstown, New Jersey, on January 10 to find subzero temperatures, snow, frozen pipes, and no heat. They spent about six weeks in intensive training, which included lectures, drills, and watching films. Exactly one month later, members of the Harvard University Unit received word that only 37 of their officers (including Dr. Thomas Quigley), along with 60 nurses and 275 enlisted personnel, would actually be assigned to the 5th General Hospital. The remaining officers, including Major Cave, Major Thorndike, and Dr. Carter Rowe, would be assigned to the 34th Infantry Division, which was in need of medical officers. This news frustrated members of the Harvard unit because the Surgeon General's Office had promised to keep the unit together while serving overseas. After all efforts to include the remaining officers in the 5th General Hospital failed, these officers were assigned to the Army Medical Center in Washington, DC, and later to the 105th General Hospital, which was also associated with Harvard.

Deployment to Belfast, Ireland

The convoy carrying their personnel embarked on February 19 from New York City. However, the bulk of the personnel did not arrive at its destination in Belfast, Northern Ireland, until May 12 due to mechanical issues with the ship they were

Box 64.6. Commendation for the 6th General Hospital and the MGH Board of Trustees

> (Reprinted from Faxon 1959, 462.)
>
> Headquarters
> Mediterranean Theater of Operations
> United States Army
> APO 512
>
> October 16, 1945.
>
> AG 201.22/034-P
> SUBJECT: Commendation
> TO: The Chairman of the Board of Trustees:
> Massachusetts General Hospital,
> Boston, Massachusetts
>
> With the inactivation of the Sixth General Hospital after long overseas service in this command, it is fitting to extend to the Board of Trustees and the Staff of the Massachusetts General Hospital my appreciation and commendation of this unit.
>
> Established at Casablanca, French Morocco, in the early phases of the North African Campaign the Sixth General Hospital formed the nucleus of medical service in the Atlantic Base Section, North African Theater of Operations. The busy period at Rome, Italy, and the subsequent establishment at Bologna, Italy, continued to demonstrate the high standards of professional work maintained by its competent officers.
>
> Credit is reflected on the officers and Nurses of the Sixth General Hospital as individuals; the unit as a whole has brought great credit to the Massachusetts General Hospital.
>
> Joseph T. McNarney,
> General, US Army
> Commanding

on, which required them to return home and await new transportation arrangements. Once rejoined, members of the 5th assumed their duties on May 21 at what had been the British 31st General Hospital in Musgrave Park.

The hospital encompassed an old three-story brick building (previously a boys' reform school), 10 Nissen huts, and various other structures. Although it had a total potential capacity of 800 beds—300 in the brick building and 500 in the huts—at the time of the 5th General Hospital's arrival, only three wards were functioning, serving 47 patients. After only two weeks of operation, the 5th had opened nine more wards and had increased capacity to treat at least 400 patients. Many other services were housed in the brick building, including operating rooms, a pharmacy, kitchens, the radiography department, a receiving office, the registrar, and a dental clinic. The facility was woefully inadequate according to American medical standards and required much cleaning, painting, and modification to meet the needs of the Hospital. They requested construction of additional patient wards and staff quarters, which was eventually begun but never completed as capacity needs soon declined.

Major Quigley served as the head of orthopaedics in the 5th General Hospital at Belfast from the time it began operations until December of 1942, as well as an unofficial consultant for all of Northern Ireland. He emphasized the importance to patient outcomes of having a well-trained team of professionals—including nurses, physiotherapists, plasterers, and occupational therapists. Without such support, patient recovery was slowed or hindered. After the war, Quigley was to describe his service in Belfast as being just as challenging as serving an internship for Harvey Cushing.

By June of 1942, they needed additional bed capacity, and the 5th General Hospital, in collaboration with the Northern Island Base Section Surgeon, agreed to open and manage a convalescent ward with a capacity of 900 beds in the newly constructed British hospital in nearby Waringfield. Patient census for two the sites together peaked at 1,500 on August 25 and then declined to 549 on December 1, at which time the remaining patients were transferred to the United States and all operations of the Hospital at this station ceased. While in Belfast, the 5th cared for a total of 7,487 patients.

Deployment to Odstock, England

The personnel of the 5th General Hospital—then consisting of 31 officers, 66 nurses, and 268 enlisted men, along with other support people—flew in batches to a hospital facility in Odstock, England, near Salisbury, on December 12. The facility, similar to the one in Belfast, consisted of a brick building and Nissen huts and had initial capacity for 600 beds, which was later expanded to 1,000 beds. It consisted of over 20 wards, including two large wards for officers, one isolation ward, and special wards. The latter were organized for providing care for tuberculosis; care for eyes, ears, nose, and throat conditions; nursing care; and physiotherapy.

The facility was in desperate need of repair. It lacked heat and electricity, had leaky roofs, and its living and bathing quarters were compromised by drainage of water. All members of the 5th were involved in repair of the facility for several months. Finally, the new facility opened for operations on March 1, 1943. It continued to operate until May 12, 1944, during which time it served 10,004 patients. Besides providing general care of the wounded, the 5th also specialized in treating soldiers with combat fatigue.

Deployment to Normandy, France

The 5th General Hospital was next deployed to Normandy, France. Personnel—which now consisted of 58 officers, 100 nurses, and 500 enlisted men—arrived at Omaha Beach on July 6th, one month following D-day. Its designated site still being occupied by the Germans, the 5th instead chose a field near Carentan and camped for three weeks with the 7th Field Hospital. It began operations on July 31, without lights or electricity. The low-lying area flooded easily and swarmed with mosquitoes. Its maximum capacity was 1,500 beds, and by August 15, its census was up to 1,400. Because it was located near the front, the 5th cared for many soldiers experiencing combat

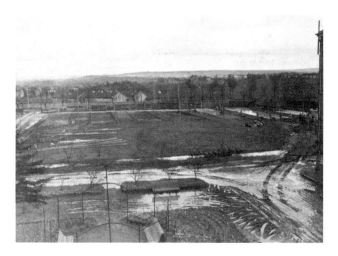

Aerial view of the construction of the 5th General Hospital. U.S. National Library of Medicine.

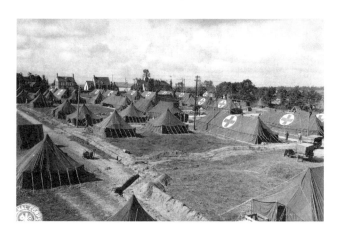

Partial view of the 5th General Hospital in the vicinity of Carentan; east of Saint-Hilaire-Petitville, in northwest Normandy, France. August 1944. Conseil Régional de Basse-Normandie/National Archives and Records Administration.

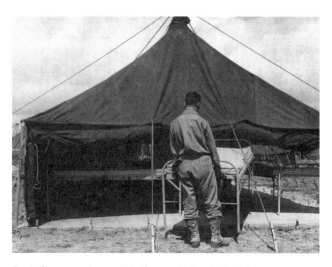

Beds for a ward tent, 5th General Hospital, 1944. U.S. National Library of Medicine.

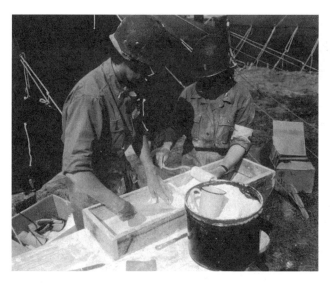
Nurses preparing plaster bandages at the 5th General Hospital. U.S. National Library of Medicine.

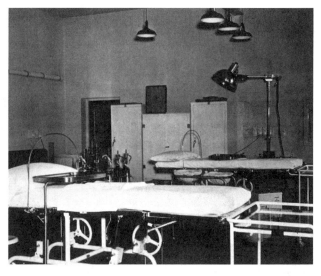
Operating room in the 5th General Hospital. U.S. National Library of Medicine.

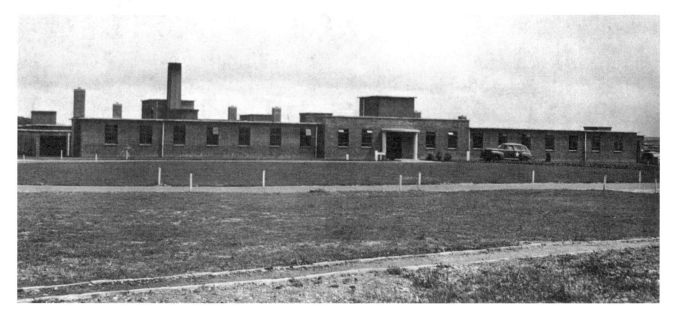
General view of the 5th General Hospital. U.S. National Library of Medicine.

fatigue and those suspected of inflicting wounds on themselves, along with lightly wounded soldiers whom the army wanted to return to duty in short order, if possible. The 5th cared for a total of 4,238 patients that August.

Closing of the 5th General Hospital

The 5th General Hospital officially closed on May 12, 1944. In addition to being an area station hospital, the 5th General Hospital was the first hospital to treat soldiers with combat exhaustion or self-inflicted wounds, and return them to duty in one to two weeks. All efforts were made to preserve manpower on the continent.

105th General Hospital

After some of the officers in the 5th General Hospital were separated and left behind in the US,

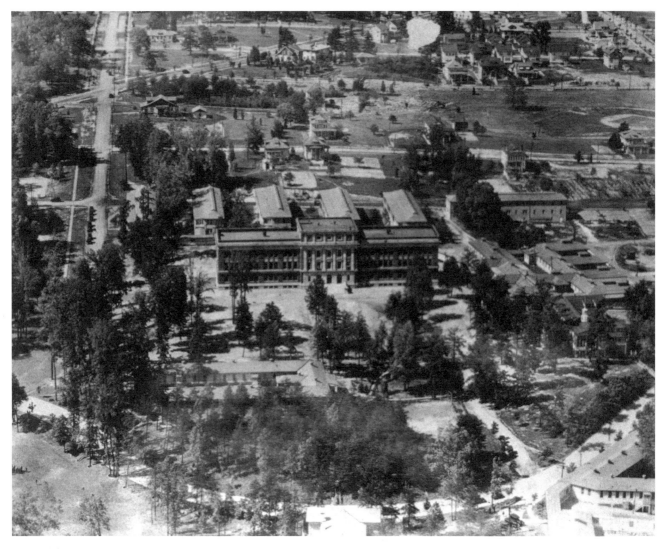
Aerial view of US Army Walter Reed General Hospital. U.S. National Library of Medicine.

while the others were deployed to Ireland (thus splitting the Harvard/MGH unit); those left behind were activated in the 105th General Hospital in Washington, DC on April 20, 1942, at Walter Reed Hospital. It became one of Harvard University's two reserve hospitals. The hospital unit, after one week at Fort Mason, Washington, was transported by train to San Francisco (the port of embarkation). After 10 days, they sailed on the USS *West Point*. The ship was a large troop transport that had been converted from a luxury liner. In addition to the 105th, it carried personnel from the 42nd General Hospital (composed of the unit from the University of Maryland), the 118th General Hospital (composed of half of the unit from the Johns Hopkins Hospital), and several station hospitals, as well as many enlisted personnel.

US Military Hospitals in Australia

Throughout the war in the Pacific, the US military had a large presence in Australia, particularly in Brisbane, a city of 350,000, where the US had about 9,000 hospital beds. The first military hospital that the US set up in Queensland was the 153rd Station Hospital. It was located at the Gatton Agricultural College, which was 90 km away from Brisbane in order to be a safe distance from any conflicts with the Japanese there. However, it operated at this location for only a few months before being moved to the Gold Coast (Southport School) and then to New Guinea.

Deployment to Gatton, Australia

The ship with personnel from the 105th General Hospital sailed uninterrupted and without convoy to Australia. The ocean journey was 7,000 miles. "The ship had passed slowly under the [Golden] Gate – a landmark which was later to become a symbol for all homesick service men in the Pacific as the Statue of Liberty was for those in the Atlantic" (Millard 1944). After arriving in Melbourne in late May or June, 1942, the unit was transported by train 1,300 miles north to Gatton, Australia, which was about 90 km west of Brisbane (on the Gold Coast). On July 11, the 105th General Hospital took over operation from the 153rd Station Hospital, and within two weeks they had the hospital running smoothly. The facility was located at the Agricultural College of Gatton on 84 acres of land. Patients were quartered in tents in the beginning but later were moved to huts constructed by the Australian Civil Constitution Corps (CCC).

Most of the year of 1942 was spent in building new wards, huts, barracks, roads, tents and fortifications (mainly by the CCC); and subsequently "the specialist medical staff from the prestigious Harvard University felt underutilized, out of the way and forgotten" during these early months in Gatton (Cave 1944). The 4th and 5th Portable Hospitals, however, organized just two months after the personnel from the 105th General Hospital arrived in Gatton. These portable hospitals included six surgical and two medical officers from the 105th (including Jonathan Cohen; see chapter 23), and "the excellent and creditable performance of each Portable Hospital during the Burma campaign is well known" (Harrison 1944).

Late in 1942, the 105th General Hospital cared for many injured soldiers in the battle of Buna-Gona. The following year was very busy because

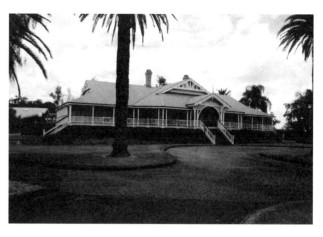

Gatton Agricultural College Campus of the University of Queensland; just east of Gatton, Australia. Queensland Heritage Register, © The State of Queensland 2021.

there were steep casualties from the New Guinea campaigns. Throughout 1942 and into 1943, the surgeons, nurses, and staff of the 105th worked diligently to keep up with the ever-increasing patient population. By mid-1943, this influx had stabilized, even in light of the mass patient evacuations and admissions that sometimes happened. By summer of 1943 the 105th had treated 10,000 patients, and the staff had gained experience and confidence. Dr. Carter Rowe narrates his experience in **Box 64.7**.

Earlier that year (mid-February), Lt. Col. Augustus Thorndike, the first chief of surgery, became commanding officer of the 105th. The staff "welcomed Colonel Thorndike as the new Commanding Officer, particularly in view of [his] excellent job in organizing the hospital originally" (Post Record Staff 1944). Major Edwin F. Cave, then chief of the orthopaedic service, replaced him, becoming chief of the surgical service. Dr. Carter R. Rowe, a member of the orthopaedic staff, was then promoted to chief of the section of orthopaedic surgery, which was the largest section in the 105th. Captains Lester B. K. Yee, Eric R. Sanderson, John J. Kneisel, Rogert C. Nydegger, Felix Schwartz, and Littleton L. McCharen also served on the orthopaedic staff. According to Harrison (1944): "The evaluation and treatment

Box 64.7. Dr. Carter Rowe: First Year at the 105th General Hospital

> "In Australia, for the first year, we were unable to send seriously wounded personnel back to the United States as we had no ships and practically no air transportation. This lack necessitated large rehabilitation programs on site, conditioning patients to return to their units, or to some type of limited duty. The majority were returned to their original stations. It was during this period, in addition to combat injuries, Dr. Cave and I were faced with a large number of recurrent dislocations of the shoulder. The technique we had used in the past was the Nicola procedure, which promptly proved inadequate for combat duty. Our Australian colleagues recommended the Bankart procedure which was new to us. We quickly reviewed the Bankart technique, made necessary additions, and designed our instruments to carry this out with the help of an air corps technician (the cutting forceps, curved spike and head retractor). With our new instruments, the avulsed capsule could be securely reattached and double-breasted along the glenoid rim with sufficient strength to tolerate combat duty. With its success, we continued to use the Bankart procedure after the war in professional and collegiate contact sports."
>
> (Rowe 1996)

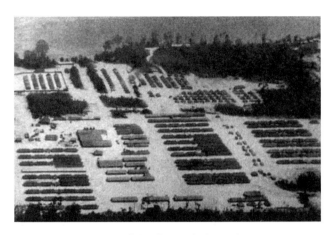

Completed hospital—105th General Hospital.
Lest We Forget: Orthopaedics at the Massachusetts General Hospital, 1900–1995 by Carter R. Rowe. Dublin, New Hampshire: William L. Bauhan, 1996. Courtesy of Bauhan Publishing.

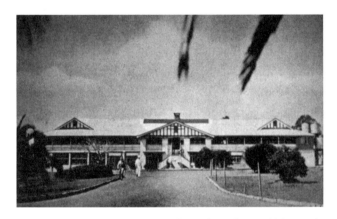

Sheldon Hall Surgical Building of the 105th General Hospital.
Lest We Forget: Orthopaedics at the Massachusetts General Hospital, 1900–1995 by Carter R. Rowe. Dublin, New Hampshire: William L. Bauhan, 1996. Courtesy of Bauhan Publishing.

of back pain, abnormalities of the feet, arthritis, and psychoneurosis giving rise to symptoms of an orthopedic nature are some of the more common problems of the Orthopedic Section." He also noted the most common surgical procedures included: "Arthrotimies [*sic*] of the knee joint, open reduction and internal fixation of fractures of the extremities, bone grafts for malunion and nonunion and repair of recurrent dislocation of the shoulder" (Harrison 1944).

From 1943 to 1944, before the Philippines was retaken, the US military had over 9,000 hospital beds in Brisbane: 1,200 at the 105th General Hospital at Gatton, 3,000 at the 42nd General Hospital at Holland Park, 2,600 beds at the 109th Naval Fleet Hospital at Camp Hill, and the remainder at two evacuation hospitals, two surgical hospitals, and eight portable surgical hospitals. Colonel Thorndike had been Commander of the hospital for 11 months when he was called back to the United States, and "he had every reason to be proud of what had been accomplished under his command" (Cave 1944). At the 105th General Hospital, "[one] of the most important innovations [by Colonel Thorndike] was the establishment of the Patients' Reconditioning Program… Included in the schedule were graded exercises, games, drill, indoctrination and entertainment"

(Quoted in Post Record Staff 1944). At the time, "the 105th was performing its mission in World War II of salvaging great masses of diseased and damaged humanity by cure and rehabilitation" (Quoted in Post Record Staff 1944). He returned to the US to serve in the surgeon general's office as a consultant/leader of the rehabilitation or reconditioning program for injured soldiers (see Thorndike, chapter 12). Lt. Col. Cave replaced Colonel Thorndike as Commanding Officer.

Deployment to Biak Island

By 1944 the Allied offensive "pierced the outer perimeter of Japanese defenses at multiple points, [and] the 105th received patients from far distant battlefronts…New Britain, the Admiralty Islands, the north shore of New Guinea and the Philippines" (Quoted in Post Record Staff 1944). By that spring, the 105th General Hospital moved to Biak Island from Australia. Their mission here was to treat soldiers wounded during combat in the Philippines, Leyte, and various other islands in the Pacific Southwest where Allied troops were engaged in "island-hopping" in pursuit of the enemy (**Box 64.8**).

The hospital treated about 19,000 patients in two years. In the Pacific southwest theatre, malaria was often a greater threat than combat, as it removed about 65% of US and Australian soldiers from active duty. Dysentery, scrub typhus, and dengue fever were responsible for incapacitating an additional 25% of soldiers, meaning that a combined 90% were removed from active duty due to non–combat-related illness, although the majority returned to service. These rates are in stark contrast to combat casualties, which killed 10% of all troops and wounded another 20%. Quinine was often unavailable; sulfanilamide powder was used throughout the war and penicillin was introduced during the latter part of the war.

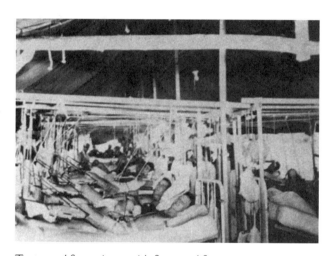

Tent ward for patients with fractured femurs.
Lest We Forget: Orthopaedics at the Massachusetts General Hospital, 1900–1995 by Carter R. Rowe. Dublin, New Hampshire: William L. Bauhan, 1996. Courtesy of Bauhan Publishing.

Box 64.8. Dr. Carter Rowe's Experience at Biak Island

> "Biak was a coral island on which was little standing water and consequently few mosquitoes and malaria. When we were reassigned to the Philippine Islands, however, we encountered new diseases such as bush typhus (Tsutsuga-mushi fever), liver flukes, filariasis, and malignant malaria. After one year, we had begun preparation to move to the northern tip of Luzon for the projected invasion of Japan when fortunately, V-J Day, August 19, 1945, ended World War II, and our three and a half years of overseas combat duty."
>
> (Rowe 1996)

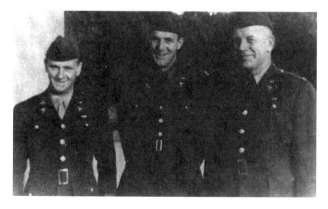

Major Edwin Cave, Captain Carter Rowe and Colonel Augustus Thorndike Jr. shortly after landing in Queensland, Australia, 1952.
Lest We Forget: Orthopaedics at the Massachusetts General Hospital, 1900–1995 by Carter R. Rowe. Dublin, New Hampshire: William L. Bauhan, 1996. Courtesy of Bauhan Publishing.

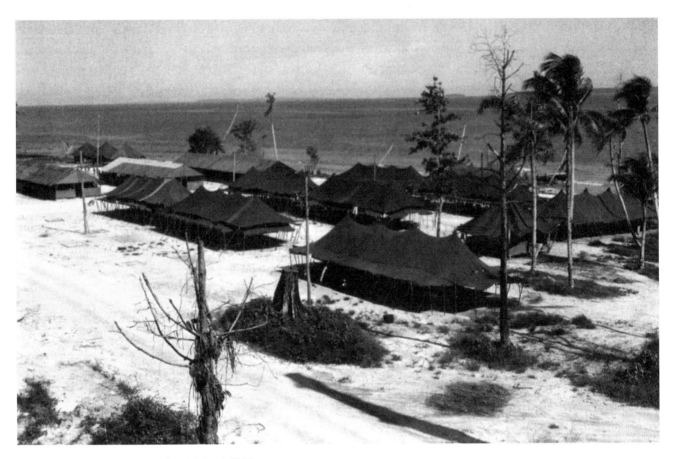

Hospital tents on the beach of Biak Island, 1945. U.S. National Library of Medicine.

Lucy Diggs, a second lieutenant in the US Army Nurse Corps, wrote two songs that exemplified the camaraderie of the 105th General Hospital. In the "The Harvard Hero," a child questions their father, a medical officer, about his service in the war. The child learns of the bravery of those serving in the army medical corps and of their mission—to keep injured soldiers alive in the face of overwhelming odds—an objective as important to the war effort as sinking enemy submarines or protecting the US at home through the US Coast Guard and the Naval Reserves. The second song, "The Chant of the 105th," sung to the tune of "The Man on the Flying Trapeze," celebrates the beginnings of the 105th and the unit's service in Gatton—including their tolerance of both bugs and heat during the Australian summer and unappetizing field rations. Despite this celebration, however, the point of the song is clear: the unit shares a longing for home after years overseas. Both of these songs were sung at the 1944 Officers and Nurses Dinner.

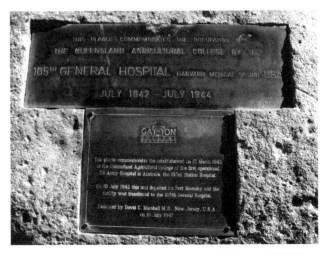

Plaque commemorating the 105th General Hospital (HMS), July 1942–July 1944. Queensland War Memorials Register, © The State of Queensland 2021.

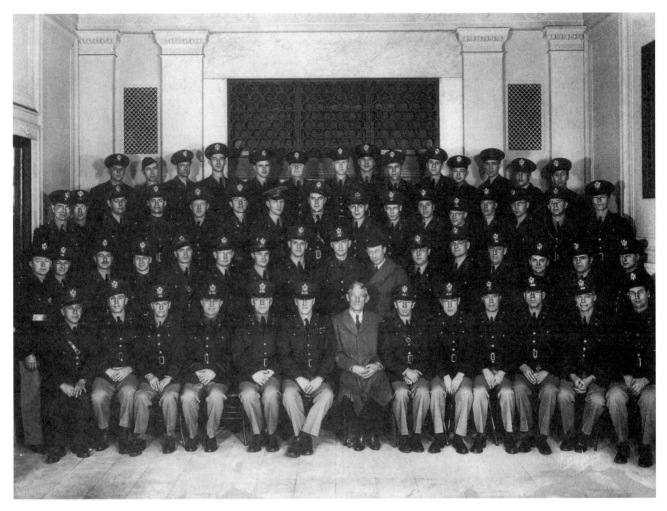

Medical Staff (Harvard Unit) of the 5th General Hospital, 1942.
The Teaching Hospital: Brigham and Women's Hospital and the Evolution of Academic Medicine by Peter V. Tishler, Christine Wenc, and Joseph Loscalzo. McGraw-Hill Education, 2014. Brigham and Women's Hospital Archives.

Closing of the 105th General Hospital

The 105th General Hospital closed on November 21, 1945. Over the course of the war, "the contribution of the Massachusetts General Hospital to the armed forces [in the European, Mediterranean and Pacific-Asian Theatres] was 40 per cent of its Active Staff, 48 per cent of its graduates, 33 per cent of the nursing staff, and 11 per cent of its nonprofessional employees" (Faxon 1959). Over a five-year period, only seven of the military staff members at MGH died while serving. As one of the largest subspecialties relied upon during the fight, World War II firmly established orthopaedics as an accepted and respected surgical specialty.

Index

Illustrations are indicated by page numbers in *italics*. Page numbers followed by *t* and *b* indicate tables and boxes.

Page numbers are formatted as: Volume: page

A

AAOS. *See* American Academy of Orthopaedic Surgeons (AAOS)
AAOS Council on Education, 4: 173
AAOS Diversity Committee, 1: 239
AAST. *See* American Association for the Surgery of Trauma (AAST)
Abbott, Edward Gilbert, 1: 59; 2: 87–88
Abbott, Josephine Dormitzer, 2: 97
Abbott, LeRoy C., 1: 189, 197; 2: 77, 110, 160, 183; 3: 180, 229; 4: 473
Abbott Frame, 4: 232, *232*
"Abscesses of Hip Disease, The" (Lovett and Goldthwait), 2: *52*
abdominal surgery, 1: 81; 3: 18, 108
Abe, Isso, 2: 279
Abraham, John, 4: 190*b*
absorbable animal membrane research, 3: 166, *166*, 167, *171*
Academy of Medicine, 4: 324
Accreditation Council for Graduate Medical Education (ACGME), 1: 200, 213, 217, 237–239
acetabular dysplasia, 2: 389, *389*, 390
"Acetone" (Sever), 2: 84
ACGME. *See* Accreditation Council for Graduate Medical Education (ACGME)
Achilles tendon
 club foot and, 2: 25, 29, 145
 gastrocnemius paralysis and, 2: 150
 injury in, 3: 272
 sliding procedure and, 2: *198*
 subcutaneous release of, 2: 29, 36
 tenotomy, 1: 100–101, 106; 2: 25
achillobursitis, 2: 89
Ackerman, Gary, 1: 217*b*
acromioclavicular joint dislocation, 1: 268, 277
acromioplasty, 3: 191, 239
ACS Committee on Fractures, 3: 64; 4: 324
activating transcription factor-2 (ATF-2), 2: 330
acute ligament injuries, 1: 277
acute thigh compartment syndrome, 3: 417, *417*, 418
Adams, Frances Kidder, 3: 228
Adams, Helen Foster, 3: 228, 236
Adams, Herbert D., 3: 275
Adams, John, 1: 8–10, 14, 18
Adams, John D.
 back pain treatment, 4: 358
 Boston Dispensary and, 4: 358–359
 education and training, 4: 357–358
 HMS appointment, 4: 360
 Massachusetts Regional Fracture Committcc, 3: 64
 Mt. Sinai Hospital and, 4: 204
 New England Medical Center and, 4: 360
 occupational therapy and, 4: 358–359
 patellar turndown procedure, 4: 373–374
 private medical practice, 4: 358
 professional memberships, 4: 360
 publications and research, 4: 359, *359*
 scaphoid fracture treatment, 4: 359–360
 Tufts Medical School appointment, 4: 360
Adams, John Quincy, 1: 10
Adams, M., 3: 133
Adams, Nancy, 3: 236
Adams, Samuel, 3: 236
Adams, Samuel (1722–1803), 1: 13, 15–17
Adams, Zabdiel B. (1875–1940), 3: *228*
 AOA Commission on Congenital Dislocation of the Hip and, 3: 232, *232*, 233–234
 Base Hospital No. 6 and, 4: 433–434
 Boston Children's Hospital and, 2: 247; 3: 228
 Boston City Hospital and, 4: 305*b*
 CDH treatment, 3: 233–235
 death of, 3: 236
 early life, 3: 228
 education and training, 3: 228
 fracture management and, 3: 61
 HMS appointment, 3: 232
 Lakeville State Sanatorium and, 3: 235
 marriage and family, 3: 228, 236
 Medical Reserve Corps and, 3: 232
 memberships and, 3: 235–236
 as MGH house officer, 1: 189
 as MGH orthopaedic surgeon, 3: 228, 235, 266, 268
 military surgeon training and, 2: 42
 New England Deaconess Hospital and, 4: 225

495

publications and research,
3: 228–232
scoliosis treatment and, 2: 84,
86; 3: 229–232
World War I and, 3: 232; 4: 412
Adams, Zabdiel B. (father), 3: 228
Adam's machine, 2: 86
Affiliated Hospitals Center, Inc.,
4: 42, 113–114, 118, 120, 127,
132
Agel, Julie, 1: 287
Agency for Healthcare Research and
Quality, 2: 371
Aitken, Alexander P. (1904–1993),
4: *350*
BCH Bone and Joint Service,
4: 353, 356, 380*b*
Boston City Hospital and, 4: 350
Boston University Medical School
appointment, 4: 350
Chelsea Memorial Hospital and,
4: 350
classification of epiphyseal fractures, 4: 355–356
death of, 4: 356
education and training, 4: 350
epiphyseal injury treatment,
4: 350–352, 355–356
fracture of the proximal tibial epiphyseal cartilage case,
4: 355
fracture research and, 4: 354
hospital appointments, 4: 356
legacy of, 4: 356
Liberty Mutual Insurance Rehabilitation Clinic and, 4: 352–353, 356
Massachusetts Regional Fracture
Committee, 3: 64
Monson State Hospital and,
4: 350
private medical practice, 4: 356
professional memberships,
4: 352, 356
publications and research,
4: 350–355
rehabilitation of injured workers
and, 4: 350, 352–354
ruptured intervertebral disc treatment, 4: 350, 352–353
Tufts Medical School appointment, 4: 353
workers' compensation issues,
4: 353–354
Aitken, H. F., 1: *89*
Akbarnia, Behrooz, 2: 359, 361
Akeson, Wayne, 3: 382
Akins, Carlton M., 1: 217*b*
Alais, J., 1: *34*

Alan Gerry Clinical Professor of
Orthopaedic Surgery, 3: 224, 464*b*
Albee, F. H., 3: 157; 4: 406
Albert, E., 3: 95
Albert, Todd J., 4: 266*b*
Albert Einstein College of Medicine,
2: 408
Alden, Eliza, 2: 231
Alden, Louise, 2: 241
Alder Hey Hospital (Liverpool),
4: 401
Aldrich, Marion, 3: 164
Allen, Arthur W., 3: 60*b*, 315;
4: 208
Allen, John Michael, 2: 438
Allen, L., 3: 133
Allen Street House (MGH),
3: 17–18
Allgemeines Krankenhaus, 1: 81
Allgöwer, Martin, 2: 406
Allied Relief Fund, 4: 363
Allison, Addie Shultz, 3: 163
Allison, James, 3: 163
Allison, Marion Aldrich, 3: 164
Allison, Nathaniel (1876–1932),
3: *163, 174*; 4: *417*
absorbable animal membrane
research, 3: 166, *166*, 167, *171*
adult orthopaedics and, 2: 157
AEF splint board, 4: 416–417
American Ambulance Hospital
and, 2: 119
animal research and, 3: 165–167,
170, *171*
AOA Committee on war preparation, 2: 124
AOA preparedness committee,
4: 394
as AOA president, 3: 172
army manual of splints and appliances, 2: 126
arthroplasty research,
3: 165–166
as BCH house officer, 3: 163
on bone atrophy, 3: 170
Chicago University orthopaedics
department, 3: 175
death of, 3: 176
Department for Military Orthopedics and, 4: 405–406
Diagnosis in Joint Disease,
3: 175, 289, *290*
early life, 3: 163
education and training, 3: 163
*Fundamentals of Orthopaedic Surgery in General Medicine and
Surgery*, 2: 135–136
on hip dislocations, 3: 164, 175
HMS appointment, 3: 173

knee derangement treatment,
3: 165
legacy of, 3: 176–177
on Legg-Calvé-Perthes disease,
3: 165–166
low-back pain research, 3: 175
marriage and, 3: 164
memberships and, 3: 176, 176*b*
MGH Fracture Clinic and,
3: 60*b*, 314, 371
MGH house officers and, 1: 189
as MGH orthopaedics chief,
1: 152; 2: 133–134; 3: 11*b*,
173–174, 227
military orthopaedics and, 2: 128
New England Peabody Home for
Crippled Children and, 2: 270;
3: 174
orthopaedic research and,
3: 164–167, 170, 174–175
on orthopaedics education,
2: 134; 3: 170–173
private medical practice, 2: 146
"Progress in Orthopaedic Surgery" series, 2: 297
publications and research,
4: 102, 225–226, 372
on sacroiliac joint fusion, 3: 185
on splints for Army, 3: 167–168,
168, 169, 169*b*
synovial fluid research, 3: 174,
174, 175
Walter Reed General Hospital
and, 4: 452
Washington University orthopaedic department and, 3: 163–165, 170; 4: 419
World War I and, 3: 157,
166–169; 4: 417
Allison, Nathaniel (grandfather),
3: 163
allografts
bone banks for, 3: 386, 396,
433, 440–441
distal femoral osteonecrosis and,
3: 433
femoral heads and, 3: 442
infection and freeze-dried,
3: 440
irradiation and, 3: 435
knee fusion with, 3: 435
long-term study of, 3: 433, 435
malignant bone tumors and,
3: 389
osteoarticular, 3: 442
osteosarcomas and, 3: 433
transmission of disease through,
3: 442–443, *443*
Alman, B. A., 2: 212
Alqueza, Arnold, 4: 190*b*

Index

Alqueza, Arnold B., 3: 463*b*
Altman, Greg, 4: 285–286
Altschule, Mark D., 1: 171, 239
AMA Committee on the Medical Aspects of Sports, 1: 274, 280
AMA Council on Medical Education and Hospitals, 1: 146, 196–197, 199, 211
Amadio, Peter C., 3: 431
Ambulatory Care Center (ACC) (MGH), 3: 396
Ambulatory Care Unit (ACU) (MGH), 3: 399
American Academy for Cerebral Palsy, 2: 176, 196–198
American Academy of Arts and Sciences, 1: 29, 61
American Academy of Orthopaedic Surgeons (AAOS), 1: xxv, 213; 2: 176, 201–203; 3: 90; 4: 337
American Ambulance Field Service, 2: 118
American Ambulance Hospital (Neuilly, France), 2: *119*; 4: *386*
   Harvard Unit and, 2: 118–120; 3: 166, 180, *180*; 4: 386, *387*, 389*b*, 391
   Osgood and, 2: 117–120; 4: 386, 391–393
   Smith-Petersen and, 3: 180
American Appreciation, An (Wilson), 3: 369
American Association for Labor Legislation, 4: 325–326
American Association for the Surgery of Trauma (AAST), 3: 65, 315, *315*; 4: *319*, 349
American Association of Medical Colleges (AAMC), 1: 168–169
American Association of Tissue Banks, 3: 386, 442–443, *443*
American Board of Orthopaedic Surgery (ABOS), 1: xxv, 197–200, 211, 213, 215–216, 231; 2: 317; 4: 173, 377–379
American British Canadian (ABC) Traveling Fellow, 3: 218
American College of Rheumatology, 4: 57–58
American College of Sports Medicine, 2: *387*
American College of Surgeons (ACS), 2: 158; 3: 112, *112*, 113*b*, 131, 310, 367; 4: 102, 324, 354
American College of Surgeons Board of Regents, 3: 62–63
American Expeditionary Forces (AEF)
   base hospitals for BEF, 4: 420, 426
   Division of Orthopedic Surgery, 4: 410*b*, 417, 439, 453–454
   Goldthwait and, 4: 416
   Johns Hopkins Hospital Unit and, 2: 221
   medical care in, 4: 417
   orthopaedic treatment and, 4: 409, 410*b*
   Osgood and, 2: 124, 126, 128; 4: 417, 421*b*
   physician deaths in, 4: 425
   Shortell and, 4: 338
   splint board and, 4: 416
   standardization of splints and dressings for, 2: 124; 3: 168
   Wilson and, 3: 370
American Field Service Ambulance, 4: 386, *386*, 387, *387*, 388
American Hospital Association, 1: 211
American Jewish Committee, 4: 203
American Journal of Orthopedic Surgery, 4: 226
American Medical Association (AMA), 1: xxv, 69, 189–191, 211, 213; 2: 42, 124; 3: 35, 131
American Mutual Liability Insurance Company, 3: 314, 316
American Orthopaedic Association (AOA), 4: 463
   Barr and, 1: 158
   Bradford and, 2: 24–26, 34, 43
   Buckminster Brown and, 1: 111
   Committee of Undergraduate Training, 2: 183
   founding of, 1: 114; 2: 48, *48*, 49
   graduate education study committee, 1: 196–197
   investigation of fusion on tubercular spines, 3: 157–158
   Lovett and, 2: 51
   military surgeon training and, 2: 65
   orthopaedic surgery terminology, 1: xxiv, xxv
   orthopaedics residencies survey, 2: 160–161
   Osgood and, 1: xxii; 2: 137
   Phelps and, 1: 193
   preparedness committee, 4: 394
   scoliosis treatment committee, 2: 87–88
   World War I and, 2: 64, 124
American Orthopaedic Foot and Ankle Society (AOFAS), 2: 316
American Orthopaedic Foot Society (AOFS), 2: 316–317; 3: 295, 298
American Orthopaedic Society of Sports Medicine (AOSSM), 1: 286, 289; 2: 163, 375; 3: 360
"American Orthopedic Surgery" (Bick), 1: 114
American Pediatric Society, 2: 15
American Public Health Association, 4: 439
American Radium Society, 1: 275–276
American Rheumatism Association, 2: 137; 4: 41*b*, 57–58, 63, 169
American Shoulder and Elbow Surgeons (ASES), 2: 380; 3: 415, *415*
American Society for Surgery of the Hand (ASSH), 2: 251; 3: 316, 428, *428*, 429, *430*; 4: 168, 186
American Society for Testing and Materials (ATSM), 3: 210
American Society of Hand Therapists, 4: 168
American Surgical Association, 1: 87; 2: 43; 3: 58
American Surgical Materials Association, 3: 210
American Whigs, 1: 11
AmeriCares, 3: 416
Ames Test, 4: 171
Ammer, Christine, 2: 277
amputations
   blood perfusion in, 3: 287
   economic importance and, 4: 419
   ether and, 1: 61
   fractures and, 1: 50, 54
   geriatric patients and, 3: 330
   Gritti-Stokes, 3: 374
   guillotine, 4: *469*
   John Collins Warren and, 1: 52–53, 61
   kineplastic forearm, 4: 360
   kit for, 1: *60*
   length and, 3: 374
   malpractice suits and, 1: 50
   military wounds and, 1: 23; 4: 418–419
   mortality rates, 1: 65, 74, 84
   osteosarcoma and, 3: 391
   research in, 3: 373, *373*
   results of, 3: 374*t*
   sepsis and, 3: 373
   shoulder, 1: 23
   skin traction and, 4: *419*
   suction socket prosthesis and, 1: 273
   temporary prostheses and, 3: 374
   transmetatarsal, 4: 276
   trauma and, 3: 373
   tuberculosis and, 3: 374

without anesthesia, 1: 10, 36, 65
wounded soldiers and,
4: 446–447
Amputees and Their Prostheses (Pierce and Mital), 3: 320
AMTI, 3.224
Amuralt, Tom, 3: 463
Anatomical and Surgical Treatment of Hernia (Cooper), 1: 36
Anatomy Act, 1: 52
Anatomy of the Breast (Cooper), 1: 36
Anatomy of the Thymus Gland (Cooper), 1: 36
Anderson, Gunnar B. J., 4: 266*b*
Anderson, Margaret, 2: 170, 191–194, 264, 304, 350
Anderson, Megan E., 4: 287
Andrews, H. V., 3: 133
Andry, Nicolas, 1: xxi, xxii, xxiii, xxiv; 3: 90; 4: 233
anesthesia
  acetonuria associated with death after, 3: 305
  bubble bottle method, 4: 323
  charting in, 3: 95, 96
  chloroform as, 1: 62–63, 82
  Cotton-Boothby apparatus, 4: 320, 323
  ether as, 1: 55–58, 60–62, 63, 64–65, 82
  hypnosis and, 1: 56, 65
  nitrous oxide as, 1: 56–59, 63
  orthopaedic surgery and, 2: 15
  surgery before, 1: 6, 10, 23, 36, 74
  use at Boston Orthopedic Institution, 1: 107, 118
  use at Massachusetts General Hospital (MGH), 1: 57–62, 118
anesthesiology, 1: 61
ankle valgus, 2: 212
ankles
  arthrodesis and, 3: 330
  astragalectomy and, 2: 93–94
  athletes and, 3: 348
  central-graft operation, 3: 368
  fractures, 4: 313–315, 315, 316
  gait analysis and, 2: 406–407
  instability and Pott's fracture, 4: 317, 318
  lubrication and, 3: 324
  sports injuries and, 1: 281
  stabilization of, 2: 148
  tendon transfers and, 2: 148
  tuberculosis and, 1: 73
  weakness and, 2: 150
ankylosis, 4: 64
Anna Jacques Hospital, 2: 269, 272

Annual Bibliography of Orthopaedic Surgery, 3: 261
anterior cruciate ligament (ACL)
  direct repair of, 2: 91
  growth plate disturbances, 2: 379
  intra-articular healing of, 2: 439
  intra-/extra-articular reconstruction, 3: 448
  outpatient arthroscopic reconstructions, 4: 255
  reconstruction of, 2: 91, 378–379, 386
  skeletally immature patients and, 2: 378–379
  Tegner Activity Scale and, 2: 380
  young athletes and, 2: 385, 385, 386
Anthology Club, 1: 29
antisepsis
  acceptance in the U.S., 1: 118
  carbolic acid treatment, 1: 82–83
  Coll Warren promotion of, 1: 85
  discovery of, 1: 55
  Lister and, 1: 55, 81, 84; 3: 45
  orthopaedic surgery and, 2: 15
  prevention of infection and, 1: 84–85
  surgeon resistance to, 1: 85
  trench warfare and, 4: 385
Antiseptic surgery (Cheyne), 1: 83
AO Foundation, 3: 409, 409
AOA. *See* American Orthopaedic Association (AOA)
apothecary, 1: 184
Appleton, Paul, 3: 410; 4: 288
Arbuckle, Robert H., 4: 163, 193
Archibald, Edward W., 3: 26, 50
Archives of Surgery (Jackson), 3: 35
Arlington Mills, 2: 267
Armed Forces Institute of Pathology, 4: 126
arms
  Bankart procedure and, 3: 359–360
  Boston Arm, 2: 326
  carpal tunnel syndrome, 2: 375
  compartment syndrome, 2: 249–250
  cubitus varus deformity, 2: 229
  dead arm syndrome, 3: 359–360
  distal humerus prosthesis, 2: 250
  kineplastic forearm amputation, 4: 360
  Krukenberg procedure, 2: 425
  tendon transfers and, 3: 428
  Volkmann ischemic contracture, 2: 200–201, 249–250
  x-ray of fetal, 3: 97, 97
Armstrong, Stewart, 4: 41*b*

Arnold, Benedict, 1: 19, 33
Arnold, Horace D., 1: 250; 3: 122
arthritis. *See also* osteoarthritis; rheumatoid arthritis
  allied health professionals and, 4: 28
  experimental septic, 2: 79
  femoroacetabular impingement, 3: 189
  forms of chronic, 4: 55
  Green and, 2: 171
  growth disturbances in children, 4: 56
  hand and, 4: 96
  hip fusion for, 3: 156*b*
  hips and, 2: 380
  juvenile idiopathic, 2: 171, 350
  Lovett Fund and, 2: 82
  MGH and, 2: 82
  nylon arthroplasty and, 4: 65–66, 66*b*, 69
  orthopaedic treatment for, 2: 171; 4: 32–33
  pauciarticular, 2: 171, 350
  pediatric, 2: 349–350
  prevention and, 4: 60–61
  psoriatic, 4: 99
  rheumatoid, 2: 82, 171, 350; 3: 239
  roentgenotherapy for, 4: 64, 64
  sacroiliac joint fusion for, 3: 184–185
  synovectomy in chronic, 4: 102, 371–372
  treatment of, 4: 32–33, 43, 54–55
  Vitallium mold arthroplasty and, 3: 239
Arthritis, Medicine and the Spiritual Law (Swaim), 4: 58, 58
Arthritis and Rheumatism Foundation, 4: 39
Arthritis Foundation, 3: 279
arthrodesis procedures
  ankles and, 3: 330
  central-graft operation, 3: 368, 368
  joints and, 3: 165
  MCP joint, 4: 97
  Morris on, 2: 282
  rheumatoid arthritis and, 4: 166
  rheumatoid arthritis of the hand research, 4: 167
  sacroiliac joint and, 3: 183–185
  wrists and, 3: 191, 239; 4: 166–167
arthrogram, 3: 99
arthrogryposis multiplex congenita, 2: 274–275, 287

Index

arthroplasty. *See also* mold arthroplasty
  absorbable animal membrane research, 3: 165–167
  advances in, 4: 43
  of the elbow, 3: 64, 341; 4: 63
  hip and, 3: 181, 242, 242t, *242*, 243
  implant, 4: 99–100
  of the knee, 4: 64, 70b–71b, 93–94, 103, 179t
  metacarpophalangeal, 4: 97
  nylon, 4: 64, 65, 66, 66b, 93
  release of contractures, 4: 166
  silicone flexible implants, 4: 166, *167*, 168
  total knee, 4: 129–130, 131t
  using interpositional tissues, 4: 64
  volar plate, 2: 248
  wrist and, 3: 191
Arthroscopic Surgery Update (McGinty), 2: 279
arthroscopy
  cameras and, 2: 279
  knee injuries and, 1: 279; 4: 129
  knee simulator, 4: 173
  McGinty and Matza's procedure, 2: 279, 280b, 281
  operative, 3: 422–423
  orthopaedics education and, 1: 220, 230
Arthroscopy Association of North America, 2: 281; 3: 422, *422*
arthrotomy, 3: 165, 165b, 166, 351
Arthur H. Huene Award, 2: 403
Arthur T. Legg Memorial Room, 2: *106*, 107
articular cartilage
  allografts and, 3: 389–390
  chondrocytes and, 3: 444
  compression forces and, 3: 326
  cup arthroplasty of the hip and, 3: 244
  degradative enzymes in, 3: *401*
  dimethyl sulfoxide (DMSO) and glycerol, 3: 442
  gene transfer treatment, 3: 445
  histologic-histochemical grading system for, 3: 384, 385t, *385*
  lubrication and, 3: 326–327
  osteoarthritis and, 3: 387–388
  preservation of, 3: 442, *442*
  repair using tritiated thymidine, 3: 383
  sling procedure and, 3: 296
Aseptic Treatment of Wounds, The (Walter), 4: 106, *106*, 107b
Ashworth, Michael A., 4: 22
assistive technology, 2: 408

Association of American Medical Colleges (AAMC), 1: 211; 2: 158
Association of Bone and Joint Surgeons, 3: 436, *436*
Association of Franklin Medal Scholars, 1: 31
Association of Residency Coordinators in Orthopaedic Surgery, 1: 238
astragalectomy (Whitman's operation), 2: 92–94
Asylum for the Insane, The, 1: 294
athletic injuries. *See* sports medicine
Athletic Injuries. Prevention, Diagnosis and Treatment (Thorndike), 1: 265, *266*
athletic training. *See also* sports medicine
  dieticians and, 1: 258
  football team and, 1: 248, 250–253, 255–256, 258
  over-training and, 1: 251, 265
  scientific study of, 1: 250–251, 265–266
athletics. *See* Harvard athletics
Atsatt, Rodney F., 1: 193; 2: 140
ATSM Committee F-4 on Medical and Surgical Materials and Devices, 3: 210
Attucks, Crispus, 1: 14
Au, Katherine, 2: 425
Aufranc, Otto E. (1909–1990), 3: *236*, *245*, *273*, *300*
  AAOS and, 2: 215
  accomplishments of, 3: 241–242
  Boston Children's Hospital and, 3: 237
  Boston City Hospital internship, 3: 237
  Bronze Star and, 3: 240, 240b, *240*
  Chandler and, 3: 277
  Children's Hospital/MGH combined program and, 3: 237
  Constructive Surgery of the Hip, 3: 244, *246*
  on Coonse, 4: 372–373
  death of, 3: 247
  early life, 3: 236–237
  education and training, 3: 237
  Fracture Clinic and, 3: 60b, 241–242, 245
  "Fracture of the Month" column, 3: 243, *243*
  hip nailing and, 3: 237
  hip surgery and, 3: 238–243; 4: 187
  HMS appointment, 3: 241–242
  as honorary orthopaedic surgeon, 3: *398b*

  honors and awards, 3: 245b
  Knight's Cross, Royal Norwegian Order of St. Olav, 3: *245*
  kyphosis treatment, 3: 239–240
  legacy of, 3: 247
  MGH Staff Associates and, 3: 241
  as MGH surgeon, 1: 203–204; 2: 325; 3: 74, 192, 217, 238–239, 241, 246
  mold arthroplasty and, 3: 192, 218, 238–239, 241–243, 243b, 244, 292b, 456b
  New England Baptist Hospital and, 3: 246–247
  Newton-Wellesley Hospital, 3: 240
  patient care and, 3: 244
  PBBH and, 4: 373
  private medical practice, 3: 238–240; 4: 158
  publications and research, 1: 286; 3: 191–192, 218, 239–244, 246, 302; 4: 161, 373
  rheumatoid arthritis research, 2: 137; 3: 239
  6th General Hospital and, 4: *476*, 482, 483b
  Smith-Petersen and, 3: 237–240
  Tufts appointment, 3: 247
  World War II service, 3: 239–241
Aufranc, Randolph Arnold, 3: 247
Aufranc, St. George Tucker, 3: 247; 4: 163, 193
Augustus Thorndike Professor of Orthopaedic Surgery, 3: 450, 464b
Augustus White III Symposium, 4: 265, 266b
Austen, Frank F., 4: 42, 114, 119, 128, 132
Austen, R. Frank, 4: 68–69
Austen, W. Gerald, 3: 256, 287, 397
Austin Moore prosthesis, 3: 213, 241, 354b
Australian Civil Constitution Corps (CCC), 4: 489
Australian Orthopaedic Association, 3: 360
Avallone, Nicholas, 4: 190b
Avicenna Hospital, 2: 421
Awbrey, Brian J., 3: 460b, 464b
Axelrod, Terry S., 3: 431
Aycock, W. Lloyd, 2: 82
Ayres, Douglas K., 4: 287

B

Babcock, Warren L., 4: 429, 433, 437
Bach, Bernard R., Jr., 1: 284, 288–289; 3: 379
back disabilities. *See also* sciatica
   industrial accidents and, 2: 92; 4: 358
   laminectomy and, 3: 204, 206–208
   low-back pain, 2: 371–372, 396; 3: 175, 204–206, 250*b*–252*b*
   lumbago and, 3: 203
   lumbar spinal stenosis, 2: 373–374
   MRI and, 3: 255
   Norton-Brown spinal brace and, 3: 318, *318tg*, 319
   Ober Test and, 2: 151–152
   psychiatric investigation and, 3: 258
   ruptured intervertebral disc, 3: 204, *204*, 205–207, *207*, 208; 4: 352–353
   sacroiliac joint and, 3: 184
   Sever on, 2: 92
   spine fusion and, 3: 207–208
   treatment of, 3: 203
Back Problems Guideline Panel, 2: 371
"Back Strains and Sciatica" (Ober), 2: 151–152
Bader Functional Room, 2: *106*
Bae, Donald S., 2: *417*, 418–419, *419t*, *419*; 4: 190*b*
Baer, William S., 2: 126; 3: 158, 166–167; 4: 416
Baetzer, Fred H., 3: 87
Bailey, Fred Warren, 2: 78
Bailey, George G., Jr. (unk.–1998)
   Boston City Hospital and, 4: 360
   death of, 4: 360
   education and training, 4: 360
   kineplastic forearm amputation case, 4: 360
   Mt. Auburn Hospital and, 4: 360
   professional memberships, 4: 360
   publications and research, 4: 360
Baker, Charles, 2: 39
Baker, Frances Prescott, 3: 308
Balach, Franklin, 4: 41*b*
Balch, Emily, 3: 142
Balch, Franklin G., Jr., 4: 193
Balkan Frame, 3: 317, 357*b*
Ball, Anna, 1: 95
Ballentine, H. Thomas, 3: 314
Bancroft, Frederic, 3: 316
Bankart, A. S. Blundell, 3: 449

Bankart procedure, 3: 351–354, 357–358, 358*t*, *359*, 360, 450
Banks, Henry H. (1921–), 1: 202, 205, 207; 4: 72, 342
   AAOS and, 2: 314
   Aufranc and, 3: 247
   on BCH residencies, 4: 377
   BIH Board of Consultants, 4: 262–263
   Boston Children's Hospital and, 1: 204–206; 2: 233, 301; 4: 72
   Boston City Hospital and, 4: 297
   on Carl Walter, 4: 108
   cerebral palsy research and treatment, 2: 196–200; 4: 74, 76–77
   education and training, 4: 72
   flexor carpi ulnaris transfer procedure, 2: 188
   on Green, 2: 168, 204–205
   Grice and, 1: 206
   hip fracture research, 4: 74–78
   Little Orthopaedic Club and, 4: 74
   on Mark Rogers, 4: 229–230
   metastatic malignant melanoma fracture case, 4: 77–78
   MGH and, 1: 203–204
   on Ober, 2: 149
   Orthopaedic Surgery at Tufts University, 4: 77
   on osteochondritis dissecans, 2: 195
   PBBH and, 1: 204–205; 4: 19–20, 22, 72, 73*b*–74*b*, 128
   as PBBH chief of orthopaedics, 4: 22, 43, 76, 116*b*, 196*b*
   on PBBH research program, 4: 75*b*
   professional memberships, 4: 76–77
   publications and research, 4: 72, 75–77
   on Quigley, 1: 276–277, 282
   RBBH and, 4: 36, 40
   residency training under Green, 1: 202–203
   as Tufts University chair of orthopaedics, 4: 22, 76–77, 116
   US Army Medical Corps and, 4: 72
   on Zimbler, 4: 250
Bar Harbor Medical and Surgical Hospital, 2: 312
Barber, D. B., 2: 172
Barlow, Joel, 1: 292–293
Barnes Hospital, 3: 165; 4: 125
Barr, Dorrice Nash, 3: 247

Barr, Joseph S. (1901–1964), 1: *205*; 2: *249*, *278*, *286*, *290*, *320*; 3: 142, *201*, 213
   as AAOS president, 3: 210
   appointments and positions, 3: 202*b*
   on audio-visual aids in teaching, 1: 161
   back pain and sciatica research, 3: 203–208
   Brigham and Women's Hospital and, 4: 195*b*
   as chair of AOA research committee, 3: 209, *209*
   as clinical professor, 1: 158
   Committee of Undergraduate Training, 2: 183
   death of, 3: 214
   development of research at MGH, 1: 180
   early life, 3: 201
   education and training, 3: 201
   Ferguson and, 2: 188
   Glimcher and, 2: 321–322
   on herniated disc and sciatica, 3: 184
   HMS appointment, 2: 223; 3: 202; 4: 61
   John Ball and Buckminster Brown Professorship, 3: 202, 453*b*, 464*b*; 4: 195*b*
   Joint Committee for the Study of Surgical Materials and, 3: 210
   leadership of, 3: 453, 453*b*–456*b*
   legacy of, 3: 212–214
   Marlborough Medical Associates and, 2: 146, 269, 299
   marriage and family, 3: 214
   memberships and, 3: 212–213
   as MGH orthopaedics chief, 3: 11*b*, 202, 227, 241, 277
   MGH residents and, 3: *212*, *217*, *238*, *254*, *278*, *285*, *323*, *377*, *456*; 4: *161*, *245*
   MGH Staff Associates and, 3: 241
   as MGH surgeon, 3: 187, 201
   New England Peabody Home for Crippled Children and, 3: 209
   New England Society of Bone and Joint Surgery, 4: 347
   orthopaedic research and, 3: 210–212
   on orthopaedics curriculum, 1: 207
   PBBH 50th anniversary, 4: 21
   polio research, 3: 209, 331–333
   private medical practice, 3: 454*b*
   as professor of orthopaedic surgery, 1: 158, 179–180

Index

publications and research, 2: 152, 250; 3: 202–211, 302, 331
rehabilitation planning and, 1: 272
resident training by, 1: 199, 203, 206–207
retirement of, 2: 325
ruptured intervertebral disc research, 3: 204; 4: 352
scoliosis treatment, 2: 396; 3: 208–209
on shoulder arthrodesis, 2: 154
slipped capital femoral epiphysis research, 4: 237
on the surgical experiment, 3: 210
US Navy and, 3: 201
Barr, Joseph S., Jr. (1934–), 3: *247*, *461*
  ankle arthrodesis case, 3: 330
  Boston Interhospital Augmentation Study (BIAS) and, 3: 248–249
  Boston Prosthetics Course and, 1: 217
  Children's Hospital/MGH combined program and, 3: 248
  early life, 3: 247
  education and training, 3: 248
  Faulkner Hospital and, 3: 248
  Glimcher and, 3: 248
  Halo Vest, 3: 321
  HMS appointment, 3: 248
  on Leffert, 3: 413
  on low-back pain, 3: 250*b*–252*b*
  as MGH clinical faculty, 3: 464*b*
  as MGH surgeon, 3: 214, 248, 398*b*
  professional memberships and, 3: 249
  publications and research, 3: 249
  sailing and, 3: 249, 252
  Schmidt and, 3: 248
  spine treatment and, 3: 460*b*
  US Naval Medical Corps and, 3: 248
Barr, Mary, 3: 214
Barrell, Joseph, 3: 9
Barrett, Ian, 2: 400
Barron, M. E., 4: 199
Bartlett, John, 1: 41; 3: 3, 5
Bartlett, Josiah, 1: 293
Bartlett, Marshall K., 3: 241; 4: 475, 482*b*
Bartlett, Ralph W., 2: 34
Barton, Lyman G., Jr., 2: 119; 4: 389*b*
Baruch, Bernard M., 1: 272
Baruch Committee, 1: 272–273

base hospitals. *See also* military reconstruction hospitals; US Army Base Hospitals
  AEF and, 4: 417, 419–420
  amputations and, 4: 418
  Boston-derived, 4: 420*t*
  Camp Devens, 4: 452
  Camp Taylor, 4: 452
  field splinting and, 4: 408
  Harvard Units and, 4: 419–420, 437–438
  injuries and mortality rates in, 4: 424
  organization of American, 4: 419–420
  orthopaedics surgery and, 4: 406, 412, 417–419, 440, 443, 445, 451–453
  training in, 4: 420–421
  US and British medical staff in, 4: 422
  wounded soldiers and, 4: 385, 414, 416–417
basic fibroblast growth factor (bFGF), 3: 445
Bateman, James E., 2: 317; 3: 295
Bates, Frank D. (1925–2011)
  Boston Children's Hospital and, 2: 301
  Brigham and Women's Hospital and, 4: 193
  Korean War and, 2: 218
  PBBH and, 4: 20, 22, 116, 128
  Winchester Hospital and, 3: 299
Battle of Bunker Hill, 1: *17*, 18, *18*, 19, 22
Battle of Lexington and Concord, 1: 17–18, 22
"Battle of the Delta, The," 1: 245–247
Baue, Arthur, 1: 90
Bauer, Thomas, 4: 174
Bauer, Walter, 2: 82, 171; 3: 335
Bayne-Jones, Stanhope, 4: 405*b*
Beach, Henry H. A., 2: 24; 3: 40
Bean, Harold C., 2: 230
Bearse, Carl, 4: 208
Beattie, George, 2: 300
Beauchamp, Richard, 2: 351, *351*
Bedford Veterans Administration Hospital, 3: 314
Beecher, Henry K., 1: 171, 239; 3: 96
Begg, Alexander S., 1: 88
Bell, Anna Elizabeth Bowman, 2: 219
Bell, Emily J. Buck, 2: 220
Bell, Enoch, 2: 219
Bell, J. L., 1: 24
Bell, John, 1: 37

Bell, John F. (1909–1989)
  Boston Children's Hospital and, 2: 299
  club foot treatment, 2: 208
  Crippled Children's Clinic and, 2: 221
  Crotched Mountain Foundation, 2: 221
  death of, 2: 221
  disabled children and, 2: 221
  education and training, 2: 219, 220*b*
  Journal of Bone and Joint Surgery editor, 2: 221
  marriage and family, 2: 220
  Ober and, 2: 220
  Palmer Memorial Hospital and, 2: 219–220
  PBBH and, 2: 220
  pediatric orthopaedics and, 2: 221
  publications of, 2: 208, 220–221
  University of Vermont and, 2: 220–221
  Vermont Department of Health and, 2: 221
Bell, Joseph, 1: 84
Bell, Sir Charles, 1: 37, 73, 76
Bellare, Anuj, 4: 194
Bellevue Medical College, 2: 63
Bemis, George, 1: 307, 317
Bender, Anita, 4: 81
Bender, Ralph H. (1930–1999), 4: *80*
  on back pain, 4: 80
  Beth Israel Hospital and, 4: 247
  death of, 4: 81
  education and training, 4: 80
  hospital appointments, 4: 80
  marriage and family, 4: 81
  private medical practice, 4: 80
  professional memberships, 4: 81
  RBBH and, 4: 41*b*, 68, 80, 102
  US Air Force and, 4: 80
Benet, George, 4: 389*b*
Bennet, Eban E., 2: 72, 74–75
Bennett, G. A., 3: 335
Bennett, George E., 2: 77–78, 119; 4: 473
Benz, Edward, 2: 331
Berenberg, William, 2: 196, 213, 354, 406, 408
Bergenfeldt, E., 4: 356
Berlin, David D.
  Beth Israel Hospital and, 4: 361
  Boston City Hospital and, 4: 361
  education and training, 4: 361
  publications and research, 4: 361
  scaphoid fracture treatment, 4: 361

Tufts Medical School appointment, 4: 361
Bernard, Claude, 1: 82; 3: 142
Bernard, Francis, 1: 8, 13
Bernese periacetabular osteotomy, 2: 391–392
Bernhardt, Mark, 4: 263
Bernstein, Fredrika Ehrenfried, 4: 220
Bernstein, Irving, 4: 220
Bernstein, J., 1: 168
Berry, George P., 1: 180; 2: 183, 324; 3: 202, 334; 4: 113, 303
Bertody, Charles, 1: 60
Berven, Sigurd, 3: *278*
Beth Israel Deaconess Medical Center (BIDMC)
    Augustus White III Symposium, 4: 265, 266*b*
    Bierbaum and, 1: 233–234
    CareGroup and, 4: 281
    Carl J. Shapiro Department of Orthopaedics, 4: 288
    East Campus, 4: *213, 287*
    Emergency Department, 4: 286
    financial difficulties, 4: 283–284
    formation of, 4: 214, 223, 270, 281, 283
    HCORP and, 4: 284, 288
    as HMS teaching hospital, 4: 214
    Kocher and, 2: 377
    orthopaedics department, 1: 171; 4: 284–288
    orthopaedics department chiefs, 4: 289*b*
    orthopaedics residencies, 1: 223–224, 234, 236, 242; 4: 285–288
    West Campus, 4: *213, 280*
Beth Israel Hospital Association, 4: 204–205
Beth Israel Hospital (BIH)
    affiliation with Harvard Medical School, 4: 213–214, 251
    affiliation with Tufts Medical School, 4: 213–214, 214*b*, 228
    Brookline Avenue location, 4: 211, *211*, 228
    continuing medical education and, 4: 208
    establishment of new location, 4: 210, 210*b*, 211
    facilities for, 4: 207–208, 210
    financial difficulties, 4: 210–211, 281
    founding of, 4: 199
    growth of, 4: 209–210
    HCORP and, 1: 218; 4: 247–248
    HMS courses at, 1: 158
    house officers at, 4: 209*b*
    immigrant care in, 4: 283
    infectious disease fellowship, 1: 91
    internships at, 1: 196
    Jewish patients at, 4: 199, 205–206, 223
    Jewish physician training at, 1: 158; 4: 199, 283
    leadership of, 4: 206–211
    medical education and, 4: 213
    merger with New England Deaconess Hospital, 4: 214, 223, 270, 281, 283
    Mueller Professorship, 4: 263
    non-discrimination and, 4: 199
    opening of, 4: 205, 223
    operating room at, 4: *212, 228*
    Orthopaedic Biomechanics Laboratory, 4: 262
    orthopaedic division chiefs, 4: 223, 289*b*
    orthopaedic residencies at, 4: 247–248, 251
    orthopaedics department at, 4: 213, 247, 262–263
    orthopaedics department chiefs, 4: 289*b*
    orthopaedics surgery at, 2: 377; 3: 325; 4: 208, 208*b*
    sports medicine and, 4: 255
    surgeon-in-chiefs at, 4: 283, 283*t*
    surgical departments at, 4: 208
    Townsend Street location, 4: 205, *205, 206, 207*
Beth Israel Medical Center (NY), 2: 408; 4: 206
Bettman, Henry Wald, 3: 86
Bhashyam, Abhiram R., 3: 463*b*
Bianco, Anthony, Jr., 2: 304
Bick, Edgar M., 1: 101, 114; 4: 88
Bicknell, Macalister, 3: 192
BIDMC. *See* Beth Israel Deaconess Medical Center (BIDMC)
Bierbaum, Benjamin
    as BIDMC chief of orthopaedics, 1: 233–234, 236; 4: 284–286, 289*b*
    Boston Children's Hospital and, 2: 286, 438
    Brigham and Women's Hospital and, 4: 193
    Crippled Children's Clinic and, 2: 314
    hip surgery and, 4: 284
    HMS appointment, 4: 284–285
    New England Baptist Hospital and, 1: 233; 4: 284
    PBBH and, 4: 22, 116, 128, 163
    Tufts Medical School appointment, 4: 284
Biesiadecki, Alfred, 1: 82
Bigelow, Henry Jacob (1818–1890), 1: *137*; 3: *23*, 30, *32, 46*
    as accomplished surgeon, 3: 39–41
    bladder stones treatment, 3: 41–42
    cellular pathology and, 3: 34
    Charitable Surgical Institution, 3: 30
    Chickahominy fever and, 3: 44
    Civil War medicine and, 3: 43–44
    code of conduct, 3: 47*b*, 48
    controversy over, 3: 44–45
    disbelief in antisepsis, 3: 45
    discounting of Warren, 3: 32–34, 36
    "Discourse on Self-Limited Diseases, A," 3: 12–13
    drawings of femur malunions, 3: *42*
    early life, 3: 23
    education and training, 3: 23–25
    ether and anesthetics, 3: 27–29, 31–34
    European medical studies, 3: 25
    excision of the elbow, 3: 34
    femoral neck fractures, 3: 38–39, *39*
    hip dislocations and, 3: 34–36, 38
    hip joint excision, 3: 34
    as HMS professor of surgery, 1: 137; 3: 34, 42–43, *43*, 44
    home in Newton, 3: *48*
    house on Tuckernuck Island, 3: *49*
    on the importance of flexion, 3: 38
    injury and death of, 3: 49–50
    "Insensibility During Surgical Operations Produced by Inhalation," 3: 27, *27*
    legacy of, 3: 45–48
    Manual of Orthopedic Surgery, 3: 25–26, *26*
    marriage and family, 3: 30, 34
    Mechanism of Dislocation and Fracture of the Hip, 3: 35, *35*, 38
    memberships and, 3: 48
    as MGH surgeon, 1: 84; 3: 15, 25–27, 30–31, *31*
    as MGH surgeon emeritus, 3: 45–46
    New England Peabody Home for Crippled Children and, 2: 230

Index

nitrous oxide and, 1: 56
orthopaedic contributions,
  3: 34–36, 37b, 38–39
orthopaedics curriculum and,
  1: 140
posthumous commemorations of,
  3: 50, 50b, 51, 51b
reform of HMS and, 1: 139;
  3: 44–45
resistance to antisepsis techniques, 1: 85
as senior surgeon at MGH,
  1: 86; 2: 20
on spinal disease, 2: 57
support for House of the Good
  Samaritan, 1: 124
surgical illustrations and, 3: 25
surgical instruments and,
  3: 40–41
Tremont Street Medical School
  and, 3: 26, 42
ununited fractures research,
  3: 34–35
on use of ether, 1: 57, 59, 61–62
Bigelow, Jacob, 1: 60, 296, 299–300, 302; 3: 12, 23, 42
Bigelow, Mary Scollay, 3: 23
Bigelow, Sturgis, 1: *61*
Bigelow, Susan Sturgis, 3: 30, 34
Bigelow, W. S. (William Sturgis),
  3: 23, 34, 40–41, 47b, 48, 50
Bigelow Building (MGH), 3: 15–17
Bigelow Medal, 3: *49*, 50
Bigelow's septum, 3: 39
Bigos, Stanley, 2: 371
BIH/Camp International Visiting
  Lecture, 4: 263
Billroth, Theodor, 1: 81–82
Binney, Horace, 3: 237; 4: 420
Biochemistry and Physiology of Bone
  (Bourne), 3: 337
bioethics, 4: 324
Biography of Otto E. Aufranc, A,
  3: *246*
Biomaterials and Innovative Technologies Laboratory, 3: 463, 464b
biomechanics
  backpack loads and, 2: 408
  bone structure property relations,
    2: 410
  collagen in the intervertebral
    discs and, 2: 328
  CT arthrography and, 2: 410
  early study of, 1: xxii
  Harrington rods and, 2: 325
  hips and, 2: 407
  laboratory for, 3: 220
  orthopaedics education and,
    1: 220, 230, 241

osteoarthritis and, 3: 322,
  326–328, 383–384
posterior cruciate ligament injury
  and, 3: 448
subchondral bone with impact
  loading, 3: 326–327
"Biomechanics of Baseball Pitching"
  (Pappas), 2: *288*
Biomotion Laboratory, 3: 463, 464b
biopsy, 3: 390–391
Bird, Larry, 2: 369
birth abnormalities, 2: 275, 334, *334*
birth fractures, 2: 172. *See also* congenital pseudarthrosis of the tibia
birth palsies research, 2: 415, 417,
  417, 418–420
Black, Eric, 4: 190b
Blackman, Kenneth D., 1: 178
bladder stones, 3: 41–42
Blake, John Bapst, 4: 291
Blake, Joseph A., 2: 118; 4: 416
Bland, Edward, 4: 482b
Bland, Edward F., 3: 241; 4: 22
Blazar, Philip, 3: 410; 4: 194
Blazina, M. E., 1: 279
blood poisoning, 2: 299
blood transfusions, 1: 23; 3: 313
Bloodgood, Joseph C., 3: 137
bloodletting, 1: 9, 23, 74
Bloomberg, Maxwell H., 4: 208b
Blount, Walter, 2: 176, 335
Blumer, George, 2: 158
Boachie-Adjei, Oheneba, 4: 266b
Bock, Arlie V., 1: 265; 2: 253
Bock, Bernard, 1: 217b
body mechanics, 3: 81, 91;
  4: 82–83, 233, 236
Body Mechanics in Health and Disease
  (Goldthwait et al.), 3: 91; 4: 53,
  62
Body Snatchers, 1: *32*
Bohlman, Henry H., 4: 266b
Böhm, Max, 3: 67, 71, 265–266
Boland, Arthur L. (1935–), 1: *283*,
  285
  awards and honors, 1: 288–289
  Brigham and Women's Hospital
    and, 1: 284; 4: 163, 193
  Children's Hospital/MGH combined program and, 1: 283
  on concussions, 1: 286–287
  education and training,
    1: 283–284
  Harvard University Health Service and, 1: 284
  as head surgeon for Harvard athletics, 1: 284–288; 3: 399
  as HMS clinical instructor,
    1: 166, 284
  knee injuries and, 1: 287

  as MGH clinical faculty, 3: 464b
  as MGH surgeon, 3: 399
  PBBH and, 4: 116, 128, 163
  publications of, 1: 286, 288
  sports medicine and, 1: 284–289; 2: 384; 3: 448, 460b
  women basketball players and,
    1: 285–286
Boland, Jane Macknight, 1: 289
Bonar, Lawrence C., 2: 324
bone and joint disorders
  arthrodesis and, 3: 165
  atypical multiple case tuberculosis, 2: 257
  bone atrophy and, 3: 170
  chondrosarcoma, 3: 406
  conditions of interest in, 3: 82b
  fusion and, 3: 368
  Legg and, 2: 110
  lubrication and, 3: 324–327
  mobilization of, 4: 27b
  PBBH annual report, 4: 13, 13t,
    16
  sacroiliac joint treatment,
    3: 183–184
  schools for disabled children,
    2: 37
  subchondral bone research,
    3: 326–327, *327*
  total disability following fractures,
    3: *373*
  tubercular cows and, 2: 16
  tuberculosis in pediatric patients,
    2: 308–309
  tuberculosis of the hip, 3: 148
  tuberculosis treatment, 2: 11,
    25; 3: 166, 289
  use of x-rays, 3: 101–103
bone banks, 3: 386, 388, 396, 433
bone cement, 4: 129, 133, 171
bone grafts
  arthrodesis procedures, 3: 368
  Boston approach and, 2: 392
  chemotherapy and, 2: 423
  chronic nonunions of the
    humerus and, 2: *96*
  early study of, 1: xxiii
  flexion injuries and, 3: 348
  Grice procedure and, 2: 209–210
  injured soldiers and, 3: 336, *337*
  kyphosis and, 2: 343
  modified Colonna reconstructive
    method, 3: 194
  non-union fractures and, 2: 238;
    3: 59
  posterior spinal fusion and,
    2: 341
  radioactive calcium tracers in,
    2: 237, 240
  spinal fusion and, 3: 208, 425

503

tibial pseudarthrosis in neurofibromatosis case, 2: 175–176
  total hip replacement and, 3: 279
bone granuloma, 2: 171
bone growth
  activating transcription factor-2 (ATF-2) and, 2: 330
  Digby's method for measuring, 2: 170, 170*t*
  distal femur and proximal tibia, 2: 191–192, *192*, 193
  effects of irradiation on epiphyseal growth, 3: 331
  epiphyseal arrest and, 2: 192, 192*t*, 193
  Green and, 2: 170, 191–194
  Green-Andersen growth charts, 2: 193, *193*, 194
  Moseley's growth charts, 2: 194
  orthoroentgenograms and, 2: 192–193
  Paley multiplier method, 2: 194
  research in, 2: 191–194
  skeletal age in predictions, 2: 192
bone irradiation, 2: 237
Bone Sarcoma Registry of the American College of Surgeons, 4: 102
bone sarcomas, 3: 136–137, 137*t*, 138–140, 140*b*, 141–142
bones and teeth
  apatite crystals and, 2: 321
  collagen in, 2: 327–328
  electron microscopes and, 2: 323, *324*
  Haversian systems in, 2: 241
  hydroxylysine and, 2: 327–328
  mineralized crystals, 2: 325–326
  research in, 2: 322–324
  research in lesions, 2: 236
Bonfiglio, Michael, 3: 303
Boothby, Walter M., 4: 216, 323, 389*b*, 422*b*
Boott, Francis, 1: 59
Borden Research Award, 2: 319
Borges, Larry, 3: 420
Boron Neutron Capture Synovectomy, 4: 136
Bosch, Joanne P., 4: 183
Bost, Frederick C., 2: 274; 4: 60
Boston, Mass.
  annual Christmas tree from Halifax, 3: 135, *135*
  cholera epidemic, 1: 295; 4: 293
  colonial economy in, 1: 10
  Committee of Correspondence in, 1: 16
  Fort Warren, 1: 20
  Halifax Harbor explosion aid, 3: 134–135
  infectious disease in, 1: 7–9; 2: 4

  inoculation hospitals, 1: 8–9
  Irish Catholics in, 4: 200
  Irish immigration to, 4: 293
  Jewish immigration to, 4: 199–200, 220
  Jewish physicians in, 4: 199–200
  Jewish Quarter, 4: 200, *200*
  malnutrition in, 2: 4
  maps, 1: *7*, *114*, *296*
  military reconstruction hospital and, 4: 444
  need for hospital in, 1: 41; 3: 3; 4: 293–294, 294*b*
  orthopaedics institutions in, 1: 189–190
  Stamp Act protests in, 1: 11–13
  tea party protest and, 1: 15–16
  Townshend Act protests, 1: 13–14
  Warren family and, 1: 4*b*
Boston Almshouse, 1: 29; 3: 3
  HMS clinical teaching at, 1: 28, 40; 3: 4–5
  house pupils at, 1: 80
  inadequacy of, 1: 41; 3: 3–4
  John Ball Brown and, 1: 96
  medical care at, 2: 20; 3: 3–4
Boston Arm, 2: 326, *326*; 3: 287
Boston Association of Cardiac Clinics, 1: 129
Boston Ballet, 2: 384, *384*
Boston brace, 2: 339–340, *340*, 358–359, *359–360*, *361*, 423, *424*
Boston Brace Instructional Courses, 2: 358
Boston Bruins, 3: 348, 356–357, 357*b*, 397, 399, 448; 4: 342
Boston Children's Hospital (BCH), 1: *194*; 2: *177*, *437*, *438*
  Act of Incorporation, 2: 7, *7*
  astragalectomy at, 2: 93–94
  bedside teaching at, 2: *435*
  Berlin polio epidemic team, 2: 260, 264
  Boston brace and, 2: 339–340, 423
  Boston Concept and, 2: 392
  cerebral palsy cases, 2: 171–172
  Cerebral Palsy Clinic, 2: 402, 406, 409
  charitable surgical appliances, 2: *14*
  children with poliomyelitis and, 1: 191; 2: 163
  children's convalescence and, 2: 9
  clinical service rotations, 1: 198
  clinical surgery curricula at, 1: 141, 143, 147, 151, 155–157, 162
  cows and, 2: 429

  decline in skeletal tuberculosis admissions, 2: 16, 16*t*
  Department of Medicine, 2: 427
  Department of Orthopaedic Surgery, 1: 171–172, 189–190; 2: 10–13, 15–16, 40, *98*, *133*, *156*, *177*, *200*, *222*, *252*, *255*, *283*, *293*, 354–355, 427, 434, 438–439, 439*b*; 3: 67
  Department of Surgery, 2: 427
  endowed professorships, 2: 438, 439*b*
  founding of, 1: 123; 2: 3–9
  Growth Study (Green and Anderson), 2: 193
  HCORP and, 1: 213, 215
  hip disease and, 2: 52
  House of the Good Samaritan merger, 1: 130; 2: 433
  house officers at, 1: 184, 189
  house officer's certificate, 2: *41*
  impact of World War II on, 4: 468
  Infantile Paralysis Clinic, 2: 79
  innovation and change at, 2: 427–428, 430–434, 436–439
  internships at, 1: 196
  Massachusetts Infantile Paralysis Clinics, 2: 188–189
  military surgeon training at, 1: 151, 191; 4: 396
  Myelodysplasia Clinic, 2: 359, 402
  named funds, 2: 436, 439*b*
  nursing program at, 2: 13–14
  objections to, 2: 8–9
  organizational models, 2: 436–437
  orthopaedic admissions at, 2: 15*t*, 40, 40*t*
  orthopaedic chairpersons, 2: 15*b*
  orthopaedic surgeries, 2: 9–12, 12*t*, 13, *13*, 14–15, 39–40, 337–338, 338*t*
  orthopaedics residencies, 1: 186–187, 199, 202–207, 211, 217–218, 224–225; 2: *413*
  outpatient services at, 1: 190; 2: 11–12
  patient registry, 2: *10*
  PBBH and, 4: 10, 14
  pediatrics at, 2: 3
  polio clinics at, 2: 78–79, 188
  private/public system in, 2: 313, 337, 339
  psoas abscesses and, 2: 54
  radiology at, 2: 16, *16*, 17, 17*t*, 431
  Report of the Medical Staff, 2: 9

resident salaries, 1: 206, *206*
scoliosis clinic at, 2: 35–36, 84–86
Sever-L'Episcopo procedure, 2: 417
Spanish American War patients, 4: *311*
specialization in, 2: 11
Spinal Surgery Service, 2: 359
spinal tuberculosis and, 2: 11, 308–309
sports medicine and, 2: 287, 384
Statement by Four Physicians, 2: 6–7
surgeon-scholars at, 2: 217, 357
surgical procedures for scoliosis, 2: *369*
surgical training at, 1: 188–189
teaching clinics at, 1: 194; 2: *62*
teaching fellows, 1: 192–193
tuberculosis patients, 2: 275
20th century overview of, 2: 427–428, 430–434, 436–439
use of radiographs, 2: 54
Boston Children's Hospital (BCH). Facilities
   appliance shop at, 2: 22, *22*, *431*
   Bader building, 2: 432, *432–433*
   Bader Solarium, 2: *432*
   Boy's Ward, 2: *14*
   expansion of, 2: 9–11, 13, *433*, *434t*
   Fegan building, 2: 433
   Functional Therapy Room, 2: *432*
   gait laboratory, 2: 107, 406
   Girl's Surgical Ward, 2: *15*
   gymnasium, 2: *433*
   Hunnewell Building entrance, 2: *429*
   on Huntington Ave., 2: 11, *11*, 12, *12*, 427–428, *428*
   Ida C. Smith ward, 2: *431*
   Infant's Hospital, 2: *431*
   lack of elevators in, 2: 430, *430*
   on Longwood Avenue, 2: 64, 428, 430–431
   Medical Center and Prouty Garden, 2: *436*
   orthopaedic research laboratory, 2: 234
   Pavilion Wards, 2: *435*
   research laboratories, 2: 234–236, 285, 434, 438–439
   standard ward in, 2: *144*, *429*
   Ward I, 2: *434*
   at Washington and Rutland Streets, 2: *11*
   in the winter, 2: *430*

Boston Children's Hospital/Massachusetts General residency program, 1: 210; 2: 144
Boston City Base Hospital No. 7 (France), 4: 301–302
Boston City Hospital (BCH), 4: *306*, *379*
   affiliation with Boston University Medical School, 4: 296–297, 303, 380
   affiliation with Harvard Medical School, 4: 296, 298, 302–303, 379–380
   affiliation with Tufts Medical School, 4: 228, 296–297, 303
   Base Hospital No. 7 and, 1: 256; 4: 301–302, 420t, 438–439
   Bone and Joint Service, 4: 306–307, 328, 333–334, 357, 377, 377t, 380b
   Bradford and, 2: 21; 4: 298, 303, 307
   Burrell and, 4: 298–299, *299*, 300–301, 307
   Centre building, 4: *295*
   clinical courses for Harvard students at, 4: 380t–381t
   compound fracture therapy at, 4: *335*, 337
   construction of, 4: 295
   end of Harvard Medical School relationship, 4: 380
   ether tray at, 4: *298*
   examining room, 4: *300*
   fracture treatment and, 4: 362
   Harvard Fifth Surgical Service at, 4: 275, 277, 297, 302–303, 305–306
   Harvard Medical Unit at, 4: 296–297, 303
   house officers at, 4: 305, 305b
   intern and residency training programs, 4: 303–306
   internships at, 1: 189, 196
   Joseph H. Shortell Fracture Unit, 4: *342*, *342*, 357
   medical school affiliations, 4: 370–371
   merger with Boston University Medical Center Hospital, 4: 297
   Nichols and, 1: 174, 252; 4: 301–302
   opening of, 4: 295–296
   operating room at, 4: *298*, *301*
   orthopaedic residencies at, 1: 186, 199; 3: 237; 4: 377–380
   orthopaedic surgery at, 4: 307

   Outpatient Department, 4: *300*, *357*
   Pavilion I, 4: *295*
   physical therapy room, 4: *308*
   planning for, 4: 293–295
   plot plan for, 4: *293*, *307*
   Relief Station, 4: *305*
   specialty services at, 4: 306–307
   staffing of, 4: 296
   surgeon-scholars at, 1: 174; 4: 333, 357
   Surgical Outpatient Department Building, 4: *295*
   surgical services at, 4: 297–303, 307, 370–371
   Surgical Ward, 4: *295*
   teaching clinics at, 1: 141, 143
   Thorndike Building, 4: *296*
   Thorndike Memorial Laboratory, 4: 297
   treatment of children in, 2: 4
   Tufts University Medical Service and, 4: 297
   undergraduate surgical education, 4: 303
   Ward O, 4: *296*
   wards in, 4: *301*
   West Roxbury Department, 4: 447–448
   women in orthopaedics at, 1: 200
Boston City Hospital Relief Station, 2: 269
Boston Concept, 2: 391, *391*, 392
Boston Dispensary, 1: 40, 96; 2: 20, 306; 3: 3; 4: 48, 311, *311*, 358
Boston Dynamics, 4: 173
Boston Hospital for Women, 4: 42–43, 69, 113–114, 119
Boston Infant's Hospital, 2: 242
Boston Interhospital Augmentation Study (BIAS), 3: 248–249
Boston Lying-in-Hospital, 1: 123; 4: 113–114
Boston Massacre, 1: 14–16
Boston Medical and Surgical Journal, 4: 293, 294b
Boston Medical Association, 1: 25, 38; 3: 25
Boston Medical Center (BMC), 4: 89, 297
Boston Medical Library, 1: 39, 59; 2: 271
Boston Medical Society, 4: 200, 202
Boston Organ Bank Group, 3: 386
Boston Orthopaedic Group, 4: 251, 285–286, 288
"Boston Orthopaedic Institution, The" (Cohen), 1: 114

Boston Orthopedic Club, 2: 171, 230, 294, 329; 3: 289; 4: 66
Boston Orthopedic Institution
  attraction of patients from the U.S. and abroad, 1: 99
  Buckminster Brown and, 1: 107, 118, 120–122
  closing of, 1: 121–122; 3: 30
  founding of, 1: xxiv, 99
  John Ball Brown and, 1: 99–100, 107, 113–114, 118–122
  long term treatment in, 2: 25
  origins and growth of, 1: 114–118
  scholarship on, 1: 114
  treatment advances in, 1: 118–120
  use of ether, 1: 107, 118
Boston Orthopedique Infirmary, 1: 99–100, 113. *See also* Boston Orthopedic Institution
Boston Pathology Course, 1: 216, 218
Boston Prosthetics Course, 1: 220
Boston Red Sox, 1: 258; 2: 288; 3: 348; 4: 345
Boston Rugby Football Club, 2: 383, *383*, 400
Boston School of Occupational Therapy, 4: 30, 32
Boston School of Physical Education, 3: 84
Boston School of Physical Therapy, 4: 30, 32
Boston Shriner's Hospital, 1: 123
Boston Society for Medical Improvement, 1: 61; 3: 44, 48, 150
Boston Surgical Society, 2: 69; 3: 50, 65
Boston University School of Medicine, 1: 239; 2: 273–274; 4: 67–68, 296
Boston Veterans Administration Hospital, 1: 71, 90; 3: 298
Bottomly, John T., 3: 116
Bouillaud, J. B., 4: 93
Bourne, Geoffrey, 3: 337
Bouvé, Marjorie, 4: 444
Bouvier, Sauveur-Henri Victor, 1: 106
Bowditch, Charles Pickering, 1: 82; 3: 142
Bowditch, Henry I., 1: 53, 73, 82, *82*; 2: 306; 3: 9, 97–98; 4: 3
Bowditch, Henry P., 2: 48; 3: 94
Bowditch, Katherine Putman, 3: 142
Bowditch, Nathaniel, 3: 15, 142, 146
Bowen, Abel, 1: *29*
Bowker, John H., 3: 299

Boyd, A. D., Jr., 4: 136
Boyd, Robert J. (1930–), 3: *254*, 256
  Barr and, 3: 255
  Children's Hospital/MGH combined program and, 3: 253
  education and training, 3: 253
  hip surgery and, 3: 253
  HMS appointment, 3: 254
  Lemuel Shattuck Hospital and, 3: 253
  Lynn General Hospital and, 3: 253
  MGH Staff Associates and, 3: 256
  as MGH surgeon, 3: 253, 256, 398*b*
  private medical practice, 3: 256
  Problem Back Clinic at MGH and, 3: 254
  problem back service and, 3: 388*t*
  publications and research, 3: 253–255, *255*
  Scarlet Key Society and, 3: 253
  Sledge and, 4: 127
  spine and trauma work, 3: 254–255, 420, 460*b*
  Trauma Management, 3: 62, 253
Boyes, Joseph, 3: 427
Boylston, Thomas, 3: 5
Boylston Medical School, 1: 138
Boylston Medical Society, 3: 25–26, 48
Bozic, Kevin J., 1: 225; 4: 266*b*
brachial plexus injuries, 2: 90–91, 96; 3: 412–414
Brachial Plexus Injuries (Leffert), 3: 414
brachioradialis transfer, 2: 153–154, *154*
Brackett, Elliott G. (1860–1942), 3: *147, 157*; 4: *394*
  Advisory Orthopedic Board and, 3: 157
  AOA meeting and, 2: 137
  Beth Israel Hospital and, 4: 208*b*
  Boston Children's Hospital and, 2: 13, 34, 40, 247, 264; 3: 147–148, 153
  Boston City Hospital and, 4: 305*b*, 308*b*, 406
  Bradford and, 3: 147, 150–151
  on Buckminster Brown, 3: 150
  chronic hip disease and, 3: 147, 151
  Clinical Congress of Surgeons in North America and, 3: 116

Department for Military Orthopedics and, 4: 405–406
  early life, 3: 147
  education and training, 3: 147
  on functional inactivity, 2: 110
  on fusion in tubercular spines, 3: 148–149, 157–158, 158*b*
  on gunshot injuries, 3: 156, 156*b*
  HMS appointment, 3: 154
  HMS Orthopaedic surgery and, 1: 171
  hot pack treatment and, 2: 264
  House of the Good Samaritan and, 2: 114; 3: 148
  interest in the hip, 3: 148
  Journal of Bone and Joint Surgery editor, 3: 157–159, 160*b*, 161, 344
  legacy of, 3: 161–162
  marriage and, 3: 154
  memberships and, 3: 161
  as MGH orthopaedics chief, 2: 129–130; 3: 11*b*, 155, 227
  as MGH surgeon, 2: 99; 3: 153
  military surgeon training and, 2: 42; 4: 393, 395–396
  pathological findings in tubercular spine specimens, 3: 154–155
  Pott's Disease treatment, 3: 148–150
  private medical practice, 3: 154
  publications and research, 2: 56, 61; 3: 148, 151, 153–155
  RBBH and, 4: 406
  rehabilitation of soldiers and, 4: 396, 439, 444
  on sacroiliac joint fusion, 3: 185
  schools for disabled children, 2: 36; 3: 151, 161
  scoliosis treatment and, 2: 35, 56; 3: 151–152
  Section of Orthopaedic Surgery and, 4: 412
  treatment by Bradford, 3: 147
  US Army Medical Corps and, 4: 405
  use of orthopaedics apparatus, 3: 150–151
  Volunteer Aid Association and, 3: 152–153
  World War I and, 3: 156–157; 4: 404–405, 411
Brackett, Katherine F. Pedrick, 3: 154
Bradford, Charles F., 2: 19
Bradford, Charles Henry (1904–2000)
  Battle of Corregidor, 4: 363–364

Index

BCH Bone and Joint Service, 4: 367
Boston City Hospital and, 4: 362
Boston University Medical School appointment, 4: 366
Britten hip fusion technique and, 4: 363
civil defense and, 4: 364–366
Combat Over Corregidor, 4: *364*
Cotting School and, 4: 367
death of, 4: 368
education and training, 4: 361–362
Faulkner Hospital and, 4: 362
fracture treatment and, 4: 362
hospital appointments, 4: 364
legacy of, 4: 366–368
marriage and family, 4: 361
Massachusetts Medical Society lecture, 4: *365*, 366*b*, 367, 367*b*
Mt. Auburn Hospital and, 4: 362
poetry writing and, 4: 364
professional memberships, 4: 368
publications and research, 4: 352, 363, 365, *365*, 368
tibial spine fracture case, 4: 365
Tufts Medical School appointment, 4: 366
US Army Medical Corps and, 4: 363–364
World War II medical volunteers and, 4: 362–363
Bradford, Charles Hickling, 2: 42–43
Bradford, Edith Fiske, 2: 42; 4: 361
Bradford, Edward H. (1848–1926), 2: *19*, *39*, *44*
AOA address, 2: 24–26
as AOA president, 2: 43
as BCH surgeon-in-chief, 2: 39–40, *41*
Boston Children's Hospital and, 2: 10–11, 13, 15–16, 21, 29, 39–40
Boston City Hospital and, 4: 298, 303, 307
Boston City Hospital appointments, 2: 21, 24
Bradford Frame and, 2: 27, *27*, 30–31, *31*, 32
Buckminster Brown and, 2: 20; 3: 150
on Burrell, 4: 298–299
CDH treatment, 2: 32–33, *33*, 34
club foot apparatus, 2: 22–23, *23*
club foot treatment, 2: 22–24, 28, *28*, 29
curative workshops and, 4: 403

as dean of HMS, 1: 172–174; 2: 15, 41–42; 4: 324
death of, 2: 43–44
early life, 2: 19
education and training, 2: 19–20
European medical studies, 1: 186; 2: 20
first craniotomy performed, 2: 24–25
FitzSimmons and, 2: 255
general surgery and, 2: 24
hip disease treatment, 2: 21–22, 32
HMS appointment, 2: 21, 40–41, 428; 4: 213
House of the Good Samaritan and, 1: 128–130; 2: 21
influences on, 2: 20, 22
knee flexion contracture appliance, 2: *20*, *21*
knee valgus deformity, 2: *21*
legacy of, 2: 42–44
loss of eyesight, 2: 43
Lovett and, 2: 49
marriage and family, 2: 42
on medical education, 4: 299–301
memberships and, 2: 43
method of reducing the gibbus, 3: *149*
as MGH surgeon, 3: 266
nose and throat clinic creation, 2: 40–41
orthopaedic brace shop, 2: *22*, *22*
as orthopaedic chair, 2: 15*b*
Orthopaedic Journal Club, 3: 369
orthopaedic surgery advances, 2: 27, 36, 39–40
Orthopedic Surgery, 4: 318
osteotomies and, 2: 29, 34
poliomyelitis treatment, 2: 264
on Pott's Disease, 3: 148
on preventative measures, 2: 36
private medical practice and, 1: 176
as professor of orthopaedic surgery, 1: 69, 111, 141, 143, 171
"Progress in Orthopaedic Surgery" series, 2: 43, 297
schools for disabled children, 2: 36–39, 67, 97, 308; 3: 151
scientific study and, 1: 256
scoliosis treatment, 2: *35*, *35*, *36*, 58
Sever and, 2: 92
Soutter and, 2: 292, 297
as surgical house officer at MGH, 2: 20

teaching hospitals and, 1: 174, 187–188
Treatise on Orthopaedic Surgery, A, 1: 108, 143; 2: 29–30, 43, 50, *50*, 51
treatment of Brackett, 3: 147
tuberculosis treatment, 2: 32
Bradford, Edward H., Jr., 2: 42
Bradford, Edward, Jr., 4: 361
Bradford, Eliza Edes Hickling, 2: 19
Bradford, Elizabeth, 2: 42; 4: 361, 368
Bradford, Gamaliel, 1: 96
Bradford, Mary Lythgoe, 4: 361
Bradford, Robert Fiske, 2: 42
Bradford, William, 2: 19
Bradford Frame, 2: 27, *27*, 30–31, *31*, 32
Bradlee, Helen C., 3: 18
Bradlee, J. Putnam, 3: 18
Bradley, Alfred E., 4: 416
Bradley, John, 3: 289
Braintree HealthSouth Hospital, 4: 194
Brase, D. W., 4: 167
Braswell, Margaret, 2: 349
Braunwald, Eugene, 4: 119
Brazelton, T. Berry, 2: 385
Breed's Hill (Bunker Hill), 1: 18, *18*
Breene, R. G., 4: 93
Bremer, John L., 4: *6*
Brendze, R., 3: *461*
Brengle, Fred E., 3: 463
Brengle, Joan, 3: 463
Brewster, Albert H. (1892–1988), 2: *222*
AAOS and, 4: 337
Boston Children's Hospital and, 2: 222–223, 231, 252, 274; 4: 60, 338
countersinking the talus, 2: 228, 283
Crippled Children's Clinic and, 2: 230, 287
death of, 2: 231
donations to Boston Medical Library, 2: 271
education and training, 2: 221
foot deformity treatment, 2: 228–229
grand rounds and, 2: 230
HMS appointment, 2: 222–223; 4: 60
Marlborough Medical Associates and, 2: 269, 299
marriage and family, 2: 231
New England Peabody Home for Crippled Children and, 2: 230–231
Osgood tribute, 2: 136

PBBH and, 2: 222; 4: 16–18, 20, 110
private medical practice, 2: 146, 230, *230*
professional memberships and, 2: 230
publications of, 2: 79, 223, 225, 227–229; 4: 240
scoliosis treatment, 2: 223–228
on supracondylar fractures of the humerus, 2: 229
turnbuckle jacket and, 2: 223–224, *224*, 225, 227
World War I service and, 2: 221–222
Brewster, Albert H., Jr., 2: 231
Brewster, Elsie Estelle Carter, 2: 231
Brewster, Nancy, 2: 231
Brezinski, Mark, 4: 194
Brick, Gregory W., 4: 193, 195*b*
Brickley-Parsons, D., 2: 328
Bridges, Miss, 3: 133
Brigham, Elizabeth Fay, 4: vii, 1*b*, 23*b*, 24, 39*b*
Brigham, John Bent, 4: 1*b*
Brigham, Peter Bent, 4: 1, 1*b*, 2, 2*b*, 4–5, 22
Brigham, Robert Breck, 4: vii, 22, 23*b*, 24, 39*b*
Brigham, Uriah, 4: 1*b*
Brigham and Women's Hospital (BWH), 4: vii, *120, 122, 192, 196*
  acute rehabilitation service, 4: 191
  Administrative Building, 4: *191*
  Ambulatory building, 4: *193*
  Ambulatory Care Center, 4: *193*, 194
  Bornstein Family Amphitheater, 4: *191*
  capitellocondylar total elbow replacements, 4: 146–147
  Carl J. and Ruth Shapiro Cardiovascular Center, 4: *195*
  carpal tunnel syndrome study, 2: 375
  Cartilage Repair Center, 4: 195*b*
  Center for Molecular Orthopaedics, 4: 194, 195*b*
  clinical and research faculty, 4: 195*b*
  Faulkner Hospital, 4: 194, *194*
  Foot and Ankle Center, 4: 194
  formation of, 4: 43, 113–114, 119–120, 127
  fundraising for, 4: 118
  HCORP and, 1: 213, 215
  Mary Horrigan Conner's Center for Women's Health, 4: *194*
  modernization of, 4: 191–196
  Musculoskeletal (MSK) Research Center, 4: 195*b*
  naming of, 4: 119, 123
  new facility construction, 4: 118–119, 122, 132
  opening of, 4: 121, *123*
  Orthopaedic and Arthritis Center, 4: 121, 123, 195*b*
  orthopaedic biomechanics laboratory, 4: 137–138
  orthopaedic chairmen at, 4: 196*b*
  orthopaedic grand rounds in, 4: 191
  orthopaedic research laboratory and, 4: 194
  orthopaedic surgery department, 1: 171; 4: 43, 113–115, 121
  orthopaedics fellowships, 1: 241
  orthopaedics residencies, 1: 217–218, 223–224, 241–242
  professional staff committee, 4: 132
  professorships at, 4: 195*b*
  RBBH as specialty arthritis hospital in, 4: 122–123
  research at, 4: 121
  Skeletal Biology Laboratory, 4: 195*b*
  staffing of, 4: 193–196
  surgeon-scholars at, 4: 143, 163, 193–194, 195*b*
  surgical caseloads at, 4: 194–195
  Tissue Engineering Laboratory, 4: 195*b*
  Total Joint Replacement Registry, 4: 141, *172*, 173
  transition period at, 4: 113–118, 132
  work with prosthetic devices at, 4: 122
Brigham and Women's Physician Organization (BWPO), 4: 192
Brigham and Women's/Mass General Health Care Center (Foxboro), 4: 194
Brigham Anesthesia Associates, 4: 22
Brigham Family, 4: 1*b*
Brigham Orthopaedic Foundation (BOF), 4: 123, 172, 191–192
Brigham Orthopedic Associates (BOA), 4: 123, 172, 191–192
British 31st General Hospital, 4: 485
British Base Hospital No. 12 (Rouen, France), 3: 166
British Expeditionary Forces (BEF)
  American Medical Corps and, 4: 420
  American medical volunteers and, 4: 405*b*, 425
  Base Hospital No. 5 and, 4: 420
  Harvard Unit and, 1: 256; 4: 10, 391, 438
  physician deaths in, 4: 425
  use of AEF base hospitals, 4: 420
British hospitals
  American surgeon-volunteers in, 4: 409
  documentation and, 4: 407
  general scheme of, 4: *414*
  increase in military, 4: 454
  orthopaedic surgery and, 4: 409
  registrars in, 4: 12
  World War I and, 4: 407, 409, 454
British Orthopaedic Association, 1: xxiv; 2: 137; 3: 345, 360; 4: 363, *404*
British Red Cross, 4: 399, 401
British Royal Army Medical Corps, 4: 393
British Society for Surgery of the Hand, 4: 95
Broderick, Thomas F., 3: 209, 332–333
Brodhurst, Bernard Edward, 1: 83, 106
Brodie, Sir Benjamin Collins, 1: 106
bronchitis, 2: 4
Bronfin, Isidore D., 4: 206, 209
Brooks, Barney, 3: 165–167, 170, *171*; 4: 178
Brooks, Charles, 1: 239
Brostrom, Frank, 2: 78, 110
Browder, N. C., 1: 259
Brower, Thomas D., 1: 162; 3: 382
Brown, Anna Ball, 1: 95
Brown, Arnold Welles, 1: 98
Brown, Buckminster (1819–1891), 1: *105*
  advancement of Harvard Medical School and, 1: 111
  advocacy for disabled children, 1: 107, 109, 126
  Boston Dispensary and, 2: 306
  Boston Orthopedic Institution and, 1: 107, 118, 120–122
  congenital hip dislocation treatment, 1: 108
  death of, 1: 111
  Edward H. Bradford and, 2: 20, 22
  European medical studies, 1: 105–106, 186
  forward-thinking treatment of, 1: 107–108
  House of the Good Samaritan and, 1: 107, 121–122, 125–128; 2: 49
  long-term treatment and, 2: 25
  marriage and, 1: 107

Index

orthopaedic specialization of, 1: 99, 107–108
orthopaedic treatment advances, 1: 118; 2: 26–27, 32
Pott's Disease and, 1: 97, 105, 109
publications of, 1: 110*b*, 120, *120*, 121
scoliosis brace and, 1: 109
Brown, Charles H., Jr., 4: 193, 195*b*
Brown, Douglas, 2: 163
Brown, Francis Henry
Boston Children's Hospital and, 2: 5, *5*, 6, 9–10, 21
on hospital construction, 2: 5
orthopaedics expertise, 2: 9
Brown, George, 1: 98
Brown, Jabez, 1: 95
Brown, John Ball (1784–1862), 1: *95, 102*
apparatus used for knee contracture, 1: *98*
Boston dispensary and, 1: 293
Boston Orthopedic Institution and, 1: 99–100, 107, 113–122; 3: 30
club foot treatment, 2: 36
correction of spine deformities, 1: 97–98, 100
death of, 1: 103, 122
early telemedicine by, 1: 100
education and training, 1: 95–96
establishment of orthopaedics as specialty, 1: 95–96, 98–99, 119
founding of Boston Orthopedic Institution, 1: xxiv
George Parkman and, 1: 296
legacy of, 1: 102–103
marriage and family, 1: 96–98
opening of orthopaedic specialty hospital, 1: 99
orthopaedic surgery and, 1: 99–102, 113; 2: 25–26
publications of, 1: 102*b*, 120, *120*, 121
Remarks on the Operation for the Cure of Club Feet with Cases, 1: 100
Report of Cases in the Orthopedic Infirmary of the City of Boston, 1: *120*
surgical appointments, 1: 96–97
Brown, John Warren, 1: 97
Brown, Larry, 4: 364
Brown, Lloyd T. (1880–1961), 4: *81*
on body mechanics and rheumatoid disease, 4: 82–83
Boston Children's Hospital and, 4: 82

Boston City Hospital and, 4: 406
Burrage Hospital and, 4: 226
Children's Island Sanitorium and, 4: 87
chronic disease treatment and, 4: 52
club foot treatment, 4: 84
congenital club foot and, 4: 81–82, *83*, 87
death of, 4: 39, 87*b*
education and training, 4: 81–82
HMS appointment, 2: 223; 4: 60, 86
hospital appointments, 4: 83
marriage and family, 4: 83, 87
medical officer teaching, 4: 84
MGH and, 4: 82, 84, 86
military surgeon training and, 2: 42
orthopaedics surgery and, 2: 66; 3: 268
Orthopedics and Body Mechanics Committee, 4: 235
posture research and, 4: 84, *84*, 85–86, 233
private medical practice, 4: 82
professional memberships, 4: 87, 87*b*
publications and research, 2: 297; 3: 91; 4: 82–84, 87
RBBH and, 3: 257; 4: vii, 25, 31–34, 36, 45, 79, 86–87, 93, 111, 406
RBBH Emergency Campaign speech, 4: 32, 32*b*
rehabilitation of soldiers and, 4: 444
retirement and, 4: 36
Brown, Marian Epes Wigglesworth, 4: 83
Brown, Percy E., 2: 16, 54; 3: 99
Brown, Rebecca Warren, 1: 96, 98
Brown, Sarah Alvord Newcomb, 1: 107
Brown, Sarah Tyler Meigs, 3: 257, 263
Brown, T., 3: 209, 214
Brown, Thornton (1913–2000), 1: *203*; 3: *257, 263, 461*
as AOA president, 3: 262, *262*, 263
back pain research and, 3: 257–258, *258*, 259–260
on Boston and orthopaedics, 1: 93; 2: 324
on changes at MGH Orthopaedic Service, 3: 453*b*–458*b*
Children's Hospital/MGH combined program and, 3: 257
death of, 3: 263

early life, 3: 257
education and training, 3: 257
Journal of Bone and Joint Surgery editor, 3: 260–262, 346
marriage and family, 3: 257
Massachusetts General Hospital, 1955–1980, The, 3: 299
as MGH orthopaedics chief, 3: 11*b*, 202, 227, *259*, 459
MGH residents and, 3: *259, 260, 459*
as MGH surgeon, 3: 257, 398*b*
Milton Hospital and, 3: 257
on Mt. Sinai Hospital, 4: 201–202
Norton-Brown spinal brace, 3: 317–319
"Orthopaedics at Harvard," 1: 195; 2: 271
private medical practice, 1: 203
publications and research, 3: 257–260, 317, 455*b*
RBBH and, 4: 37, 40
World War II service, 3: 257
Brown University Medical School, 3: 400–401
Browne, Hablot Knight, 1: *21*
Browne & Nichols School, 2: 83, 97
Brubacher, Jacob W., 3: 463*b*
Brugler, Guy, 2: 214
Brunschwig, Hieronymus, 4: 469
Bruschart, Thomas, 3: 431
Bryant, Henry, 3: 30
Bryant, Thomas, 1: 83
Buchanan, J. Robert, 3: 391
Buchbinder, Rachelle, 3: 437
Buchman, Frank N. D., 4: 57
Buchmanism, 4: 57
Bucholz, Carl Hermann (1874–unk.), 3: *264*
back pain research and, 3: 203
education and training, 3: 264
on exercise treatment of paralysis, 3: 265
HMS appointment, 3: 265
legacy of, 3: 269
as MGH surgeon, 3: 268
publications and research, 2: 136, 297
Therapeutic Exercise and Massage, 3: 269
World War I and, 3: 268
Zander's medico-mechanical department and, 3: 71, 264–266, 266*t*, 267, 268*b*
Buck, Emily Jane, 2: 220
Buck's traction, 1: 80
Budd, J. W., 4: 102
Bulfinch, Charles, 1: 28, 41; 3: 10–11

Bulfinch Building (MGH), 1: *41*; 3: *9*, *13*, 15, *16*, 22, *60*, 70*b*
Bull, Charles, 3: 77
Bullard, S. E., 2: 244
Bunker Hill Monument Committee, 1: 68
Bunnin, Beverly D., 4: 101
Burgess, Earnest M., 3: 248
Burke, Dennis W., 3: 398, 460*b*, 464*b*
Burke, John, 3: 62, 253, 458*b*
burn care, 3: 336
Burne, F., 2: 98
Burnett, Joseph H. (1892–1963)
    BCH Bone and Joint Service, 4: 307, 328, 369, 371
    Boston City Hospital and, 4: 347, 368, 370–371
    Boston University Medical School appointment, 4: 368
    carpal scaphoid fracture case, 4: 368
    death of, 4: 371
    education and training, 4: 368
    football injury research, 4: 370, *370*
    HMS appointment, 4: 368
    marriage and, 4: 371
    professional memberships, 4: 371
    publications and research, 4: 368–370, *370*
    scaphoid fracture research, 4: 360, 368–369
    sports medicine and, 4: 368–370
Burnett, Margaret Rogers, 4: 371
Burns, Frances, 2: 260, 264
Burns, John, 3: *458*
Burns, Mary, 2: 214
Burrage Hospital, 4: 226, *227*
Burrell, Herbert L., 4: 298–299, *299*, 300–301, 307
Burrell-Cotton operation, 4: 329
Burwell, C. Sidney, 1: 131, 158, 179, 272; 4: 362
Burwell, Sterling, 4: 472
Buschenfeldt, Karl W., 3: 317
Butler, Allan M., 3: 301
Butler, Fergus A., 4: 53
BWH. *See* Brigham and Women's Hospital (BWH)
Bygrave, Elizabeth Clark, 2: 92, 97
Byrne, John, 2: 250
Byrne, John J., 4: 303

C

Cabot, Arthur Tracy, 2: 11; 3: 53–54, 56
Cabot, Richard C., 2: 320
Cabot, Samuel, 3: 25, *31*

Cadet Nursing Corps, 4: 467
calcaneal apophysitis (Sever's Disease)
    case study of, 2: 89
    characteristics of, 2: 89
    heel pain in children, 2: 89
    Sever's study of, 2: 88–90, 100
    x-ray appearance of, 2: *88*
calcaneovalgus deformity, 2: 92
calcar femorale, 3: 39, *39*
Calderwood, Carmelita, 3: 303
Calderwood's Orthopedic Nursing (Larson and Gould), 3: 303
Caldwell, Guy A., 1: 162; 2: 183
Calhoun, John C., 1: 307
Calvé, Jacques, 2: 103–104
Cambridge Hospital, 1: 220; 3: 396–397, 399
Camp, Walter, 1: 248, *248*
Camp Blanding Station Hospital, 4: 475
Camp Devens (Mass.), 4: 426, 437, 452
Camp Kilmer (N.J.), 4: 475
Camp Taylor (Kentucky), 4: 452
Camp Wikoff (Montauk Point, LI), 4: 310–311
Campbell, Crawford J., 1: 216; 3: 385–386, 392, 461, *462*
Campbell, Douglas, 3: 431
Campbell, W., 2: 91
Campbell, Willis, 2: 105, 294
Campbell Clinic, 4: 356
Canadian Board of Certification for Prosthetics and Orthotics, 2: 347
Canadian Orthopaedic Association, 2: 137, 183
Canadian Orthopaedic Research Society, 3: 262
Cannon, Bradford, 3: 336
Cannon, Walter B., 4: 6, 299, 420
Cannon, Walter W., 3: 97
capitellocondylar total elbow prosthesis, 4: 145, *145*, 146–147
carbolic acid treatment, 1: 82–83, *84*
CareGroup, 1: 233; 4: 281, 284
Carlos Otis Stratton Mountain Clinic, 3: 311
Carnett, John B., 4: 235–236
Carney Hospital, 3: *78*
    adult orthopaedic clinic at, 2: 101; 3: 78
    Goldthwait and, 3: 78, 80; 4: 45
    internships at, 1: 186, 189
    Lovett and, 2: 49
    MacAusland and, 3: 308; 4: 45
    orthopaedics residencies, 4: 378
    Painter and, 4: 44–45, 224
    posture clinic at, 4: 86
    Rogers (Mark) and, 4: 224
    Sullivan and, 4: 343

    testing of foot strength apparatus, 2: 102
    treatment of adults and children in, 2: 4
    Tufts clinical instruction at, 4: 45
Carothers, Charles O., 4: 356
carpal bones, 3: 101–102
carpal tunnel syndrome
    computer use and, 4: 186
    familial bilateral, 3: 321
    genetics in, 4: 186
    research in, 2: 375; 3: 402
    self-assessment of, 4: 184–185
    wrist position and, 3: 403
Carpenter, G. K., 2: 438
Carr, Charles F., 3: 363–364
Carrie M. Hall Nurses Residence, 4: 20
Carroll, Norris, 2: 305
Carroll, Robert, 2: 251
Carter, Dennis, 3: 397
cartilage transplantation, 2: 294
Case Western Reserve University School of Medicine, 3: 337
Casemyr, Natalie E.J., 3: 463*b*
Casino Boulogne-sur-Mer, 4: *426*, *427*, *428*
Caspari, Richard B., 2: 279
Casscells, Ward, 3: 446
Cassella, Mickey, 2: 178–180, 182
Castle, A. C., 1: 314–317
Castleman, Benjamin, 2: 320; 3: 205, 259
Catastrophe, The, 1: *78*
Catharina Ormandy Professorship, 2: 438, 439*b*
Cats-Baril, William L., 3: 379, *379*
Cattell, Richard B., 4: 275–276
Cave, Edwin F. (1896–1976), 1: *270*; 3: *270*, *271*, *273*; 4: *491*
    on Achilles tendon injury, 3: 272
    AOA presidential address and, 3: 274, *274*
    Bankart procedure and, 3: 351, *351*
    on Barr's orthopaedic research, 3: 211
    Children's Hospital/MGH combined program and, 3: 270
    death of, 3: 276, 448
    early life, 3: 270
    education and training, 3: 270
    endowed lectures and, 3: 275
    femoral neck fracture treatment, 3: 185–186, *186*
    5th General Hospital and, 4: 484
    as Fracture Clinic chief, 3: 60*b*, 241, 272

Index

Fractures and Other Injuries, 3: 273, *273*; 4: 356
hip nailing and, 3: 237
HMS appointment, 2: 223; 3: 272; 4: 60–61
Joint Committee for the Study of Surgical Materials and, 3: 210
knee arthrotomy research, 3: 351
marriage and family, 3: 271, 276
on measuring and recording joint function, 3: 270
as MGH surgeon, 3: 187, 192, 270–271
New England Peabody Home for Crippled Children and, 2: 270
105th General Hospital and, 4: 489
orthopaedics education and, 3: 272–274
private medical practice, 3: 271–272
professional honors, 3: 275*b*, 276
publications and research, 2: 297; 3: 270, 272, 366
Scudder Oration on Trauma, 3: 63
Smith-Petersen and, 3: 270
34th Infantry Division and, 4: 484
torn ligaments in the knee research, 3: 272
on trauma, 3: 275–276
Trauma Management, 3: 62, 253, 273
on Van Gorder, 3: 368
World War II service, 1: 270; 3: 271; 4: 17
Cave, Joan Tozzer Lincoln, 3: 276
Cave, Louise Fessenden, 3: 271, 276
cavus feet, 2: 228–229
CDH. *See* congenital dislocated hips (CDH)
celastic body jackets, 2: 178
Center for Human Simulation, 4: 173
Center of Healing Arts, 3: 423
Central States Orthopedic Club, 4: 393
cerebral palsy
   Banks and, 2: 196–200
   Boston Children's Hospital and, 2: 171–172
   children and, 2: 171–172, 196–198, 300–301
   experimental approaches to, 3: 164
   foot surgery in, 2: 229
   Green and, 2: 171–172, 196–200
   Grice procedure and, 2: 212
   hamstring lengthening and, 2: 172
   Lovett and, 2: 51
   research in, 2: 196, 401
   sensory deficits in children's hands, 2: 300–301, *301*
   spinal deformities in, 2: 370
   surgery for, 2: 197–198
   treatment of, 2: 172, 196–200, 300–301
   triple arthrodesis (Hoke type) and, 2: 172
Cerebral Palsy and Spasticity Center (Children's Hospital), 2: 406
Cerebral Palsy Clinic (Children's Hospital), 2: 402, 406, 409
cerebrospinal meningitis, 2: 4
"Certain Aspects of Infantile Paralysis" (Lovett and Martin), 2: *70*
Cervical Spine Research Society, 3: *249*, 321; 4: 265, 269
Chandler, Betsy McCombs, 3: 280
Chandler, Fremont A., 2: 176, 183
Chandler, Hugh P. (1931–2014), 3: *277–278*, 280, *461*
   Aufranc Fellowship and, 3: 277
   Bone Stock Deficiency in Total Hip Replacement, 3: 278–279
   Children's Hospital/MGH combined program and, 3: 277
   death of, 3: 280
   direct lateral approach to the hip and, 3: 277–278, *278*
   early life, 3: 277
   education and training, 3: 277
   marriage and family, 3: 280
   as MGH surgeon, 3: 244, 277, 398*b*
   pelvic osteolysis with acetabular replacement case, 3: 279
   publications and research, 3: 278
   recognition of, 3: 279–280
   sailing and, 3: 280
Channing, Walter, 1: 296, 299, 302
Chanoff, David, 4: *265*
Chapin, Mrs. Henry B., 1: 129
Chaplan, Ronald N., 4: 163, 193
Chapman, Earle, 3: 241
Chapman, Mabel C., 3: 304
Charcot, Jean-Martin, 3: 142
Charitable Surgical Institution, 3: 30
Charleston Naval Hospital, 3: 191; 4: 246
Charnley, John, 2: 239
Charnley, Sir John, 3: 218–220
Chase, Henry, 3: 101
Cheal, Edward, 4: 263
Cheever, Charles A., 1: 96
Cheever, David W., 4: *297*
   on Bigelow, 3: 39, 44
   Boston City Hospital and, 4: 298, 303–304
   as Boston City Hospital surgeon-in-chief, 4: 298, 306–307
   British Expeditionary Forces and, 4: 9–10
   on Goldthwait, 3: 79
   HMS appointment, 3: 94; 4: 298, 307
   PBBH and, 4: 5, 10–11, 17
Chelsea Memorial Hospital, 2: 102; 3: 314
Chelsea Naval Hospital, 4: 47–48, 97
chemotherapy, 2: 422–423
Chen, Chien-Min, 3: 368
Chernack, Robert, 4: 194, 195*b*
Cheselden, William, 1: 6, 36
Chessler, Robert, 1: xxii
Chest Wall and Spinal Deformity Study Group, 2: 361–362
Cheyne, W. Watson, 1: *83*
Chicago Polyclinic, 2: 50
Chicago Shriner's Hospital, 2: 355
Chicago University, 3: 175
Chickahominy fever, 3: 44
Child, C. Gardner, 4: 303
children
   bone granuloma and, 2: 171
   cerebral palsy and, 2: 171–172, 196–198, 300–301
   club foot and, 1: xxii, 118–119; 2: 12*t*, 15*t*, 22–23, 145
   development of hospitals for, 2: 3–4
   early treatment of, 1: xxii
   growth disturbances with chronic arthritis, 4: 56
   heel pain in, 2: 89
   hip disease and, 2: 52
   juvenile idiopathic arthritis and, 2: 164, 171, 350
   kyphosis and, 2: 343–345
   mortality, 2: 4–5, 15
   muscle atrophy in, 2: 110
   national health initiatives, 4: 235–236
   orthopaedic rehabilitation and, 1: 107, 121
   osteochondritis dissecans in, 2: 194–195
   osteomyelitis in, 2: 169
   physical therapy and, 2: 61, 107
   poliomyelitis and, 1: 191; 2: 61, 189–191, 210, 213
   posture and, 4: 233–234, *234*, 235, *236*
   rheumatic heart disease and, 1: 130

schools for disabled, 2: 36–39, 97
spinal deformities and, 1: xxi, xxii, 97–98, 123
spinal tuberculosis and, 1: 108
Sprengel deformity, 2: 195, *196*
state clinics for crippled, 2: 107, 221
trauma and, 2: 359, 365, 368, 378, 385
use of ether, 1: 63
children, disabled. *See* disabled children
Children's Convalescent Home, 2: 84
Children's Hospital (Boston, Mass.), 2: 4–16. *See also* Boston Children's Hospital (BCH)
Children's Hospital Medical Center, 4: 113–114. *See also* Boston Children's Hospital (BCH)
Children's Hospital of Philadelphia (CHOP), 2: 3–5, 424
Children's Infirmary, 2: 3
Children's Island Sanitorium, 4: 87
Children's Medical Center (Wellesley), 2: 314
Children's Memorial Hospital (Chicago), 2: 302
Children's Sports Injury Prevention Fund, 2: 439*b*
Children's Sunlight Hospital (Scituate), 3: 307
Childress, Harold M., 4: 335
Chiodo, Christopher, 4: 190*b*, 194
Chipman, W. W., 3: 113*b*
chloroform, 1: 62–63, 82; 3: 15, 31
Choate, Rufus, 1: 307
Choate Hospital, 2: 256
cholera epidemic, 1: 295; 4: 293
chondrocytes, 3: 327, 442, 444–445, 449
chondrodysplasia, 4: 218–220
chondrosarcoma, 2: 237; 3: 390, 406
Christian, Henry A., 1: 173–174, 176; 4: 4, 6, 9, 16, 79, 104
Christophe, Kenneth, 4: 40, 89
chronic diseases
anatomy and, 3: 91
body mechanics and, 3: 81, 91
bone and joint disorders, 1: 153; 3: 85, 90
faulty body mechanics and, 3: 91
Goldthwait and, 4: 39*b*, 52
orthopaedic surgeons and, 4: 46, 53
posture and, 4: 52, 86
prevention of, 3: 90

RBBH and, 4: 25*b*, 27, 30, 30*b*, 32*b*, 33, 36, 39*b*, 45, 86
rheumatoid arthritis and, 4: 36
travel abroad and, 1: 72
chronic regional pain syndrome (CRPS), 2: 68
Chronicle of Boston Jewry, A (Ehrenfried), 4: 220
Chuinard, Eldon G., 1: 162
Chung, Kevin C., 3: 410
Church, Benjamin, 1: 15–16
Churchill, Edward D., 1: 198–199; 2: 322; 3: 1; 4: 302, 470–471, *472*
Churchill, Edward H., 2: 79
Churchill, Winston, 4: 479
chymopapain, 3: 254–255, 397, 419, *421*
Civale, Jean, 3: 41
Clark, Charles, 4: 174
Clark, Dean A., 4: 158
Clark, H. G., 3: *31*
Clark, John G., 3: 113*b*, 122, 355
Clarke, Joseph Taylor, 4: 448
Clay, Lucius D., 2: 260, 264
Clayton, Mack, 4: 243
cleidocranial dysostosis, 2: 254
Cleveland, Grover, 2: 72
Cleveland, Mather, 3: 196
Clifford, John H., 1: 307
Clifton Springs Sanatorium, 3: 88; 4: 52–53
Cline, Henry, 1: 33–34, 37
Clinical Biomechanics of the Spine (White and Panjabi), 4: 262
Clinical Congress of Surgeons in North America, 3: 116, 123
Clinical Orthopaedic Examination (McRae), 1: 167
Cloos, David W., 4: 163, 193
clover leaf rod, 3: 272
club foot
apparatus for, 1: 98, 100, 106; 2: *23*, 24; 4: *83*
Bradford and, 2: 22–24, 28–29
correction of, 1: *98*, 100, *100*, *101*, 106; 2: 36
correction of bilateral, 2: *29*
Denis Browne splint, 2: 208
early diagnosis and treatment for, 1: 100; 2: 28–29
medial deltoid ligament release, 2: 145
nonoperative treatment of, 2: 28; 4: 216
Ober and, 2: 145
osteotomies and, 2: 29
pathological findings and, 3: 54
plantar fasciotomy and, 2: 24

Stromeyer's subcutaneous tenotomy for, 1: 118, *118*
tarsectomy and, 2: 23
tenotomy and, 1: 106, 118; 2: 25–26
Cobb, John, 2: 225–226
Cochran, Robert C., 4: 438–439
Cochrane, William A., 3: 244, 302, 371, *371*, 372
Codman, Amory, 2: 182
Codman, Catherine, 1: 50, *129*, 130
Codman, Elizabeth Hand, 3: 93
Codman, Ernest A. (1869–1940), 3: *93, 103, 105, 115, 143*
abdominal surgery and, 3: 108
as anatomy assistant at HMS, 2: 114
anesthesia and, 3: 95, *95*, 96
bone sarcomas and, 3: 136–140, 140*b*, 141–142, 145; 4: 102
on brachial plexus injury, 2: 96
Camp Taylor base hospital and, 4: 452
cartoon of Back Bay public, 3: 121, *121*, 122, *122*
clinical congress meeting, 3: 116
Committee on Standardization of Hospitals and, 3: 112, 113*b*, 115–116, 123–124
death of, 2: 116; 3: 145–146
dedication of headstone, 3: *145*, 146
on diagnosis with x-rays, 3: 99
duodenal ulcer and, 3: 108
early life, 3: 93
education and training, 3: 93–95
End-Result Idea, 1: 194; 2: 135; 3: 110–111, *111*, 112, 114, 116, *116*, 118–119, 119*b*, 120, 122–126, *126*, 127*b*, 128–131, 136; 4: 12, 141
fluoroscope and, 2: 307
forward-thinking of, 3: 135–136
Fracture Course and, 3: 62
fracture treatment and, 3: 101–102
Halifax Harbor explosion and, 3: 132–135
Harvard Medical Association letter, 3: 119*b*
HMS appointment, 3: 96, 99
Hospital Efficiency meeting, 3: 120–122
interest in hunting and fishing, 3: 94, 143–145
interest in sprains, 3: 100–102
interest in subacromial bursitis, 3: 104–105, 107–109

Index

interest in subdeltoid bursa, 3: 95, 98, 103–104, *104*, 105, 108
legacy of, 3: 145–146
life history chart, 3: *106*
marriage and, 3: 142–143
memberships and, 3: 65
MGH internship and, 3: 95–96
as MGH surgeon, 1: 190, 194; 3: 99, 112, 118, 142, 266
on monetary value of surgeon services, 3: 129–130
operating in the Bigelow Amphitheatre, 3: *107*
personal case documentation, 3: 126, 128–130
Philadelphia Medical Society address, 3: 117*b*–118*b*
private hospital ideals, 3: 114*b*, 115
private hospital of, 3: 112, 114, 116, 118, 135
private practice and, 3: 136
publication of x-rays, 3: 97, *97*, 98, *99*
publications and research, 3: 99–104, *104*, 108–112, 115–116, 125, 136, 139–142
resolution honoring, 3: 144*b*, 146
on safety of x-rays, 3: 99–100
Shoulder, 2: 239; 3: 105, 115, 122, 140*b*
shoulder and, 3: 103–105, 107–110, 354
as skiagrapher at BCH, 2: 16, 114; 3: 96–99, 142
Study in Hospital Efficiency, 3: 125, *125*, 127*b*, 128–131
surgical scissor design, 3: *138*
Treatment of Fractures, 3: 56
World War I and, 3: 132, 135
Codman, John, 3: 94, 108, 142
Codman, Katherine Bowditch, 3: 142–143, 144*b*, 145
Codman, William Combs, 3: 93
Codman Center for Clinical Effectiveness in Surgery, 3: 146
Codman Hospital, 3: 112, 114, 116, 118, *126*, 135
Codman's Paradox, 3: 105
Cohen, Jonathan, 1: 114
Cohen, Jonathan (1915–2003), 2: *179*
as assistant pathologist, 2: 234
on Barr, 3: 206–207
bone irradiation research, 2: 237, *237*
bone lesions and tumor research, 2: 236

book reviews by, 2: 239, 240*b*
Boston Children's Hospital and, 2: 233–236, 301; 4: 126, 245
Boston Orthopedic Institution and, 1: 121
death of, 2: 241
education and training, 2: 231
Farber and, 2: 235–236
Fourth Portable Surgical Hospital (4PSH) and, 2: 232–233
Fourth Portable Surgical Hospital's Service in the War against Japan, 2: 232–233
Green and, 2: 234–235
HMS appointment, 2: 233
Jewish Hospital (St. Louis) and, 2: 231
Journal of Bone and Joint Surgery editor, 2: 238–240; 3: 346
marriage and family, 2: 241
metal implants and, 2: 237–238
MGH and, 2: 233
mobile army surgical hospitals (MASHs) and, 2: 231
105th General Hospital and, 4: 489
orthopaedic research laboratory and, 2: 234
orthopaedic surgery and, 2: 235
professional memberships, 2: 240–241
publications and research, 2: 233–234, 236, 239, *239*; 3: *216*; 4: 102
publications of, 2: 236*b*
World War II service, 2: 231–233
Cohen, Louise Alden, 2: 241
Cohen, Mark S., 3: 431
Cohnheim, Julius, 1: 82
Coleman, Sherman, 2: 302
college athletes. *See also* Harvard athletics
Arthur L. Boland and, 1: 286
Augustus Thorndike and, 1: 274
Bill of Rights for, 1: 274, 280, 280*b*
Coller, Fred A., 2: 119; 4: 389*b*
Colles fracture, 2: 47; 3: 99
Collins, Abigail, 1: 24
Collins, John, 1: 24, 31
Collis P. Huntington Memorial Hospital for Cancer Research, 1: 87
Colonna, Paul C., 2: 183; 3: 208
Colton, Gardner Quincy, 1: 56
Colton, Theodore, 3: 253
Combat Over Corregidor (Bradford), 4: *364*
Combined Jewish Philanthropies (CJP), 4: 168

Committee F-4 on Surgical Implants, 3: 210
Committee for International Activities (POS), 2: 425
Committee of Correspondence, 1: 16
Committee of the Colonization of Society, 1: 239
Committee of Undergraduate Training (AOA), 2: 183
Committee on Education of the American Medical Association, 2: 41
Committee on Industrial Injuries, 3: 63
Committee on Recording Lateral Curvature, 2: 247
Committee on Staff Reorganization and Office Building (King Committee). *See* King Report (MGH)
Committee on Standardization of Hospitals, 3: 112, 113*b*, 115–116, 123–125, 131
Committee on Surgical Implants, 2: 238
Committee on Trauma, 2: 131; 3: 63
compartment syndrome, 2: 249–250; 3: 417–418
Compere, Edward, 2: 300
compound fractures
amputation and, 1: 54, 68
Boston City Hospital outcomes, 4: *335*, 337
Committee on Fractures and, 3: 64
fracture boxes and, 1: 80
immobilization methods, 4: 399
Lister's antisepsis dressings and, 1: 84–85; 3: 59
military orthopaedics and, 2: 120; 3: 64; 4: 391, 399, 409, 423*b*, 434
orthopaedic treatment for, 4: 464
surgery and, 4: 320, 321*b*–322*b*
computed tomography (CT), 2: 365, 389, 410–411; 3: 254
Conant, William M. (1856–1937), 1: 248
Concord, Mass., 1: 17–18
concussions
athletes and, 2: 385
football and, 1: 247, 254, 274–275
signs and symptoms of, 1: 287*t*
three knockout rule, 1: 275
treatment of, 1: 286–287
congenital dislocated hips (CDH)
Allison and, 3: 164, 175
AOA Commission on, 3: 234

Bradford and, 2: 32–34
Buckminster Brown and, 1: 108
closed manipulation, 2: 33–34
Guérin's method for, 1: 106–107
open reductions, 2: 33;
   3: 233–234
reduction procedures, 3: 234–235
reductions reviewed by the AOA Commission, 3: 232–233, 233*t*
treatment of, 2: 32–33
use of shelf procedure, 2: 151
congenital pseudarthrosis of the tibia, 2: 172–176
congenital torticollis, 2: 256, 258
Conn, A., 2: 334–335
Conn, Harold R., 4: 473
Conquest of Cancer by Radium and Other Methods, The (Quigley), 1: 275
Conservational Hip Outcomes Research (ANCHOR) Group, 2: 392, *393*
Constable, John D., 3: 321
Constructive Surgery of the Hip (Aufranc), 3: 244, *246*
Continental Hospital (Boston), 1: 24
Converse, Elizabeth, 3: 339
Converse, Frederick S., 3: 339
Conway, James, 2: 305
Conwell, H. Earle, 3: 191
Cook, Robert J., 2: 438
Cooke, John, 3: 193*b*, 238
Cooksey, Eunice, 2: 247
Coonse, G. Kenneth (1897–1951)
   Aufranc and, 4: 372–373
   BCH Bone and Joint Service, 4: 373
   death of, 4: 375
   education and training, 4: 371
   HMS appointment, 3: 237; 4: 371, 373
   hospital appointments, 4: 371
   humerus fracture treatment, 4: 372
   legacy of, 4: 375–376
   marriage and family, 4: 375
   Massachusetts Regional Fracture Committee, 3: 64
   MGH and, 4: 371–372
   Newton-Wellesley Hospital and, 4: 371, 373, 375
   patellar turndown procedure, 4: 373–374
   PBBH and, 4: 373
   professional memberships, 4: 371, 375, 375*b*
   publications and research, 4: 371–374
   synovectomy in chronic arthritis research, 4: 102, 371–372
   treatment of shock, 4: 373, *373*
   University of Missouri appointment, 4: 372–373
   World War I service, 4: 371, 373
Coonse, Hilda Gant, 4: 375
Cooper, Maurice, 4: 373
Cooper, Reginald, 1: 234; 3: 303
Cooper, Sir Astley, 1: *34*
   anatomy lectures, 1: 34–35, 37
   Bigelow on, 3: 36
   dislocations and, 1: 44–45
   as Guy's Hospital surgeon, 1: 35–36
   influence on John Collins Warren, 1: 36–37
   publications of, 1: 35–36
   surgical advances by, 1: 35
   Treatise on Dislocations and Fractures of Joints, 1: *35*, 42, 43
Cooper, William, 1: 33–34
Coordinating Council on Medical Education (CCME), 1: 211
Cope, Oliver, 3: 336
Cope, Stuart, 4: 116, 128, 163, 193
Copel, Joseph W. (1917–1985), 4: *88*
   Beth Israel Hospital and, 4: 89, 247, 262
   Boston University appointment, 4: 89
   Brigham and Women's Hospital, 4: 163
   death of, 4: 89
   education and training, 4: 88
   HMS appointment, 4: 89
   marriage and family, 4: 88–89
   private medical practice, 4: 89
   publications and research, 4: 88–89
   RBBH and, 4: 35, 38, 68, 89, 93
   US Army and, 4: 88
Copel, Marcia Kagno, 4: 89
Copley, John Singleton, 1: *3*, 11
Corey Hill Hospital, 3: *88*, 89; 4: 224
Corkery, Paul J., 4: 295
Corliss, Julie, 4: 183
Cornell Medical School, 4: 109
Cornwall, Andrew P., 3: 268
Cotrel, Yves, 2: 342
Cotting, Benjamin E., 2: 10
Cotting, Frances J., 2: 38
Cotting, W. F., 4: 338
Cotting, W. P., 2: 438
Cotting School, 2: 38, 308, *312*; 3: 151; 4: 367
Cotton, Frederic J. (1869–1938), 1: *202*; 4: *309*, 323, 331
   ACS founder, 4: 324
   ankle fractures and, 4: 313–315
   bacteriology research, 4: 310
   BCH Bone and Joint Service, 4: 307, 328, 333, 380*b*
   BCH residencies and, 4: 377
   Beth Israel Hospital and, 4: 207, 220
   board certification efforts, 4: 324
   bone and joint treatment, 4: 313, 323, 328
   book of x-ray photographs and, 3: 57
   Boston Children's Hospital and, 4: 311
   Boston Children's Hospital skiagrapher, 3: 56
   Boston City Hospital and, 4: 217, 242, 307, 312–313, 328
   Boston Dispensary and, 4: 311
   bubble bottle anesthesia method, 4: 323
   calcaneus fracture treatment, 4: 313, *313*, 314*b*
   clinical congress meeting, 3: 116
   as consulting surgeon, 4: 323–324
   Cotton's fracture and, 4: 313–315, *315*, 316
   death of, 4: 330
   Dislocations and Joint Fractures, 3: 371; 4: 307, 314, 316–317, *317*, 318
   education and training, 4: 309
   on fracture management, 4: 320, *320*, 321*b*–322*b*, 339*b*–340*b*
   George W. Gay Lecture, 4: 324
   hip fracture treatment, 4: 318–320
   HMS appointments, 4: 323, 323*b*, 329
   honors and awards, 4: 312, 324, 329
   on industrial accidents, 4: 325–327, 338
   lectures of, 4: 329
   legacy of, 4: 329–331
   marriage and family, 4: 330
   Massachusetts Regional Fracture Committee, 3: 64
   medical illustration, 3: 56, *58*
   as mentor, 3: 237
   MGH and, 4: 310
   military reconstruction hospitals and, 4: 444–445, 449–451
   Mt. Sinai Hospital and, 4: 204, 220, 312
   named procedures, 4: 329

Index

New England Regional Committee on Fractures, 4: 341
orthopaedics education and, 4: 323
Orthopedic Surgery, 4: 318
os calcis fracture research, 4: 313
PBBH teaching and, 4: 10
Physicians' Art Society and, 4: 329–330
professional memberships, 4: 324, 329–330
publications and research, 4: 310–313, 316–320, 323, 325–326, 329
Reverdin method and, 4: 216
roentgenology and, 2: 56
sling device to reduce kyphosis, 4: *317*
Spanish American War service, 4: 310–311
test to determine ankle instability, 4: *317*, 318
Treatment of Fractures, 4: 312
trigger knee research, 4: 311–312
Tufts Medical School appointment, 4: 329
US General Hospital No. 10 and, 4: 452
worker health care advocacy, 4: 325–327
workers' compensation advocacy, 4: 325, 444
World War I service, 4: 327
Cotton, Isabella Cole, 4: 309
Cotton, Jane Baldwin, 4: 330
Cotton, Jean, 4: 330
Cotton, Joseph Potter, 4: 309, 316
Cotton advancement operation, 4: 329
Cotton osteotomy, 4: 329
Cotton-Boothby anesthesia apparatus, 4: *320*, 323
Cotton's Fracture, 4: 313–315, *315*, 316
Cotton's Hammer, 4: *319*, 320
Council of Medical Specialty Societies, 1: 211
Council of Musculoskeletal Specialty Societies (AAOS), 4: 186
Councilman, William T., 2: 32; 4: 4, *6*
Coventry, Mark, 3: 261–262, 433
Cowell, Henry, 2: 239
Cox, Edith I., 4: 389*b*
coxa plana, 2: 102–106. *See also* Legg-Calvé-Perthes disease
Cozen, Lewis N., 3: 70*b*, 74, 187; 4: 383, 471
Cracchiolo, Andrea, 2: 317

Craig, John, 2: 234
Crandon, LeRoi G., 4: 207, 216, *217*
Crane, Carl C., 3: 266
craniotomy, 2: 24–25
Crawford, Alvin, 4: 246, 266*b*
Crawford, Dorothy, 2: 313
Crenshaw, Andrew H., Jr., 4: 168, 356
crew, 1: 250–251, 258
Crile, George, 3: 104
Crippled Children's Clinics (Massachusetts Dept. of Health), 2: 221, 230, 287, 299, 314; 4: 376
Crippled Children's Service (Vermont Dept. of Health), 2: 208, 220–221; 3: 209
Crockett, David C., 2: 322; 3: 259
Cronkhite, Leonard, 2: 285
Crosby, L. M., 3: 133
Crotched Mountain Foundation, 2: 221
Crothers, Bronson, 2: 171–172
Crowninshield, Annie, 1: 76
cubitus varus deformity, 2: 229
Cudworth, Alden L., 2: 326
Cullis Consumptive Home, 4: 275
curative workshops
    King Manuel II and, 4: 400–403
    rehabilitation of soldiers and, 4: 401–403, *403*, 404, 442, 448, *448*, 449
    Shepherd's Bush Military Hospital and, 4: 399, 401
    trades practiced in, 4: 402*b*
    US Army and, 4: 403–404
Curley, James M., 3: 120
Curran, J. A., 1: 185
Curtis, Burr, 2: 351
Curtiss, Paul H., Jr., 2: 238; 3: 398*b*, 461, *461*–462
Cushing, Ernest W., 4: 23
Cushing, Harvey W., 3: *180*
    American Ambulance Hospital and, 4: 9–10, *388*, 389*b*, *390*
    anesthesia charting and, 3: 96
    Base Hospital No. 5 and, 4: 420, 420*t*, 422*b*, *422*
    Boston Children's Hospital and, 2: 12
    Codman and, 3: 94–95
    on Dane's foot plate, 2: 245
    development of orthopaedics department, 1: 177
    Harvard Unit and, 2: 119, 125; 3: 369, *370*; 4: 419
    honors and awards, 3: 94
    as MGH surgeon, 3: 95
    on organization of surgery, 4: 13–14

PBBH and, 1: 174, 204; 2: 168, 269; 4: 4–6, *6*, 8–9, 12–13, 16, 79
    Quigley and, 1: 276
    Sever and, 2: 92
    Surgeon's Journal, 3: 369
    Thorndike and, 1: 263
Cutler, Elliott C., 4: *106*, *472*
    American Ambulance Hospital and, 4: 389*b*, 390–391
    Base Hospital No. 5 and, 4: 420, 422*b*
    Carl Walter and, 4: 104–105
    death of, 4: 18
    Harvard Unit and, 2: 119; 4: 17
    HMS appointment, 1: 179
    on medical education, 4: 16
    Moseley Professor of Surgery, 1: 268
    as PBBH chief of surgery, 1: 269–270; 4: 8, 10, 15–16, 18, 79, 110
    publications and research, 1: 153–154
    specialty clinics and, 4: 15–16
    support for orthopaedic surgery specialization, 4: 16–17
    Surgical Research Laboratory, 3: 237
    on wounded soldier care, 4: 389–390
    as WWII surgery specialist, 4: 471
Cutler, Robert, 4: 20
Cutler Army Hospital (Fort Devens), 2: 358

D

Dabuzhaky, Leonard, 4: 279
Daland, Florence, 3: 159, 347
Dalton, John Call, Jr., 1: 60
Dana Farber Cancer Institute, 1: 91; 2: 331
Dandy, Walter, 3: 204
Dane, Eunice Cooksey, 2: 247
Dane, John H. (1865–1939), 2: *241*
    Boston Children's Hospital and, 2: 242, 307
    Boston Dispensary and, 2: 247
    Boston Infant's Hospital and, 2: 242
    clinical congress meeting, 3: 118
    death of, 2: 247
    education and training, 2: 241–242
    flat feet research and treatment, 2: 242, *242*, 243, *243*, 244–246
    foot plate, 2: 244–246

HMS appointment, 2: 242, 247
House of the Good Samaritan
 and, 2: 242
Lovett and, 2: 242, 246–247
Marcella Street Home and,
 2: 242, 247
marriage and family, 2: 247
professional memberships, 2: 246
publications of, 2: 246–247
Thomas splint modification,
 2: 247, *247*
US General Hospital No. 2 and,
 4: 452
World War I service, 2: 247
Dane, John H., Jr., 2: 247
Danforth, Murray S.
 on importance of examination
  and diagnosis, 3: 185
 Journal of Bone and Joint Surgery
  editor, 3: 161, 344; 4: 50
 MGH and, 3: 268
 military orthopaedics and,
  4: 406, 444
 publications and research,
  2: 136, 297
 rehabilitation of soldiers and,
  4: 444
 Walter Reed General Hospital
  and, 4: 452
Danforth, Samuel, 1: 15, 25, 40
D'Angio, G. J., 2: 237
Darling, Eugene A. (1868–1934),
 1: 250–251
Darrach, William, 4: 473
Darrach procedure, 3: 191
Darrow, Clarence, 1: 276
*Dartmouth Atlas of Health Care in
 Virginia, The* (Wennberg et al.),
 2: 374, *374*, 375
Dartmouth Medical School, 2: 371;
 3: 363
Dartmouth-Hitchcock Medical Center, 2: 371
David S. Grice Annual Lecture,
 2: 215–216, 216*t*
Davies, John A. K., 4: 194, 195*b*,
 263
Davies, Robert, 4: 262
Davis, Arthur G., 3: 344
Davis, G. Gwilym, 3: 157; 4: 406
Davis, Henry G., 2: 22–23, 26
Davis, Joseph, 2: 219
Davis, Robert, 4: 286
Davy, Sir Humphrey, 1: 56
Dawbarn, Robert H. M., 3: 105
Dawes, William, 1: 17
Dawson, Clyde W., 3: 74
Dawson, David M., 4: 168
Day, Charles, 1: 169; 4: 287
Day, George, 4: 307

Day Nursery (Holyoke), 2: 256
De Forest, R., 3: 210
De Machinamentis of Oribasius,
 3: *149*
De Ville, Kenneth Allen, 1: 47
Deaconess Home and Training
 School, 4: 273
Deaconess term, 4: 274*b*
dead arm syndrome, 3: 359–360
*Death of General Warren at the Battle
 of Bunker's Hill, The* (Trumbull),
 1: *19*
Deaver, George, 4: 76
DeBakey, Michael, 4: 469
debarkation hospitals, 4: 451–452
deep vein thrombosis (DVT),
 3: 218; 4: 251–252
DeHaven, Ken, 3: 448
Deland, F. Stanton, Jr., 4: 114, 120
Deland, Jonathan, 1: 217*b*
Delano, Frederick, 2: 72
DeLorme, Eleanor Person, 3: 281,
 287
DeLorme, Thomas I., Jr. (1917–
 2003), 3: *281*, 285
 awards and, 3: 281–282
 blood perfusion research, 3: 287
 Children's Hospital/MGH combined program and, 3: 285
 death of, 3: 287
 early life, 3: 281
 education and training, 3: 281
 Elgin table and, 3: *287*
 expansion of MGH orthopaedics
  and, 3: 286
 Fracture course and, 3: *273*
 Gardiner Hospital and, 3: 282,
  284
 heavy-/progressive resistance
  exercises and, 3: 282, *282*,
  283–286
 HMS appointment, 3: 287
 legacy of, 3: 287
 Legon of Merit medal, 3: 284,
  284
 as Liberty Mutual Insurance
  Company medical director,
  3: 286–287
 Marlborough Medical Associates
  and, 2: 146, 269, 299
 marriage and family, 3: 281
 as MGH surgeon, 3: 285
 Milton Hospital and, 3: 287
 physical therapy and, 3: 284
 PRE (Progressive Resistance Exercise), 3: 286
 publications and research,
  3: 282–283, 285–286; 4: 91
 rehabilitation and, 3: 459, 461

resistance training in recovery,
 3: 282
spinal surgeries and, 3: 287
US Army Medical Corps and,
 3: 282
weightlifting and, 3: 281
West Roxbury Veterans Hospital
 and, 3: 285
DeLorme table, 3: 284
Delpech, Jacques-Mathieu, 1: xxiii,
 106
Delta Upsilon fraternity, 4: 258, *258*
Denis Browne splint, 2: 208
dentistry, 1: 56–57
Denucé, Maurice, 3: 233–235
Derby, George, 4: 307
Description of a Skeleton of the Mastodon Giganteus of North America
 (J. C. Warren), 1: *52*
Deshmukh, R. V., 4: 178
Detmold, William Ludwig, 1: 100–
 101; 2: 25–26
DeWolfe, C. W., 3: 133
Dexter, Aaron, 1: 25, 95–96
Deyo, Richard, 2: 371
diabetes, 3: 408, 413, 438
Diagnosis in Joint Disease (Allison
 and Ghormley), 3: 175, 289, *290*
Diao, Edward, 1: 217*b*
diarrheal disease, 2: 4
diastematomyelia, 2: 236, 399–400
Dickinson, Robert L., 3: 120, 123
Dickson, Frank D., 2: 78
Dickson, Fred, 2: 77
Dieffenbach, Johann Friedrich, 1: 76
Digby, Kenelm H., 2: 170
Diggs, Lucy, 4: 492
Dignan, Beth A., 2: 277
Dillon Field House, 1: 274, *284*,
 285
Dines, Robert, 4: 247
Dingle, J., 4: 127
diphtheria, 2: 4
disabled adults
 back problems and, 3: 207
 hip disease and, 2: 294; 3: 155
 MGH rehabilitation clinic and,
  1: 273; 3: 455
 orthopaedic care for, 2: 132
 polio and, 3: 286
 soldiers and veterans, 1: 271–
  273; 2: 65, 67; 3: 44
disabled children. *See also* cerebral
 palsy; club foot
 advocacy for, 1: 107
 Crippled Children's Clinic and,
  2: 221
 House of the Good Samaritan
  and, 1: 123
 industrial training and, 2: 97

Index 517

orthopaedic care for, 2: 132
polio and, 2: 191
schools for, 2: 36–41, 67–68, 97, 308, 310–311, *312*
"Discourse on Self-Limited Diseases, A" (Bigelow), 3: 12–13
Diseases of the Bones and Joints (Osgood, Goldthwait and Painter), 2: 117; 3: 81–82; 4: 45
dislocations. *See also* congenital dislocated hips (CDH); hip dislocations
chronic posterior elbow, 3: 366
patella and, 2: 294–296; 3: 79, 79*b*, 80, *81*
shoulders and, 3: 352, *352*, 353, 355–356, *356*
Treatise on Dislocations and Fractures of Joints, 1: *35*, *42*, *43*
use of ether, 1: 62
voluntary, 3: 355–356, *356*
Dislocations and Joint Fractures (Cotton), 3: 371; 4: 307, 314, 316–317, *317*, 318
distal humerus, 2: 250
Division of Orthopaedic Surgery in the A.E.F., The (Goldthwait), 4: 473
Dixon, Frank D., 3: 173
Dixon, Robert B., 4: 23
Doctor's Hospital, 1: 276
Dodd, Walter J., 2: 114, 116; 3: 20, *20*, 21, 96, 99, 192, 266; 4: 389*b*
Dodson, Tom, 3: 1
Donaghy, R. M., 3: 205
Doppelt, Samuel, 1: 167; 3: 386, 396, 398, 440, 460*b*, 461
Dowling, John Joseph, 4: 420*t*, 438
Down syndrome, 2: 368, 370
Dr. John Ball Brown (Harding), 1: *95*
Dr. Robert K. Rosenthal Cerebral Palsy Fund in Orthopaedics, 2: 439*b*
Draper, George, 2: 72, 75–76, 78
Drew, Michael A., 4: 163, 193, 279
Drinker, C. K., 2: 81
Drinker, Philip, 2: 78, *78*, 191
Dubousset, Jean, 2: 342
Dudley, H. Robert, 4: 102
Duggal, Navan, 4: 288
Duhamel, Henri-Louis, 1: xxi
Dukakis, Kitty, 3: 419
Dukakis, Michael, 3: 419, 423
Dunlop, George, 4: 279
Dunn, Beryl, 2: 180–181
Dunn, Naughton, 2: 92–94, 150, 181
Dunphy, J. Englebert, 2: 220; 4: 303
Dunster House (Harvard University), 2: *388*
Duocondylar prostheses, 4: 178

duodenal ulcer, 3: 108
duopatellar prosthesis, 4: 130
Dupuytren, Guillaume, 1: 73–75
Duthie, J. J. R., 4: 33
Dwight, Edwin, 4: *302*
Dwight, Thomas, 1: 87–88, 127; 2: *97*, 247, 296; 3: 33, 94, 231; 4: 82, 310
Dwyer, Allen, 2: 336
Dwyer instrumentation, 2: 336, *336*, 342
Dwyer procedure, 2: 328
Dyer, George, 4: 190*b*

E

Eames, Charles, 4: *470*
Eames, Ray, 4: *470*
Eames molded plywood leg splint, 4: *470*
early onset scoliosis (EOS), 2: 360–361
Early Orthopaedic Surgeons of America, The (Shands), 1: 114
Earp, Brandon, 3: 410; 4: 190*b*
Easley, Walter, 3: 282
East Boston Relief Station, 2: 254
Eastern States Orthopaedic Club, 4: 87
Eaton, Richard G. (1929–), 2: *200*, 249
animal model of compartment syndrome, 2: 248
Boston Children's Hospital and, 2: 248, 250
Children's Hospital/MGH combined program and, 2: 248
education and training, 2: 248
hand surgery education, 2: 248, 250–251
HMS appointment, 2: 248
on ischemia-edema cycle, 2: 200–201, *201*
Joint Injuries of the Hand, 2: 250, *250*
Peter Bent Brigham Hospital and, 4: 22
professional memberships, 2: 251
publications and research, 2: 248–250; 3: 309
Roosevelt Hospital and, 2: 248, 250–251
US Army active duty, 2: 248
Ebert, Robert H., 1: 210–211; 2: 203; 4: 113, 119, 123
École de Médicine (University of Paris), 1: 73
Eddy, Chauncey, 1: 103
Edison, Thomas, 3: 96

Edith M. Ashley Professorship, 3: 202, 464*b*
Edsall, David L., 4: *6*
Allison and, 1: 152
Beth Israel Hospital and, 4: 213
clinical research at MGH and, 3: 211
as dean of HMS, 1: 174–177; 2: 81–82; 4: 213, 275, 297, 302
on departmental organization, 1: 176–178
on faculty governance, 1: 175–178
on faculty rank, 1: 178
HMS reforms and, 1: 147
on MGH and HMS relations, 1: 174
postgraduate education and, 2: 160
Edwards, Thomas, 4: 262–263
Effects of Chloroform and of Strong Chloric Ether as Narcotic Agents (J. C. Warren), 1: 62
Ehrenfried, Albert (1880–1951), 4: *215*
attempts at resignation from Beth Israel, 4: 209, 209*b*, 210
Beth Israel Hospital and, 4: 205–210, 220
Boston Children's Hospital and, 4: 215
Boston City Hospital and, 4: 217–218
Chronicle of Boston Jewry, 4: 220
civic and professional engagements, 4: 221*b*
clinical congress meeting, 3: 116
club foot research and, 4: 216
death of, 4: 221
education and training, 4: 215
hereditary deforming chondrodysplasia research, 4: 218–219, *219*, 220
HMS appointment, 4: 218
insufflation anesthesia apparatus, 4: 215–216
Jewish Memorial Hospital and, 4: 215
on military service, 4: 220–221
military surgeon training and, 4: 218
Mt. Sinai Hospital and, 4: 202–205, 215
on need for total Jewish hospital, 4: 205
publications and research, 4: 216–219, *219*, 220–221
pulmonary tuberculosis treatment, 4: 215

Reverdin method and,
4: 216–217
Surgical After-Treatment,
4: 217, *217*
vascular anastomosis and, 4: 216
Ehrenfried, George, 4: 215, 220
Ehrenfried, Rachel Blauspan, 4: 215
Ehrenfried's disease (hereditary deforming chondrodysplasia), 4: 218–220
Ehrlich, Christopher, 3: 401
Ehrlich, Michael G. (1939–2018), 3: *400*, *461*
　Brown University Medical School appointment, 3: 400–401
　death of, 3: 401
　early life, 3: 400
　education and training, 3: 400
　gait laboratory and, 3: 397
　honors and awards, 3: 400
　idiopathic subluxation of the radial head case, 3: 401
　marriage and family, 3: 401
　as MGH surgeon, 3: 385–386, 395, 398b, 413
　Miriam Hospital and, 3: 401
　pediatric orthopaedics and, 3: 388t, 400–401, 460b
　publications and research, 3: 400–401
　Rhode Island Hospital and, 3: 401
Ehrlich, Nancy Band, 3: 401
Ehrlich, Timothy, 3: 401
Ehrlichman, Lauren, 3: 463b
Eiselsberg, Anton, 1: 264
elbow
　arthroplasty of, 3: 64, 341; 4: 63
　basket plaster treatment, 2: *122*
　brachioradialis transfer and, 2: 153
　capitellocondylar total prosthesis, 4: 145, *145*, 146–147
　chronic posterior dislocations, 3: 366
　early arthrogram of, 3: *99*
　excision of, 3: 34, 309, 368
　external epicondyle fracture of, 2: 46
　flexion contracture of, 2: 418
　fusion and, 3: 368
　hinged prostheses, 4: 147
　idiopathic subluxation of the radial head, 3: 401
　intra-articular radial nerve entrapment, 3: 410–411
　nonconstrained total prosthesis, 4: 145
　non-hinged metal–polyethylene prosthesis, 4: 145–146
　total replacement of, 4: 129
electromyogram, 3: 320
electron microscopes, 2: 323, *324*, 325
Elgin table, 3: *287*
Eliot, Charles W., 1: *139*
　educational reforms and, 1: 139, 140b, 146–147; 2: 19, 41; 3: 44–45, 94
　medical education and, 1: 141; 4: 2
　on medical faculty organization, 1: 173
　on medical leadership, 4: 4
　on medical student caliber, 1: 131, 140
　opposition to football, 1: 253
Elks' Reconstruction Hospital, 4: 447–448
Ellen and Melvin Gordon Professor of Medical Education, 4: 264
Elliott, J. W., 2: 306
Elliott G. Brackett Fund, 3: 161
Ellis, Daniel S., 3: 241
Elliston, Harriet Hammond, 4: 90, 92
Elliston, William A. (1904–1984), 4: 41b, *90*
　Boston Children's Hospital and, 2: 313
　Brigham and Women's Hospital and, 4: 193
　death of, 4: 92
　education and training, 4: 90
　hip arthroplasty follow-up, 4: 40
　HMS appointment, 4: 90
　life and community service in Weston, 4: 91–92
　marriage and family, 4: 90, 92
　on nylon arthroplasty of the knee, 4: 91
　PBBH and, 4: 18, 20
　publications and research, 4: 90–91
　RBBH and, 4: 32, 35, 38, 41, 68, 89–90, 93, 132
　US Army Medical Corps and, 4: 90
　Veterans Administration Hospital and, 4: 90–91
Elliston, William Rowley, 4: 90
Emans, John (1944–), 2: *357*
　Boston brace and, 2: 358–359, *359*
　Boston Children's Hospital and, 2: 338, 354, 358–359
　Brigham and Women's Hospital and, 4: 163, 193
　Chest Wall and Spinal Deformity Study Group, 2: 361–362
　Core Curriculum Committee and, 1: 216
　Cutler Army Hospital and, 2: 358
　education and training, 2: 358, 388
　Hall and, 2: 347, 358
　HMS appointment, 2: 358
　honors and awards, 2: 363
　Myelodysplasia Program, 2: 359
　nutritional status research, 2: 361–362
　Parker Hill Hospital and, 2: 358
　professional memberships, 2: 363, 363b
　publications and research, 2: *358*, 359–363
　scoliosis treatment, 2: 339, 344
　Spinal Surgery Service, 2: 359
embarkation hospitals, 4: 451–452
Emergency Care and Transportation of the Sick and Injured (MacAusland), 3: 310, *311*
Emerson, Ralph Waldo, 1: 57
Emerson, Roger, 3: 396, 399
Emerson Hospital, 3: 317, 319
Emmons, Nathaniel H., 2: 6
Emory University Hospital, 4: 158
Enders, John, 2: 189
End-Result Idea (Codman)
　accountability and, 3: 119b
　bone sarcomas and, 3: 136–138
　Boston Children's Hospital and, 1: 194
　cards recording outcomes, 3: *111*, 113b
　Codman Hospital and, 3: 112, 114, *126*
　Codman's personal cases, 3: 126, 128–129
　Codman's promotion of, 3: 126
　as experiment, 3: 119–120
　filing system for, 3: *116*
　Halifax YMCA Emergency Hospital and, 3: 134
　hospital efficiency and, 3: 127b
　opposition to, 3: 118–120, 122–123
　PBBH and, 4: 12
　performance-based promotions and, 3: 123–124
　promotion of, 3: 116, 118, 123
　Robert Osgood and, 2: 135
　spread of, 3: 125
　treatment outcomes reporting, 3: 110–111
　young surgeons and, 3: 130–131

Enneking, William, 1: 218–220; 3: 382
Entrapment Neuropathies (Dawson, et al.), 4: 168
Epidemic Aid Team, 2: 260
epiphyseal arrest, 2: 170–171, 192, 192*t*, *192*, 193
epiphyseal injuries, 2: 321; 4: 350–351, *351*, 352, 355
Erickson, A. Ingrid, 1: 217*b*
Ernest A. Codman Award, 3: 146
Ernst, Harold C., 1: 171; 4: 6
Erving, W. G., 4: 394
Esposito, Phil, 3: 357, 357*b*
Essentials of Body Mechanics (Goldthwait et al.), 3: *90*, 91
Estok, Dan M., II, 4: 193, 195*b*
ether
  asthma and, 1: 56
  commemoration of first use, 1: *61*, *64*, *65*; 3: 32
  composition of, 1: 61
  deaths and, 3: 31
  discovery rights of, 1: 60
  ethical use of, 1: 58
  Morton's inhaler, 1: *58*
  use as anesthesia, 1: 55–62, *63*, 64–65, 82
  use at MGH, 1: 57–63, 85; 3: 15, 22, 27–28, 28*b*, 29, 29*b*, 30–34
  use at social events, 1: 56
  use on children, 1: 63
  use outside the U.S., 1: 59
Ether Day 1846 (Prosperi and Prosperi), 1: *59*
Ether Dome (MGH), 1: *59*, *63*, 84; 3: *14*, 16
Ether Monument, 1: *64*, *65*; 3: 32, 32*b*
Etherization (J. C. Warren), 1: 62, *62*; 3: 33
Evans, Christopher, 2: 82, 166; 3: 462; 4: 194, 195*b*
Evans, D. K., 2: 211
Evans, Frances, 4: 41*b*
Evarts, C. M. "Mac," 1: 234
Ewald, Frederick C. (1933–), 4: *144*
  Brigham and Women's Hospital, 4: 163
  Brigham Orthopedic Associates (BOA) and, 4: 123
  capitellocondylar total elbow prosthesis, 4: 145, *145*, 146, *146*, 147
  Children's Hospital/MGH combined program and, 4: 144
  education and training, 4: 144
  giant cell synovitis case, 4: 148
  Helen Fay Hunter orthopaedic research fellowship, 4: 144
  HMS appointment, 4: 144
  Knee Society president, 4: 150
  legacy of, 4: 150
  PBBH and, 4: 116, 129, 144–145, 161
  professional memberships, 4: 150
  publications and research, 4: 130, *130*, 134, 144–146, *146*, 147, *147*, 148–149, *149*, 150, 189
  RBBH and, 4: 129, 132, 144–145, 150
  roentgenographic total knee arthroplasty-scoring system, 4: 150
  total knee arthroplasty and, 4: 130–131, 131*t*, 145
  total knee prosthesis research, 4: 147–148, *148*, 149–150
  West Roxbury Veterans Administration Hospital and, 4: 144
Ewing, James, 3: 137
Experience in the Management of Fractures and Dislocations (Wilson), 3: 376
"Extra-Articular Arthrodesis of the Subastragalar Joint" (Grice), 2: *208*, 209
extracorporeal shockwave therapy (ESWT), 3: 437–438

F

Fahey, Robert, 4: 341
Fallon, Anne, 2: 260, *260*
Falmouth Hospital, 4: 89
Faraday, Michael, 1: 56
Farber, Sidney, 2: 171, 215, 234–236; 4: 72
Farnsworth, Dana, 1: 277, 284
fasciotomies, 1: 35; 2: 201, 250; 3: 417–418. *See also* Ober-Yount fasciotomy
fat embolism syndrome, 2: 397, *397*, 398
Faulkner Hospital, 3: 248, 314, 331; 4: 194, *194*
Faxon, Henry H., 4: 482
Faxon, John, 1: 42, 44
Faxon, Nathaniel W., 3: 70*b*; 4: 475, 482
Fearing, Albert, 2: 5
Federated Jewish Charities, 4: 205
Federation of Jewish Charities, 4: 200
Federation of Spine Associations, 4: 265
Federation of State Medical Boards (FSMB), 3: 424
Felch, L. P., 3: 269
Feldon, Paul, 4: 98
Fell, Honor B., 4: 126
femoral heads
  acetabular dysplasia case, 2: 390
  acetabular replacement and, 3: 279
  avascular necrosis of, 4: 154–156, 238
  blood supply to, 1: 36; 2: 392
  bone allografts and, 3: 442
  excision of, 3: 155
  flattening of, 2: *103*
  fractures of, 1: 49; 3: 38–39
  hip dislocations and, 2: 352–353, 401, 418
  hip joint excision and, 3: 34
  histologic-histochemical grading system for, 3: 384
  Legg-Calvé-Perthes disease, 2: 105, 351
  osteoarthritis and, 3: 221
  osteonecrosis of, 2: 328–329, 394; 3: 434; 4: 156–157
  palpating, 1: 48
  replacement of, 3: 213
  sclerosis of, 3: 441
  slipped capital femoral epiphysis (SCFE) and, 2: 176
  tuberculosis and, 2: 108
  wear on, 3: 224
femoral neck fractures. *See also* hip fractures
  AAOS study of, 3: 191
  Bigelow and, 3: 38–39
  calcar femorale and, 3: 39, *39*
  experience among AAOS members, 3: 190*t*
  fracture research and, 3: 377
  osteoarthritis and, 3: 383–384
  roentgenology and, 3: 377
  Smith-Petersen and, 3: 62, 181, 185–186, *186*, 189, 189*b*, 190
  tissue response at, 4: 76
  treatment of, 3: 367
  triflanged nail for, 3: 62, 185–186, *186*, 189, 189*b*, 190
femoral spurs, 3: 39
femoroacetabular impingement, 3: 188–189
femur fractures
  Buck's traction and, 1: 80
  Gaucher's disease, 3: 434
  growth disturbances in, 2: 400
  immediate reamed nailings of, 3: 416
  malunions, 3: *42*

sepsis after intramedullary fixation, 2: 248; 3: 309–310
triflanged nail for, 3: 62, 185, *186*, 189, 189*b*
wartime treatment of, 4: 408
Ferguson, Albert B., Jr. (1919–2014), 4: *109*
  death of, 4: 111
  education and training, 4: 110
  HMS appointment, 4: 111
  muscle dynamics research, 4: 111
  Orthopaedic Surgery in Infancy and Childhood, 2: 188, 239, 303
  PBBH and, 1: 204; 2: 188; 4: 19, 21, 36, 79, 110–111
  professional memberships, 4: 111
  publications and research, 4: 102
  RBBH and, 4: 93, 111
  spiral femur fracture case, 4: 110
  University of Pittsburgh appointment, 2: 188; 3: 382–383; 4: 73*b*, 111
  US Marine Corps and, 4: 110
Ferguson, Albert B., Sr., 4: 109–110
Ferguson, Jeremiah, 4: 109
Fernandez, Diego L., 3: 409, 431
Fessenden, Louise, 3: 271
Fifth Portable Surgical Hospital, 4: 489
Fine, Jacob, 4: 283*t*
Fink, Edward, 4: 279–280
Fink, Mitchell P., 4: 283*t*
Finkelstein, Clara, 2: 319
Finney, John M. T., 4: 324
Finton, Frederick P., 1: *80*
First Operation Under Ether (Hinckley), 1: *55*, 59
Fischer, Josef E., 4: 287, 289*b*
Fisher, Bob, 1: 255
Fisher, Josef E., 1: 234; 2: 397
Fisher, Roland F., 3: 167
Fisher, Thomas J., 3: 431
Fiske, Eben W., 4: 389*b*, 394
Fiske, Edith, 2: 42
Fiske Prize, 2: 52
Fitchet, Seth M. (1887–1939), 2: *252*
  Boston Children's Hospital and, 2: 222, 252, 274; 4: 338
  cleidocranial dysostosis, 2: 254
  death of, 2: 254
  education and training, 2: 251
  Harvard Department of Hygiene and, 2: 253
  HMS appointment, 2: 252
  MGH and, 2: 252
  military service, 2: 251
  Morris and, 2: 282
  private medical practice, 2: 252

public health and, 2: 253
publications and research, 1: 263; 2: 253–254
ruptures of the serratus anterior, 2: 253
Stillman Infirmary and, 2: 253
Fitton-Jackson, Sylvia, 4: 126
Fitz, Reginald Heber, 1: 179; 3: 94
Fitz, Wolfgang, 4: 194
FitzSimmons, Elizabeth Grace Rogers, 2: 258
FitzSimmons, Henry J. (1880–1935), 1: *187*; 2: *254*, 255, 258
  on atypical multiple bone tuberculosis, 2: 257
  Boston Children's Hospital and, 1: 187; 2: 252, 254–256, 258, 274, 282; 4: 338
  Boston University and, 2: 258
  Camp Devens base hospital and, 4: 452
  congenital torticollis research, 2: 256, 258
  death of, 2: 258
  East Boston Relief Station and, 2: 254
  education and training, 2: 254
  European medical studies, 2: 255
  HMS appointment, 2: 223, 256, 258; 4: 59–60
  marriage and family, 2: 258
  military surgeon training and, 2: 42
  Ober on, 2: 256, 258
  orthopaedics internship under Bradford, 2: 255
  orthopaedics internship under Lovett, 2: 144
  Osgood on, 2: 258–259
  professional memberships, 2: 258, 258*b*
  publications and research, 2: 256, 258
  ton Children's Hospital and, 1: 188
  World War I service, 2: 258
5005th USAF Hospital (Elmendorf), 3: 215
Flagg, Elisha, 3: 67
Flatt, Adrian, 4: 97
Fleisher, Leon, 3: 414
Flexner, Abraham, 1: 146–147; 3: 165
Flexner Report, 1: 146–147
flexor carpi ulnaris transfer procedure, 2: 172, 188, 198–199, *199*, 200
Fliedner, Theodor, 4: 274*b*
Flier, Jeffrey, 1: 242
Floating Hospital for Children, 2: 306, 370

flow cytometry, 3: 388
Floyd, W. Emerson, 3: 410
Floyd, W., III, 2: 417
Flugstad, Daniel, 3: 433
fluoroscope, 2: 307; 3: 96–97
Flynn, John, 3: 433
Foley, T. M., 4: 451
Folkman, Judah, 4: 182
Foot and Ankle, The (Trott and Bateman), 2: 317
foot problems. *See also* club foot
  ankle valgus, 2: 212
  arches and, 2: 317
  arthritis and, 4: 61
  astragalectomy (Whitman's operation), 2: 92–93
  athletes and, 3: 348
  Batchelor technique, 2: 212
  Brewster and, 2: 228–229
  calcaneovalgus deformity, 2: 92–93
  cavus feet, 2: 229
  cerebral palsy treatment, 2: 229
  congenital flatfoot, 4: 63
  correction of fixed deformities, 4: 62, 62*t*, 63
  countersinking the talus, 2: 228–229, 283
  Dane and, 2: 242–246
  design of shoes for, 2: 54–56
  evaluation through glass, 2: 54–55, *55*
  extra-articular arthrodesis of the subtalar joint, 2: 210–211, *211*, 212
  flat feet, 2: 54–56, 101–102, 107–108, 242–243, *243*, 244–246
  gait analysis and, 2: 407
  Green-Grice procedure, 2: 212
  heel cord contractures, 2: 265
  hindfoot pain, 4: 188
  Hoke's stabilization requirements, 2: 282–283
  John Brown's device for, 1: 106
  Lambrinudi stabilization, 2: 229
  Morton's neuroma, 2: 287
  nurses and, 2: 54–56
  Osgood on, 2: 123–124
  paralytic flat foot deformities, 2: 210–212
  planovalgus deformity, 4: 188
  poliomyelitis and, 2: 210
  radiography and, 2: 56
  rheumatoid arthritis and, 4: 188
  shoe fit and design, 2: 293, 317, 407
  skeletal anatomy and, 2: 247
  sling procedure and, 3: 294, *294*, 295, 296*b*–297*b*

Index

stabilization of, 2: 282–284
treatment of, 2: 54–56, 107–108
triple arthrodesis, 2: 172, 228–229
valgus deformity treatment, 2: 197, 209–212
weakness/paralysis in, 2: 150–151
wire drop foot splints, 2: *123*
football
acromioclavicular joint dislocation in, 1: 268, 277
athletic training and, 1: 248, 250–253, 255–256, 258
Bloody Monday game, 1: 245
Boston Game, 1: 247
collegiate reform and, 1: 253–254
concussions in, 1: 247, 254, 274–275
establishment of rules in, 1: 247–248
Hampden Park, Springfield, 1: *249*
Harvard game, 1906, 1: *257*
Harvard Rose Bowl game, 1920, 1: *259*
injuries in, 1: 247–248, 252–255, 255t, 256, 258–262, 288
preventative strappings, 1: *269*
protective padding and helmets in, 1: 255, *267*
ruptures of the serratus anterior, 2: 253
secondary school injuries in, 4: 370, *370*
sports medicine and, 1: 248, 250, 254–256
team photo, 1890, 1: *249*
Forbes, A. Mackenzie, 2: 87–88; 3: 231; 4: 233, 394
Forbes, Andrew, 3: 437
Forbes, Elliot, 2: 277
Fort Bragg (Fayetteville, N.C.), 4: 484
Fort Leonard Wood (Missouri), 3: 432
Fort Oglethorpe (Georgia), 4: 338
Fort Ord US Army Hospital, 4: 259
Fort Riley (Kansas), 4: 452–453
Fort Totten (Queens, NY), 4: *422*
Fort Warren (Mass.), 1: 20
Foster, Charles C., 1: 109, 111
Foster, Charles H. W., 3: 123
Foster, Helen, 3: 228
Foultz, W. S., 2: 237
Fourth Portable Surgical Hospital (4PSH), 2: 232–233; 4: 489
Fourth Portable Surgical Hospital's Service in the War against Japan, The (Cohen), 2: 232–233

fracture boxes, 1: 80–81
Fracture Clinic (MGH), 2: 130; 3: 60, 60b, 61–62, 241–242, 245, 273, *273*, 313–315, 371, 373, 378, 456b
Fracture Committee of the American College of Surgeons, 2: 131; 3: 61
fractures. *See also* compound fractures; femoral neck fractures; femur fractures; hip fractures
amputations and, 1: 50, 54
ankle, 4: 313–315, *315*, 316
Austin Moore prosthesis, 3: 213
bandaging care and, 1: 76
basket plasters for, 2: *122*
bilateral comminuted patellar, 3: 56b
birth, 1: 264
calcaneus treatment by impaction, 4: *313*, 314b
cervical spine, 3: 340–341
clinics for, 2: 130–131
conference on treatment for, 2: 131
Cotton's, 4: 313–315, *315*, 316
displaced supracondylar humerus, 2: 379
distal femoral physeal, 2: 400
distal radius treatment, 3: 408–409
elderly patients and, 3: *353*, 354, 354b; 4: 341
fender, 4: 242
Gartland type 3 supracondylar humeral, 2: 368
general and orthopaedic surgeon collaboration on, 4: 463–465
hip nailing and, 3: 237
hips and, 3: 213; 4: 74–75, 159b–160b, 318–320, 341
of the humerus, 3: 323–324; 4: 372
impaction treatment for, 4: 319–320
increase in, 1: 63
intercondylar T humeral, 2: 397, *397*
intra-articular, 3: 408
lateral tibial plateau, 4: *312*
leg length and, 2: 350
long-bone, 3: 60–61
malpractice suits and, 1: 50–51; 3: 63
managing pediatric, 2: 379
metastatic breast disease and, 2: 411
metastatic pathological, 3: *376*, 377–378
olecranon, 3: 309

open anterior lumbosacral dislocation, 3: 420
open treatment of, 3: 55–56, 58–62, 64
open-bone, 4: *400*
orthopaedic treatment of, 4: 463
os calcis, 4: 313, 314b, 335–336
outcomes of, 1: 50; 3: 339
plaster casts for, 2: *122*
portable traction device, 2: 297
Pott's, 4: *317*, 318
proximal humerus, 2: 96, *122*
pseudofracture of tibia, 3: 341, *342*
of the radial head, 2: 396–397; 3: 322–323
risk prediction research, 2: 411, *411*
scaphoid, 3: 101–102; 4: 359–361
scientific study of, 1: 264
shoulders, 3: 339
supracondylar humerus, 2: 229, 345, 379
Swiss method of treating, 2: 406
table for, 2: *121*
tibial spine, 4: 365
tibial tuberosity, 2: 91
total disability following joint, 3: *373*
traction treatment for, 2: 23
treatment for compound, 4: 335, 337, 392
treatment of, 1: 80–81; 3: 35, 60, 101; 4: 339b–340b, 362
triflanged nail for, 3: 62, 185–186, *186*, 189, 189b
ununited, 3: 34–35
vanadium steel plates and, 4: 340, *342*
wire arm splint for, 2: *122*
Fractures (Wilson), 3: 315
Fractures and Dislocations (Stimson), 1: 147
Fractures and Dislocations (Wilson and Cochrane), 3: 371, *371*
Fractures and Other Injuries (Cave), 3: 273, *273*; 4: 356
Fractures of the Distal Radius (Fernandez and Jupiter), 3: 409, *409*
Francis A. Countway Library of Medicine, 1: 59, 66; 2: 271; 4: 20
Frank R. Ober Research Fund, 2: 165
Franklin, Benjamin, 1: 12, 14
Fraser, Somers, 4: 438–439
Frazier, Charles H., 4: 299
Frederick and Joan Brengle Learning Center, 3: 463

Frederick W. and Jane M. Ilfeld Professorship, 2: 438, 439*b*
Fredericks, G. R., 3: 442
Free Hospital for Women, 4: 113–114
Freedman, K. B., 1: 168
Frei, Emil, III, 2: 422
Freiberg, Albert H., 2: 77–78, 87; 3: 157, 229; 4: 406, 451
Freiberg, Joseph A., 1: 193; 2: 79; 4: 59
Friedenberg, Z., 2: 214
Friedlaender, Gary, 3: 393, 440; 4: 266*b*
Friedman, Richard, 1: 217*b*
Frost, Eben H., 1: 60
Frost, Gilbert, 3: 97
frozen shoulder, 1: 277–278
Frymoyer, J. W., 3: 205
Fuldner, Russell, 3: 74
Fundamentals of Orthopaedic Surgery in General Medicine and Surgery (Osgood and Allison), 2: 135–136
Funsten, Robert, 3: 303
Furbush, C. L., 4: 439, 440*b*

G

Gage, M., 3: 210
Gage, Thomas, 1: 16
gait
    backpack loads and, 2: 408
    cerebral palsy and, 2: 406–407
    clinical analysis and, 2: 408
    hip abductor weakness and, 2: 33
    impact of shoes on, 2: 293, 407
    low back disorders and, 2: 408
    nonmechanical treatment of, 2: 244
    nonoperative treatment of, 2: 271
    Ober-Yount fasciotomy and, 2: 153
    physical therapy and, 2: 107
    shelf procedure and, 2: 151
    stroke and, 2: 408
    total knee replacement and, 2: 408
    Trendelenburg, 2: 33, 108, 151
    use of cameras to analyze, 2: 406
gait laboratory, 2: 107, 406, 424; 3: 397
Galante, Jorge, 3: 220, 222
Galeazzi method, 2: 227
Gall, Edward, 3: 331
Gallie, William E., 1: 197; 2: 160; 4: 443
Galloway, Herbert P. H., 3: 233; 4: 411, 426, 454, 464
Gambrill, Howard, Jr., 4: 40

Gandhi, Mohandas Karamchand, 4: 262
Ganz, Reinhold, 2: 390–392
Garbino, Peter, 2: 438
Gardiner Hospital, 3: 282, 284
Gardner, George E., 2: 215
Garg, Sumeet, 2: 378
Garland, Joseph E., 3: 12
Garrey, W. E., 1: 267
Gartland, John, 3: 308–309
Gates, Frank D. (1925–2011), 2: *218*
    Boston Children's Hospital and, 2: 218
    death of, 2: 218–219
    education and training, 2: 218
    HMS appointment, 2: 218
Gates, Frederick T., 1: 146
Gatton Agricultural College, 4: 489, *489*
Gaucher's disease, 3: 433–434
Gauvain, Sir Henry, 4: 363, 367
Gay, George H., 1: 308; 3: *31*
Gay, George W., 4: 324
Gay, Martin, 1: 306
Gay, Warren F., 3: 68, 266
Gaynor, David, 3: 463
Gebhardt, Mark C.
    as Beth Israel chief of orthopaedics, 4: 289*b*
    as BIDMC chief of orthopaedics, 4: 287
    Boston Children's Hospital and, 2: 439*b*
    Boston Pathology Course and, 1: 216
    Frederick W. and Jane M. Ilfeld Professorship, 2: 439*b*
    HCORP and, 1: 218, 224–225, 227
    on Mankin, 3: 393
    as MGH clinical faculty, 3: 464*b*
    orthopaedic chair at BIDMC, 1: 234, 242
    orthopaedic oncology and, 3: 460*b*
    publications and research, 3: 433
    tumor treatment and, 3: 397
Geiger, Ronald, 2: 277, 290
Gelberman, Richard H. (1943–), 3: *402*
    avascular necrosis of the lunate case, 3: 403
    Core Curriculum Committee and, 1: 216
    education and training, 3: 402
    flexor tendon research, 3: 403, *403*
    hand and microvascular service, 3: 402–403

    HCORP and, 3: 403–404
    HMS appointment, 3: 403
    honors and awards, 3: 403–405
    as MGH chief of Hand Service, 3: 403
    as MGH surgeon, 3: 399
    Operative Nerve Repair and Reconstruction, 3: 404
    publications and research, 3: 402, *402*, 403–404
    Smith Day lectures, 3: 431
    tissue fluid pressures research, 3: 404, *404*
    University of California in San Diego and, 3: 402
    Washington University School of Medicine and, 3: 404–405
gene therapy, 2: 82
General Leonard Wood Army Community Hospital, 3: 432
General Leonard Wood Gold Medal, 4: 337
genu valgum, 1: *117*
genu varum, 1: *117*
George III, King, 1: 11
George W. Gay Lecture, 4: 324
George Washington University, 2: 351
Georgia Warm Springs Foundation, 2: 77–78, 107, 264, *264*, 270
Gerald, Park, 2: 234
Gerbino, Peter, 2: 439*b*
Gerhart, Tobin, 1: 217*b*; 4: 251, 262–263, 286, 288
German Orthopaedic Association, 2: 43
Ghivizzani, Steve, 4: 194
Ghogawala, Zoher, 4: 272*b*
Ghormley, Jean McDougall, 3: 288, 290
Ghormley, Ralph K. (1893–1959), 3: *288*
    death of, 3: 290
    Diagnosis in Joint Disease, 3: 175, 289, *290*
    early life, 3: 288
    education and training, 3: 288
    HMS appointment, 3: 288; 4: 59
    on joint disease, 3: 288–289, *289*
    as joint tuberculosis expert, 3: 289
    leadership of, 3: 289–290
    marriage and family, 3: 288
    Mayo Clinic and, 3: 289
    memberships and, 3: 290, 290*b*
    as MGH surgeon, 3: 288
    military orthopaedics and, 4: 453

New England Peabody Home for Crippled Children and, 2: 270; 3: 288
private medical practice, 2: 146; 3: 288
publications and research, 3: 288–289
triple arthrodesis and, 2: 150
tuberculosis research and, 3: 288–289
US Army Medical Corps and, 3: 288
Giannestras, Nicholas, 2: 317; 3: *293*
Gibney, Virgil P., 2: 27, 43, 48, 52; 4: 463
Gilbreth, Frank B., 3: 120
Gill, A. Bruce, 2: 78, 183
Gill, Madeline K., 4: 59
Gill, Thomas J., 1: 167; 3: 462, 464*b*
Gilles, Hamish G., 4: 163, 193
Giza, Eric, 1: 217*b*
glanders, 2: 46
Glaser, Robert J., 4: 113
Glazer, Paul, 4: 286
Gleich operation, 4: 313
glenohumeral deformity, 2: 418–419, 419*t*
Glick, Hyman, 4: 251, 262–263, 286, 288
Glickel, Steven Z., 3: 430
Glimcher, Aaron, 2: 319
Glimcher, Clara Finkelstein, 2: 319
Glimcher, Laurie, 2: 330–331
Glimcher, Melvin J. (1925–2014), 1: *208, 210, 285*; 2: *319, 320, 330*; 3: *455*
  activating transcription factor-2 (ATF-2) and, 2: 330
  BIH Board of Consultants, 4: 262–263
  bone research, 2: 321–330
  Boston Arm development, 2: 326
  Boston Children's Hospital and, 1: 180; 2: 320, 327, 329; 4: 127
  Brigham and Women's Hospital and, 4: 163, 193
  Children's Hospital/MGH combined program and, 2: 320
  as Children's orthopaedic surgeon-in-chief, 2: 15*b*, 286, 326–327, 337, 406, 422, 434
  death of, 2: 331
  on DeLorme's blood perfusion research, 3: 287
  as Edith M. Ashley Professor, 3: 464*b*

education and training, 2: 319–321
electron microscopes and, 2: 323, *324*, 325
epiphyseal injuries after frostbite case, 2: 321–323
gait laboratory, 2: 406
Hall and, 2: 336
as Harriet M. Peabody Professor, 2: 327, 337, 439*b*
HCORP and, 4: 247
HMS appointment, 2: 321, 327
as honorary orthopaedic surgeon, 3: 398*b*
honors and awards, 2: 319, 324–325, 327–331
leadership of, 3: 453, 455*b*–457*b*
legacy of, 2: 330–331; 3: 458*b*
marriage and family, 2: 331
MGH Orthopaedic Research Laboratories and, 2: 321–324
as MGH orthopaedics chief, 1: 210; 2: 325; 3: 11*b*, 202, 228, 245, 385, 458*b*, 459; 4: 126
MGH residents and, 2: *327*; 3: *457*
orthopaedic research and, 3: 211
orthopaedics curriculum and, 1: 164; 3: 457*b*
osteonecrosis of the femoral head research, 2: 328, *328*, 329; 4: 156
PBBH and, 4: 163
professional memberships, 2: 329, 331
publications and research, 2: 321, *321*, 322, 324–330
research laboratories, 2: 434, 439; 3: 455*b*, 458*b*
Glowacki, Julie, 4: 194, 195*b*
gluteus maximus
  modification of use of sacrospinalis, 2: 146–147
  Ober operation and, 2: 148, 153
  paralysis of, 2: 146–147
  posterior approach to the hips, 2: 353
Goddu, Louis A. O., 3: 268; 4: 204
Godfrey, Ambrose, 1: 56
Godfrey, Arthur, 3: 198–199
Goethals, Thomas R., 4: 474, 482*b*
Goetjes, D. H., 2: 91
Goff, C. F., 4: 313
Gokaslan, Ziya L., 4: 272*b*
Goldberg, Michael, 2: 368
Goldring, Steve, 4: 280
Goldstone, Melissa, 3: 328
Goldthwait, Ellen W. R., 4: 27
Goldthwait, Francis Saltonstall, 3: 89

Goldthwait, Jessie Sophia Rand, 3: 79, 89
Goldthwait, Joel C., 4: 37–38
Goldthwait, Joel E. (1866–1961), 3: *77, 89, 91*; 4: *24*, 398
  adult orthopaedics and, 2: 101; 3: 78–79
  AOA preparedness committee, 4: 394
  back pain research and, 3: 203–204
  Beth Israel Hospital and, 4: 247
  Body Mechanics in Health and Disease, 3: 91
  Boston Children's Hospital and, 1: 187; 2: 13, 40, 247; 3: 78
  Boston City Hospital and, 1: 187; 4: 305*b*
  Boston School of Physical Education and, 3: 84
  Brigham Hospital and, 3: 81, 84, 91–92
  Carney Hospital and, 3: 78, 80; 4: 45, 86
  chronic disease treatment and, 4: 52
  clinical congress meeting, 3: 118
  Corey Hill Hospital and, 3: 89; 4: 224
  curative workshops and, 4: 402–403
  death of, 3: 92; 4: 38
  Diseases of the Bones and Joints, 2: 117; 3: 81–82
  dislocation of the patella case, 3: 79, 79*b*, 80, *81*
  Division of Orthopedic Surgery in the A.E.F., 4: 473
  early life, 3: 77
  education and training, 3: 77–78
  Essentials of Body Mechanics, 3: *90*, 91
  etiology of orthopaedic impairments and diseases, 3: 81–82
  on faulty body mechanics, 3: 91
  founding of AAOS, 3: 90
  on hip disease, 2: 52, *52*
  HMS appointment, 3: 80, 84
  Hospital Efficiency meeting, 3: 120
  House of the Good Samaritan and, 2: 114; 3: 78
  on importance of posture, 3: 81, 83, 87–89; 4: 53, 62, 82, 233
  interest in visceroptosis, 3: 83–84, 84*b*, 86–88
  iron bars, 3: 89, *89, 149*
  legacy of, 3: 91–92
  Marcella Street Home and, 2: 247

marriage and family, 3: 79, 89
on medical research, 3: 2
memberships and, 3: 92
MGH biochemistry laboratory, 2: 322; 3: 455b–456b
as MGH orthopaedics chief, 3: 11b, 67–68, 80–81, 227
military orthopaedics and, 2: 127–128; 3: 156; 4: 406, 443
military reconstruction hospitals and, 4: 440, 444–445
military surgeon training and, 2: 65
New England Deaconess Hospital and, 3: 78; 4: 274
orthopaedic surgery, 2: 116
patellar tendon transfer, 2: 294
on patient evaluation, 3: 90
on polio, 2: 77
private medical practice, 4: 62
publications and research, 3: 78–84, 90, 90, 91
RBBH and, 3: 81, 84, 91–92; 4: 23–25, 25b, 26–28, 31, 36–38, 39b, 79, 93, 111
rehabilitation of soldiers and, 4: 396, 402, 411
resolution in honor of, 4: 38, 39b
Robert Jones Lecture, 3: 90
Shattuck Lecture, 3: 84–85, 85, 86
surgical records from, 2: 115b
US Army Distinguished Service Medal, 3: 83, 83
US Medical Reserve Corps, 3: 89
on variations in human anatomy, 3: 85–86, 86t
World War I and, 2: 124–125; 4: 402–403
World War I volunteer orthopaedic surgeons and, 4: 398–399, 399, 404, 406–407, 411
Goldthwait, Mary Lydia Pitman, 3: 77
Goldthwait, Thomas, 3: 77
Goldthwait, William Johnson, 3: 77
Goldthwait Research Fund, 4: 27–28
Goldthwait Reservation, 3: 92, 92
Good Samaritan Hospital, 1: 107. See also House of the Good Samaritan
Goodnow, Elisha, 4: 293
Goodridge, Frederick J., 3: 266
Goodsir, John, 1: xxii
Gordon, Leonard, 3: 431
Gordon Hall, 1: 86

Gordon Research Conference on Bioengineering and Orthopaedic Sciences, 3: 445, 445
Gorforth, Helen R., 3: 365
Gorgas, William C., 4: 411, 429, 447
Gould, Augustus Addison, 1: 60
Gould, Marjorie, 3: 303
Gould, Nathaniel D., 1: 309; 3: 293
Grabias, Stanley L., 1: 217b; 3: 460b
Graffman, Gary, 3: 414
Graham, Henry, 2: 168
Grand Palais (Paris), 4: 401
Grandlay, J., 3: 210
Great Britain, 1: 11–16; 4: 393, 399, 432, 476. See also British Expeditionary Forces (BEF); British hospitals
Great Ormond Street Hospital, 2: 5
Greater Boston Bikur Cholim Hospital, 4: 212
Greater Hartford Tuberculosis Respiratory Disease Association, 2: 267
Green, Daniel, 4: 239
Green, David, 4: 98
Green, Elizabeth, 2: 168
Green, Gladys Griffith, 2: 168
Green, Janet, 2: 168
Green, Jean, 2: 167
Green, Neil, 2: 351, 351
Green, Robert M., 1: 89
Green, Samuel A., 3: 46
Green, William T. (1901–1986), 1: 200, 204, 207; 2: 167, 169, 177, 179, 180, 204
  as AAOS president, 2: 201–202, 202, 203
  on arthritis, 2: 171
  birth palsies research, 2: 415, 417
  on bone granuloma, 2: 171
  on bone growth and leg length discrepancy, 2: 170, 191–193
  Boston Children's Hospital and, 1: 158, 179–180; 2: 168–169, 176–178, 191, 274, 301; 3: 277, 293; 4: 72
  CDH treatment, 3: 235
  cerebral palsy treatment, 2: 171–172, 196–200, 229
  Children's Hospital/MGH combined program and, 4: 68, 158
  on clinical staff, 1: 201
  Cohen and, 2: 234–235
  on congenital pseudarthrosis of the tibia, 2: 172–176
  contributions to pediatric orthopaedics, 2: 168

  Crippled Children's Clinic and, 2: 287
  death of, 2: 205
  early life, 2: 167
  education and training, 2: 167–168
  Epidemic Aid Team, 2: 260
  as first Harriet M. Peabody Professor, 2: 183, 203, 439b
  flexor carpi ulnaris transfer procedure, 2: 172, 188, 198–200
  grand rounds and, 2: 178–181, 181, 182, 230, 271
  on Grice, 2: 215
  Growth Study, 2: 193, 193, 194, 304, 432
  hamstring contractures and, 2: 198
  Harriet M. Peabody Professor of Orthopaedic Surgery, 3: 202
  Harvard Infantile Paralysis Clinic and, 2: 176, 188
  HCORP and, 1: 200–210
  HMS appointment, 2: 168, 176, 183, 223, 270; 4: 61
  honorary degrees, 2: 203
  Infantile Paralysis Clinic and, 2: 79
  on Kuhns, 4: 66
  legacy of, 2: 203–205
  marriage and family, 2: 168
  McGinty and, 2: 279
  meticulousness and, 2: 178–179, 182–183
  on muscle grades, 2: 180
  Ober and, 2: 163, 168
  as orthopaedic chair, 2: 15b
  orthopaedic research laboratory and, 2: 234
  on orthopaedics curriculum, 1: 159, 162–164, 200–201; 2: 202
  orthopaedics education and, 2: 183–186, 188, 203, 205
  orthopaedics leadership, 2: 176–178, 191, 197
  on osteochondritis dissecans, 2: 194–195
  on osteomyelitis, 2: 169–170
  PBBH and, 4: 16, 18–22, 73b, 79, 108, 110
  as PBBH chief of orthopaedic surgery, 4: 196b
  Pediatric Orthopaedic Society and, 2: 351
  polio research and, 2: 189–190; 3: 332
  polio treatment, 2: 188–191
  private medical practice and, 1: 179; 2: 313

Index

professional memberships, 2: 204
as professor of orthopaedic surgery, 1: 158, 176, 198; 2: 176
publications and research, 2: 169, 188, 194–200, 229, 249, 264, 350
RBBH and, 4: 40, 68
rehabilitation planning and, 1: 272
on residency program, 1: 208
resident training by, 1: 199, 202–203, *203*, 204–206
on slipped capital femoral epiphysis (SCFE), 2: 176
on Sprengel deformity, 2: 195
surgery techniques, 2: 177
Tachdjian and, 2: 301–304
tibial osteoperiosteal graft method, 2: *228*
Trott and, 2: 317–318
Unit for Epidemic Aid in Infantile Paralysis (NFP), 2: 188–189
on Volkmann ischemic contracture, 2: 200–201, *201*
Green, William T., Jr., 2: 168, 182, 204–205
Green Dragon Tavern, 1: *11*, 12, *12*, 17, 24
Green-Andersen growth charts, 2: 193, *193*, 194, 304
Greenberg, B. E., 4: 199
Green-Grice procedure, 2: 212
Greenough, Francis, 2: 9
Greenough, Robert B., 2: 119, 157–158; 3: 118; 4: 389*b*
Greer, James A., 3: 398*b*
Gregory, Ernest, 4: 226
Grenfell, Sir William, 3: 91
Grenfell Mission, 2: 111
Grice, David S. (1914–1960), 2: *207*
AAOS and, 2: 215
Banks and, 1: 202, 205
Boston Children's Hospital and, 2: 208, 299
club foot treatment, 2: 208
education and training, 2: 207–208
extra-articular arthrodesis of the subtalar joint, 2: *208*, 209–212
HMS appointment, 2: 208, 210, 213
legacy of, 2: 214–216
marriage and family, 2: 214
Massachusetts Infantile Paralysis Clinic and, 2: 208, 212, 314
memorial funds for, 2: 215
orthopaedics education and, 2: 213–214
orthopaedics leadership, 2: 191

paralytic flat foot operative technique, 2: 210–212
PBBH and, 2: 208; 4: 18–19, 110
poliomyelitis treatment, 2: 208, 212–213, 213*b*, 315
private medical practice and, 2: 313
professional memberships, 2: 215
publications of, 2: 189, 208, 220
residency training by, 2: 213–214
Simmons College and, 2: 213
University of Pennsylvania and, 2: 213–214
University of Vermont and, 2: 208
valgus deformity treatment, 2: 198, 209–210
Grice, Elizabeth Fry, 2: 207
Grice, John, 2: 207
Grice, Mary Burns, 2: 214
Griffin, Bertha Mae Dail, 2: 349
Griffin, Jesse Christopher, 2: 349
Griffin, Margaret Braswell, 2: 349
Griffin, Paul P. (1927–2018), 2: *349*, *350*, *356*
arthritis treatment, 2: 350
BIH Board of Consultants, 4: 262
Boston Children's Hospital and, 2: 301, 338, 349, 351, 354–355, 434
Chicago Shriner's Hospital and, 2: 355
Crippled Children's Clinic and, 2: 314
death of, 2: 356
education and training, 2: 349
George Washington University and, 2: 351
HMS appointment, 2: 349–351, 354
Laboratory for Skeletal Disorders and Rehabilitation and, 2: 413
as orthopaedic chair, 2: 15*b*, 286
orthopaedics appointments, 2: 351
PBBH and, 4: 20, 22
Pediatric Orthopaedic International Seminars program, 2: 304
Pediatric Orthopaedic Society and, 2: 351
pediatric orthopaedics, 2: 354–355
private medical practice and, 2: 313
publications and research, 2: 349–351, *351*, *354*

traumatic hip dislocation case, 2: 352–353
Griffith, Gladys, 2: 168
Griffiths, Maurice, 4: 92
Grillo, Hermes C., 1: 184
Gritti-Stokes amputation, 3: 374
Gross, Richard, 2: 354–355, 438
Gross, Robert E., 2: 215
Gross, Samuel D., 1: 79
Gross, Samuel W., 3: 142
Groves, Ernest W. Hey, 2: 91; 3: 209
Gucker, Harriet, 2: 266
Gucker, Thomas III (1915–1986), 2: *259*, *260*
Berlin polio epidemic and, 2: 260, 264
Boston Children's Hospital and, 2: 260, 264
contributions to orthopaedic rehabilitation, 2: 266
death of, 2: 266
education and training, 2: 259–260
Georgia Warm Springs Foundation and, 2: 264
marriage and family, 2: 266
on patient reaction to polio, 2: 261*b*–263*b*
poliomyelitis and, 2: 259, 264, 266
professional memberships, 2: 264–265
publications and research, 2: 264–266
on pulmonary function, 2: 265–266
tendon transfers and, 2: 265
University of Pennsylvania and, 2: 265
University of Southern California and, 2: 266
Guérin, Jules, 1: 54, 98, 106; 3: 26
gunshot injuries, 2: 66, 119, 161, 233; 3: 43, 156, 156*b*; 4: 437, 441
Gupta, Amit, 3: 431
Guthrie, Douglas, 1: 183
Guy's and Old St. Thomas hospitals, 1: *34*
Guy's Hospital (London), 1: 6, 33–35, 37, 83

H

Haggert, G. Edmund, 2: 165; 4: 344–345, 378
Hale, Worth, 1: 176–177
Hale Hospital, 3: 331

Halifax Harbor explosion, 3: 132, *132*, 133–135
Halifax YMCA Emergency Hospital, 3: *133*, 134
Hall, Caroline Doane, 2: 267
Hall, Col. John, 3: 282, 284
Hall, Emmett Matthew, 2: 333
Hall, Francis C., 3: 338
Hall, Francis N. Walsh, 2: 333, 337, 348
Hall, H. J., 2: *55*
Hall, Isabelle Mary Parker, 2: 333
Hall, John E. (1925–2018), 2: *333*, 346
    as BCH Orthopaedic chair, 2: 15*b*, 338–339, 384, 434, 436
    BIH Board of Consultants, 4: 262
    Boston Children's Hospital and, 2: 61, 279, 337–339, 399, 439*b*
    Brigham and Women's Hospital and, 2: 337; 4: 163, 193
    Cerebral Palsy Clinic and, 2: 402
    as clinical chief, 2: 286, 422
    death of, 2: 348
    Dwyer instrumentation and, 2: 342
    education and training, 2: 333
    Harrington Lecture, 2: 344, *344*
    Hospital for Sick Children and, 2: 334–336
    kyphosis and, 2: 343–345
    marriage and family, 2: 333, 337
    as mentor, 2: 345–347
    military service, 2: 333
    New England Baptist Hospital and, 2: 338
    orthopaedics leadership, 2: 347
    orthopaedics residents and, 2: *413*
    PBBH and, 4: 163
    pediatric orthopaedics, 2: 345, *345*
    private medical practice, 2: 338
    professional memberships, 2: 347
    Prosthetic Research and Development Unit, 2: 335
    publications and research, 2: *336*, 340–344, *344*, 345, 385, 391–392
    Relton-Hall frame, 2: 334–335, *335*
    Royal National Orthopaedic Hospital and, 2: 333–334
    scoliosis treatment, 2: 328, 334–336, 339–340, *340*, 341–345; 4: 127
    Seal of Chevalier du Tastevin, 2: 348
    spinal surgery at BCH and, 2: 337–338
    sports medicine and, 2: 287
    Tachdjian and, 2: 304
    Toronto General Hospital and, 2: 334
Hall, Leland, 3: 364
Hall, Llewellyn (ca.1899–1969), 2: 267, *267*
Hall, Marshall, 1: xxii
Hallett, Mark, 4: 168
hallux valgus deformities, 4: 40, 94
Halo Vest, The (Pierce and Barr), 3: 321
halo-vest apparatus, 4: 153
Halsted, William, 1: 185–186; 4: 105
Hamann, Carl A., 3: 104
Hamilton, Alice, 3: 142
Hamilton, F. A., 4: 204
Hamilton, Frank H., 1: 50–51
Hamilton, Steward, 4: 482*b*
Hamilton Air Force Base, 3: 337
Hammersmith Hospital, 4: *398*, 401
Hammond, Franklin, 4: 90
Hammond, George, 3: 275
Hammond, Harriet, 4: 90
Hampden Park (Springfield, Mass.), 1: *249*
hamstring contractures, 2: 197–198, *198*
Hancock, John, 1: 17–18
Hand, The (Marble), 3: 316
Hand Division of the Pan American Medical Association, 2: 251
Hand Forum, 3: 411
Handbook of Anatomy Adapted for Dissecting and Clinical References from Original Dissections by John Warren (Green), 1: 89
Handbook of Anatomy (Aitken), 1: *89*
hands. *See also* wrists
    arthritis and, 4: 96
    boutonniere deformities, 4: 98
    epiphyseal injuries after frostbite, 2: 321–323
    extensor tendon ruptures, 4: 97
    factitious lymphedema of, 3: 429
    focal scleroderma of, 4: 183
    IP joint hyperextension, 4: 97
    neuromas in, 2: 248
    opera-glass deformity, 4: 99
    osteochondritis in a finger, 3: 363
    pianists and, 3: 414
    proximal interphalangeal joint and, 2: 251
    reconstructive surgery of, 4: 98–99
    rheumatoid arthritis and, 4: 96–98, *98*
    sarcoidosis, 4: 98
    soft tissues and, 4: 98
    swan neck deformity, 4: 98
    systemic lupus erythematosus (SLE), 4: 98
    systemic sclerosis, 4: 98
    tendon transfers and, 3: 428
    treatment of, 2: 248
    volar plate arthroplasty and, 2: 248
Hands (Simmons), 4: 183
Hand-Schüller-Christian disease, 2: 171
Hanelin, Joseph, 3: 294; 4: 91, 237–238
Hanley, Daniel F., 2: 372
Hanley, Edward, 3: 249
Hannah, John, 3: 357
Hansen, Robert L., 3: 258, 317
Hansen, Sigvard T., 3: 416
Hansjörg Wyss/AO Foundation Professor of Orthopaedic Surgery, 3: 409, 464*b*
Harborview Medical Center, 3: 416
Harding, Chester, 1: *95*
Harmer, Torr W., 1: 264; 3: 60; 4: 208
Harold and Anna Snider Ullian Orthopaedic Fund, 2: 439*b*
Harrast, J. J., 4: 173
Harriet M. Peabody Professor of Orthopaedic Surgery (HMS), 2: 183, 203, 327, 337, 438, 439*b*; 3: 202
Harrington, F. B., 2: 245; 3: 96, 110–111
Harrington, Paul, 2: 316, 335
Harrington, T. F., 1: 23
Harrington rods, 2: 316, *317*, 325, 335, 340
Harris, C. K., 2: 285
Harris, Mathew, 2: 439
Harris, Mitchel, 4: 194
Harris, Robert, 1: 204
Harris, W. Robert, 4: 351, 355–356
Harris, William H. (1927–), 3: 215, *217*
    adult reconstruction and, 3: 460*b*
    AMTI and, 3:224
    as Alan Gerry Clinical Professor of Orthopaedic Surgery, 3: 464*b*
    awards and, 3: 224, 224*b*
    biomechanics laboratory director, 3: 464*b*

biomechanics research and, 3: 220
bone-ingrowth type prostheses, 3: 222–223
Children's Hospital/MGH combined program and, 3: 215
early life, 3: 215
education and training, 3: 215
fellowships and, 3: 216, 218
Harris Hip Score and, 3: 219, *219*
on Haversian systems in bone, 2: 241; 3: *216*
hip research and surgery, 3: 217–225, 244, 388*t*
HMS appointment, 3: 216–217, 219–220, 224
innovation and, 3: 216–217, 224
knee arthroplasty and, 4: 129
Knee Biomechanics and Biomaterials Laboratory, 3: 464*b*
legacy of, 3: 224–225
memberships and, 3: 224–225
as MGH clinical faculty, 3: 464*b*
as MGH surgeon, 3: 216, 219–220, 398*b*; 4: 126
MIT appointment, 3: 219–220
mold arthroplasty and, 3: 218–219
on osteolysis after hip replacement, 3: 220, *220*, 221
publications and research, 3: 215–216, 218–220, 243, 398; 4: 135, *135*
on Smith-Petersen, 3: 216–217
Vanishing Bone, 3: 225, *225*
Harris Hip Score, 3: 219, *219*
Harris Orthopaedic Biomechanics and Biomaterials Laboratory, 3: 220, 463
Harris S. Yett Prize in Orthopedic Surgery, 4: 251
Harris-Galante Prosthesis (HGP), 3: 222
Hartwell, Harry F., 3: 68
Harvard Athletic Association, 1: 253, 258–259, 263
Harvard Athletic Committee, 1: 250; 4: 85
Harvard athletics
  athlete heart size, 1: 262, 267, 288
  Athlete's Bill of Rights and, 1: 279, 280*b*, 281
  basketball and, 1: 285–286
  crew team, 1: 250–251, 258
  dieticians and, 1: 258
  fatigue and, 1: 264–265
  football development, 1: 245, 247–248
  football injuries and, 1: 247–248, 252–262
  football team, 1: *249*, 251, *257*
  ice hockey, 1: 275, 286
  injury prevention and, 1: 279, 285–286
  knee joint injuries in, 1: 267–268, 268*t*
  musculoskeletal injuries, 1: 288
  physical therapy and, 1: 258
  protective padding and helmets in, 1: 255, *267*, 275
  sports medicine and, 1: 245–269, 274–282, 284–286; 2: 287; 3: 399
  Varsity Club logo, 1: *274*
  women athletes, 1: 285–286
Harvard Cancer Commission, 1: 256
Harvard Club, 1: 181, *181*
Harvard College. *See also* Harvard University
  anatomical society at, 1: 21, 133
  faculty in 1806, 1: 40
  football at, 1: 245
  medical examination of freshmen, 4: 84
  normal and abnormal posture in freshmen, 4: *84*
  Spunkers and, 1: 21, 32, 133
  vote to send Harvard Medical School surgeons to WWI service, 4: 386
Harvard Combined Orthopaedic Residency Program (HCORP)
  accreditation of, 1: 232–233, 239–241
  ACGME Orthopaedic RRC Committee review of, 1: 217–220
  Beth Israel Deaconess Medical Center and, 4: 284, 288
  Boston Pathology Course, 1: 216, 218
  Boston Prosthetics Course, 1: 220
  case sessions in, 1: 229*t*
  clinical curriculum, 1: 223–225
  combined grand rounds, 1: 232
  conference schedule for, 1: 221*t*
  core curriculum and, 1: 215–217, 227–232, 241–242
  development of, 1: 192–200
  directors of, 1: 243*b*
  distribution of residents and staff, 1: 227*t*
  diversity in, 1: 239
  early surgical training, 1: 183–186
  educational resources for, 1: 217
  evolution of, 1: 183
  funding for, 1: 206
  Green and, 1: 200–210
  growth of, 1: *240*
  Herndon and restructuring, 1: 222–243
  independent review of, 1: 234–237
  leadership of, 1: 181, 210–211
  Mankin and, 1: 211–220, 239; 3: 387, 397
  orthopaedic research in, 1: 218
  Pappas and, 1: 208–209
  program length and size, 1: 214–215, 218–220, 222–223, 239
  program review, 1: 238, 242–243
  reorganization of, 1: 211–216
  resident evaluations and, 1: 237–238
  resident salaries, 1: 206
  rotation schedule, 1: 225–226, 226*t*, 227, 227*t*
  specialty blocks in, 1: 228, 229*t*
  weekly program director's conference, 1: 230*b*
  women in, 1: 239; 3: 208
Harvard Community Health Physicians at Beth Israel Hospital, 4: 263
Harvard Community Health Plan, 1: 225
Harvard Corporation, 1: 25, 27, 40, 133, 178; 3: 4
Harvard Department of Hygiene, 2: 253
Harvard Fifth Surgical Service, 4: 275, 277, 279, 297, 302–303, 305–306
Harvard Fourth Medical Service, 4: 296
Harvard Hall, 1: 25, 134, *135*
Harvard Health Services, 3: 310
Harvard Infantile Paralysis Clinic, 2: 79, 107, 109, 176, 191, 432
Harvard Infantile Paralysis Commission, 2: 68, 70, 72, 99, 189
Harvard Medical Alumni Association, 1: 264; 2: 306
Harvard Medical Association, 3: 116, 119*b*
Harvard Medical Faculty Physicians (HMFP), 4: 214
Harvard Medical Meetings, 1: 174
Harvard Medical School (HMS), 1: *135*, 298. *See also* Holden Chapel; orthopaedics curriculum
  admission requirements, 1: 138, 141
  admission tickets to lectures, 1: *27*, 300
  Almshouse and, 3: 4

attendance certificates, 1: *28*
Beth Israel Hospital and, 4: 213–214
Bigelow and, 1: 137; 3: 34, 42–44
Boylston Medical Society, 3: 25–26
Brigham Orthopaedic Foundation staff and, 4: 192
budget and, 1: 158, 174
calendar reform, 1: 140
Cheever Professor of Surgery, 4: 303
classes and faculty, 1834, 1: *297*
clinical courses at BCH, 4: 380*t*–381*t*
Coll Warren and, 1: 85
construction in 1904, 1: *86*
continuing medical education and, 3: 396
curricular reform, 1: 140
deans of, 1: 68–69
departmental organization, 1: 172–175
diversity in, 1: 239
educational reforms and, 1: 139, 140*b*, 141, 146–147; 2: 41; 3: 44–45, 94
Ellen and Melvin Gordon Professor of Medical Education, 4: 264, 266
Epidemic Aid Team, 2: 260
faculty at, 1: 40, 176
faculty salaries, 1: 178–179
financial structure reform, 1: 140
floor plan, 1: *304*
founding of, 1: 6, 25–29, 133–134
George W. Gay Lecture, 4: 324
human dissections and, 1: 26, 38
Jack Warren and, 1: 21, 25–29, 40
John Ball and Buckminster Brown chair, 2: 63–64
John Collins Warren and, 1: 38–40, 66, 68–69; 3: 30
John Homans Professor of Surgery, 4: 298
Laboratory for Skeletal Disorders and Rehabilitation, 2: 413
Laboratory of Surgical Pathology and, 2: 90
locations of, 1: 134*t*, 135, 141
military hospitals and, 1: 270
military orthopaedic surgery course, 4: 455–462
military surgeon training at, 2: 42, 65–66
minority admissions to, 1: 138*b*

move from Cambridge to Boston, 1: 40–41; 2: 3
musculoskeletal medicine in, 1: 169
nose and throat clinic, 2: 40–41
orthopaedic clinic, 1: 173–174
orthopaedic curriculum, 1: 133–170
orthopaedic research and, 1: 193
orthopaedics as specialty course, 1: 141–143
PBBH and, 4: 1–4, 12, *12*, 13–14
postgraduate education and, 2: 157
preclinical and clinical departments, 1: 182*b*
qualifications for professors, 1: 26
radiology at, 2: 16
School for Health Officers, 2: 42, 65–66
Sears Surgical Laboratory, 4: 303
student evaluation of curricula, 1: 157–158, 167
surgery curriculum, 1: 140–141
surgical illustrations and, 3: 25
Surgical Research Laboratory, 4: 105, *106*, 107–108
teaching departments, 1: 157
Warren family and, 1: 71
women students and, 1: 138, 138*b*, 239; 3: 44
World War I volunteer orthopaedic surgeons, 2: 117–119, 124–127, 145; 3: *180*
World War II surgeons, 2: 232
Harvard Medical School (HMS). Department of Orthopaedic Surgery. *See also* Harvard Combined Orthopaedic Residency Program (HCORP)
advisory councils, 1: 182
as branch of Division of Surgery, 1: 171
chairperson of, 1: 180–182
curricular reform and, 1: 177
evolution of, 1: 171–182
faculty governance and, 1: 175–178
faculty rank and, 1: 178
faculty salaries, 1: 178–180
Harriet M. Peabody Professor of Orthopaedic Surgery, 2: 183, 203, 327, 337
John Ball and Buckminster Brown Chair of Orthopaedic Surgery, 1: 111, 177; 2: 63–64

John E. Hall Professorship in Orthopaedic Surgery, 2: 347
Lovett as chief of, 2: 64
organization of, 1: 171–182, 182*b*
teaching hospitals and, 1: 172–176, 180–181
Harvard Orthopaedic Journal, 1: 231–232
Harvard Orthopaedic Residency Program, 1: 167
Harvard Second Medical Service, 4: 296
Harvard Unit (1st), 3: 180, *180*
Harvard Unit (5th General Hospital), 1: 270, 277; 3: 271; 4: 17, *17*, 484–485
Harvard Unit (105th General Hospital), 1: 270–271; 2: 231–232; 3: 271, 351; 4: 488–489
Harvard Unit (American Ambulance Hospital), 2: 119–121, 123–124; 3: *180*, 369, *370*; 4: 388, *388*, 389*b*, *390*, 391, 393. *See also* American Ambulance Hospital (Neuilly, France)
Harvard Unit (Base Hospital No. 5), 1: 270; 2: 125, 145; 4: 405, 419–421, 421*b*, *421*, 422–424, *428*
Harvard Unit (Walter Reed General Hospital), 4: 488
Harvard University. *See also* Harvard athletics; Harvard College
Dunster House, 2: *388*
establishment of medical school, 1: 6, 25–29, 133–134
Kirkland House, 2: 358, *358*
posture research and, 4: 84, *84*, 85–86, 234, *234*
public service ideal and, 2: 64
World War I and, 2: 64
Harvard University Health Services, 1: 274, 277, 284; 3: 450
Harvard Vanguard Medical Associates, 4: 194, 195*b*, 288
Harvard Varsity Club, 1: *272*, *282*, 289
Harvard/MGH Sports Medicine Fellowship Program, 3: 448
Hasty Pudding Club, 1: 32
Hatcher, Howard, 3: 382
Hatt, R. Nelson, 3: 368; 4: 378
Hauck, Charles, 4: 41*b*
Haus, Brian, 3: 409
Haverhill Clinic, 2: 107
Haversian system, 1: xxii
Hawkes, Micajah, 1: 42, 44, 49
Hayes, Helen, 2: 315
Hayes, Mabel, 4: 97

Index

Hayes, Wilson C. (Toby), 4: 262–264, 271, 284–285
Hayward, George, 1: 54, 60, *60*, 61–62, 65, 137, 296, 302; 3: 12, 27, 34, 112
HCORP. *See* Harvard Combined Orthopaedic Residency Program (HCORP)
Head, William, 4: 116, 129, 161–162, 193
head surgery, 3: 18
Health, William, 1: 18
health care
    disparities for minorities, 4: 264–265
    humanitarianism and, 2: 413, 421
    injured workers and, 4: 327
    issues in, 2: 375
    managed care movement, 3: 397
    medical costs, 3: 379, 379t
    physician profiling and, 2: 373–374
    policy and, 2: 371
    polio courses for, 2: 189
    prospective payment system (PPS), 3: 397
    resource utilization, 2: 372
Health Security Act, 2: 374–375
Heard, J. Theodore, 4: 23
Heary, Robert F., 4: 272b
heavy-resistance exercise, 3: 282, *282*, 283–285
Hebraic debility, 4: 203
Heckman, James, 1: 233; 2: 240; 3: 463, 464b; 4: 173–174
Hedequest, Daniel, 2: 344
Hektoen, Ludvig, 2: 78
Helems, Don, 4: 129
Helen Hallett Thompson Fund, 2: 107
Helmers, Sandra, 2: 342
Henderson, M. S., 3: 166; 4: 394
Hendren, Hardy, 2: 182, 399
Henry, William B., Jr., 3: 398b
Henry Ford Hospital, 2: 167–168; 3: 328
Henry J. Bigelow Medal, 2: 69; 3: 135
Henry J. Bigelow Operating Theater, 1: 84
Henry J. Mankin Orthopaedic Research Professorship, 3: 392
Hensinger, Robert, 2: 302
heparin, 3: 362
Hérard, Françoise, 3: 48
Herder, Lindsay, 3: 410
Hermann, Otto J. (1884–1973), 4: *334*
    AAOS and, 4: 337

BCH Bone and Joint Service, 4: 307, 328, 333–334, 337, 380b
BCH compound fracture therapy research, 4: *335*, 337
BCH residencies and, 4: 377–378
Boston City Hospital and, 3: 237; 4: 242, 333–334
Boston University Medical School appointment, 4: 335
Cotton and, 4: 334
death of, 4: 337
education and training, 4: 333
HMS appointment, 4: 334–335
honors and awards, 4: 337
lectures and presentations, 4: 334–335, 337
Massachusetts Regional Fracture Committee, 3: 64
New England Regional Committee on Fractures, 4: 341
os calcis fractures research, 4: 335–336
professional memberships, 4: 334
publications and research, 4: 335, *335*, 337
Scudder Oration on Trauma, 3: 63
Tufts Medical School appointment, 4: 335
Herndon, Charles, 2: 195
Herndon, James H., 1: *222*
    Brigham and Women's Hospital and, 4: 195b
    congenital kyphosis case, 2: 399
    dedication of Codman's headstone, 3: *145*
    fat embolism syndrome research, 2: 397
    on Frank R. Ober, 2: 149
    on Glimcher, 2: 325
    on Hall, 2: 347
    Harvard Orthopaedic Journal, 1: 232
    leadership of, 1: 236
    as MGH clinical faculty, 3: 464b
    military service, 2: 399
    Pittsburgh Orthopaedic Journal, 1: 232
    as residency program director, 1: 222
    restructuring of HCORP, 1: 222–243
    on Riseborough, 2: 398–399
    Scoliosis and Other Deformities of the Axial Skeleton, 2: 398, *398*
    Smith Day lectures, 3: 431
    on Watts, 2: 421–422
    William H. and Johanna A. Harris Professor, 3: 464b

on William T. Green, 2: 169, 178–179
Herndon, William, 2: 359
Herodicus Society, 2: *387*
Herring, Tony, 2: 346, 438
Hersey, Ezekiel, 1: 25, 133
Heuter, Carl, 3: 181
Hey, William, 1: xxii
Heymann, Emil, 4: 215
Heywood, Charles Frederick, 1: 60
Hibbs, Russell A., 3: 155, 203; 4: 343, 394
Hibbs spinal fusion procedure, 2: 164; 3: 155; 4: 343
Hickling, Harriet Fredrica, 1: 299
Hildreth, Dr., 1: 97
Hilibrand, Alan S., 4: 266b
Hill, Walter, 4: 401
Hillman, J. William, 1: 162
Hinckley, Robert C., 1: 55, 59; 3: *30*
hip abduction splint, 1: *127*
hip dislocations. *See also* congenital dislocated hips (CDH)
    bilateral, 1: 126–127; 3: 235
    diagnosis of, 1: 46
    Henry J. Bigelow and, 3: 34–36
    hip joint excision, 3: 34
    J. Mason Warren and, 1: 75
    John Collins Warren and, 1: 42, 44–46, *46*, 47–50, 68; 3: 13, 13b, 36
    Lorenz technique and, 3: 164
    relaxing the Y-ligament, 3: 35–36, 38
    traction treatment for, 1: 108, *108*; 2: 32
    traumatic hip dislocation case, 2: 352–353
    treatment of, 1: 68, 74–75
hip disorders. *See also* total hip replacement
    abduction contracture, 2: 153, *153*
    acetabular dysplasia, 2: 389, *389*, 390
    anterior supra-articular subperiosteal approach to, 3: 181, 182b
    antisepsis technique, 2: 52
    bacterial infections and, 2: 108
    bilateral bony ankylosis, 3: *196*
    biomechanics research, 2: 407
    Bradford and, 2: 21–22, 32
    congenital hip dysplasia, 2: 302
    direct anterior approach to, 3: 181
    direct lateral approach and, 3: 277–278
    displacement of proximal femoral epiphysis, 3: 372

Down syndrome and, 2: 368
fascia lata arthroplasty and,
   3: 181
femoroacetabular impingement,
   3: 188–189
flexion/adduction contractures,
   2: 293–294
hip abductor paralysis treatment,
   2: 149–150
hip fusion for severe disabling
   arthritis, 3: 156*b*
importance of anticoagulation in,
   3: *218*
lateral approach, 3: 219
Legg-Calvé-Perthes disease,
   2: 351
Lovett and, 2: 32, 53
Lovett and Shaffer's paper on,
   2: 49, *49*, 52
metastatic malignant melanoma
   fracture case, 4: 77–78
Millis and, 2: 392
mold arthroplasty and, 3: *196*,
   218–219, 241, 244
nailing fractured, 3: 237
Ober-Yount fasciotomy, 2: 172
osteoarthritis and, 2: 389;
   3: 155, *222*
poliomyelitis contracture treatment, 2: 294, 295*b*
posterior approach to, 2: 146
prophylactic antibiotics in surgery, 3: 253
prostheses and, 2: 407
radiography in, 2: 54
septic arthritis of, 2: 380
slipped capital femoral epiphysis
   (SCFE), 2: 176
splints for, 2: 247
subtrochanteric osteotomy,
   2: 293–294
traction treatment for, 2: 21–22,
   53, *54*; 3: 148
transient synovitis of, 2: 380
Trendelenburg gait and, 2: 33
Trumble technique for fusion of,
   3: 367
tuberculosis and, 2: 21–22,
   52–53, *54*; 3: 148
vastus slide and, 3: 278
hip fractures. *See also* femoral neck
   fractures
   antibiotic use, 3: 253, 255
   anticoagulation in, 3: *218*
   Austin Moore prosthesis for,
      3: 213
   Banks and, 4: 74–75
   Britten hip fusion technique,
      4: 363
   elderly patients and, 4: 341

hospitalization for, 2: 372
MGH approach to,
   4: 159*b*–160*b*
mold arthroplasty and, 3: 218
pathophysiology and treatment
   of, 4: 43
reduction and impaction of,
   4: 318–320, 322*b*
Hip Society, 2: 407; 3: 224; 4: 141
Hippocratic Oath, 2: 1
Hirohashi, Kenji, 4: 145
Hirsch, Carl, 4: 259–260
*History of the Massachusetts General
   Hospital* (Bowditch), 3: 15
*History of the Orthopedic Department
   at Children's Hospital* (Lovett),
   2: 247
HMS. *See* Harvard Medical School
   (HMS)
Ho, Sandy, 2: 405
Hochberg, Fred, 3: 414
Hodge, Andrew, 3: 397–398
Hodgen, John T., 1: 188
Hodges, Richard M., 3: 44, 51
Hodgkins, Lyman, 2: 244
Hodgson, Arthur R., 2: 336, 398
Hoffa, Albert, 2: 33
Hogan, Daniel E., 4: 263
Hoke, Michael, 2: 77–78, 282–283
Holden Chapel, 1: *135*
   anatomy lectures in, 1: 26, 29,
      38
   floor plan, 1: *26*
   human dissections and, 1: 26, 38
   medical instruction in, 1: 134
Holland, Daniel, 3: 241
Holmes, Donald, 4: 117
Holmes, George, 3: 192
Holmes, Oliver Wendell, 1: *291*
   as anatomy professor at HMS,
      1: 66; 4: 298
   on anesthesia, 1: 56, 61
   on Bigelow, 3: 13, 27, 38, 51
   Boston Dispensary and, 2: 306
   European medical studies, 1: 73
   on George Hayward, 1: 302
   on George Parkman, 1: 291,
      294, 296
   on hip dislocation case, 1: 46
   on invention of stethoscope,
      1: 74
   on J. Mason Warren, 1: 77
   on John Warren, 1: 27, 69;
      3: 33–34
   on medical studies, 1: 138
   as MGH consulting surgeon,
      3: 14
   as MGH surgeon emeritus, 3: 46
   on need for clinics, 3: 3

reform of HMS and, 1: 139–
   140; 3: 45
Tremont Street Medical School,
   3: 42
trial of John Webster and,
   1: 308–309
Holmes, Timothy, 1: 81, 83
Holyoke, Augustus, 1: 95
Holyoke, Edward A., 1: 21
Homans, John, 2: 10, 306; 3: *38*,
   94, 118, 145; 4: 5, 9
Hooton, Elizabeth, 1: 9
Hoover, Herbert, 4: 235
Hôpital de Bicêtre, 1: 73
Hôpital de la Charité, 1: 37, 73–74
Hôpital de la Pitié, 1: 73–74
Hôpital de la Salpêtrière, 1: 73
Hôpital des Enfants Malades, 1: 73,
   106
Hôpital Saint-Louis, 1: 73, 82
Hormell, Robert S. (1917–2006),
   4: *92*
   Boston Children's Hospital and,
      4: 93
   chronic arthritis research,
      4: 92–93
   on congenital scoliosis, 4: 65, 93
   death of, 4: 94
   education and training, 4: 92
   HMS appointment, 4: 93
   knee arthroplasty and, 4: 93–94
   PBBH and, 4: 35
   publications and research,
      4: 92–94
   RBBH and, 4: 38, 41*b*, 68, 89,
      93–94
   study of hallux valgus, 4: 40, 94
Horn, Carl E., 2: *271*
Hornicek, Francis J., 3: 390, 462,
   464*b*
Hosea, Timothy, 4: 262
Hospital for Joint Diseases, 3: 382–
   383, 385, 389, 413, 427
Hospital for Sick Children (Toronto),
   2: 334–336
Hospital for Special Surgery, 1: 89;
   2: 27; 3: 376; 4: 130, 134
Hospital for the Ruptured and
   Crippled, 2: 27, 43, 52, 225–226;
   3: 376
Hospital of the University of Pennsylvania, 4: 465
hospitals. *See also* base hospitals; military reconstruction hospitals
   Boston development of, 3: 3–7,
      9–12
   consolidation of, 4: 20
   debarkation, 4: 451–452
   embarkation, 4: 451–452
   end results concept, 1: 112

exclusion of poor women from,
  1: 123
F.H. Brown on construction of,
  2: 5
government and, 2: 138b–139b
internships in, 1: 186
military field, 1: 272; 2: 118;
  4: *414*, 468
military hospitals in Australia,
  4: 488–489
mobile army surgical hospitals (MASHs), 2: 231–232;
  4: 468–469, *470*
orthopaedics services in, 4: 451
portable surgical, 4: 468–469,
  489
prejudice against Jewish physicians in, 1: 158
reserve units for army service,
  4: 429
standardization of, 3: 112, 113b,
  115–116, 123–125, 131
unpopularity of, 1: 41
Hôtel-Dieu, 1: 37, 73–74, 82
Hough, Garry de N., Jr., 2: 230
House of Providence, 2: 256
House of the Good Samaritan,
  1: *128*; 2: 4
  Anne Smith Robbins and,
    1: 123–125; 2: 114
  attraction of patients from the
    U.S. and abroad, 1: 125
  BCH merger, 1: 130; 2: 433
  Bradford and, 2: 21, 25, 28–29
  Buckminster Brown and, 1: 107,
    121–122, 125–128; 2: 28
  Children's Ward, 1: *123*
  closure of orthopaedic wards,
    1: 129–130
  disabled children and, 2: 306
  founding of, 1: 123–124
  hip disease treatment at,
    1: 128–129
  Lovett and, 2: 49
  orthopaedic wards in, 1: 123,
    125–126, 129; 2: 20
  orthopaedics residencies, 1: 186
  Osgood and, 2: 114
  poor women and, 1: 123–124
  rheumatic heart disease treatment
    at, 1: 130
  surgical records from, 2: 114,
    115b
  training of orthopaedic surgeons,
    1: 127, 129
  treatment of adults and children
    in, 2: 4
house pupils (pups), 1: 80, 184, *185*;
  2: 20; 3: 4, 16
Howard, Herbert B., 3: 120

Howard University, 1: 239
Howorth procedure, 4: 243
Hresko, M. Timothy (1954–),
  2: *364*
  Boston Children's Hospital and,
    2: 364, 366–368, 439b
  education and training, 2: 364
  HMS appointment, 2: 364
  latent psoas abscess case, 2: 365
  Medical Student Undergraduate
    Education Committee, 1: 166
  orthopaedics appointments,
    2: 364
  orthopaedics curriculum, 1: 167
  pediatric orthopaedics, 2: 365
  publications and research,
    2: 366, *366*, 367, *367*, 368
  scoliosis and spinal deformity
    research, 2: 364–367
  on trauma in children, 2: 365,
    368
  University of Massachusetts and,
    2: 364
Hse, John, 2: 266
Hsu, Hu-Ping, 4: 194
Hubbard, Leroy W., 2: 77–78
Huddleston, James, 3: 254, 256
Huffaker, Stephen, 4: 190b
Hugenberger, Arthur, 2: 268
Hugenberger, Elizabeth, 2: 268
Hugenberger, Franklin, 2: 268
Hugenberger, Gordon, 2: 272
Hugenberger, Helen, 2: 268
Hugenberger, Herman, 2: 268
Hugenberger, Janet McMullin,
  2: 272
Hugenberger, Joan, 2: 269, 271–272
Hugenberger, Paul W. (1903–1996),
  2: *268*, *271*
  Boston Children's Hospital and,
    2: 233, 269–272, 301
  Boston City Hospital and, 2: 269
  donations to Boston Medical
    Library, 2: 271
  education and training, 2: 268
  famous patients of, 2: 271–272
  Georgia Warm Springs Foundation and, 2: 270
  grand rounds and, 2: 271
  HMS appointment, 2: 269–270
  Marlborough Medical Associates
    and, 2: 146, 269, 299
  marriage and family, 2: 272
  MGH and, 2: 268
  New England Peabody Home
    for Crippled Children and,
    2: 269–270
  Ober and, 2: 269, 271
  orthopaedics appointments,
    2: 270

  orthopaedics internships, 2: 269
  PBBH and, 2: 269; 4: 16,
    18–20, 22, 110, 116, 128
  private medical practice, 2: 269
  professional memberships,
    2: 270, 272
  publications and research,
    2: 268–269, 271
  Salem Hospital and, 2: 270–272
Hugenberger Orthopaedic Library,
  2: 272
Huggins Hospital (Wolfeboro, NH),
  2: 218
Hughes, Mable, 3: 362
human anatomy
  anatomical atlas and, 1: 89
  Astley Cooper and, 1: 34
  Harvard courses in, 1: 6, 25,
    133–134, 136–138, 140–141
  HMS courses in, 1: *229*, 230
  legalization of human dissection,
    1: 52
  military surgeon training and,
    2: 66
  orthopaedic chronic disease and,
    3: 85
  skeleton, 1: *136*
  variations in, 3: 85–86, 86t
human dissections
  grave robbing and, 1: 32, 34
  legalization of, 1: 52
  in medical education, 1: 26–27,
    34, 38, 40, 51–52
  in military hospitals, 1: 24
Human Limbs and Their Substitutes
  (Wilson and Klopsteg), 3: 376
humeral fractures
  displaced supracondylar, 2: 379
  Gartland type 3 supracondylar,
    2: 368
  intercondylar T fractures, 2: 397,
    397
  nonunion of the humerus, 2: 96,
    96, 250
  pins used in, 2: 379
  proximal, 2: 96, *122*
  resorption of the humerus, 2: 97,
    97
  supracondylar, 2: 229, 345, 379
Hunter, John, 1: xxi, 33, 36–37
Hunter, William, 1: 6, *133*
Hussey, Phyllis Ann, 4: 153
Hussey, Robert W. (1936–1992),
  4: *151*
  Brigham and Women's Hospital,
    4: 163
  Children's Hospital/MGH combined program and, 4: 151
  death of, 4: 153
  education and training, 4: 151

HMS appointment, 4: 152
marriage and family, 4: 153
Medical College of Virginia appointment, 4: 153
PBBH and, 4: 116, 128–129, 151, 163
publications and research, 4: *151*, 152–153
Rancho Los Amigos fellowship, 4: 129, 151
spinal cord injury research and treatment, 4: 151, *151*, 152–153
US Navy and, 4: 151
VA Medical Center (Richmond, VA), 4: 153
West Roxbury Veterans Administration Hospital and, 4: 129, 152
Hutchinson, Thomas, 1: 16
Hyatt, George, 3: 439
hydroxylysine, 2: 327–328
Hylamer metal-backed polyethylene acetabular components, 4: 172
Hynes, John, 4: 303
hypnosis, 1: 56

I

ice hockey, 1: 275, 286
Ida C. Smith ward (BCH), 2: 431
Ilfeld, Fred, 3: 317
iliofemoral ligament, 3: 35–36, 38
iliotibial band
    ACL reconstruction and, 2: 378–379, *386*; 3: 448
    contractures and, 3: 209
    hip abductor paralysis treatment, 2: 149–150
    knee flexion contracture and, 3: 374
    modification of sacrospinalis and, 2: 147
    Ober Operation and, 2: 153
    tendon transplantations and, 2: 109
    tightness in, 2: 151–152
IMSuRT. *See* International Medical-Surgical Response Team (IMSuRT)
inclinometers, 2: 366, *367*
industrial accidents
    back disabilities and, 2: 92; 4: 358
    BCH Relief Station and, 4: 305, *305*
    carpal tunnel syndrome and, 4: 184–186
    Cotton and, 4: 323, 325, 327
    defects in patient care, 4: 325, 352–354
    fracture care and, 4: 338, 339*b*–340*b*
    insurance and, 2: 92; 4: 325, 339*b*, 341
    intervertebral disc surgery in, 3: 316
    kineplastic forearm amputation case, 4: 360
    Maria Hospital (Stockholm) and, 1: 263
    os calcis fractures and, 4: 325
    ruptured intervertebral discs and, 4: 352
    Sever and, 2: 92
    workers' compensation issues, 4: 184–186, 253, 325, 352–353
Industrial School for Crippled and Deformed Children (Boston), 2: 36–37, *37*, 38, 97, 308; 3: 151, 161
Industrial School for Crippled Children (Boston), 2: 38, *38*
infantile paralysis (poliomyelitis). *See* poliomyelitis
infections
    allografts and, 3: 435, 440, 442
    amputations and, 1: 23, 74, 84
    antisepsis dressings and, 1: 84–85
    carbolic acid treatment, 1: 82–83, *83*, *84*
    hand-washing policy and, 1: 193
    infantile paralysis (poliomyelitis) and, 2: 261
    mortality due to, 1: 74, 81, 84
    postoperative, 3: 253
    resection and, 1: 81
    Revolutionary War deaths and, 1: 22
    tubercular cows and, 2: 16
    use of ultraviolet light for, 4: 164, 164*t*
infectious diseases, 1: 7–9; 2: 4–5, 15
influenza, 1: 4, 7; 3: 135
Ingalls, William, 1: 32; 2: 5, 9, 11
Ingersoll, Robert, 4: 376
Ingraham, Frank, 2: 215
Insal, John, 4: 130
insane, 3: 3–4, 6
"Insensibility During Surgical Operations Produced by Inhalation" (Bigelow), 3: 27, *27*
Inside Brigham and Women's Hospital, 4: *123*
Institute for Children with Thalidomide Induced Limb Deformation, 2: 413
Institute Pasteur, 1: 91
institutional racism, 3: 15–16
Instituto Buon Pastore, 4: *480*, 481
insufflation anesthesia apparatus, 4: 215–216
"Interior of a Hospital Tent, The" (Sargent), 4: *424*
International Arthroscopic Association, 3: 422
International Association of Industrial Accident Boards and Commission, 2: 92
International Federation of Societies for Surgery of the Hand, 2: 251
International Hip Society, 3: 224
International Journal of Orthopaedic Surgery, 2: 80
International Knee Documentation Committee (IKDC), 1: 287; 2: 381
International Medical-Surgical Response Team (IMSuRT), 3: 417–418
International Pediatric Orthopedic Think Tank (IPOTT), 2: 304, *304*
International Society of Orthopaedic Surgery and Traumatology (SICOT), 2: 80–81, *81*, 137
interpedicular segmental fixation (ISF) pedicle screw plate, 3: 420–421
Interurban Orthopaedic Club, 2: 230
Ioli, James, 4: 193, 195*b*
Iowa Hip Score, 3: 219
Ireland, Robert, 1: 317
iron lung, 2: *79*
    Berlin polio epidemic and, 2: 260, 264
    Boston polio epidemic and, 2: 314
    Drinker and, 2: 78, *78*
    infantile paralysis (poliomyelitis) and, 2: 261*b*–262*b*, 266
    invention of, 2: 191
    Massachusetts Infantile Paralysis Clinic and, 2: 212
    poliomyelitis and, 2: 78, *190*
ischemia-edema cycle, 2: 200–201, *201*
ISOLA implants, 2: *370*, 371
Isola Study Group, 2: 371
Istituto Ortopedico Rizzoli (Bologna, Italy), 3: 435–436

J

J. Collins Warren Laboratory, 1: 87
J. Robert Gladden Orthopaedic Society, 4: *265*
Jackson, Charles T., 1: 57, 60, 306

Index

Jackson, G. H., 3: 35
Jackson, George H., Jr., 2: 140
Jackson, Henry, 2: 20
Jackson, J. B. S., 1: 67
Jackson, James
   founding of MGH, 1: 31,
      40–42; 3: 5, 5, 6b–7b, 12–13
   on George Hayward, 1: 302
   George Parkman and, 1: 296
   Harvard Medical teaching, 1: 299
   John Collins Warren and, 1: 37,
      40, 66
   medical studies in London, 1: 37
   publications of, 1: 38–39
   support for House of the Good
      Samaritan, 1: 124
Jackson, James, Jr., 1: 73
Jackson, Robert W., 2: 279; 3: 446
Jaffe, Henry, 3: 382, 385, 392
Jaffe, Norman, 2: 422
Jagger, Thomas A., 3: 338
James, J. I. P., 2: 333–335, 399
James H. Herndon Resident Teaching and Mentoring Award, 3: 463
James Lawrence Kernan Hospital, 4: 157
Janeway, Charles A., 2: 215
Jasty, Murali, 3: 398, 460b, 464b
JDW (Jigme Dorji Wangchuk)
   National Referral Hospital, 3: 418
Jeffries, John, 1: 292
Jenkins, Roger, 4: 281
Jennings, Ellen Osgood, 2: 138
Jennings, L. Candace (1949–)
   cancer fatigue and, 3: 405–406
   education and training, 3: 405
   HCORP and, 3: 405
   Hospice and Palliative Medicine
      fellowship, 3: 407
   as MGH surgeon, 3: 405
   orthopaedic oncology and,
      3: 405, 460b
   publications and research,
      3: 405–406
   ulnar nerve compression case,
      3: 405–406
Jette, Alan, 3: 391
Jewish Hospital (St. Louis), 2: 231
Jewish Memorial Hospital and Rehabilitation Center, 4: 212
Jewish Memorial Hospital (Boston), 4: 212, 215
Jewish patients
   "Hebraic Debility" and, 4: 202,
      203b, 203
   hospital formation for, 4: 200–
      202, 223
   limited medical care for,
      4: 199–200

   in-patient care for observant,
      4: 199, 204–206
Johansson, S., 3: 189
John Ball and Buckminster Brown
   Clinical Professor of Orthopaedic
   Surgery, 1: 111, 177; 2: 63–64,
   64, 133, 147, 157; 3: 202, 464b;
   4: 195b
John E. Hall Professorship in Orthopaedic Surgery (HMS), 2: 347,
   438, 439b
Johns Hopkins Base Hospital Unit,
   2: 221; 3: 288, 291
Johns Hopkins Hospital, 1: 185;
   4: 429
Johns Hopkins Medical School
   departmental organization at,
      1: 175–176
   Flexner Report and, 1: 146–147
   governance and, 1: 177
   trust for, 4: 1, 3
Johnson, Howard, 2: 272
Johnson, J. A., 2: 77–78
Johnson, Lanny, 3: 446
Johnson, Robert W., Jr., 4: 239
Joint Commission on Accreditation of Healthcare Organizations
   (JCAHO), 3: 146
Joint Commission on Hospital
   Accreditation, 3: 131
joint disease. *See* bone and joint
   disorders
Joint Injuries of the Hand (Eaton),
   2: 250, *250*
Joint Kinematics Laboratory, 3: 463,
   464b
Jones, Arlene MacFarlane, 3: 291
Jones, Daniel F., 3: 60b, 313, 371;
   4: 274–276
Jones, Deryk, 4: 190b
Jones, Ezra A., 2: 78
Jones, Howard, 4: 347
Jones, Neil, 3: 431
Jones, Sir Robert, 4: *394*
   on active motion, 2: 68
   BEF Director of Military Orthopedics, 4: 405
   on femur fracture treatment,
      4: 408
   on importance of American surgeons, 4: 412b–413b
   Lovett and, 2: 63, 80–81
   MGH and, 3: 299
   military orthopaedics and,
      2: 124, 127; 4: 392–394, 401,
      407
   Notes on Military Orthopaedics,
      4: 442, *442*, 443
   orthopaedic surgery and, 4: 463
   Orthopedic Surgery, 2: 69, *69*

   Osgood and, 2: 116, 124–125,
      125, 126
   on prevention of deformity,
      4: 409
   request for American orthopaedic
      surgeons, 4: 393, 398
   SICOT and, 2: 81
Jones, William N. (1916–1991),
   3: *291*, *461*
   death of, 3: 293
   early life, 3: 291
   education and training, 3: 291
   evolution of the Vitallium mold,
      3: 292b, 293
   "Fracture of the Month" column,
      3: 243, 291
   as MGH surgeon, 3: 398b
   mold arthroplasty and,
      3: 291–292
   orthopedic arthritis service,
      3: 388t
   publications and research,
      3: 291; 4: 187
   US Army Medical Corps and,
      3: 291
Jones splints, 4: 389, 411
Joplin, Robert J. (1902–1983),
   3: *293*
   AOFS and, 3: 295, 298
   Boston Children's Hospital and,
      2: 274; 3: 293
   Boston VA Hospital and, 3: 298
   death of, 3: 298
   early life, 3: 293
   education and training, 3: 293
   on epiphyseal injuries, 4: 356
   foot surgery and, 3: 294–295,
      296b–297b, 298
   HMS appointment, 3: 293, 298
   legacy of, 3: 298
   memberships and, 3: 298
   as MGH surgeon, 3: 293–294,
      298
   publications and research,
      3: 293–294, *294*, 295, 341;
      4: 63
   RBBH and, 3: 293; 4: 36, 93,
      111
   sling procedure and, 3: 294, *294*,
      295, 296b–297b
   Slipped Capital Femoral Epiphysis,
      3: 294, 333
   slipped capital femoral epiphysis
      research, 4: 237–238
Jorevinroux, P., 2: 340
Joseph O'Donnell Family Chair
   in Orthopedic Sports Medicine,
   2: 438, 439b
Joseph S. Barr Memorial Fund,
   3: 214

Joseph S. Barr Visiting Consultantship, 3: 213
Joseph Warren, about 1765 (Copley), 1: *3, 11*
Josiah B. Thomas Hospital, 2: 252
Joslin, Elliott P., 4: 274
Joslin and Overholt Clinic, 4: 279
Journal of Bone and Joint Surgery (JBJS)
    American issues of, 3: 345, 347
    Annual Bibliography of Orthopaedic Surgery, 3: 261
    as British Orthopaedic Association's official publication, 3: 345
    budget deficits and, 3: 345–346
    Charles Painter as acting editor, 4: 50
    David Grice as associate editor, 2: 214
    Elliott Brackett as editor, 2: 130; 3: 157–159, 160*b*, 161
    expansion of editorial board positions, 3: 345
    Frank Ober as associate editor, 2: 165
    H. Winnett Orr as editor, 2: 125
    James Heckman as editor, 1: 233; 2: 240
    John Bell as associate editor, 2: 221
    Jonathan Cohen as editor, 2: 238–239
    as the journal of record, 3: 261–262
    logo for, 3: *261*
    name changes of, 1: xxiv
    ownership reorganization, 3: 346–347
    standards for, 3: 261
    Thornton Brown as editor, 3: 260–262
    Zabdiel Adams as associate editor, 3: 235
Journal of Pediatrics, 2: 7
Joyce, Michael, 1: 217*b*; 4: 189
Judet hip prosthesis, 3: 293
Junghanns, Herbert, 4: 262
Jupiter, Beryl, 3: 411
Jupiter, Jesse B. (1946–), 3: *407, 461*
    Cave Traveling Fellowship and, 1: 217*b*
    Children's Hospital/MGH combined program and, 3: 408
    education and training, 3: 407–408
    fracture treatment and, 3: 408–409

    Fractures of the Distal Radius, 3: 409, *409*
    Hand Forum president, 3: 411
    as Hansjorg Wyss/AO Foundation Professor, 3: 464*b*
    HMS appointment, 3: 408–409
    honors and awards, 3: 409
    intra-articular radial nerve entrapment case, 3: 410–411
    memberships and, 3: 411
    as MGH clinical faculty, 3: 464*b*
    MGH hand service and, 3: 396, 410, 460*b*
    as MGH surgeon, 3: 408
    MGH trauma unit and, 3: 399, 408
    named lectures and, 3: 410–411
    public health service and, 3: 408
    publications and research, 3: 408–411
    WRIST and, 3: 410
juvenile rheumatoid arthritis, 2: 171

K

Kaden, D. A., 4: 171
Kadiyala, Rajendra, 4: 190*b*
Kadzielski, John J., 3: 463*b*
Kagno, Marcia, 4: 89
Kanavel, Allan B., 3: 113*b*
Kaplan, Ronald K., 4: 89
Karlin, Lawrence I. (1945–), 2: *369*
    Boston Children's Hospital and, 2: 369–371
    education and training, 2: 369
    HMS appointment, 2: 370
    ISOLA implants and, 2: 371
    Isola Study Group, 2: 371
    orthopaedics appointments, 2: 369
    pediatric orthopaedics, 2: 370
    professional memberships, 2: 370
    publications of, 2: 371
    Scheuermann kyphosis treatment, 2: 371
    Tufts Medical School and, 2: 369
Karp, Evelyn Gerstein, 4: 241
Karp, Meier G. (1904–1962), 4: *240*
    as Beth Israel chief of orthopaedics, 4: 241, 289*b*
    Beth Israel Hospital and, 4: 240
    Boston Children's Hospital and, 4: 240
    death of, 4: 241
    education and training, 4: 240
    HMS appointment, 4: 240–241
    marriage and family, 4: 241
    PBBH and, 4: 18–20, 110, 240
    private medical practice, 2: 313; 4: 240

    professional memberships, 4: 241
    publications and research, 2: 229; 4: 240–241
    Thayer General Hospital and, 4: 241
    US Army and, 4: 241
    West Roxbury Veterans Administration Hospital and, 4: 240
Kasser, James
    Boston Children's Hospital and, 2: 354, 364, 434, 439*b*
    Catharina Ormandy Professorship, 2: 439*b*
    on Griffin, 2: 354
    HCORP and, 1: 224–225
    John E. Hall Professorship in Orthopaedic Surgery, 2: 439*b*
    Karlin and, 2: 369
    as orthopaedic chair, 2: 15*b*, 436
    publications of, 2: 368, 380
    on Zeke Zimbler, 4: 249
Kast, Thomas, 1: 25
Katz, Eton P., 2: 324
Katz, Jeffrey N., 2: 375; 4: 184–186, 195*b*, 269
Katzeff, Miriam (1899–1989), 2: *273*
    arthrogryposis multiplex congenita case, 2: 274–275
    Boston Children's Hospital and, 2: 222, 252, 273–275
    death of, 2: 275
    education and training, 2: 273
    as first female orthopaedic surgeon in Mass., 1: 239; 2: 275
    New England Hospital for Women and Children and, 2: 274
    orthopaedics appointments, 2: 274
    Osgood tribute, 2: 275
    professional memberships, 2: 275
    publications of, 2: 275
Kawalek, Thaddeus, 3: 282
Keats, John, 1: 36
Keely, John L., 2: 220
Keen, William W., 2: 72, *73*; 3: 103; 4: 411
Keep, Nathan C., 1: 308
Keeting, Mr., 1: 97
Kehinde, Olaniyi, 4: 169
Keith, Arthur, 2: 39
Keller, Joseph Black, 2: 126
Keller, Robert B. (ca. 1937–), 2: *371*
    Boston Children's Hospital and, 2: 286, 371
    Brigham and Women's Hospital and, 4: 193
    carpal tunnel syndrome research, 2: 375; 4: 184–185

Index

Dartmouth Atlas of Health Care in Virginia, The, 2: 375
Dartmouth-Hitchcock Medical Center and, 2: 371
education and training, 2: 371
Harrington rods and, 2: 316, 371
health care policy and, 2: 371–376
Health Security Act and, 2: 374–375
HMS appointment, 2: 371
low-back pain research, 2: 371–372
Maine Carpal Tunnel Study, 2: 375
Maine Lumbar Spine Study Group, 2: 373, *373*
Maine Medical Assessment Foundation, 2: 372
Maine Medical Practice of Neurosurgery and Spine, 2: 376
MGH/Children's Hospital residency, 2: 371
PBBH and, 4: 22, 116, 128
private medical practice, 2: 371, 376
professional memberships, 2: 371, 376
publications of, 2: 372, *372*, 374–375, *375*, 376
scoliosis and spine surgery, 2: 371–374
University of Massachusetts and, 2: 371
Keller, William L., 3: 168; 4: 416
Kellogg, E. H., 1: 307
Kelly, Robert P., 4: 158
Kelsey, Jennifer, 4: 264
Kennedy, Edward, 3: 275
Kennedy, John F., 3: 191
Kennedy, Robert H., 4: 473
Kennedy Institute of Rheumatology, 4: 268, *268*
Kenzora, John E. (1940–)
avascular necrosis of the femoral head research, 4: 154–156, *156*
Beth Israel Hospital and, 4: 154
Boston Children's Hospital and, 4: 154, 157
Children's Hospital/MGH combined program and, 4: 154
education and training, 4: 153
HMS appointment, 4: 157
hospital appointments, 4: 157
hydroxylysine-deficient collagen disease case, 4: 155
as MGH research fellow, 2: 328; 4: 153–154

osteonecrosis of the femoral head research, 4: 156–157
PBBH and, 4: 154, 157, 163
publications and research, 2: 328, *328*; 4: *153*, 154–156, *156*, 157
RBBH and, 4: 154
University of Maryland appointment, 4: 157
Keogh, Alfred, 2: 68
Kermond, Evelyn Conway, 3: 299
Kermond, William L. (1928-2012), 3: *298*, 461
death of, 3: 299
early life, 3: 298
education and training, 3: 298–299
HMS appointment, 3: 299
marriage and family, 3: 299
as MGH surgeon, 3: 299, 398*b*
mold arthroplasty and, 3: 292*b*
Por Cristo volunteerism, 3: 299
private medical practice, 1: 284; 4: 169
publications and research, 3: 299
White 9 Rehabilitation Unit and, 3: 299
Winchester Hospital and, 3: 299
Kettyle, William M., 2: 277
Kevy, Shervin, 2: 234
Key, Einer, 1: 263
Key, John Albert, 1: 189; 2: 171; 4: 237, 453, 473
Kibler, Alison, 3: 328
Kidner, Frederick C., 2: 78; 4: 473
Kilfoyle, Richard, 1: 202; 2: 314; 4: 341, 378
Kim, S., 4: 251
Kim, Saechin, 4: 286
Kim, Young-Jo, 2: 390, 439*b*
Kinematic knee prosthesis, 4: 138–139, 147, 149–150
Kiner, Ralph, 4: 342
King, Donald S., 2: 195; 3: 301
King, Graham J.W., 3: 431
King, Martin Luther, Jr., 4: 262
King, Thomas V., 1: 217*b*
King Faisal Specialist Hospital, 2: 424, *425*
King Report (MGH), 3: 301–302
King's College (Nova Scotia), 2: 284, *284*
Kirk, Norman T., 4: 471, 472*b*, 473
Kirkby, Eleanor, 3: 246
Kirkland House (Harvard University), 2: *358*
Kite, J. Hiram, 4: 158
Klein, Armin (1892–1954), 4: *231*
as Beth Israel chief of orthopaedics, 4: 236, 239, 289*b*

Beth Israel Hospital and, 4: 208*b*
Chelsea Survey of posture, 4: 234–235
death of, 4: 239
education and training, 4: 231
histology laboratory and, 2: 322
HMS appointment, 4: 236
Klein's Line, 4: 238–239, *239*
legacy of, 4: 239
MGH and, 4: 231, 236
as MGH surgeon, 3: 375, 456*b*
Orthopedics and Body Mechanics Committee, 4: 236
posture research and, 4: 84, 233–235, *235–236*
private medical practice, 4: 231
professional memberships, 4: 239, 239*b*
publications and research, 2: 136–137; 4: 231–233, *236*, 237, 239
scoliosis research and, 4: 231–233
Slipped Capital Femoral Epiphysis, 3: 294; 4: 238
slipped capital femoral epiphysis research, 3: 331, 333; 4: 237–239
Tufts Medical School appointment, 4: 236
US Army Medical Corps and, 4: 231
US General Hospital No. 3 and, 4: 452
Kleinert, Harold E., 3: 408
Klein's Line, 4: 238–239, *239*
Kleweno, Conor, 4: 190*b*
Kloen, Peter, 4: 190*b*
Klopsteg, Paul E., 3: 376
Klumpke paralysis, 2: 90
Knee Biomechanics and Biomaterials Laboratory, 3: 463, 464*b*
knee flexion contracture
before and after treatment, 1: *99*, *125*
apparatus for, 1: *98*, 107
Bradford's appliance for, 2: *20*, *21*
iliotibial band and, 3: 374
iron extension hinge for, 2: *123*
leg brace for, 1: *124*
osteotomies for, 2: 117
physical therapy and, 3: 375
plaster shells for, 2: 265
prevention and, 4: 61
surgical approach to, 3: 374–375, *375*
treatment of, 1: 126–127
Knee Society, 4: 150
knees. *See also* total knee replacement

ACL injuries, 1: 277–278, 285–286
amputations and, 1: 61, 65, 84
ankylosis, 4: 64
arthroplasty of, 4: 64, 70b–71b, 103, 129–130, 131t, 179t
arthroscopic simulator, 4: 173
arthroscopy and, 1: 279; 4: 129
arthrotomy and, 3: 165, 165b, 166, 351
bilateral knee valgus deformities, 1: 125
bone tumors and, 3: 389
cautery and, 1: 73
central-graft operation, 3: 368
discoid medial meniscus tear, 3: 422
dislocated patella treatment, 2: 294–296; 3: 79, 79b, 80, 81
gait and, 2: 408
hamstring lengthening and, 2: 172
internal derangement of, 1: xxii; 4: 48
joint injuries in Harvard sports, 1: 268t
lateral tibial plateau fracture, 4: 312
ligament rupture treatment, 1: 278
meniscectomy and, 1: 279
mold arthroplasty and, 3: 291–292
nylon arthroplasty in arthritic, 4: 65, 66, 66b, 69, 91, 93–94
Osgood-Schlatter disease and, 2: 115
outcomes with duopatellar prostheses, 4: 180t
patella dislocations, 2: 294–296; 3: 79, 79b, 80, 81
patella fractures, 4: 320
patellar turndown procedure, 4: 373–374
pes anserinus transplant, 1: 279
posterior cruciate ligament (PCL) deficiency, 3: 450
resection and, 1: 81
rheumatoid arthritis and, 4: 188–189
splint for knock, 2: 247
sports medicine and, 1: 267–268, 287; 2: 387
synovectomy in rheumatoid arthritis, 4: 40, 102–103
torn ligaments in, 3: 272
torn meniscus, 1: 278
treatment of sports injuries, 1: 277–279
trigger/jerking, 4: 311–312
tuberculosis and, 1: 73; 4: 225
valgus deformity, 2: 21
Kneisel, John J., 4: 489
Knirk, Jerry L., 3: 409; 4: 194, 195b, 262–263
Kocher, Mininder S. (1966–), 2: 376
  ACL research, 2: 378–379
  Beth Israel Deaconess Medical Center (BIDMC) and, 2: 377
  Boston Children's Hospital and, 2: 377, 379, 439b
  Brigham and Women's Hospital and, 2: 377
  clinical research grants, 2: 377–378
  education and training, 2: 377
  on ethics of ghost surgery, 2: 380, 381
  on ethics of orthopaedic research, 2: 381, 381
  HCORP and, 2: 377
  hip research, 2: 380
  HMS appointment, 2: 377
  honors and awards, 2: 377, 377b, 381
  humeral fracture research, 2: 368, 379
  New England Baptist Hospital and, 2: 377
  outcomes research, 2: 379–380
  professional memberships, 2: 382b
  publications and research, 2: 378, 378, 379–381
  sports medicine and, 2: 377–378
  team physician positions, 2: 382b
Kocher, Theodor, 2: 146
Kocher approach, 2: 347
Köhler's disease, 4: 240
Kopta, Joseph, 1: 232
Korean War
  deferment during, 4: 125, 221
  physician volunteers and, 4: 220–221
  US Army physicians, 2: 218
Koris, Mark J., 4: 193, 195b
Kornack, Fulton C., 1: 217; 3: 460b, 464b
Krag, Martin, 3: 249
Kramer, D. L., 3: 420
Krane, Stephen, 2: 321; 3: 458b
Krause, Fedor, 4: 215
Krebs, David E., 3: 460b, 464b
Kreb's School, 2: 38
Krida, Arthur, 2: 111
Krisher, James, 4: 40
Kronenberg, Henry, 2: 330
Krukenberg procedure, 2: 425
Kubik, Charles, 3: 203, 204
Kuhn, George H., 2: 5
Kühne, Willy, 3: 142
Kuhns, Jane Roper, 4: 66
Kuhns, John G. (1898–1969), 4: 59
  amputations research, 3: 373, 373; 4: 60
  arthritis research and, 4: 60–61, 61, 63
  Body Mechanics in Health and Disease, 3: 90, 91; 4: 62
  Boston Children's Hospital and, 2: 222, 274; 4: 59–61
  on congenital flatfoot, 4: 63
  correction of fixed foot deformities, 4: 62, 62t, 63
  death of, 4: 66
  education and training, 4: 59
  end-results clinic, 1: 194
  on Goldthwait, 3: 82, 92
  HMS appointment, 2: 223; 4: 59–61
  HMS medical student teaching, 4: 35
  knee arthroplasty and, 4: 64
  lymphatic supply of joints research, 1: 193; 4: 59–60
  marriage and family, 4: 66
  on medical education, 1: 93
  on nylon arthroplasty in arthritis, 4: 65, 65, 66, 66b, 69
  private medical practice, 4: 62
  professional memberships, 4: 66
  publications and research, 4: 60–66, 93
  RBBH and, 3: 91, 293; 4: 31–32, 35, 38, 60–62
  as RBBH chief of orthopaedics, 4: 63–66, 79, 89, 196b
  on roentgenotherapy for arthritis, 4: 64, 64
  scoliosis treatment, 2: 223; 4: 62, 65
  on Swaim, 4: 58
Küntscher, Gerhard, 3: 272
Küntscher femoral rod, 3: 272
Kurth, Harold, 4: 360
kyphoscoliosis, 1: 97, 105; 4: 155
kyphosis, 2: 343–345, 359, 366; 3: 239–240; 4: 317

L

La Coeur's triple osteotomy, 2: 390
Laboratory for Skeletal Disorders and Rehabilitation (HMS), 2: 413
Ladd, William E., 1: 264; 3: 64
Laënnec, René, 1: 74
Lahey, Frank, 4: 275–276, 277b
Lahey Clinic, 4: 275–277, 281, 378
Lahey Clinic Integrated Orthopaedic Program, 4: 378–379

Lahey Clinic Medical Center, 4: 279
Lahey Hospital and Medical Center, 4: 214
Laing, Matthew, 2: 371
Lakeville State Hospital, 4: 378
Lakeville State Sanatorium, 2: 102; 3: 235, 365, 367
LaMarche, W. J., 3: 269
Lambert, Alexander, 4: 416
Lambert, Alfred, 1: 60
Lambrinudi stabilization, 2: 229
laminectomy, 3: 204, 206–208
Landfried, M., 3: 433
Landsteiner, Karl, 3: 313
Lane, Timothy, 1: 217*b*
Lange, Thomas, 3: 390
Langenbeck, Bernhard von, 1: 82; 2: 146
Langmaid, S. G., 2: 6, 9
Langnecker, Henry L., 3: 266
laparotomy, 3: 55
LaPrade, Robert F., 1: 287
Larson, Carroll B. (1909–1978), 3: *300, 303*
   AAOS subcommittee on undergraduate teaching, 1: 162
   Calderwood's Orthopedic Nursing, 3: 303
   Children's Hospital/MGH combined program and, 3: 301
   death of, 3: 303
   early life, 3: 300
   education and training, 3: 300
   foot deformity treatment, 2: 229
   hip arthroplasty research, 3: 302
   hip surgery and, 3: 238, 240
   Iowa Hip Score, 3: 219
   King Report and, 3: 301–302
   kyphosis treatment, 3: 239
   legacy of, 3: 303
   marriage and family, 3: 300
   as MGH surgeon, 3: 74, 192, 302
   mold arthroplasty and, 3: 238–239, 241, 302
   nursing education and, 3: 302–303
   private medical practice, 3: 301
   professional roles, 3: 303, 303*b*
   publications and research, 3: 239, 241–242, 244, 302–303
   Santa Clara County Hospital and, 3: 300
   septic wounds in osteomyelitis case, 3: 301
   Smith-Petersen and, 3: 237
   University of Iowa orthopaedics chair, 3: 303
   US Army ROTC and, 3: 300
   World War II service, 3: 301
Larson, Charles Bernard, 3: 300
Larson, Ida Caroline, 3: 300
Larson, Nadine West Townsend, 3: 300
Larson, Robert L., 1: 279
Lateral Curvature of the Spine and Round Shoulders (Lovett), 2: 79, *79*, 227
Lattvin, Maggie, 4: 80
Latvian Medical Foundation, 3: 451
laudanum, 1: 10
Laurencin, Cato T., 4: 266*b*
Lavine, Leroy S., 3: 386, 388, 462, 463
Law, W. Alexander, 3: 192, 199
law of osteoblasts, 1: xxiii
Lawrence, Amos, 2: 3–4
Lawrence, John, 2: 425
Lawrence, William P., 2: 3
Le, Hai V., 3: 463*b*; 4: 190*b*
Leach, Robert E., 4: 89, *342*, 379
Leadbetter, Guy W., 4: 473
Lee, Henry, 3: 24
Lee, Olivia, 4: 190*b*
Lee, Roger I., 4: 84, *84*, 233–234, 420
Lee, Sang-Gil P., 3: 460*b*, 464*b*
Leffert, Adam, 3: 415
Leffert, Linda Garelik, 3: 415
Leffert, Lisa, 3: 415
Leffert, Robert D. (1923–2008), 3: *412, 461*
   Brachial Plexus Injuries, 3: 414
   brachial plexus injuries and, 3: 412, *412*, 413–414
   death of, 3: 415
   diabetes presenting as peripheral neuropathy case, 3: 413
   education and training, 3: 412
   HMS appointment, 3: 413, 415
   Hospital for Joint Diseases and, 3: 413
   memberships and, 3: 415
   as MGH clinical faculty, 3: 464*b*
   as MGH surgeon, 3: 320–321, 385, 395, 398*b*, 413
   Mount Sinai Medical School and, 3: 413
   orthopaedics education and, 3: 415
   pianist hand treatment and, 3: 414
   publications and research, 3: 412–415
   rehabilitation and, 3: 386, 388*t*, 413, 461
   shoulder treatment and, 3: 386, 412–414, 460*b*
   thoracic outlet syndrome treatment, 3: 415
   US Navy and, 3: 412
leg length
   discrepancy in, 2: 170, 191, 193, 350
   distal femoral physeal fractures, 2: 400
   effects of irradiation on epiphyseal growth, 3: 331
   epiphyseal arrest, 2: 170–171
   fractures and, 2: 350
   lengthening procedures, 2: 110
   muscle strength and, 3: 332
   prediction techniques for, 2: 193
   research in, 2: 191, 350
   teleroentgenography and, 2: 170, 170*t*
   use of sympathetic ganglionectomy, 3: 332
Legg, Allen, 2: 101
Legg, Arthur T. (1874–1939), 2: *84, 105*, 255
   Boston Children's Hospital and, 2: 13, 40, 101–102, 106, 252, 274, 282; 4: 338
   Clinics for Crippled Children and, 2: 230
   as consulting orthopaedic surgeon, 2: 102
   on coxa plana research, 3: 166
   death of, 2: 112
   education and training, 2: 101
   foot research, 2: 107–108
   gait laboratory, 2: 107
   Georgia Warm Springs Foundation board and, 2: 78
   Harvard Infantile Paralysis Clinic director, 2: 107, 188
   on hip disease, 2: 108
   HMS appointment, 2: 102; 4: 59–60
   identification of coxa plana, 2: 102–106; 3: 165
   on joint disease, 2: 110
   leg lengthening and, 2: 110
   marriage and, 2: 111–112
   military surgeon training and, 2: 42, 66; 4: 396
   on muscle atrophy in children, 2: 110
   orthopaedic surgery advances, 2: 79
   pediatric orthopaedics and, 2: 101, 106–107
   Physical Therapy in Infantile Paralysis, 2: 107
   poliomyelitis treatment, 2: 107, 109

professional memberships, 2: 110–111
public health and, 2: 107
publications of, 2: 107
Section for Orthopedic Surgery (AMA), 2: 110–111
on tendon transplantation, 2: 108, *108*, 109
testing of foot strength apparatus, 2: 102
Tufts appointment, 2: 102
Legg, Charles Edmund, 2: 101
Legg, Emily Harding, 2: 101
Legg, Marie L. Robinson, 2: 111–112
Legg-Calvé-Perthes disease
case reports, 2: 103, *103*, 104
epiphyseal extrusion measurement, 2: *354*
etiology of, 2: 104
identification of, 2: 13, 102, *102*, 103–106
long-term study of, 2: 425
research in, 2: 351; 3: 165–166
treatment of, 2: 105
Legg-Perthes Study Group, 2: 425; 4: 250
legs. *See also* leg length
acute thigh compartment syndrome, 3: 417–418
correction of bowleg, 1: *101*; 2: 247
fasciotomies, 3: 417
limb deformities, 2: 23, 334, 354, 413; 3: 58
limb-salvage procedure, 2: 422, 423*b*
radiculitis in, 3: 204
Lehigh Valley Hospital, 3: 407
Leidholt, John, 2: 314
Leinonen, Edwin, 4: 244
Leland, Adams, 3: 313
Leland, George A., 1: 154; 3: 60; 4: 433
Lemuel Shattuck Hospital, 3: 246, 253
Leonard, Ralph D., 4: *359*
L'Episcopo, James B., 2: 90, 96, 417
LeRoy, Abbott, 2: 78
Lest We Forget (Rowe), 3: 61, 70*b*, 187, 347, *357*, 360
"Letter to the Honorable Isaac Parker" (J.C. Warren), 1: *45*
Letterman Army Hospital, 3: 336
Letterman General Hospital, 4: 451
LeVay, David, 4: 383
Levine, Leroy, 3: 397, 398*b*, 461
Levine, Philip T., 2: 324
Lewinnek, George, 4: 262
Lewis, Frances West, 2: 4

Lewis, William H., 1: 252
Lewis, Winslow, Jr., 1: 308
Lewis H. Millender Community of Excellence Award, 4: 168
Lewis H. Millender Occupational Medicine Conference, 4: 168
Lexington, Mass., 1: 17–18
Lhowe, David W. (1951–), 3: *416*
acute thigh compartment syndrome research, 3: 417, *417*, 418
Cambridge Hospital clinic and, 3: 399, 416
education and training, 3: 416
Harborview Medical Center and, 3: 416
HCORP and, 3: 416
HMS appointment, 3: 416
hospital appointments, 3: 416
humanitarian work and, 3: 416–418
IMSuRT and, 3: 417–418
as MGH clinical faculty, 3: 464*b*
as MGH surgeon, 3: 416
Pristina Hospital (Kosovo) and, 3: 416–417
Project HOPE and, 3: 417
publications and research, 3: 416
trauma care and, 3: 399, 416–418, 460*b*
Winchester Hospital and, 3: 417
Li, Guoan, 3: 462
Liaison Committee on Graduate Medical Education (LCGME), 1: 210–212
Liang, M. H., 4: 26
Liberating Technologies, Inc., 2: 326
Liberty Mutual Insurance Company, 3: 287; 4: 352–353
Liberty Mutual Research Center, 2: 326
Lidge, Ralph, 3: 448
Life of John Collins Warren, The (Edward Warren), 1: 46
Lifeso, Robert, 2: 424
ligatures, 1: 10, 55, 85
limb deformities
internal fixation of fractures to prevent, 3: 58
pediatric orthopaedics and, 2: 334, 354
thalidomide and, 2: 413
traction treatment for, 2: 23
limb salvage surgery, 3: 390–391, 433
Lincoln, Joan Tozzer, 3: 276
Lindbergh, Charles, 2: 232
Linenthal, Arthur J., 4: 210
Lingley, James, 3: 331

Linker, Beth, 4: 233
Linn, Frank C., 3: 324–325
Lippiello, Louis, 3: 383, 385–386
Lippman, Walter, 4: 469
Lipson, Jenifer Burns, 4: 271
Lipson, Stephen J. (1946–2013), 4: 116*b*, 163, *267*
on back surgery, 4: 270
Berg-Sloat Traveling Fellowship and, 4: 268
as Beth Israel chief of orthopaedics, 1: 233; 4: 223, 268, 270, 289*b*
as BIDMC chief of orthopaedics, 4: 268, 270–271, 281, 289*b*
BIDMC teaching program and, 1: 166–167, 220, 224, 226; 4: 286
Cave Traveling Fellowship and, 1: 217*b*
death of, 4: 271
development of multiple sclerosis, 4: 271
education and training, 4: 267
HCORP and, 4: 267
HMS appointment, 4: 271
honors and awards, 4: 268, 272
Kennedy Institute of Rheumatology and, 4: 268
legacy of, 4: 271–272
Mankin on, 4: 267–268
marriage and family, 4: 271
MGH and, 4: 267
PBBH and, 4: 268
publications and research, 4: 268–269, *269*, 270–271
spinal stenosis due to epidural lipomatosis case, 4: 269
spine research, 4: 268–271
Lisfranc, Jacque, 1: 73–74
Lister, Joseph
antisepsis principles, 1: 55, 81, 84–85; 3: 45
carbolic acid treatment, 1: 82–83, *83*, 85
treatment of compound fractures, 1: 84
Liston, Robert, 1: 76, 84
litholapaxy, 3: 41
lithotrite, 3: 41
Litterer-Siewe disease, 2: 171
Little, Moses, 1: 95
Little, Muirhead, 4: 402
Little, William John, 1: xxiii, 98, 106; 2: 26; 3: 54
Little Orthopaedic Club, 4: 74
Littlefield, Ephraim, 1: 303, *303*, 304, 309
Littler, J. William, 2: 248, 250
Lloyd, James, 1: 6, 8, 10

Lloyd Alpern–Dr. Rosenthal Physical Therapy Fund, 2: 439*b*
Locke, Edward, 4: 296
Locke, Joseph, 4: 100, *100*
Loder, Halsey B., 4: 438
Loh, Y. C., 3: 317
Long, Crawford W., 1: 56–57, 60, 63
Long Island Hospital, 2: 284
Longfellow, Frances (Fannie), 1: 297, 306
Longfellow, Henry Wadsworth, 1: 297, 302, 306
Longwood Medical Building Trust, 1: 264
Lord, J. F., 1: 177
Lorenz, Adolf, 2: 34, 242; 3: 234
Lorenz, Hans, 1: 264
Los Angeles Orthopaedic Hospital, 2: 266
Losina, Elena, 4: 195*b*
Loskin, Albert, 4: 280
Louis, Dean, 4: 168, 183
Louis, Pierre Charles Alexander, 1: 73–74
Louise and Edwin F. Cave Traveling Fellowship, 1: 217, 217*b*; 3: 274
Lovell General Hospital, 4: 482*b*
Lovett, Elizabeth Moorfield Storey, 2: 80, 230
Lovett, John Dyson, 2: 45
Lovett, Mary Elizabeth Williamson, 2: 45
Lovett, Robert Williamson (1859–1924), 1: *190*; 2: 45
   address to the American Orthopaedic Association, 2: 51
   Advisory Orthopedic Board and, 3: 157
   AOA and, 2: 48, *48*
   on astragalectomy, 2: 93–94
   Beth Israel Hospital and, 4: 208, 208*b*, 223
   birth palsies research, 2: 415
   Boston Children's Hospital and, 1: 188, 190–192; 2: 1, 10, 12–13, 40, 49, 54, 62, 64, 68
   Boston City Hospital and, 1: 141, 143; 2: 45–47; 4: 298, 305*b*
   Boston Dispensary and, 2: 49
   Bradford and, 2: 49
   Brigham and Women's Hospital and, 4: 195*b*
   "Case of Glanders," 2: 46
   cerebral palsy cases, 2: 51
   "Certain Aspects of Infantile Paralysis," 2: *70*
   clinical surgery teaching and, 1: 141, 143
   Dane and, 2: 242, 246–247
   death of, 2: 80–81
   Department for Military Orthopedics and, 4: 406
   on departmental organization, 1: 176
   diaries of, 2: 45–46, *46*, 47, *47*, 48
   on disabled soldiers, 2: 67–68
   donations to Boston Medical Library, 2: 271
   early life, 2: 45
   education and training, 2: 45
   endowment in memory of, 2: 81–82
   Fiske Prize, 2: 52
   FitzSimmons and, 2: 144
   foot treatment, 2: 54–55, *55*, 56
   Harvard orthopaedic clinic and, 1: 174
   hip disease treatment and research, 2: 32, 49, *49*, 52, *52*, 53–54
   History of the Orthopedic Department at Children's Hospital, 2: 247
   as HMS chief of orthopaedics, 2: 64, 68
   House of the Good Samaritan and, 2: 49
   on incision and drainage of psoas abscesses, 2: 53–54
   Infantile Paralysis Commission, 2: 68, 99, 107
   John Ball and Buckminster Brown Professorship, 2: 63–64, *64*; 4: 195*b*
   Lateral Curvature of the Spine and Round Shoulders, 2: 79, *79*, 227
   legacy of, 2: 80
   Lovett Board, 2: *59*
   marriage and family, 2: 80, 230
   Mellon Lecture (Univ. of Pittsburgh), 2: 66–67
   military surgeon training by, 2: 42, 65–69
   New England Peabody Home for Crippled Children and, 2: 270
   at New York Orthopaedic Dispensary and Hospital, 2: 47–48
   obituary, 1: 93
   orthopaedic apprenticeship, 1: 186
   as orthopaedic chair, 2: 15*b*
   orthopaedic surgery, 2: 34, 51
   orthopaedics contributions, 2: 69–71
   Orthopedic Surgery, 2: 69, *69*; 4: 318
   PBBH and, 4: 10, 12
   pedagogy and, 2: 68–69
   as physician to Franklin D. Roosevelt, 2: 71–73, *73*, 74, *74*, 75, *75*, 76–77, 271
   poliomyelitis treatment, 2: 61–63, *63*, 70–79, 147–148, 264
   private medical practice and, 1: 176
   professional memberships, 2: 80, 80*b*
   as professor of orthopaedic surgery, 1: 147, 151, 171
   public health and, 2: 61
   publications and research, 2: 223, 246; 4: 259, 310
   scoliosis treatment, 2: 56–61, 79–80, 86, 223–225
   SICOT and, 2: 80
   social events and, 2: 49
   spina bifida treatment, 2: 51–52
   spring muscle test, 2: 70–71
   study of spine mechanics, 2: 57, *57*, 58, *58*, 59
   Surgery of Joints, The, 2: 52
   teaching hospitals and, 1: 187
   tracheostomy results, 2: 49, 51
   Treatise on Orthopaedic Surgery, A, 1: 108, 143; 2: 29–30, 43, 50, *50*, 51
   tuberculosis treatment, 2: 32
   turnbuckle jacket and, 2: 80, 224, *224*, 225
   US Army Medical Reserve Corps and, 2: 66
   use of radiographs, 2: 54
Lovett Board, 2: *59*, 86
Lovett Fund Committee, 2: 81–82
Low, Harry C. (1871–1943)
   acetonuria associated with death after anesthesia case, 3: 305
   Boston Children's Hospital and, 3: 304
   Boston City Hospital and, 3: 304
   Burrage Hospital and, 4: 226
   Children's Sunlight Hospital and, 3: 307
   Committee on Occupational Therapy chair, 3: 304–306
   death of, 3: 307
   early life, 3: 304
   education and training, 3: 304
   European medical studies, 3: 304
   marriage and, 3: 304
   on the MGH orthopaedic outpatient clinic, 3: 304, *304*, 306*b*–307*b*

as MGH surgeon, 3: 269, 304, 306
New England Home for Little Wanderers and, 3: 307
as poliomyelitis surgeon, 3: 306–307
"Progress in Orthopaedic Surgery" series, 2: 297
publications and research, 3: 304
Low, Mabel C. Chapman, 3: 304
Lowell, Abbott Lawrence, 1: 174, 176; 2: 41–42, 64
Lowell, Charles
hip dislocation case, 1: 42, 44–49, 49*b*, 50; 3: 13, 13*b*, 36
hip dislocation close-up, 1: *49*
letter of support for, 1: *45*
malpractice suit against John Collins, 1: 44, 50–51, 68
x-ray of pelvis and hips, 1: *49*
Lowell, J. Drennan (1922–1987), 4: *158*, 161
bladder fistula case, 4: 162
Boston Children's Hospital and, 2: 384
as BWH assistant chief of orthopaedic surgery, 4: 163
BWH medical staff president, 4: 163
Children's Hospital/MGH combined program and, 4: 158
death of, 4: 164
education and training, 4: 158
Emory University Hospital and, 4: 158
Fracture course and, 3: *273*
hip fracture research, 4: *160*
HMS appointment, 4: 162
marriage and family, 4: 164
MGH and, 3: 244; 4: 158–159
on MGH approach to hip fractures, 4: 159*b*–160*b*
PBBH and, 4: 116, 116*b*, 128–129
as PBBH chief of clinical orthopaedics, 4: 161–163
private medical practice, 4: 158
professional memberships, 4: 162–163, 163*b*
publications and research, 4: 159, 161–164
RBBH and, 4: 114
reconstructive hip surgery and, 4: 159
train hobby and, 4: 160
US Army and, 4: 158
on use of ultraviolet light, 4: 162–163, *163*, 164
Lowell, Olivia, 1: 263
Lowell, Ruth, 4: 164

Lowell General Hospital, 4: 243
Lower Extremity Amputations for Arterial Insufficiency (Warren and Record), 1: 90; 3: 330
Lowry, Robert, 4: 277
LTI Digital™ Arm Systems for Adults, 2: 326
lubrication, 3: 324–325
Lucas-Championniere, Just, 1: xxiii
Ludmerer, Kenneth, 1: 146
lumbago, 3: 203
lumbar spinal stenosis, 2: 373–374
lunate dislocation, 3: 101–102
Lund, F. B., 4: 331
Lund, Fred, 4: 220
Lycée Pasteur Hospital, 4: 388, 389*b*, 390
Lynch, Peter, 2: 414
Lynn General Hospital, 3: 253
Lyon, Mary, 2: 276
Lysholm Knee Scoring Scale, 2: 380

M

MacArthur, Douglas, 2: 232
MacAusland, Andrew R., 3: 308
MacAusland, Dorothy Brayton, 3: 308
MacAusland, Frances Prescott Baker, 3: 308
MacAusland, William R., Jr. (1922–2004), 3: *308*
as AAOS president, 3: 311, *311*, 312
ABC traveling fellowship and, 3: 309
Carlos Otis Stratton Mountain Clinic and, 3: 311
Carney Hospital and, 3: 308; 4: 45
death of, 3: 312
early life, 3: 308
education and training, 3: 308
Emergency Care and Transportation of the Sick and Injured, 3: 310, *311*
emergency responder training and, 3: 310–311
HMS appointment, 3: 308
knee arthroplasty and, 4: 64
love of skiing and, 3: 311
marriage and family, 3: 308, 312
memberships and, 3: 309
as MGH surgeon, 3: 266, 398*b*
Orthopaedics, 3: 310
Orthopaedics Overseas and, 3: 310
private medical practice, 3: 308, 310

publications and research, 2: 248; 3: 308–310, *376*, 377–378
Rocky Mountain Trauma Society and, 3: 311
on sepsis after intramedullary fixation of femoral fractures, 3: 309–310
trauma research and, 3: 309
as Tufts University professor, 3: 308
US Air Force and, 3: 308
West Roxbury Veterans Administration Hospital and, 3: 312
MacAusland, William R., Sr., 3: 308
Macdonald, Ian, 4: 102
MacEwen, Dean, 2: 304
Macewen, William, 1: xxiii
MacFarlane, Arlene, 3: 291
MacFarlane, J. A., 4: 468–469, 471
MacIntosh prosthesis, 4: 69, 71*b*, 129, 188
Mackin, Evelyn J., 4: 168
Macknight, Jane, 1: 289
Maddox, Robert, 2: *121*
Magee, James, 4: 471
Magill, H. Kelvin, 4: 376
magnetic resonance imaging (MRI), 3: 255
Magnuson, Paul B., 4: 473
Maine Carpal Tunnel Study (Keller, et al.), 2: 375, *375*
Maine Carpal Tunnel Syndrome Study, 4: 184
Maine Lumbar Spine Study Group, 2: 373, *373*, 374
Maine Medical Assessment Foundation, 2: 372, 374; 4: 184–185
Maine Medical Association, 2: 372
Maine Medical Practice of Neurosurgery and Spine, 2: 376
Maine Medical Society, 1: 49
Maisonneuve, Jacques, 1: 82
malaria treatment, 4: 491
Malchau, Henrik, 3: 219
Malenfant, J., 3: 45
Mallon, William J., 3: 143, *145*
Mallory, Tracy B., 2: 254
malpractice suits
Charles Lowell and, 1: 44, 50
early concerns about, 1: 24
fractures and, 1: 50–51; 3: 63
increase in, 1: 50–51
insurance and, 1: 51
Joseph Warren on, 1: 12
orthopaedics and, 1: 50; 3: 378–379
Malt, Ronald, 3: 217
Management of Fractures and Dislocations (Wilson), 3: 62, 273

Mankin, Allison, 3: 393
Mankin, Carole J. Pinkney, 1: 218; 3: 382, 385, 393
Mankin, David, 3: 393
Mankin, Henry J. (1928–2018), 1: *210, 212*; 3: *381, 386, 393, 461*
- AAOS and, 3: 388
- articular cartilage research, 3: 383, *383*, 384, *385*, 388, 442
- BIH Board of Consultants, 4: 262–263
- breakfast meetings with residents, 1: 213, *214*
- on Chandler, 3: 279
- chordoma of the spinal column and, 3: 390
- core curriculum and, 1: 215
- death of, 3: 393
- early life, 3: 381
- Edith M. Ashley Professor, 3: 464*b*
- education and training, 3: 381–382
- establishment of the Institute of Health Professions, 3: 391–392
- femoral allograft transplantation, 3: 389, *389*, 390
- HCORP and, 1: 210–221, 239; 3: 387, 397
- histologic-histochemical grading system, 3: 384, 384*t*, 385
- HMS appointment, 3: 385
- honors and awards, 3: 392, 393*b*
- Hospital for Joint Diseases and, 3: 382–383, 385, 389
- Korean War and, 3: 382
- limb salvage surgery and, 3: 390–391
- on Lipson, 4: 267–268
- marriage and family, 3: 382, 385
- memberships and, 3: 392
- MGH Bone Bank and, 3: 386, 388, 396, 439
- as MGH clinical faculty, 3: 464*b*
- MGH operations improvement and, 3: 387, 395–399
- as MGH orthopaedics chief, 1: 180; 3: 11*b*, 219, 228, 320, 378, 385–388, 395–399, 459, 461
- MGH residents and, 3: *387, 460*
- Mount Sinai Medical School and, 3: 383, 385
- NIH and, 3: 383, 387–388, 392
- Orthopaedic Biology and Oncology Laboratories, 3: 464*b*
- orthopaedic oncology and, 3: 386, 388, 388*t*, 390, 392–393, 460*b*
- orthopaedic research support, 1: 218
- orthopaedics education and, 3: 386
- pathology course and, 3: 396
- *Pathophysiology of Orthopaedic Diseases*, 4: 226
- publications and research, 3: 383–385, 387–392, 433, 440
- as residency program director, 1: 181, 210–211, 213–221
- on rickets and osteomalacia, 3: 388
- on Rowe, 3: 360
- specialty services at MGH under, 3: 388*t*, 459, 460*t*, 461–462
- on sports medicine clinic, 2: 384
- *Such a Joy for a Yiddish Boy*, 3: 392, *392*
- University of Chicago clinics and, 3: 382
- University of Pittsburgh appointment, 3: 382–383
- US Navy and, 3: 382

Mankin, Hymie, 3: 381
Mankin, Keith, 3: 392, *392*, 393, 398*b*, 401, 460*b*, 464*b*
Mankin, Mary, 3: 381
Mankin System, 3: 384, 384*t*, 385
Mann, Robert W., 2: 326; 3: 397, 398*b*
Mansfield, Frederick L. (1947–), 3: *419*
- education and training, 3: 419
- HCORP and, 3: 419
- HMS appointment, 3: 419
- memberships and, 3: 421
- as MGH clinical faculty, 3: 464*b*
- as MGH surgeon, 3: 419
- open anterior lumbosacral fracture dislocation case, 3: 420
- orthopaedics education and, 3: 421
- publications and research, 3: 419–421
- sciatica treatment and, 3: 254
- spine surgery and, 3: 397, 419–421, 460*b*
- use of chymopapain, 3: 254, 419, *421*

Manson, Anne, 2: 277
Manson, James G. (1931–2009)
- Boston Children's Hospital and, 2: 276–277
- death of, 2: 277
- early life, 2: 275
- education and training, 2: 276
- hemophilia clinic, 2: 276
- HMS appointment, 2: 276
- marriage and family, 2: 276–277
- MGH residency, 2: *276*
- MIT Medical and, 2: 276–277, 290
- Mount Auburn Hospital and, 2: 276
- PBBH and, 4: 22

Manson, Mary Lyon, 2: 276
Manual of Bandaging, Strapping and Splinting, A (Thorndike), 1: 268
Manual of Chemistry (Webster), 1: 299, 301
Manual of Orthopedic Surgery, A (Thorndike), 2: 311, *312*
Manual of Orthopedic Surgery (Bigelow), 3: 25–26, *26*
Manuel II, King, 4: 399–401, *401*, 402–403, 442
marathon runners, 1: 250
Marble, Alice Ingram, 3: 316
Marble, Henry C. (1885–1965), 3: *312*
- AAST and, 3: 315, *315*
- American Mutual Liability Insurance Company and, 3: 314, 316
- American Society for Surgery of the Hand and, 3: 316
- anatomy education and, 3: 314
- Base Hospital No. 6 and, 4: 433–434, 436
- Bedford Veterans Administration Hospital and, 3: 314
- blood transfusion work, 3: 313
- Chelsea Memorial Hospital and, 3: 314
- death of, 3: 316
- early life, 3: 312
- education and training, 3: 312–313
- Faulkner Hospital and, 3: 314
- as Fracture Clinic chief, 3: 60*b*
- fracture research and, 3: 340
- *Fractures*, 3: 315
- *Hand, The*, 3: 316
- HMS appointment, 3: 313
- legacy of, 3: 316
- marriage and family, 3: 316
- Massachusetts Regional Fracture Committee, 3: 64
- memberships and, 3: 316
- MGH Fracture Clinic and, 3: 60, 313–315
- MGH Hand Clinic and, 3: 314
- as MGH surgeon, 3: 313–315
- orthopaedics education and, 3: 315

publications and research, 3: 314–316
Scudder Oration on Trauma, 3: 63
Surgical Treatment of the Motor-Skeletal System, 3: 316
US Army Medical Corps and, 3: 313
US General Hospital No. 3 and, 4: 452
Marcella Street Home, 2: 242, 247
March of Dimes, 2: 315
Marcove, Ralph, 3: 382
Margliot, Z., 3: 409
Marian Ropes Award, 4: 100
Marie-Strumpell disease, 3: 239
Marion B. Gebbie Research Fellowship, 4: 127
Marjoua, Youssra, 4: 190*b*
Marlborough Medical Associates, 2: 146, 269, 299
Marmor modular design prosthesis, 4: 130
Marnoy, Samuel L., 4: 208*b*
Marshall, H. W., 3: 155
Martin, Edward, 3: 112, 113*b*
Martin, Ernest, 2: 70, 70, 71
Martin, Franklin H., 3: 113*b*; 4: 324
Martin, Geraldine, 4: 389*b*
Martin, Joseph, 1: 181, 232–234; 4: 284–285
Martin, Scott D., 1: 230; 4: 193, 195*b*
Martin, Tamara, 4: 193
Marvin, Frank W., 4: 407
Mary Alley Hospital, 2: 269
Mary Hitchcock Memorial Hospital, 3: 363–364
Mary Horrigan Conner's Center for Women's Health, 4: *194*
Mary MacArthur Memorial Respiratory Unit (Wellesley Hospital), 2: 189, 315
Maslin, Robert, 2: 354
Mason, Jonathan, 1: 38
Mason, Susan Powell, 1: 37–38, 72
Masons, 1: 10–12, 29
Mass General Brigham (MGB), 3: 462
Massachusetts Agricultural Society, 1: 29
Massachusetts Arthritis Foundation, 4: 100
Massachusetts Board of Registration in Medicine, 3: 423
Massachusetts Eye and Ear Infirmary, 2: 252; 3: 331, 339; 4: 113–114

Massachusetts General Hospital, 1955–1980, The (Brown), 3: 299
Massachusetts General Hospital, Its Development, 1900–1935, The (Washburn), 3: 1
Massachusetts General Hospital (MGH)
 apothecary position, 1: 184
 arthritis research program at, 2: 82
 Base Hospital No. 6 and, 4: 420*t*, 429–432
 blood transfusions at, 3: 313
 clinical surgery curricula at, 1: 151
 End-Result Idea, 3: 112, 114
 expansion of staff, 3: 14–15
 faculty model at, 1: 174, 176
 fee structures, 3: 16, 21–22
 first orthopaedic case at, 1: 42, 44
 first patients at, 1: 42; 3: 11
 General Hospital No. 6 and, 3: 239, 362; 4: 474, 485*b*
 HMS clinical teaching at, 3: 13
 house physicians/surgeons, 1: 184
 house pupils (pups) at, 1: 80, 184, *185*; 2: 20
 impact of World War II on, 4: 467
 innovation at, 3: 216–217
 institutional racism and, 3: 15–16
 internes/externs, 1: 184–185
 James Jackson and, 1: 31, 41–42; 3: 5, *5*, 6*b*–7*b*, 12–13
 John Ball Brown and, 3: 12
 John Collins Warren and, 1: 31, 41–42, 52–55, 57–58; 3: 5, *5*, 6*b*–7*b*, 12–13
 King Report, 3: 301–302
 military surgeon training at, 4: 396
 modernization of, 3: 453
 nursing school at, 4: 467
 occupational rehabilitation and, 4: 444
 105th General Hospital and, 4: 493
 ophthalmology service at, 3: 13
 performance-based promotions at, 3: 123–124
 postgraduate education and, 2: 157–159
 rehabilitation clinic and, 1: 273
 reserve units for army service, 4: 429–430
 roentgenology department, 3: 21
 surgical residencies, 1: 184, *185*

surgical volume due to ether use, 1: 63, 64*t*
treatment categories, 1: 54, 54*t*
treatment of children in, 2: 4, 8
treatment of soldiers, 3: 21
treatment outcomes reporting, 1: 54; 3: 112
treatments and techniques at, 3: 20–22
use of ether anesthesia, 1: 57–63, 85; 3: 15, 22, 27–28, 28*b*, 29, 29*b*, 30–34
use of ligatures, 1: 85
use of radiographs, 2: 54
visiting surgeons at, 3: *31*
Warren family and, 1: 71
women surgeons at, 1: 239
World War II and, 4: 493
x-rays and, 3: 20, *20*
Massachusetts General Hospital. Facilities
 Allen Street House, 3: 17–18
 Ambulatory Care, 3: 396, 399
 Baker Memorial, 3: *73*, 75
 Bigelow Building, 3: 15–17
 Bulfinch Building, 1: *41*; 3: *9*, *13*, 15, *16*, 22, *60*, 70*b*
 Children's Ward, 3: *71*
 East Wing, 3: *14*, 15, *60*
 Ellison Tower, 3: 75
 Ether Dome, 1: *59*, *63*, 84; 3: *14*, 16
 expansion of, 3: 14, *14*, 15, *15*, 16–18, 18*b*, 20–21, 74–75
 Gay Ward (outpatient building), 3: *19*, 265
 Henry J. Bigelow Operating Theater, 1: 84
 medical school, 3: *15*
 Moseley Memorial Building, 3: 70*b*, 75
 Nerve Room, 3: 20
 Out-Patient Department, 3: *75*
 pathological laboratory, 3: 21
 Patient Ward, 3: *74*
 Pavilion Wards, 3: *17*
 Phillips House, 1: 86, 204; 3: *72*, *73*, 75
 Physical Therapy Department, 3: 269
 plot plans for, 3: *10*, *17*, *22*, *71*, *72*, *461*
 Treadwell Library, 3: 70*b*
 view in 1840, 1: *54*
 Wang ACC building, 3: 75
 Ward 5, 1: 203
 Ward A (Warren), 3: 17, *17*, 18
 Ward B (Jackson), 3: 17, *17*
 Ward C (Bigelow), 3: 17–18
 Ward D (Townsend), 3: 18, *18*

Ward E (Bradlee), 3: 18–19, *19*
Ward F (George A. Gardner building), 3: 19
wards in, 3: *12*
Warren Building, 3: 17
West Wing, 3: 15, *60*
White Building (George Robert White), 3: *74*, 75

Massachusetts General Hospital. Founding of
advocacy for, 1: 41; 3: 3–5, *5*, 6, *6b–7b*
Almshouse site, 1: 41
Bulfinch design for, 1: 41; 3: 10–11
construction of, 3: 9–10
funding for, 1: 41–42; 3: 6–7, 9, 14, 18–19, 21
grand opening of, 3: 11–12
Province House and, 3: 6–7, 9
seal of, 3: *10*, 11, *11*
state charter authorizing, 3: 6–7, *8*

Massachusetts General Hospital. Orthopaedics Department
adults and, 2: 157
approach to hip fractures, 4: 159b–160b
Biomaterials and Innovative Technologies Laboratory, 3: 463
Biomotion Laboratory, 3: 463, 464b
bone bank for allografts and, 3: 388, 396, 440–441, 443
Cambridge Hospital clinic, 3: 396, 399
Clinical and Research Programs, 3: 464b
clinical faculty, 3: 464b
clinical service rotations, 1: 198
continuing medical education and, 3: 396
creation of, 3: 67–69
expansion of, 3: 286
facilities for, 3: 68–69, 70b, 71, *72*, 73, *73*, 75, 80
femoral replacement prosthesis, 4: 129
Fracture Clinic at, 2: 130; 3: 60, 60b, 62, 241–242, 245, 273, *273*, 313–315, 371, 373, 378, 456b; 4: 464
Fracture Course at, 3: 62
Frederick and Joan Brengle Learning Center, 3: 463
gait laboratory and, 3: 397
growth in, 3: 227–228
Hand Clinic at, 3: 314
Harris Orthopaedic and Biomaterials laboratory, 3: 463
HCORP and, 1: 213–215
house officers at, 1: 189
internships at, 1: 196
Joint Kinematics Laboratory, 3: 463, 464b
Joseph S. Barr and, 3: 453, 453b–456b
Knee Biomechanics and Biomaterials Laboratory, 3: 463, 464b
Melvin J. Glimcher and, 3: 453, 455b–458b
opening of, 3: 68
Orthopaedic Biochemistry and Osteoarthritis Therapy Laboratory, 3: 464b
Orthopaedic Biology and Oncology Laboratories, 3: 463, 464b
Orthopaedic Biomechanics and Biomaterials Laboratory, 3: 464b
orthopaedic chairpersons at, 3: 11b
Orthopaedic Oncology Unit, 3: 440
orthopaedic rehabilitation and, 3: 459
Orthopaedic Research Laboratories, 2: 321–324; 3: 211–212
orthopaedic specialties, 3: 459, 460b, 461–462
orthopaedic staff in 1984, 3: 398b
orthopaedic surgery department, 1: 171, 180
orthopaedics curriculum and, 1: 136–137, 157–158, 167
orthopaedics fellowships, 1: 241
orthopaedics instruction at, 1: 190
orthopaedics residencies, 1: 186, 199, 204, 207, 217–218, 221–225, 241–242; 2: *249*, *278*, *290*, *320*, *327*; 3: 74
Orthopedic Biomechanics Laboratory, 3: 463
outpatient services and, 3: 80, 227, 304, 306b–307b
pediatric orthopaedics and, 3: 388t, 400
physical therapy and, 3: 454b
podiatry service and, 3: 396–398
Problem Back Clinic, 3: 254
professorships, 3: 464b
research activities, 3: 455b, 458b
Research Building, 3: *454*
Research Laboratory Centers, 3: 464b
Sarcoma Molecular Biology Laboratory, 3: 464b
specialty services under Mankin, 3: 388t, 396–398
sports medicine and, 3: 397
Sports Medicine Service, 3: 356, 448
surgeon-scholars at, 3: 228, 395–398, 398b, 399, *461*
surgical appliance shop, 3: 73
surgical residencies, 1: 198; 3: 455b, 457b–458b
Thornton Brown on changes at, 3: 453b–458b
transition in, 3: 461–463
Ward 1, 1: 273; 2: 116; 3: *67*, 68, *68*, 70b, 74–75, *80*
White 9 Rehabilitation Unit, 3: 286, 299, 455b, 459, 461
Zander Room (Medico-Mechanical Department), 3: 71, 227, 264–268

Massachusetts General Hospital Physicians Organization (MGPO), 3: 256
Massachusetts General Orthopaedic Group, 3: 246
Massachusetts General/Boston Children's Hospital residency program, 1: 210; 2: 144
Massachusetts Homeopathic Hospital, 3: 120
Massachusetts Hospital Life Insurance Company, 3: 9
Massachusetts Hospital School for Crippled Children, 2: 38–39, *39*, 384; 3: 319–320
Massachusetts Humane Society, 1: 29
Massachusetts Industrial Accident Board, 2: 92; 4: 325, 327
Massachusetts Infantile Paralysis Clinic, 2: 188–189, 191, 208, 212, 314
Massachusetts Institute of Technology (MIT), 2: 321; 4: 152
Massachusetts Medical Association, 1: 184
Massachusetts Medical College of Harvard University, 1: 6, 40, *40*, 41, *135*; 3: 35, 38
Massachusetts Medical Society, 1: 25–26, 29, 38, 99, 272–273, 277; 2: 164, 208, 230; 3: 35; 4: 162, 366b, 367, 367b
Massachusetts Memorial Hospital, 4: 347
Massachusetts Orthopaedic Association (MOA), 3: 421; 4: 253

Massachusetts Regional Fracture Committee, 3: 64
Massachusetts Rehabilitation Hospital, 3: 387, 396
Massachusetts Services for Crippled Children, 2: 208
Massachusetts Society of Examining Physicians, 4: 324
Massachusetts State Board of Health, 2: 61
Massachusetts State Hospital, 2: 102
Massachusetts Volunteer Aid Association, 2: 43
Massachusetts Women's Hospital, 4: 447–448
Massachusetts Workingmen's Compensation Law, 4: 325
massage
    avoidance of tender muscles, 1: 267; 2: 73
    congenital dislocated hips (CDH) and, 2: 178
    foot problems and, 2: 56, 245
    injured soldiers and, 2: 56, 67, 118, 120
    obstetrical paralysis and, 2: 90, 94
    physical therapy and, 1: 100; 3: 266, 297
    poliomyelitis and, 2: 62, 73, 109
    therapeutic, 3: 264–266
Massage (Böhm), 3: 266
Matson, Donald, 2: 301
Matza, R. A., 2: 279, 280*b*
Mayer, Leo, 1: 1, 107, 114; 2: 24, 33, 51, 70, 99, 165; 3: 156*b*, 196; 4: 291, 463
Mayfield, F. H., 3: 210
Mayo, Charles W., 4: 411
Mayo, Richard, 3: 310
Mayo, William J., 2: 69; 3: 40–41, 44–45, 50, 113*b*
Mayo Clinic, 3: 50, 289
McBride, Earl D., 3: 295
McCabe, Charles, 1: 167
McCall, M. G., 2: 212
McCall, Samuel W., 3: 134
McCarroll, H. Relton, 1: 162; 4: 237
McCarthy, Clare, 2: 178–180, 182, 204, 230, 287–288
McCarthy, E. A., 2: 230
McCarthy, Eddie, 3: 97
McCarthy, Joseph, 2: 368
McCarthy, Ralph, 4: 342
McCharen, Littleton L., 4: 489
McClellan, George, 3: 43
McCombs, Betsy, 3: 280
McCord, David, 4: 3, 9, 20

McDermott, Leo J., 2: 171–172, 229, 299, 438; 3: 74
McDermott, William, Jr., 4: 277–279, 303
McDonagh, Eileen, 1: 285
McDonald, John L., 2: 183
McDougall, Jean, 3: 288
McGibbon, Chris, 3: 460*b*
McGill University School of Medicine, 3: 253
McGinty, Beth A. Dignan, 2: 277–278
McGinty, John B. (1930–2019), 2: 278, 281
    AAOS chairman, 2: 281
    Arthroscopic Surgery Update, 2: 279
    arthroscopy and, 2: 279, 280*b*, 281; 3: 448
    Boston Children's Hospital and, 2: 278–279; 4: 22
    Brigham and Women's Hospital and, 4: 163, 193
    death of, 2: 281
    education and training, 2: 277
    Green and, 2: 178, 205, 279
    marriage and family, 2: 277–278
    Medical University of South Carolina and, 2: 281
    MGH and, 2: 278
    MGH/Children's Hospital residency, 2: 278
    military service, 2: 278–279
    Newton-Wellesley Hospital and, 2: 279
    Operative Arthroscopy, 2: 279
    Orthopaedics Today editor, 2: 281
    PBBH and, 2: 278–279; 4: 22, 116, 128, 163
    professional memberships, 2: 281
    publications and research, 2: 279
    Tufts University and, 2: 279
    Valley Forge Army Hospital and, 2: 279
    Veterans Administration Hospital and, 2: 279; 4: 22
McIndoe Memorial Research Unit, 2: 422, *422*
McKay, Douglas, 2: 304, 351
McKeever, Duncan, 4: 40
McKeever prothesis, 4: 40, 69, 70*b*–71*b*, 129–130, 177, 188–189
McKittrick, Leland S., 3: 301; 4: 276, 277*b*
McLaughlin, F. L., 3: 210
McLean, Franklin C., 3: 211
McLean Hospital, 1: 294
McMahon, Mark S., 3: 449
McMahon, Vince, 4: 252
McRae, Ronald, 1: 167

Meals, Roy, 3: 431
measles, 1: 7; 2: 4
Mechanic, Gerald L., 2: 324
Mechanism of Dislocation and Fracture of the Hip, The (Bigelow), 3: 35, *35*, 38
Medearis, Donald N., 3: 397
Medical and Orthopaedic Management of Chronic Arthritis, The (Osgood and Pemperton), 4: 32
Medical College of Virginia, 4: 153
medical degrees, 1: 6–7
medical education. *See also* Harvard Medical School (HMS); orthopaedics residencies
    admission requirements, 1: 146
    American, 1: 138, 142, 146–147
    apprenticeships and, 1: 6, 8, 15
    approved teaching hospitals, 1: 196, 198
    clinical facilities for, 1: 40
    curricular reform, 1: 169
    development of medical schools, 1: 25–28
    dressers, 1: 6, 33, 36–37
    early orthopaedic surgery training, 1: 186–189
    early surgical training, 1: 183–186
    in Edinburgh, 1: 7, 37, 76
    in England, 1: 6, 33, 37, 73, 142
    examinations for physicians, 1: 15, 21, 29
    Flexner Report and, 1: 146–147
    governance and, 1: 177
    graduate education, 1: 196, 196*b*, 197–199, 213
    graduate orthopaedic surgery, 2: 160–162, 162*b*
    hospitals and, 1: 41, 52
    human dissections and, 1: 21, 24, 26–27, 32, 34, 38, 52
    impact of World War II on, 4: 467
    inclusiveness in, 2: 146
    internships and, 1: 189–190
    leaders of, 1: 147
    military hospitals and, 1: 24
    musculoskeletal medicine in, 1: 168–170
    orthopaedics curriculum in, 1: 153–155, 159–162; 2: 183–184, 184*b*, 185, 185*b*, 186
    in Paris, 1: 34, 37, 73–76
    postgraduate, 2: 157–160
    reform of, 1: 139–140
    regulation of, 1: 196–200, 211–213
    regulations and milestones of, 1: 196*b*

specialization in, 1: 189;
4: 300–301
supervised training in,
1: 198–199
surgery in, 1: 29, 33–36
teaching program in, 1: 40; 4: 3
treating and teaching of fractures
in, 1: 161
use of audio-visual aids in, 1: 161
Veterans Administration hospitals
and, 1: 91
walkers, 1: 33
Medical Institution of Harvard
College (1782–1816), 1: 25–26.
See also Harvard Medical School
(HMS)
Medical Institution of Liverpool,
2: 135
*Medical Malpractice in Nineteenth-
Century America* (De Ville), 1: 47
Medical Research Council of Great
Britain, 2: 71
Medical University of South Carolina, 2: 281
*Medical War Manual No. 4 Military
Orthopaedic Surgery*, 4: 473, 474
Meeks, Berneda, 4: 255
Meeks, Laura, 4: 256
Meeks, Louis W. (1937–2015),
4: *254*
as Beth Israel acting chief of orthopaedics, 4: 223, 255, 289*b*
as Beth Israel chief of sports medicine, 4: 255
Beth Israel Hospital and, 4: 263
BIDMC teaching program and,
4: 286–287
community organizations and,
4: 255, 256*b*
death of, 4: 256
education and training, 4: 254
HCORP and, 4: 255
HMS appointment, 4: 263
marriage and family, 4: 255
orthopaedics education and,
4: 254–255
outpatient arthroscopic ACL
reconstructions, 4: 255
private medical practice, 4: 254
publications and research, 4: 255
US Army and, 4: 254
Meigs, Joe V., 2: 254
Meigs, Sarah Tyler, 3: 257
Meisenbach, Roland O., 4: 188
Mellon, William, 3: 135
Mellon Lecture (Univ. of Pittsburgh),
2: 66–67
Melrose Hospital, 4: 343
Meltzer, S. J., 3: 212
Merrick, Phiny, 1: 307

Merrill, Ed, 3: 224
Merrill, Janet, 2: 107; 4: 60, 396
Messner, Marie Blais, 2: 170, 191,
193–194
metal implants, 2: 237–238
metatarsalgia, 4: 188
Metcalf, Carleton R., 4: 440–441,
441*b*
methylmethacrylate (bone cement),
3: 220, 222; 4: 133, 171
Meyer, George von L., 2: 432
Meyerding, Henry W., 3: 340
MGH. See Massachusetts General
Hospital (MGH)
MGH Institute of Health Professions, 3: 391, *391*, 392, 397
MGH School of Nursing, 3: 302,
391
MGH Staff Associates, 3: 241
MGH Surgical Society Newsletter, 3: 1
Michael G. Ehrlich, MD, Fund for
Orthopedic Research, 3: 401
Micheli, Lyle J. (1940–), 2: *383*
on ACL reconstruction in young
athletes, 2: 385, *385*, 386, *386*
athletic spine problems and,
2: 385
as Boston Ballet attending physician, 2: 384
Boston Children's Hospital and,
2: 354, 383–385, 436, 439*b*
Brigham and Women's Hospital
and, 4: 163, 193
education and training, 2: 383
HMS appointment, 2: 383–384
honors and awards, 2: 387*b*
Joseph O'Donnell Family Chair
in Orthopedic Sports Medicine,
2: 439*b*
Massachusetts Hospital School
and, 2: 384
MGH/Children's Hospital residency, 2: 383
military service, 2: 383
New England Deaconess Hospital
and, 4: 280
orthopaedics appointments,
2: 384
orthopaedics leadership, 2: 387
PBBH and, 4: 163
private medical practice, 2: 338
publications and research,
2: 359, 378–379, 385
rugby and, 2: 383–385
sports medicine and, 2: 287,
384–385, 387
*Sports Medicine Bible for Young
Adults, The*, 2: 385
Sports Medicine Bible, The,
2: 385, *385*

Middlesex Central District Medical
Society, 3: 319
Miegel, Robert, 4: 194, 195*b*
Mignon, M. Alfred, 4: 102
Milch, R. A., 4: 21
Milgram, Joseph, 3: 382
Military Orthopaedic Surgery (Orthopaedic Council), 2: *68*, 69
military orthopaedics. See also base
hospitals
amputations and, 1: 23;
4: 418–419
bone and joint injuries, 4: 419
camp work, 2: 258; 4: 452–453
casualty clearing stations (CCS),
4: 414, *415*, 421, 424–425
compound fractures and, 4: 391,
392
curative workshops and, 4: 399–
403, *403*, 404, 442, 448, *448*,
449
documentation and, 4: 407–408
evacuation hospital care,
4: 417–418
expanded role of orthopaedists
and, 4: 453–454
facilities for, 4: 414–416
Goldthwait and, 2: 127–128;
4: 443
Goldthwait units, 4: 440
Harvard Medical School surgery
course, 4: 455–462
manual of splints and appliances
for, 2: 126
massage and, 2: 56, 67, 120, 188
medical categories for,
4: 412–414
Medical Officer instructions for,
4: 410*b*
necessary equipment for, 4: 393*b*
nerve lesions and, 4: 392
open-bone fractures, 4: *400*
Orthopaedic Centers and, 2: 127
Osgood and, 2: 120–128;
4: 423*b*
patient flow process and,
4: 435–436
reconstruction and occupational
aides, 4: 436*b*
reconstruction hospitals and,
4: 439–443, 447–449
rehabilitation and, 1: 270–272;
2: 121, 127; 3: 232; 4: 411,
454
standardization of equipment for,
2: 124
Thomas splint and, 2: 20
Thorndike and, 1: 270–272
trauma surgery and, 3: 274, 301;
4: 393

use of splints in, 2: 120; 4: 389, *391*, 408–409, 411, 416–417
war injuries and, 2: 124, 126, 128; 4: 391
World War I volunteer orthopaedic surgeons, 2: 117–119, 124–127, 145; 4: 386–396, 398–399, *399*, 402, 404, 406–409, 412*b*–413*b*, 425, 452
World War II and, 4: 463–464, 473, 485, 493
wound treatment and, 4: 392–393, 435–436

Military Orthopedics for the Expeditionary Forces, 3: 156

military reconstruction hospitals. *See also* Reconstruction Base Hospital No. 1 (Parker Hill, Boston)
amputation services, 4: 451
Canadian, 4: 443
Cotton on, 4: 449–451
gyms in, 4: 444
Harvard orthopaedic surgeons and, 4: 452
as models for civilian hospitals, 4: 450–451
occupational rehabilitation and, 4: 444
organization of British, 4: 441*b*
orthopaedics services in, 4: 439, 451
rehabilitation of wounded soldiers and, 4: 439–444, 447–450
in the United Kingdom, 4: 440–441

Millender, Bonnie Cobert, 4: 168

Millender, Lewis H. (1937–1996), 4: *165*
Beth Israel Hospital and, 4: 262
Brigham and Women's Hospital, 4: 163, 167
death of, 4: 168
education and training, 4: 165
Entrapment Neuropathies, 4: 168
hand therapy and, 4: 97–98, 132, 165, 168
HMS appointment, 4: 165
honors and awards, 4: 168
hospital appointments, 4: 167
marriage and family, 4: 168
Nalebuff on, 4: 167
New England Baptist Hospital and, 4: 165, 167
Occupational Disorders of the Upper Extremity, 4: 168, 183
occupational medicine and, 4: 167–168
PBBH and, 4: 116, 129, 161, 163

posterior interosseous syndrome case, 4: 165–166
publications and research, 4: 165, *165*, 166–167, *167*
RBBH and, 4: 132, 165, 167
Tufts appointment, 4: 167
US Public Health Service and, 4: 165
West Roxbury Veterans Administration Hospital and, 4: 167

Miller, Bill, 2: 339, 358, *359*
Miller, Richard H., 3: 60; 4: 475
Millet, Peter, 4: 194
Milligan, E. T. C., 4: 385

Millis, Michael B. (1944–), 2: *388*
acetabular dysplasia case, 2: 389, *389*, 390
Boston Children's Hospital and, 2: 338, 354, 388–389
Boston Concept and, 2: 391, *391*
Brigham and Women's Hospital and, 4: 163, 193
computer-simulated planning and, 2: 389
education and training, 2: 358, 388
Hall and, 2: 347, 388
HCORP and, 2: 388
hip and pelvis research, 2: 389–394
HMS appointment, 2: 388–389
honors and awards, 2: 388, 390
metacarpal phalangeal joint replacement, 4: 132
military service, 2: 388
orthopaedics appointments, 2: 389
orthopaedics education and, 2: 394
on Pappas, 2: 289
pediatric orthopaedics, 2: 394
periacetabular osteotomy research, 2: 390–394
professional memberships, 2: 392–393
publications and research, 2: 389–394

Milton Hospital, 1: 264; 3: 257, 287
Milwaukee Brace, 2: 265–266, 336
Minas, Thomas, 4: 193, 195*b*
Minot, Charles S., 3: 94; 4: 2–3, 6
Miriam Hospital, 3: 401
MIT Medical, 2: 276–277, 290
Mital, Mohinder A., 2: 234; 3: 320
Mitchell, William, Jr., 4: 286
Mixter, Charles G., 4: 283*t*, 468
Mixter, Samuel J., 2: 117; 3: *19*, 184

Mixter, William J.
back pain research and, 3: 203, *203*, 204–207
Beth Israel Hospital and, 1: 158
publications and research, 3: 302
ruptured intervertebral disc research, 3: 204; 4: 352–353
Mizuno, Schuichi, 4: 194
mobile army surgical hospitals (MASHs), 2: 231, *232*; 4: 468–469, *470*
Mock, Harry, 1: 271
Moe, John, 2: 335
Moellering, Robert, 4: 279
Mohan, Alice, 1: 62
Molasses Act, 1: 11
mold arthroplasty
evolution of the Vitallium, 3: 292, 292*b*, 293
hip surgery and, 3: 218, 242, *242*, 243–244
historical evolution of, 3: *194*
knee and, 3: 291–292
original design of, 3: 193*b*
postoperative roentgenogram, 3: *195*, *196*
preoperative roentgenogram, 3: *196*
problems with cup, 3: 241
results of, 3: 242*t*, 243*b*
Smith-Petersen and, 3: 181, 182*b*, 183, 192, *192*, 193–196, 198
Vitallium, 3: 193*b*, *195*, *196*, 238–239, 243*b*
Molloy, Maureen K., 1: 239; 3: 208
mononucleosis, 3: 324–325
Monson State Hospital, 4: 350
Montgomery, James B., 4: 407
Moody, Dwight, 4: 257
Moody, Ellsworth, 3: 165–166
Moore, Belveridge H., 2: 78, 172
Moore, Francis D.
on Banks, 4: 72
burn care and, 3: 336
as BWH chief of surgery, 3: 135
family of, 1: 90
as Moseley Professor of Surgery, 2: 421
PBBH 50th anniversary report, 4: 21*b*
PBBH and, 4: 79
as PBBH chief of surgery, 4: 8, 18, 22, 74*b*, 75
on Sledge, 4: 114
on surgery residents, 4: 19
Moore, Howard, 4: 372
Moral Re-Armament program (Oxford Group), 4: 57
Morales, Teresa, 3: 462, 464*b*
Moratoglu, Orhun, 3: 460*b*

Morgan, John, 1: 23
Morris, Katherine, 2: 284
Morris, Miriam Morss, 2: 282
Morris, Richard B., 1: 317
Morris, Robert H. (1892–1971),
2: *283*
   on arthrodesis procedures,
2: 282–283
   BCH Bone and Joint Service,
4: 380*b*
   Boston Children's Hospital and,
1: 194; 2: 222, 231, 252, 274,
284
   death of, 2: 284
   education and training, 2: 282
   Fitchet and, 2: 282
   on foot stabilization, 2: 282–284
   HMS appointment, 2: 223, 282;
4: 60–61
   King's College and, 2: 284
   Long Island Hospital and, 2: 284
   marriage and family, 2: 282, 284
   professional memberships, 2: 284
   publications of, 2: 282
   RBBH and, 4: 36, 93, 111
   World War I service, 2: 282
Morrison, Gordon M. (1896–1955),
4: *346*
   AAST president, 4: 349
   Boston City Hospital and, 4: 347
   boxing and, 4: 347
   Cotton and, 4: 330
   death of, 4: 349
   education and training,
4: 346–347
   football coaching and, 4: 347
   hip fracture treatment, 4: 319
   hospital appointments, 4: 347
   ischaemic paralysis case, 4: 348
   Joseph H. Shortell Fracture Unit,
4: 307
   Massachusetts Regional Fracture
Committee, 3: 64
   New England Society of Bone
and Joint Surgery, 4: 347
   professional memberships,
4: 347–349
   publications and research,
4: 316, 347
   Royal Flying Corps and,
4: 346–347
   on trauma treatment, 4: 349
Morrison, H., 4: 202, 203*b*, *203*
Morrison, Sidney L., 4: 64, *64*
Morrissey, Raymond, 2: 438
Morrow, Edward R., 2: 272
Morss, Miriam, 2: 282
Morton, William T. G., 1: *57*
   ether composition, 1: 61
   ether inhaler, 1: *58*, 63

   ether patent and, 1: 60
   ether use, 1: 55, 57–60, 62;
3: 27–29, 32–33
   as witness for Webster, 1: 310
Morton's neuroma, 2: 287
Moseley, William, 3: 74
Moseley's growth charts, 2: 194, *194*
Moss, H. L., 4: 261–262
Moss, William L., 3: 313
Mott, Valentine, 1: xxiv
Mount Auburn Cemetery, 3: 23;
4: 2
Mount Auburn Hospital, 2: 276;
3: 327
Mount Sinai Monthly magazine,
4: *201*, 202
Moyer, Carl, 4: 125
Mt. Sinai Hospital (Boston)
   Chambers Street location,
4: 201*b*, 202, *202*
   closing of, 4: 205, 223
   Compton Street location,
4: 201*b*, 202, *202*
   financial difficulties, 4: 203–205
   fundraising for, 4: 202
   Jewish patients at, 4: 199–200,
202
   Jewish physicians and, 4: 202,
204
   non-discrimination and, 4: 199,
201
   orthopaedic treatment at, 4: 202,
204, 204*t*
   outpatient services at,
4: 203–204
   planning for, 4: 200–201
   Staniford Street location, 4: 202
Mt. Sinai Hospital (New York)
   Jewish patients at, 4: 200
   orthopaedics residencies and,
4: 88
   World War II and, 4: 88
Mt. Sinai Hospital Society of Boston,
4: 200–201
Mt. Sinai Medical School, 3: 383,
385, 413, 435
Mueller, Maurice, 4: 263
Mueller Professorship, 4: 263
Muir, Helen, 4: 116*b*, 268
Multicenter Arthroscopy of the Hip
Outcomes Research Network
(MAHORN), 2: 380
multiple cartilaginous exostoses,
4: 218–219, *219*, 220
Mumford, E. B., 4: 452
Mumford, James, 4: 52
Muratoglu, Orhun, 3: 224
Muro, Felipe, 2: 309
Murphy, Eugene, 3: 317

Murphy, Steven, 2: 389–392;
4: 286
Murray, Martha, 2: 439
Murray S. Danforth Oration of
Rhode Island Hospital, 3: 275
Muscle Function (Wright), 2: 70
muscle training
   heavy-resistance exercise,
3: 282–285
   poliomyelitis and, 2: 62–63, 78,
109; 3: 284–285
   progressive resistance exercises,
3: 285
Muscular Dystrophy Association of
America, 2: 266
Musculoskeletal Imaging Fund,
2: 439*b*
musculoskeletal medicine
   apparatus for, 2: 27
   biomechanics and, 2: 410
   disease and, 2: 439
   early treatment, 1: xxiii
   in medical education,
1: 168–170
   orthopaedics curriculum and,
1: 168–170; 2: 184–186
   orthopaedics research and,
2: 439
   pathology and, 3: 432
   sarcomas and, 2: 424
   spinal disorders and, 2: 337
   sports injuries and, 1: 288
   surgery advances for, 2: 36
   tissue banks for, 3: 442–443
   tumors and, 3: 432–433, 436
Musculoskeletal Outcome Data Evaluation and Management System
(MODEMS), 4: 186
Musculoskeletal Tissue Banking (Tomford), 3: 443
Musculoskeletal Tumor Society,
3: 390, 436, *436*
Musnick, Henry, 4: 91
Myelodysplasia Clinic (Children's
Hospital), 2: 359, 402
Myers, Grace Whiting, 3: 10
myositis ossificans, 1: 266–267

N

Nachemson, Alf, 2: 373; 4: 262
Nadas, Alex, 2: 234
Nalebuff, Edward A. (1928–2018),
4: *94*
   art glass collection, 4: 100, *100*
   Boston Children's Hospital and,
4: 95
   Brigham and Women's Hospital,
4: 163
   death of, 4: 100

education and training, 4: 94–95
hand surgery and, 4: 96, 98–100
hand surgery fellowship,
    4: 95–96
HMS appointment, 4: 97–98
hospital appointments, 4: 99
implant arthroplasty research,
    4: 99–100
Marian Ropes Award, 4: 100
marriage of, 4: 100
metacarpal phalangeal joint
    replacement, 4: 132
MGH and, 4: 95
New England Baptist Hospital
    and, 4: 99
PBBH and, 4: 95, 116, 129,
    161, 163
professional memberships, 4: 100
publications and research, 4: 40,
    95–99, 99, 166, 167
RBBH and, 4: 38, 41b, 42,
    68–69, 95–97, 100, 102, 116b,
    131
RBBH hand clinic and, 4: 42
as RBBH hand service chief,
    4: 97–98
rheumatoid arthritis of the hand
    research and surgery, 4: 96,
    96, 97–98, 98, 131
rheumatoid thumb deformity
    classification, 4: 97
surgical procedures performed,
    4: 131t
Tufts appointment, 4: 98
Tufts hand fellowship, 2: 250;
    4: 98–99
US Air Force and, 4: 95
Veterans Administration Hospital
    and, 4: 95
Nalebuff, Marcia, 4: 100
Nathan, David, 2: 234
"Nation and the Hospital, The"
    (Osgood), 2: 137–138,
    138b–139b
National Academy of Medicine,
    3: 405
National Academy of Sciences,
    3: 405
National Birth Defects Center,
    2: 370
National Collegiate Athletic Association (NCAA), 1: 248, 253
National Foundation for Infantile
    Paralysis, 2: 188–189, 191, 260
National Foundation for Poliomyelitis, 2: 188, 191
National Institute of Arthritis and
    Metabolic Diseases, 3: 323
National Institutes of Health (NIH),
    3: 383, 387–388, 392; 4: 38–39

National Intercollegiate Football,
    1: 253
National Rehabilitation Association,
    2: 266
National Research Council,
    2: 215–216
Natural History of Cerebral Palsy, The
    (Crothers and Paine), 2: 172
Naval Fleet Hospital No. 109, 4: 490
Naval Medical Research Institute,
    3: 439, 440
Navy Regional Medical Center
    (Guam), 3: 446
necks, 2: 256
Nélaton, Auguste, 1: 82
nerve injuries, 2: 67, 120, 140, 393;
    3: 157, 353
Nerve Injuries Committee (Medical
    Research Council of Great Britain),
    2: 71
Nesson, H. Richard, 2: 272
Nestler, Steven P., 1: 215, 218, 220,
    232–233; 3: 435–436, 436
neuritis, 3: 324–325
neurofibromatosis, 2: 172, 174–175
Neusner, Jacob, 4: 220
New England Baptist Hospital
    (NEBH)
    affiliation with BIDMC, 4: 214
    affiliation with New England
        Deaconess Hospital, 4: 280
    Aufranc and, 3: 246–247
    Ben Bierbaum and, 1: 233–234,
        236
    Bone and Joint Institute Basic
        Science Laboratory, 4: 271,
        286
    Brackett and, 3: 153
    Edward Kennedy and, 3: 275
    Emans and, 2: 358
    Fitchet and, 2: 252
    Hall and, 2: 338
    Hresko and, 2: 364
    Kocher and, 2: 377
    Morris and, 2: 284
    Nalebuff and, 4: 98–100
    New England Bone and Joint
        Institute, 4: 280
    orthopaedics residencies, 3: 247
    Painter and, 4: 47
    Pathway Health Network and,
        4: 280
    Pedlow and, 3: 426
    Potter and, 4: 69, 116
    purchase of RBBH buildings and
        land, 4: 26, 114, 121
    reconstructive hip surgery and,
        3: 246
    Runyon and, 2: 290
    Schiller and, 2: 369

    Smith-Petersen and, 3: 362
    Swaim and, 4: 58
New England Bone and Joint Institute, 4: 280
New England Deaconess Association,
    2: 219–220
New England Deaconess Home and
    Training School, 4: 273
New England Deaconess Hospital
    (NEDH), 4: 273, 274, 275
    admissions and occupancy at,
        4: 279
    bed allocation at, 4: 277t
    early history of, 4: 275, 276t
    foot and ankle service, 4: 279
    founding of, 4: 273
    Harvard Fifth Surgical Service
        and, 4: 279
    Lahey Clinic and, 4: 275–277
    long-range planning at, 4: 278b
    maps of, 4: 276
    medical and surgical (sub) specialties in, 4: 274
    merger with Beth Israel Hospital,
        4: 214, 223, 270, 281, 283
    orthopaedics department at,
        4: 279–280
    Palmer Memorial Hospital and,
        4: 275–276
    Pathway Health Network and,
        4: 280
    physician affiliations at, 4: 277,
        277t, 278
    relationship with HMS,
        4: 277–279
    as a specialized tertiary-care facility, 4: 279
New England Dressings Committee
    (Red Cross Auxiliary), 4: 10
New England Female Medical College, 2: 273; 4: 296
New England Home for Little Wanderers, 3: 307
New England Hospital for Women
    and Children, 2: 274
New England Journal of Medicine,
    1: 39
New England Medical Center,
    4: 249, 311
New England Medical Council,
    2: 157–158
New England Muscular Dystrophy Association Clinic Directors,
    2: 403
New England Organ Bank, 3: 443
New England Orthopedic Society,
    3: 319
New England Patriots, 3: 348, 397,
    399, 448

Index 549

New England Peabody Home for Crippled Children, 2: 37, 165, 183, 191, 230–231, 269–270; 3: 174, 202, 209, 329, 362
New England Pediatric Society, 2: 13
New England Regional Committee on Fractures, 4: 341, 347
New England Rehabilitation Center, 1: 272
New England Revolution, 3: 348, 450
New England Society of Bone and Joint Surgery, 4: 347
New England Surgical Society, 1: 90; 2: 136; 3: 63
New York Bellevue Hospital, 2: 111
New York Hospital for the Ruptured and Crippled, 1: 89
New York Orthopaedic Dispensary and Hospital, 2: 20, 47–48
New York Orthopaedic Hospital, 2: 47
Newcomb, Sarah Alvord, 1: 107
Newhall, Harvey F., 3: 266
Newhauser, E. B. D., 2: 215
Newman, Erik T., 3: 463*b*; 4: 190*b*
Newton-Wellesley Hospital (NWH), 1: 225; 2: 279; 3: 240, 331, 334, 426
Nichol, Vern, 3: 248
Nichols, Edward H. (1864–1922), 1: *252*; 4: *302*
  Base Hospital No. 7 and, 1: 256; 4: 301–302, 438–439
  Boston Children's Hospital and, 2: 247, 307
  Boston City Hospital and, 1: 174, 252; 4: 301–302
  death of, 1: 256–257
  as football team surgeon, 1: 252–256
  Harvard baseball team and, 1: 251–252
  HMS appointment, 4: 302
  HMS Laboratory of Surgical Pathology and, 2: 90
  legacy of, 1: 257
  offices of, 4: *302*
  orthopaedic research and, 1: 252
  osteomyelitis research and, 4: 301
  PBBH teaching and, 4: 10, 12
  as professor of surgery, 1: 174
  study of football injuries, 1: 254–256
  Surgery of Joints, The, 2: 52
  tuberculosis treatment, 2: 32
  vascular anastomosis and, 4: 216
  World War I medical unit, 1: 256; 4: 391
Nichols, Emma, 4: 438
Nickel, Vernon, 2: 315; 3: 249, 319, 321
Nightingale, Florence, 2: 5; 4: 274*b*
nitrous oxide, 1: 56–59, 63; 3: 15
Noall, Lawrence, 3: 208
Noble, Nick, 3: 94
non-hinged metal–polyethylene prosthesis, 4: 145–146
Nordby, Eugene J., 3: 255
North Charles General Hospital, 4: 157
North Shore Children's Hospital, 2: 269
Northwestern University, 2: 302
Norton, Margaret, 3: 320
Norton, Paul L. (1903–1986)
  adjustable reamer and, 3: 317
  Children's Hospital/MGH combined program and, 3: 317
  Clinics for Crippled Children and, 2: 230; 3: 317
  death of, 3: 320
  early life, 3: 317
  education and training, 3: 317
  Emerson Hospital and, 3: 317, 319
  HMS appointment, 3: 317
  as honorary orthopaedic surgeon, 3: 398*b*
  legacy of, 3: 320
  marriage and family, 3: 320
  Massachusetts Hospital School and, 3: 319–320; 4: 378
  memberships and, 3: 319
  as MGH surgeon, 3: 70*b*, 192, 317
  New England Orthopedic Society president, 3: 319
  Norton-Brown spinal brace, 3: 317–319
  paraplegia research and, 3: 319
  publications and research, 3: 258–259, 317–320, 455*b*; 4: 95
Norton-Brown spinal brace, 3: 317–319
Norwalk train wreck, 1: 77, *78*
nose reconstructions, 1: 71, 75–76
Notes on Military Orthopaedics (Jones), 4: 442, *442*, 443
Nuffield Orthopaedic Centre (Oxford), 3: 412
Nursery and Child's Hospital (New York), 2: 3, 5
Nursery for Children (New York), 2: 3
nursing
  Cadet Nursing Corps, 4: 467
  Children's Island Sanitorium and, 4: 87
  Deaconess training and, 4: 274*b*
  early training in, 1: 41; 2: 6–8, 13–14
  foot problems, 2: 54–56
  impact of World War II on, 4: 467
  for Jewish women, 4: 208
  Larson and, 3: 302–303
  MGH School of Nursing and, 3: 302, 391
  New England Deaconess Hospital and, 4: 273
  reforms in, 3: 142
nutrition, 2: 361–362
Nydegger, Rogert C., 4: 489

O

Ober, Ernest, 2: 144, 166
Ober, Frank R. (1881–1960), 1: *188, 195*; 2: *143, 147*, 255
  AAOS and, 4: 337
  as AOA president, 2: 161
  "Back Strains and Sciatica," 2: 151–152
  Barr and, 3: 201
  Base Hospital No. 5 and, 4: 420, *422*
  Bell and, 2: 220
  on biceps-triceps transplant, 2: 154
  Boston Children's Hospital and, 1: 153, 155, 158, 178, 188, 195–196, 198–199; 2: *143*, 144–147, 149, 163, 217, 252, 274, 282; 4: 338, 468
  brachioradialis transfer for triceps weakness, 2: 153–154, *154*
  Brigham and Women's Hospital and, 4: 195*b*
  Children's Hospital/MGH combined program and, 1: 210
  club foot treatment, 2: 145
  death of, 2: 166
  on diagnosis, 2: 155–156
  education and training, 2: 143–144
  expert testimony and, 2: 164–165
  on FitzSimmons, 2: 256, 258
  Georgia Warm Springs Foundation board and, 2: 78, 165
  graduate education in orthopaedic surgery and, 2: 160–162, 162*b*
  graduate education review, 1: 196–197

Green and, 2: 168
Harvard Unit and, 4: 419
HCORP and, 1: 192, 195–199
Hibbs spinal fusion procedure, 2: 164
hip abductor paralysis treatment, 2: 149–150
hip and knee contractures, 2: 153, *153*
HMS appointment, 2: 144, 146–147, 156; 4: 59
honorary degrees, 2: 165
Hugenberger and, 2: 269, 271
iliotibial band tightness and, 2: 151–152
John Ball and Buckminster Brown Professorship, 2: 147, 157; 4: 195*b*
Journal of Bone and Joint Surgery editor, 2: 165
lectures at Tuskegee Institute, 2: 146
Lovett and, 2: 144
Lovett Fund Committee and, 2: 82
Marlborough Medical Associates and, 2: 299
marriage and, 2: 144
Massachusetts Medical Society and, 2: 164
Massachusetts Regional Fracture Committee, 3: 64
medical education, 2: 155
military orthopaedics and, 4: 473
military surgeon training and, 2: 42
modification of use of sacrospinalis, 2: 146–147
Mount Desert Island practice, 2: 143–145
New England Peabody Home for Crippled Children and, 2: 270
as orthopaedic chair, 2: 15*b*
on orthopaedic problems in children, 2: 164
orthopaedics education and, 2: 155–157, 163
on orthopaedics training at Harvard, 1: 195–196
Orthopedic Surgery revisions, 2: 166
on Osgood, 2: 148
on paralysis of the serratus anterior, 2: 154–155
PBBH and, 4: 18
poliomyelitis treatment, 2: 147–148, 154–155
posterior approach to the hip joint approach, 2: 146
postgraduate education and, 2: 157–159, 164
private medical practice and, 1: 176; 2: 146, 313; 3: 454*b*
professional memberships, 2: 165
publications of, 2: 227
RBBH and, 4: 15
rehabilitation planning and, 1: 273
Roosevelt and, 2: 77
surgery techniques, 2: 177
teaching department plan, 1: 157
on tendon transplantation, 2: 108, 147–148, *148*, 149
triple arthrodesis and, 2: 149
use of shelf procedure for CDH, 2: 151
Vermont poliomyelitis rehabilitation program, 2: 149
on wartime medical education, 4: 397
weakness/paralysis of the foot and ankle treatment, 2: 150–151
World War I and, 2: 125–126
"Your Brain is Your Invested Capital" speech, 2: 156, 158*b*–159*b*
Ober, Ina Spurling, 2: 144, 166
Ober, Melita J. Roberts, 2: 143
Ober, Otis Meriam, 2: 143
Ober abduction sign, 2: 151
Ober Research Fund, 2: 436
Ober Test, 2: 151–152
Ober-Yount fasciotomy, 2: 153, 172
Objective Structure Clinical Examination (OSCE), 1: 168
O'Brien, Michael, 4: 287
O'Brien, Paul, 4: 333, 378
obstetrical paralysis
 brachial plexus injuries, 2: 91, *91*
 Lange's theory, 2: 91
 massage and exercise for, 2: 90
 Sever-L'Episcopo procedure, 2: 90, 100
 Sever's study of, 2: 90, *90*, 94–96
 subscapularis tendon, 2: 95, *95*
 tendon transfers and, 2: 96
 treatment of, 2: 89–90, 94–95, *95*, 96
Occupational Disorders of the Upper Extremity (Millender et al.), 4: 168, 183
occupational therapy, 4: 28, *29*, 358–359
O'Connor, Frank, 4: 116*b*
O'Connor, Mary I., 4: 266*b*
O'Connor, Richard, 3: 446
O'Donoghue, Don, 3: 272

O'Donovan, T., 4: 167
Ogden, John, 2: 302
O'Hara, Dwight, 1: 273
Ohio State Medical Association, 3: 58
Ohio State University School of Medicine, 2: 407–408
O'Holleran, James, 4: 190*b*
Okike, Kanu, 2: *381*
Olcott, Christopher W., 4: 180
Oliver, Henry K., 1: 47, 49–50
Oliver Wendell Holmes Society, 4: 264
Ollier, Louis Xavier Edouard Leopold, 1: xxiii
O'Malley, Peter, 4: 264
O'Meara, John W., 2: 230
Omni Med, 3: 379
Oneida Football Club, 1: 247
O'Neil, Edward, Jr., 3: 379
O'Neil, Eugene, 4: 371
O'Neill, Eugene, 2: 272
Ontario Crippled Children's Center, 2: 334–335
opera-glass hand deformity, 4: 99
Operative Arthroscopy (McGinty et al.), 2: 279
Operative Hand Surgery (Green), 4: 98
Operative Nerve Repair and Reconstruction (Gelberman), 3: 404
ophthalmology, 1: 138; 3: 13
optical coherence tomography (OCT), 4: 194
Order of St. John of Jerusalem in England, 4: 401
Orr, Bobby, 3: 357, 357*b*
Orr, H. Winnett, 2: 125; 3: 159, 235, 340; 4: 383, 393, 400, 409
Orthopaedia (Andry), 1: xxi
Orthopaedic Biochemistry and Osteoarthritis Therapy Laboratory, 3: 464*b*
Orthopaedic Biology and Oncology Laboratories, 3: 463, 464*b*
Orthopaedic Biomechanics and Biomaterials Laboratory, 3: 464*b*
Orthopaedic Centers (Great Britain), 2: 127, 127*b*
Orthopaedic Fellow Education Fund, 2: 439*b*
Orthopaedic In-Service Training Exam (OITE), 1: 231
Orthopaedic Journal at Harvard Medical School, The, 1: 231–232
Orthopaedic Journal Club, 3: 369
orthopaedic oncology
 allografts and, 3: 389
 bone sarcomas and, 3: 136–137, 137*t*, 138–140, 140*b*, 141–142

Index

chondrosarcoma of bone, 3: 406
data digitization and, 3: 392–393
flow cytometry and, 3: 388
giant-cell tumors and, 3: 390
limb salvage surgery and,
   3: 390–391
Mankin and, 3: 386, 388
osteosarcoma and, 2: 422;
   3: 391
sacrococcygeal chordoma, 3: 390
Orthopaedic Research and Education Foundation, 2: 241; 3: 213, 215, 360
Orthopaedic Research Laboratories (MGH), 2: 321–324; 3: 211–212
Orthopaedic Research Society, 2: 240, 316, 327; 3: 262
orthopaedic surgeons
   advancement of the field, 2: 26, 50, 81, 99
   assistive technology and, 2: 408
   blue blazers and, 3: 30
   board certification of, 4: 324, 377
   diagnostic skills, 2: 155–156
   education and training, 2: 133–135
   evaluation and treatment, 2: 48
   extremity injuries and, 2: 122
   fracture care and, 4: 463–464
   general surgery foundations and, 2: 24
   graduate education and, 1: 197–199
   on hip disease, 2: 52
   interest in visceroptosis, 3: 83–84, 84b, 86–88
   logical thinking and, 2: 155
   military and, 2: 42, 65–68, 118–120
   minimum requirements for, 2: 134
   observational skills, 2: 155
   orthopaedic physician versus, 4: 47b
   recruitment of, 2: 39–40
   scientific study and, 2: 32
   as surgeon-scholars, 2: 217, 357; 3: 228, 395; 4: 43, 79, 143, 163, 193–194, 195b
   transformation of profession, 2: 130b–131b
   volunteer wartime, 2: 124–127
   war injuries and, 2: 124
   x-rays and, 2: 56
orthopaedic surgery
   advances in, 2: 14–15, 20, 25–28
   approved teaching hospitals, 1: 198

Boylston Medical School and, 1: 138
certification in, 1: 189, 196–198, 200, 231
characteristics of, 2: 132
computer-simulated planning, 2: 389
conditions for, 4: 451
development of, 2: 78
early 20th century, 2: 36
early training in, 1: 186–189
founding of, 1: xxiii; 2: 26–27
growth-sparing, 2: 360–361
Harvard athletics and, 1: 284
knee joint resections, 1: 81
in London, 1: 106
minimal requirements for specialization, 1: 191–192
naming of, 1: xxiv
orthopaedics curriculum and, 1: 141, 143, 147, 158, 162
outcomes of, 2: 372
personalities in early, 2: 99
public reporting of, 1: 102
rehabilitation and, 2: 172
residencies, 1: 186–187, 198–199; 2: 160–161
seminal text on, 2: 29–30, 50
tracing of deformities, 2: 53
traction treatment for, 2: 21–23, 25, 27
training in, 1: 101
transformation of, 2: 130b–131b
trauma and, 3: 275; 4: 393
in the United States, 1: 100–101, 107; 2: 23; 4: 393
use of traction, 2: 27
women in, 1: 200, 239
World War I and, 2: 119–126
World War II and, 4: 463–464, 473, 485, 493
Orthopaedic Surgery at Tufts University (Banks), 4: 77
Orthopaedic Surgery in Infancy and Childhood (Ferguson), 2: 188, 303
"Orthopaedic Surgery in the United States of America" (Mayer), 1: 114
Orthopaedic Surgical Advancement Fund, 2: 439b
Orthopaedic Trauma Association Visiting Scholars Program, 3: 418
orthopaedic wards
   Boston Children's Hospital and, 1: 205
   Boston City Hospital and, 2: 24
   House of the Good Samaritan, 1: 123, 125–130; 2: 25

   Massachusetts General Hospital and, 1: 193, 203, 273; 2: 116, 322; 3: 62, 68, 272, 304, 343
"Orthopaedic Work in a War Hospital" (Osgood), 2: 120
orthopaedics
   18th century history of, 1: xxi, xxii
   19th century history of, 1: xxii, xxiii, xxiv
   20th century specialty of, 1: 189–192
   advances in, 4: 466–467
   diversity initiatives in, 4: 264–265
   established as separate specialty, 1: 83, 95–96, 98–99, 119
   first case at MGH, 1: 42, 44
   impact of World War I on, 4: 453–454, 463–464
   impact of World War II on, 4: 473, 493
   malpractice suits and, 1: 50
   mechanical devices and, 1: 107–108, *108*
   opening of first specialty hospital, 1: 99
   radiology and, 2: 16–17
   rehabilitation and, 4: 454
   respect for field, 4: 453, 463–464
   scientific study of, 2: 51
   specialization in, 1: 187, 193; 4: 300–301
   as specialty course at HMS, 1: 141–143
   spelling of, 1: xxiv, xxv, *177*
   standards of practice and, 4: 463–464
Orthopaedics (MacAusland and Mayo), 3: 310
orthopaedics apparatus
   Abbott Frame, 4: 232, *232*
   Adam's machine, 2: 86
   adjustable reamer, 3: 317
   Austin Moore prosthesis, 3: 213
   Balkan Frame, 3: 317, 357b
   basket plasters, 2: *122*
   Boston Arm, 2: 326, *326*; 3: 287
   Boston brace, 2: 339–340, 358–359, *360*, *361*, 423
   brace shop, 2: 22
   braces, 3: 318–319
   Bradford Frame, 2: 27, *27*, 30–31, *31*, 32
   Bradford's method of reducing the gibbus, 3: *149*
   Buckminster Brown and, 1: 105–107

celastic body jackets, 2: 178
celluloid jackets, 2: 85
charitable surgical appliances, 2: 14
clover leaf rod, 3: 272
club foot device, 1: 98, 100, 106; 2: 23, *23*, 24
De Machinamentis of Oribasius, 3: *149*
Denis Browne splint, 2: 208
fluoroscope, 2: 307
foot strength tester, 2: 101–102
fracture table, 2: *121*
Goldthwait irons, 3: 89, *89*, *149*
Harrington rods, 2: 316, *317*, 325, 335
hyperextension cast, 3: *69*
inclinometers, 2: 366, *367*
interpedicular segmental fixation (ISF) pedicle screw plate, 3: 420
iron extension hinge, 2: *123*
iron lung, 2: 78, *79*, *190*, 191, 260, 264, 314
ISOLA implants, 2: *370*
Jewett nail-plate, 3: 320
knee flexion contracture appliance, 2: *20*
Küntscher femoral rod, 3: 272
Lovett Board, 2: *59*, 86
MacIntosh prosthesis, 4: 69, *71b*
McKeever prothesis, 4: 40, 69, *70b–71b*
McLaughlin side plate, 3: 320
metal implants, 2: 237–238
Milwaukee Brace, 2: 265–266, 336
Norton-Brown spinal brace, 3: 317–319
pedicle screws, 2: 343; 3: 420
pelvic machine design, 2: 86
Pierce Collar, 3: 321
Pierce Fusion, 3: 321
Pierce Graft, 3: 321
plaster casts, 2: *122–123*
portable traction device, 2: 297
pressure correction apparatus (Hoffa-Schede), 3: *151*, *152*
Relton-Hall frame, 2: 334–335, *335*
Risser cast, 2: 178
rocking beds, 2: 314, *315*
Sayre jacket, 1: 107
for scoliosis, 2: 35, *35*, 36, *36*, 296
scoliosis jackets, 2: 59–61, 85–87
scoliosometer, 2: 36
Smith-Petersen Vitallium mold, 3: *195*, *196*
for spinal deformities, 1: 107; 2: *31*
splints, 3: 167, *167*, 168
spring muscle test, 2: *70*
Steinmann pin, 2: 237–238
surgical scissors, 3: *138*
Taylor back brace, 2: 247
Thomas splint, 2: *123*, *247*; 3: *168*
triflanged nail, 3: 62, 185–186, *186*, 187, 189, 189b, 190, 320
turnbuckle jacket, 2: 80, 223–224, *224*, 225, *225*, 226–227, 316, *336*; 3: 209
VEPTR (Vertical Expandable Prosthetic Titanium Rib), 2: 360, *362*
wire arm splints, 2: *122*
wire drop foot splints, 2: *123*
World War I and, 2: 124
Zander chair, 3: *153*
Zander tilt table, 3: *152*
Zander's medico-mechanical equipment, 3: *69*, *71*, 264, *264*, 265, *265*, 266–267, *267*, 268b
"Orthopaedics at Harvard" (Brown), 1: 195
orthopaedics curriculum
 Allison on, 2: 134; 3: 171–173
 anatomy lectures in, 1: 134, 136
 cadaver dissection, 1: *142*
 case method and, 4: 299
 case-based discussions, 1: 167
 competency examinations, 1: 168
 development of, 1: 140–141
 early medical instruction, 1: 134, 136–138
 electives in, 1: 143, 144t, 148–151, 164–166
 evolution of, 1: 143, 147, 148b–151b, 152–170
 examination questions, 1: 140–141, 144b
 fractures in, 1: 154
 graduate training, 2: 187b
 Jack Warren and, 1: 40, 134
 John Collins Warren and, 1: 40, 136–137
 Massachusetts General Hospital (MGH) and, 1: 136–137
 medical education and, 2: 183–184, 184b, 185, 185b, 186
 military orthopaedic surgery course, 4: 455–462
 musculoskeletal medicine in, 1: 168–170; 2: 184–186
 ophthalmology and, 1: 138
 orthopaedic clerkship in, 1: 167–169
 orthopaedic surgery in, 1: 141, 143, 147, 158, 162
 recommendations for, 1: 162–163
 reform of, 1: 140
 required courses, 1: 143
 sample curriculum for, 1: 159–161
 sports medicine elective, 1: 165–166
 surgical pedagogy, 1: 137–138
 teaching clinics, 1: 155–157, 163, 170, 194
 teaching modalities, 3: 172
 for third- and fourth-year students, 1: 144t–146t
 undergraduate, 2: 183–186, 202
Orthopaedics Overseas, 3: 310
orthopaedics residencies. *See also* Harvard Combined Orthopaedic Residency Program (HCORP)
 ABOS board and, 4: 377–379
 AOA survey on, 2: 160–161
 approved hospitals for, 1: 196–200
 BCH and, 2: 413; 4: 377–379
 BCH Bone and Joint Service, 4: 377
 Carney Hospital and, 4: 378
 certification examinations and, 1: 198, 231
 core competencies in, 1: 238–239
 examinations for, 1: 210, 231
 grand rounds, 1: 189, 203, *203*, 204, *204*, 205, 218, 232
 history of, 1: 183–186
 hospital internships and, 1: 186–188
 internal review of, 1: 239
 Lahey Clinic and, 4: 378
 Lakeville State Hospital and, 4: 378
 Massachusetts General/Boston Children's Hospital residency program, 1: 210; 2: 144
 MGH and, 2: 249, 276, 278, 290, 320, 327
 minimum surgical case requirements for, 3: 435–436, *436*
 pediatric, 1: 210–211
 program length and, 1: 215–216, 218–220, 222–223
 restructuring at MGH, 1: 198–199
 RRC for, 1: 211–213, 215, 217–220, 224, 232–233, 241–242

West Roxbury Veterans Administration Hospital and, 4: 378–379
Orthopaedics Today, 2: 281
Orthopedic Nursing (Funsten and Calderwood), 3: 303
Orthopedic Surgery (Bradford and Lovett), 4: 318
Orthopedic Surgery (Jones and Lovett), 2: 69, *69*, 166
Orthopedic Treatment of Gunshot Injuries, The (Mayer), 3: 156*b*
L'Orthopédie (Andry), 3: 90
orthoroentgenograms, 2: 171
os calcis fractures, 4: 313, 314*b*, 335–336
Osgood, John Christopher, 2: 113
Osgood, Margaret Louisa, 2: 138
Osgood, Martha E. Whipple, 2: 113
Osgood, Robert B. (1873–1956), 1: *193, 194*; 2: 113, 118, 125, 140, 222, 255; 4: 404, 417
  adult orthopaedics and, 2: 157
  on AEF medical care organization, 4: 417
  AEF splint board, 4: 416
  American Ambulance Hospital and, 2: 117–123; 4: 386, 389*b*, *390*, 392–393
  on Andry's *Orthopaedia*, 1: xxii
  AOA preparedness committee, 4: 394
  on arthritis and rheumatic disease, 4: 58
  back pain research and, 3: 203
  Base Hospital No. 5 and, 4: 420, 421*b*, 422, 422*b*, *422*
  Beth Israel Hospital and, 4: 208*b*, 247
  Boston Children's Hospital and, 1: 192; 2: 16, 40–41, 114, 132–133, 140, 247, 274, 282; 3: 99
  Brigham and Women's Hospital and, 4: 195*b*
  British Expeditionary Forces and, 4: 420
  Burrage Hospital and, 4: 226
  Carney Hospital and, 2: 116
  as chief at MGH, 1: 151, 192
  chronic disease treatment and, 4: 52
  as clinical professor, 1: 158
  curative workshops and, 4: 403–404
  death of, 2: 140
  Department for Military Orthopedics and, 4: 405
  Diseases of the Bones and Joints, 2: 117; 3: 81–82
  education and training, 2: 113–114
  on Edward H. Bradford, 2: 44
  elegance and, 2: 138–140
  end-results clinics and, 1: 194
  European medical studies, 2: 116
  faculty salary, 1: 177, 179
  on FitzSimmons, 2: 258–259
  on foot problems, 2: 56, 123–124
  foot strength apparatus and, 2: 101–102
  Fundamentals of Orthopaedic Surgery in General Medicine and Surgery, 2: 135–136
  George W. Gay Lecture, 4: 324
  Georgia Warm Springs Foundation and, 2: 78
  hand-washing policy, 1: 193
  Harvard Unit and, 2: 119–121, 123–124; 3: 180, 369, *370*; 4: 386–387, 421*b*
  HCORP and, 1: 192–195
  as head of HMS orthopaedic surgery department, 1: 174–175, 177, 192
  HMS appointment, 2: 116, 133–135
  honorary degrees, 2: 137
  House of the Good Samaritan and, 2: 113–114
  identification of Osgood-Schlatter disease, 2: 115, *116*, 117
  John Ball and Buckminster Brown Professorship, 2: 133; 4: 195*b*
  Journal of Bone and Joint Surgery editor, 2: 130
  Katzeff and, 2: 275
  King Manuel II and, 4: 401
  on Legg-Calve-Perthes disease, 2: 105
  Lovett Fund and, 2: 82
  marriage and family, 2: 138
  MGH and, 2: 116–117, 129–134; 3: 67
  MGH crystal laboratory, 2: 322
  MGH Fracture Clinic and, 3: 313; 4: 464
  as MGH orthopaedics chief, 3: 11*b*, 227, 266, 268; 4: 472*b*
  MGH surgical intern, 1: 189
  military orthopaedics and, 2: 124–128; 4: 403, 406–407, 412, 417–419, 423*b*, 453
  on mobilization of stiffened joints, 4: 27*b*
  "Nation and the Hospital, The," 2: 137–138, 138*b*–139*b*
  New England Surgical Society president, 2: 136
  Ober on, 2: 148
  as orthopaedic chair, 2: 15*b*
  orthopaedic research support, 1: 193, 195
  orthopaedic surgery and, 1: xxiii; 2: 79, 106, 116–117, 132, 140
  "Orthopaedic Work in a War Hospital," 2: 120
  orthopaedics education and, 1: 152; 2: 133–136
  Orthopedics and Body Mechanics Committee, 4: 235
  poetry of, 2: 128–129, 129*b*, 140
  poliomyelitis treatment, 2: 77, 264
  on preventative measures, 2: 122–123
  private medical practice and, 1: 176; 3: 338
  professional memberships, 2: 136–137
  as professor of orthopaedic surgery, 1: 172
  "Progress in Orthopaedic Surgery" series, 2: 43, 297
  publications and research, 2: 135–137; 4: 32, 65, 421*b*
  as radiologist, 2: 114–115
  RBBH and, 4: 25–26, 28, 31, 56
  on rehabilitation of wounded soldiers, 4: 451
  roentgenograms and, 2: 54, 116
  on sacroiliac joint fusion, 3: 184–185
  scoliosis treatment, 2: 87
  on synovial fluid diagnosis, 3: 175
  on transformation of orthopaedic surgeons, 2: 130*b*–131*b*, *132*
  treatment of fractures, 3: 61
  US Army Medical Corps and, 3: 61
  on visceroptosis, 3: 87–88
  war injury studies and, 2: 128–129
  World War I and, 2: 65, 117–128; 3: 157, 166; 4: 403, 406–407, 412, 417, 421*b*
  World War II volunteers and, 4: 363
Osgood Visiting Professors, 2: 141*b*
Osgood-Schlatter disease, 2: 89, 115, *116*, 117
Osler, Sir William, 1: 1, 185, 275; 3: 2; 4: vii, 6
osteoarthritis

articular cartilage structure research, 3: 383–384, *385*
bilateral, 3: 244, 279
biomechanical factors in, 3: 322, 326–328, 383
etiology of, 3: 327
femoral neck fractures and, 3: 383–384
hip surgery and, 3: 155
histologic-histochemical grading systems, 3: 384, 384*t*, 385
knee arthroplasty and, 4: 70*b*–71*b*
Mankin System and, 3: 384, 384*t*
mold arthroplasty and, 3: 195–196
nylon arthroplasty in, 4: 65
periacetabular osteotomy and, 2: 389
total hip replacement and, 3: 221, *222*
total knee replacement and, 4: 177
Osteoarthritis Cartilage Histopathology Assessment System (OARSI), 3: 384–385
osteoarthrosis, 3: 328
osteochondritis, 3: 363
osteochondritis deformans juvenilis, 2: 103–104. *See also* Legg-Calvé-Perthes disease
osteochondritis dissecans, 2: 194–195
osteogenic sarcoma, 4: 102
osteolysis
after total hip replacement, 3: 220, *220*, 221–222, *222*, 223, 225
associated with acetabular replacement, 3: 279
rapid postoperative in Paget Disease, 3: 441
osteomalacia, 3: 388
osteomyelitis
in children, 2: 169
following intramedullary nailing of femoral shaft fractures, 2: 249
Green and, 2: 169–170
in infants, 2: 169–170
of the metatarsals and phalanges, 1: 120
orthopaedic research and, 1: 193, 252, 256
pyogenic spinal, 3: 254
radical removal of diseased bone and, 1: 252
septic wounds in, 3: 301
Staphylococcus and, 2: 169

Streptococcus and, 2: 169
treatment of, 2: 169–170
osteonecrosis
acetabular, 2: 392–394
of the femoral head, 2: 328–329; 3: 434; 4: 156–157
osteoarticular allografts and, 3: 433
pinning of the contralateral hip and, 2: 380
osteosarcoma
adjuvant therapy and, 3: 432
allografts and, 3: 433
amputations and, 3: 136, 391, 432
chemotherapy and, 2: 422
hip disarticulation for, 1: 78
limb salvage surgery and, 3: 391, 432–433
of the proximal humerus, 2: 398
wide surgical margin and, 3: 433
osteotomies
Bernese periacetabular, 2: 391–392
Boston Concept, 2: 391–392
Chiari, 2: 345
club foot and, 2: 28–29, 36
Cotton, 4: 329
derotation, 2: 34
derotational humeral, 2: 419
femoral derotation for anteversion, 2: 33–34
hips and, 4: 171
innominate, 2: 345
for knee flexion contractures, 2: 117
knee stabilization and, 1: 279
kyphosis and, 3: 239–240
La Coeur's triple, 2: 390
lateral epicondyle, 3: 441
leg lengthening and, 2: 110
Meisenbach's procedure, 4: 188
metatarsal, 4: 188
paralytic flat foot deformities, 2: 210
periacetabular, 2: 389–394
Salter innominate, 2: 390–391
scoliosis treatment, 2: 342
subtrochanteric femur, 1: 68
subtrochanteric hip, 2: 293
total hip replacement and, 3: 221
trochanteric, 4: 133, 145
Van Nes rotational, 2: 345
VCR procedure, 2: 362
Wagner spherical, 2: 390–392
Osterman, A. Lee, 3: 431
Otis, James, 1: 13, 15
Ottemo, Anita, 4: 266
Otto Aufranc Award, 3: 224

Outline of Practical Anatomy, An (John Warren), 1: 88
Oxland, Thomas R., 4: 266*b*
Ozuna, Richard, 1: 230; 4: 193, 195*b*

P

Pace, James, 2: 379
Paget, James, 1: 81; 2: 172, 194; 3: 25
Paget Disease, 3: 441
Paine, R. S., 2: 172
Painter, Charles F. (1869–1947), 4: *44*
as AOA president, 2: 64; 4: 46–47
back pain research and, 3: 203
Beth Israel Hospital and, 4: 208*b*
bone and joint disorders, 3: 82
on Brackett, 3: 150, 161
Burrage Hospital and, 4: 226
Carney Hospital and, 2: 102; 4: 44–45
clinical congress meeting, 3: 116
death of, 4: 51
Diseases of the Bones and Joints, 2: 117; 3: 81; 4: 45
education and training, 4: 44
HMS appointment, 4: 44
hospital appointments, 4: 48
internal derangement of knee-joints case, 4: 48
Journal of Bone and Joint Surgery editor, 3: 161, 344; 4: 50
Massage, 3: 266
on medical education, 4: 49, 49*b*, *49*, 50
MGH and, 4: 45
on orthopaedic surgeon versus physician, 4: 47*b*
on physical therapy, 3: 266*b*
private medical practice, 2: 116
professional memberships, 4: 50*b*, 51
publications and research, 4: 44–46, 48, 50
RBBH and, 4: 25–26, 28, 31, 39*b*, 45, 56, 79, 406
as RBBH chief of orthopaedics, 4: 45–48, 79, 196*b*
rehabilitation of soldiers and, 4: 444
sacroiliac joint treatment, 3: 183
Tufts Medical School appointment, 4: 44–45, 48
World War I and, 4: 47
Paley multiplier method, 2: 194
Palmer Memorial Hospital, 2: 219, *219, 220*; 4: 275, *275*, 276

Index

Panagakos, Panos G., 4: 22, 116, 128, 193
Pancoast, Joseph, 1: 79
Panjabi, Manohar M., 4: 260–262
Papin, Edouard, 3: 233–234
Pappano, Laura, 1: 285
Pappas, Alex, 2: 285
Pappas, Arthur M. (1931–2016), 2: *286, 288*
    athletic injury clinic and, 2: 287
    "Biomechanics of Baseball Pitching," 2: *288*
    Boston Children's Hospital and, 2: 277, 285–287
    Boston Red Sox and, 2: 288
    Brigham and Women's Hospital and, 4: 193
    on combined residency program, 1: 192, 210
    community organizations and, 2: 289
    Crippled Children's Clinic and, 2: 287
    death of, 2: 289
    education and training, 2: 285
    famous patients of, 2: 288
    as interim orthopaedic surgeon-in-chief, 2: 285–286
    MGH/Children's Hospital residency, 2: 285
    military service, 2: 285
    as orthopaedic chair, 2: 15*b*, 371
    Pappas Rehabilitation Hospital, 2: 39
    PBBH and, 2: 285; 4: 22, 116, 128
    private medical practice and, 2: 313
    professional leadership positions, 2: 289, 289*b*
    publications of, 2: 285, *287*, 288, 368
    on residency program, 1: 208
    sports medicine and, 2: 287–288
    on sports medicine clinic, 2: 384
    University of Massachusetts and, 2: 286–288, 371
    Upper Extremity Injuries in the Athlete, 2: 288
Pappas, Athena, 2: 285
Pappas, Martha, 2: 289
Pappas Rehabilitation Hospital, 2: 39
paralysis. *See also* obstetrical paralysis; poliomyelitis
    brachial plexus, 2: 96
    Bradford frame and, 2: 30
    of the deltoid muscle, 2: 148, 230
    exercise treatment for, 3: 265
    foot and ankle treatment, 2: 150–151
    of the gluteus maximus, 2: 146
    hip abductor treatment, 2: 149–150
    nerve lesions and, 2: 120
    Pott's Disease and, 3: 148–149
    radial nerve, 3: 64
    Roosevelt and, 2: 71–78
    spinal cord injury, 3: 347
    spinal tuberculosis and, 2: 309
    treatment of spastic, 2: 36, 172, 196
Paraplegia Hospital (Ahmadabad, India), 3: 423
Paré, Ambrose, 1: 55; 3: 48
Parfouru-Porel, Germaine, 3: 369–370
Park Prewett Hospital, 4: 363
Parker, Isaac, 1: 45–46
Parker Hill, 4: 23*b*, *24*, 35
Parker Hill Hospital, 2: 358; 4: 327, *328*
Parkman, Francis, 1: 298, 307
Parkman, George (1790–1849), 1: *292*
    care of the mentally ill, 1: 293–295
    dental cast, 1: *308*
    disappearance of, 1: 298, 303–304
    education and training, 1: 292–293
    Harvard Medical School and, 1: 296
    home of, 1: *313*
    on John Collins Warren, 1: 296
    John Webster and, 1: 302–303
    money-lending and, 1: 297, 302–303
    murder of, 1: 291, 304–312, 315, *315*, 318; 3: 40
    philanthropy and, 1: 295–297
    remains found, 1: 304, *305*, 306, *306*, 307–308
Parkman, George F., 1: *313*, 314
Parkman, Samuel (businessman), 1: 292
Parkman, Samuel (surgeon), 1: 60, 62; 3: 15
Parkman Bandstand, 1: *313*, 314
Parks, Helen, 4: 389*b*
Parran, Thomas, Jr., 4: 467
Parsons, Langdon, 3: 301
Partners Department of Orthopaedic Surgery, 1: 181
Partners Healthcare, 3: 462; 4: 192–194
Partners Orthopaedics, 4: 284
Partridge, Oliver, 1: 13
Pasteur, Louis, 1: 82
Patel, Dinesh G. (1936–), 3: *421*, 424, *461*
    arthroscopic surgery and, 3: 422–423, 448
    Center of Healing Arts and, 3: 423
    Children's Hospital/MGH combined program and, 3: 422
    discoid medial meniscus tear case, 3: 422
    early life, 3: 421
    education and training, 3: 422
    HCORP and, 1: 230; 3: 423
    HMS appointment, 3: 422, 424
    honors and awards, 3: 424
    hospital appointments, 3: 422
    Massachusetts Board of Registration in Medicine and, 3: 423
    as MGH clinical faculty, 3: 464*b*
    as MGH surgeon, 3: 398*b*, 423
    Patient Care Assessment (PCA) Committee, 3: 423
    professional memberships and, 3: 422–423
    publications and research, 3: 424
    sports medicine and, 3: 388*t*, 396, 422, 448, 460*b*
Patel, Shaun, 4: 190*b*
patella. *See* knees
Pathophysiology of Orthopaedic Diseases (Mankin), 4: 226
Pathway Health Network, 4: 280
Patient Care Assessment (PCA) Committee, 3: 423
patient-reported outcomes (PRO), 4: 186
Patton, George S., 4: 478
pauciarticular arthritis, 2: 171, 350
Paul, Igor, 2: 407; 3: 326–328
Pauli, C., 3: 384
Payson, George, 3: 237
PBBH. *See* Peter Bent Brigham Hospital (PBBH)
Peabody, Francis, 2: 72; 3: 244; 4: 297
Peale, Rembrandt, 1: *23*
Pearson, Ruth Elizabeth, 1: 276
Pediatric Orthopaedic International Seminars program, 2: 304
Pediatric Orthopaedic Society (POS), 2: 304, 351
Pediatric Orthopaedic Study Group (POSG), 2: 351, 425
pediatric orthopaedics. *See also* Boston Children's Hospital (BCH)
    ACL reconstruction and, 2: 385–386
    Bradford Frame and, 2: 30

children's convalescence and, 2: 9
children's hospitals and, 2: 3–9
congenital dislocated hips (CDH) and, 2: 34
congenital kyphosis and, 2: 366
"Dark Ages" of, 2: 15
early medical literature on, 2: 7
flat feet treatment, 2: 107–108
Goldthwait and, 2: 101
Green and, 2: 168
hip disease and, 2: 108
Hresko and, 2: 365
infant and neonatal mortality, 2: 15
Karlin and, 2: 370
leg lengthening and, 2: 110
Legg and, 2: 101, 106–107
managing fractures, 2: 379
polio treatment, 2: 109–110
societies for, 2: 351
sports injuries and, 2: 287, 385–387
Tachdjian and, 2: 300–304
trauma and, 2: 365, 368, 385
tuberculosis of the spine and, 2: 11
valgus deformity treatment, 2: 209
Pediatric Orthopedic Deformities (Shapiro), 2: 403, *404*
Pediatric Orthopedic Society of North America (POSNA), 2: *346*, 347, 351, *351*, 363, *363*, 364, 403, 425
Pediatric Orthopedics (Tachdjian), 2: 188, 303, *303*
pedicle screws, 2: 343; 3: 420
Pedlow, Francis X, Jr. (1959–), 3: *424*
  anterior vertebral reconstruction with allograft research, 3: 426, *426*
  early life, 3: 424–425
  education and training, 3: 425
  HCORP and, 3: 426
  HMS appointment, 3: 426
  as MGH clinical faculty, 3: 464*b*
  as MGH surgeon, 3: 426
  open anterior lumbosacral fracture dislocation case, 3: 425
  professional memberships and, 3: 426
  publications and research, 3: 426
  spinal surgeries and, 3: 425–426, 460*b*
Pedlow, Francis X, Sr., 3: 424
Pedlow, Marie T. Baranello, 3: 424
Pedrick, Katherine F., 3: 154

Peking Union Medical College, 3: 365
Pellicci, Paul, 4: 134–135
Peltier, L. F., 1: 106
Pemperton, Ralph, 4: 32
Peninsular Base Station (PBS), 4: 481–482
Pennsylvania Hospital, 1: 183
periacetabular osteotomy, 2: 389–391
Perkins, Leroy, 2: 159–160
Perkins Institution and the Massachusetts School for the Blind, 1: 273
Perlmutter, Gary S., 1: 166–167; 3: 415, 460*b*, 464*b*
Perry, Jacqueline, 3: 248
Pershing, John J., 3: 168
Person, Eleanor, 3: 281
Perthes, George, 2: 103, 105; 3: 165
Perthes disease. *See* Legg-Calvé-Perthes disease
Peter Bent Brigham Hospital Corporation, 4: 2–3
Peter Bent Brigham Hospital (PBBH), 4: *2, 7, 8, 9, 11, 15, 117*
  Administrative Building, 4: *115, 191*
  advancement of medicine and, 4: 5
  affiliation with RBBH, 4: 34, 36, 39
  annual reports, 4: 6, 16, 18
  Banks on, 4: 73*b*–74*b*
  Base Hospital No. 5 and, 4: 420*t*
  blood bank, 4: 107
  board of overseers, 4: 132
  bone and joint cases, 4: *16*
  Boston Children's Hospital and, 4: 10, 14
  Brigham Anesthesia Associates, 4: 22
  cerebral palsy cases, 2: 172
  Clinical Research Center floor plan, 4: *21*
  construction of, 4: 4, *4*, 5
  faculty group practice, 4: 13, 21–22
  faculty model at, 1: 176
  50th anniversary, 4: 20–21, 21*b*
  founding of, 2: 42; 4: 2–3
  fracture treatment and, 4: 18–19, 22, 108
  Francis Street Lobby, 4: *119*
  general surgery service at, 4: 8–10, 14, 16
  grand rounds and, 4: 118
  growth of, 4: 20, 22
  history of, 4: 1

  HMS and, 4: 1–4, 12, *12*, 13–14
  Industrial Accident Clinic, 4: 21–22
  industrial accidents and, 4: 19, 21
  internships at, 1: 189, 196
  leadership of, 4: 4–5, 9–11, 14–19, 22, 99, 127
  opening of, 4: *6*
  orthopaedic service chiefs at, 4: 43
  orthopaedic surgeons at, 4: 116–117
  orthopaedic surgery at, 1: 171; 4: 8, 11, 16–18, 22, 115–116
  orthopaedics as specialty at, 4: 1, 18
  orthopaedics diagnoses at, 4: 6–8
  orthopaedics residencies, 1: 199, 204, 207; 4: 19
  outpatient services at, 1: 173; 4: 5–6, 14, 20, 22
  patient volume at, 4: 124*t*, 129
  Pavilion C (Ward I), 4: *8*
  Pavilion F, 4: *7*
  Pavilion Wards, 4: *115*
  plans for, 4: *7*
  professors of surgery at, 1: 174
  report of bone diseases, 4: 13, 13*t*
  research program at, 4: 75*b*
  Spanish Flu at, 4: *11*
  staffing of, 4: 5, 9, 18–19, 21–22, 128–129, 161–163
  surgeon-scholars at, 4: 43, 79
  surgery specialization at, 4: 10–12, 15–16, 18–20
  surgical research laboratory, 4: 12, *12*
  surgical residencies, 1: 90
  teaching clinics at, 1: 155, 157–158, 194; 4: 14
  transition to Brigham and Women's Hospital, 4: 42, 69, 113–114, 116, 116*b*, 117–119, 121, 127, 132
  trust for, 4: 1, 3
  World War I and, 4: 9–10, 79
  World War II and, 4: 17–18
  Zander Room at, 4: 14
Peter Bent Brigham Hospital Surgical Associates, 4: 21–22
Peters, Jessica, 3: 328
Petersdorf, Robert G., 4: 121
Peterson, L., 3: 210
Petit Lycée de Talence, 4: *429, 430,* 432
Pfahler, George E., 3: 142
Pharmacopoeia of the United States, 1: 300
Phelps, A. M., 2: 99
Phelps, Abel, 4: 463
Phelps, Winthrop M., 1: 193; 2: 294

Phemister, D. B., 2: 170–171, *192*
Phillips, William, 1: 41; 3: 5, 75
Phillips House (MGH), 1: 86, 204; 3: *72, 73,* 75
phocomelia, 2: 334
Phoenix Mutual Insurance Company, 2: 267
phrenicectomy, 4: 215
physical therapy
    athletic training and, 1: 258, 266; 3: 348
    DeLorme table and, 3: 284
    early 20th century status of, 3: 266, 266*b*
    Elgin table, 3: 284, *287*
    knee flexion contracture and, 3: 375
    Legg and, 2: 107
    massage and, 1: 100; 3: 266, 297
    medical schools and, 4: 396–397
    for paralyzed children, 2: 61, 107
    RBBH patient in, 4: *28, 29*
    rehabilitation equipment for, 2: 107
    Roosevelt and, 2: 74
    sports medicine and, 2: 287
    tenotomy and, 1: 100
    Zander's medico-mechanical equipment, 3: 71, *71*
Physical Therapy in Infantile Paralysis (Legg and Merrill), 2: 107
physicians
    bleeding and, 1: 9
    board certification of, 4: 324, 377
    18th century demand for, 1: 7–8
    examinations for, 1: 15, 21, 29
    Jewish, 1: 158; 4: 199–200, 202
    licensing of, 1: 184, 190
    medical degrees and, 1: 6–7, 26–28
    standards for, 1: 26
    surgical training and, 1: 184
Physicians' Art Society of Boston, 4: 329–330
Pierce, Donald S. (1930–), 3: *461*
    Amputees and Their Prostheses, 3: 320
    Cervical Spine Research Society president, 3: 321
    early life, 3: 320
    education and training, 3: 320
    electromyogram use, 3: 320
    familial bilateral carpal tunnel syndrome case, 3: 321
    Halo Vest, 3: 321
    HMS appointment, 3: 320
    marriage and, 3: 321
    as MGH clinical faculty, 3: 464*b*
    as MGH surgeon, 3: 248, 320, 398*b*
    orthopaedics treatment tools and, 3: 321
    on pressure sores management, 3: 321
    publications and research, 3: 320–321, 355
    rehabilitation and, 3: 388*t*, 459, 461
    spine surgery and, 3: 460*b*
    Total Care of Spinal Cord Injuries, The, 3: 321
Pierce, F. Richard, 1: 264
Pierce, Janet, 3: 321
Pierce, R. Wendell, 1: 284; 3: 299
Pierce, Wallace L., 4: 39*b*
Pierce Collar, 3: 321
Pierce Fusion, 3: 321
Pierce Graft, 3: 321
Pierson, Abel Lawrence, 1: 60, 62
Pilcher, Lewis S., 4: 318
Pinel, Philippe, 1: 293–294
Pinkney, Carole, 3: 382
Pio Istituto Rachitici, 2: 36
Pittsburgh Orthopaedic Journal, 1: 232
plantar fasciitis, 3: 437–438
plantar fasciotomy, 2: 24
Plaster-of-Paris Technique in the Treatment of Fractures (Quigley), 1: 277
plastic surgery
    development of, 1: 76
    introduction to the U.S., 1: 71–72, 77
    orthopaedics curriculum and, 1: 150, 218
Plath, Sylvia, 2: 272
Platt, Sir Harry, 1: 114; 3: 369; 4: 464
Ploetz, J. E., 3: 440
pneumonia, 1: 74; 2: 4, 306
Poehling, Gary G., 2: 279
Polavarapu, H. V., 1: 186
poliomyelitis
    Berlin epidemic of, 2: 260, 264
    Boston epidemic of, 2: 213, 314–315
    calcaneus deformity, 2: 189–190
    children's hospitals and, 3: 307
    circulatory changes in, 2: 316
    electricity and, 2: 62
    epidemics of, 1: 191; 2: 61
    ganglionectomy in, 3: 332
    Green and, 2: 188–191
    Grice and, 2: 208
    Harrington rods, 2: 316, *317*
    heavy-resistance exercise and, 3: 284–285
    hip contracture treatment, 2: 294, 295*b*
    hot pack treatment, 2: 264
    importance of rest in, 2: 63, *63*
    intraspinal serum, 2: 72
    iron lung and, 2: 78, *190*, 191, 260, 264, 314
    Legg and, 2: 107, 109
    Lovett and, 2: 61–63, *63*, 70–72, 74–75, 77, 147–148
    massage treatment for, 2: 62, 73
    moist heat treatment for, 2: 264
    muscle training for, 2: 62–63, 78
    muscle transfers, 2: 154
    nonstandard treatments and, 2: 77
    Ober and, 2: 147–148
    orthopaedic treatment for, 2: 78
    paralysis of the serratus anterior, 2: 154–155
    paralytic flat foot deformities, 2: 210–212
    patient evaluation, 2: 315
    patient reaction to, 2: 261*b*–263*b*
    prevention of contractures, 2: 78
    research in, 3: 209
    rocking beds, 2: 314, *315*
    Roosevelt and, 2: 71–78
    second attacks of, 1: 276
    shoulder arthrodesis, 2: 154
    spinal taps and, 2: 72, 78
    spring muscle test, 2: 70, *70*, 71
    study of, 2: 61–62
    tendon transfers and, 2: 96, 108, *108*, 109, 147–149; 3: 332–333
    treatment of, 2: 61–63, 71–79, 109–110, 188–191
    Trott and, 2: 314, *314*, 315
    unequal limb length and, 3: 331–332
    vaccine development, 2: 189, 191, 264, 315
    Vermont epidemic of, 2: 61–62, 71
Polivy, Kenneth, 3: 254
Pongor, Paul, 4: 279
Pool, Eugene H., 3: 338
Pope, Malcolm, 2: 371
Porter, C. A., 3: 313
Porter, Charles A., 3: 116
Porter, G. A., 1: 174
Porter, John L., 2: 78; 3: 157; 4: 406, 464
Porter, W. T., 4: 216
Poss, Anita, 4: 174
Poss, Robert (1936–), 4: *169*
    ABOS board and, 4: 173

Ames Test and, 4: 171
Brigham and Women's Hospital and, 4: 163, 172, 193, 195*b*
Brigham Orthopaedic Foundation (BOF) and, 4: 172
Brigham Orthopedic Associates (BOA) and, 4: 123, 172
as BWH orthopaedics chief, 4: 143, 193, 196*b*
Children's Hospital/MGH combined program and, 4: 169
Deputy Editor for Electronic Media at *JBJS*, 4: 173–174
education and training, 4: 169
hip arthritis research, 4: 170
hip osteotomy research, 2: 390; 4: 171
HMS appointment, 4: 171–172
on Hylamer acetabular liner complications, 4: *171*, 172
marriage and family, 4: 174
MIT postdoctoral biology fellowship, 4: 169–170
PBBH and, 4: 163
private medical practice, 4: 169
professional memberships, 4: 174
publications and research, 4: 169–170, *170*, 171–172, 174
RBBH and, 4: 132, 134, 169–171
on total hip arthroplasty, 3: 223; 4: 134, 170–172, 174
US Navy and, 4: 169
Post, Abner, 4: 307
posterior cruciate ligament (PCL)
avulsion of, 2: 386
biomechanical effects of injury and repair, 3: 448
pediatric orthopaedics and, 2: 381
retention in total knee replacement, 4: 130, 138–139, 147, 180–181
robotics-assisted research, 3: 450
posterior interosseous syndrome, 4: 165–166
posterior segment fixator (PSF), 3: 420
posture. *See also* body mechanics
body types and, 4: 235, *236*
Bradford on, 2: 36
chart of normal and abnormal, 4: *84*, *234*
Chelsea Survey of, 4: 234–235
children and, 2: 36; 3: 83
contracted iliotibial band and, 2: 152
Goldthwait and, 3: 80–81, 83, 85–91; 4: 53

Harvard study in, 4: 84, *84*, 85–86, 234, *234*
high-heeled shoes and, 2: 317
impact on military draft, 4: 233
medical conflict and, 3: 83
Ober operation and, 2: 153
research in, 4: 233–235, *235*
school children and, 4: 233–234, *234*, 235, *236*
scoliosis and, 1: 109
standards for, 4: *236*
Swaim on, 4: 52–54
types of, 4: 85–86
Potter, Constance, 4: 69
Potter, Theodore A. (1912–1995), 4: *67*
arthritis treatment, 4: 67
Boston University appointment, 4: 67
Children's Hospital/MGH combined program and, 4: 68
death of, 4: 69
education and training, 4: 67
HMS appointment, 4: 69
knee arthroplasty and, 4: 64, *65*, 68–69, 70*b*–71*b*
marriage and family, 4: 69
on McKeever and MacIntosh prostheses, 4: 189
nylon arthroplasty in arthritic knees, 4: 65–66, 69
orthopaedic research and, 4: 38
private medical practice, 4: 67
professional memberships, 4: 69
publications and research, 4: 67, *68*, 69, 96
RBBH and, 4: 35, 37–38, 67–68, 89, 93, 116*b*, 187
as RBBH chief of orthopaedics, 4: 40, 41*b*, 63, 66–69, 79, 102, 196*b*
Tufts appointment, 4: 69
Pott's Disease, 1: xxiii, 97, *97*, 105, 108–109; 2: 25, *31*, 247; 3: 148, *149*, 154, 155
Pott's fracture, 4: *317*, 318
Prabhakar, M. M., 3: 423
Practical Biomechanics for the Orthopedic Surgeon (Radin et al.), 3: 328
PRE (Progressive Resistance Exercise) (DeLorme and Watkins), 3: *286*
Presbyterian Hospital, 2: 74–75
Prescott, William, 1: 18
press-fit condylar knee (PFC), 4: 180, 180*t*
pressure correction apparatus (Hoffa-Schede), 3: *151*, *152*
pressure sores, 3: 321
Preston, Thomas, 1: 14

Price, Mark, 4: 190*b*
Price, Mark D., 3: 463*b*
Priestley, Joseph, 1: 56
Principles of Orthopedic Surgery for Nurses, The (Sever), 2: 92, *93*
Principles of Orthopedic Surgery (Sever), 2: 92, *93*
Pristina Hospital (Kosovo), 3: 416–417
Pritchett, Henry S., 1: 147
Problem Back Clinic (MGH), 3: 254
"Progress in Orthopaedic Surgery" series, 2: 43, 297
progressive resistance exercises, 3: 285–286
Project HOPE, 3: 417, *417*
prospective payment system (PPS), 3: 397
Prosperi, Lucia, 1: *59*
Prosperi, Warren, 1: *59*
Prosser, W.C.H., 4: 482*b*
prostheses
all-plastic tibial, 4: 148
Austin Moore, 3: 213, 241, 354*b*
biomechanical aspects of hip, 2: 407
bone ingrowth, 3: 220–223
Brigham and Women's Hospital and, 4: 122
Buchholz shoulder, 2: 423
capitellocondylar total elbow, 4: 145, *145*, 146–147
Cohen and patents for, 2: 237
distal humerus, 2: 250
Duocondylar, 4: 178
duopatellar, 4: 130, 180*t*
electromyographic (EMG) signals and, 2: 326
femoral replacement, 4: 69
femoral stem, 3: *293*
hinged elbow, 4: 147
hip replacement, 2: 407
internal, 2: 423
Judet hip, 3: *293*
Kinematic knee, 4: 138–139, 147, 149–150
knee arthroplasty and, 3: 292
LTI Digital™ Arm Systems for Adults, 2: 326
MacIntosh, 4: 69, 71*b*, 129, 188
Marmor modular design, 4: 130
McKeever, 4: 40, 69, 70*b*–71*b*, 129–130, 177, 188–189
metal and polyethylene, 4: 148
metallic, 3: 433
myoelectric, 2: 326
nonconstrained total elbow, 4: 145
non-hinged metal–polyethylene, 4: 145–146

PFC unicompartmental knee, 4: 177
press-fit condylar knee (PFC), 4: 180, 180t
suction socket, 1: 273
temporary, 3: 374
total condylar, 4: 130
total knee, 4: 137
unicompartmental, 4: 176, 178
used in knee arthroplasty, 4: 179t
Prosthetic Research and Development Unit (Ontario Crippled Children's Center), 2: 335
Province House, 3: 6–7, 9, *9*
psoas abscesses, 2: 53–54; 4: 225
psoriatic arthritis, 4: 99
Ptasznik, Ronnie, 3: 437
public health, 2: 61, 107, 425
Pugh, J., 3: 327
pulmonary embolism (PE), 3: 196, 218, 362
pulmonary function
    anterior and posterior procedures, 2: 360
    corrective casts and, 2: 265
    Milwaukee Brace and, 2: 265–266
    scoliosis and, 2: 343
    spine fusion and, 2: 265
    thromboembolism pathophysiology, 1: 82
pulmonary tuberculosis, 1: 56; 2: 9, 16; 3: 25, 128
Pulvertaft, Guy, 3: 427; 4: 95
Putnam, George, 1: 312–313, 317
Putnam, Israel, 1: 18
Putnam, James Jackson, 2: 20
Putti, Vittorio, 2: 80; 3: 203; 4: 14, 65
pyloric stenosis, 3: 49–50

Q

Quain, Jones, 2: 242
Quain's Anatomy (Quain et al.), 2: 242
Queen Victoria Hospital, 2: *421*, 422
quiet necrosis, 2: 194
Quigley, Daniel Thomas, 1: 275
Quigley, Ruth Elizabeth Pearson, 1: 276, 282
Quigley, Thomas B. (1908–1982), 1: *275*, *281*; 4: *342*
    on acromioclavicular joint dislocation in football, 1: 268
    AMA Committee on the Medical Aspects of Sports, 1: 280
    Athlete's Bill of Rights and, 1: 280–281
    athletic injury clinic and, 2: 287
    Boston City Hospital and, 4: 297
    on Dr. Nichols, 1: 257
    education and training, 1: 276
    5th General Hospital and, 4: 484
    Harvard athletics surgeon, 1: 276–279
    Harvard University Health Service and, 1: 277
    as HMS professor, 1: 277
    legacy of, 1: 282–283
    PBBH and, 1: 204, 276–277; 2: 279; 4: 18–21, 116
    pes anserinus transplant, 1: 279
    Plaster-of-Paris Technique in the Treatment of Fractures, 1: 277
    publications of, 1: 268, 276–282; 2: 220
    sports medicine and, 1: 277–283
    US General Hospital No. 5 and, 4: 485
    WWII active duty and, 1: 270, 277; 4: 17
Quinby, William, 4: 11
Quincy, Josiah, 1: 14
Quincy City Hospital, 2: 256

R

Rabkin, Mitchell, 4: 255, 281
radiation synovectomy, 4: 64, 136
Radin, Crete Boord, 3: 328
Radin, Eric L. (1934–2020), 3: *322*, *323*, *328*
    Beth Israel Hospital and, 3: 325
    biomechanics research, 3: 326–328
    Boston Children's Hospital and, 3: 325
    Children's Hospital/MGH combined program and, 3: 322
    death of, 3: 328
    early life, 3: 322
    education and training, 3: 322
    fracture research and, 3: 322–324
    on Glimcher, 2: 326
    on Green, 2: 177
    Henry Ford Hospital and, 3: 328
    HMS appointment, 3: 325, 327
    joint lubrication research, 3: 324–325, *325*, *326*, *326*, 327
    marriages and family, 3: 328
    MIT appointment, 3: 325
    Mount Auburn Hospital and, 3: 327
    neuritis with infectious mononucleosis case, 3: 324–325
    Practical Biomechanics for the Orthopedic Surgeon, 3: 328
    publications and research, 2: 396, *396*, *397*, 406; 3: 322–326, *326*, 327–328
    subchondral bone research, 3: 326–327, *327*
    Tufts Medical School and, 3: 328
    University of Michigan appointment, 3: 328
    US Air Force Hospital and, 3: 323
    West Virginia University School of Medicine and, 3: 328
Radin, Tova, 3: 328
radiography
    diagnostic value of, 2: 56
    growth calculation and, 2: 194
    Harvard Athletic Association and, 1: 258
    in hip disease, 2: 54
    leg-length discrepancy and, 3: 299
    scoliosis treatment, 2: 366
radiology. *See also* roentgenograms
    Boston Children's Hospital and, 2: 16, *16*, 17, 17t
    HMS and, 2: 16
    Osgood and, 2: 114–116
Radius Management Services, 4: 212
Radius Specialty Hospital, 4: 212
Ragaswamy, Leela, 2: 439b
Ralph K. Ghormley Traveling Scholarship, 3: 290
Ramappa, Arun, 4: 287
Ranawat, Chit, 4: 130, 134
Rancho Los Amigos, 4: 129, 151, *151*
Rand, Frank, 4: 279–280
Rand, Isaacs, 1: 25
Rand, Jessie Sophia, 3: 79
Ranvier, Louis Antoine, 1: 82; 3: 142
Rappleye, W. C., 1: 189
Ratshesky, Abraham, 3: 134–135
Ray, Robert D., 1: 162
RBBH. *See* Robert Breck Brigham Hospital (RBBH)
Ready, John, 1: 167
Ready, John E., 4: 193, 195b
Rechtine, G. R., 3: 420
Reconstruction Base Hospital No. 1 (Parker Hill, Boston), 4: *328*, *445*, *446*. *See also* US General Hospital No. 10
    Benevolent Order of Elks funding for, 4: 447
    development of, 4: 444–445
    physiotherapy at, 4: *447*
    RBBH and, 4: 447–448

rehabilitation goals and,
  4: 446–447
Record, Emily, 3: 330
Record, Eugene E. (ca.1910–2004),
  3: *329*
  as AAOS fellow, 2: 215
  amputation research, 3: 330
  ankle arthrodesis case, 3: 330
  Boston Children's Hospital and,
    2: 299; 3: 329
  Children's Hospital/MGH combined program and, 3: 329
  death of, 3: 330
  early life, 3: 329
  education and training, 3: 329
  Lower Extremity Amputations for Arterial Insufficiency, 1: 90;
    3: 330
  Marlborough Medical Associates and, 2: 269
  marriage and family, 3: 330
  as MGH surgeon, 1: 203;
    3: 329
  New England Peabody Home for Crippled Children and, 3: 329
  private medical practice, 2: 146;
    3: 329
  publications and research, 3: 330
  US Army Reserve and, 3: 329
Record, Eugene E., Jr., 3: 329
Redfern, Peter, 1: xxii
Reed, John, 1: 307; 3: 347
reflex sympathetic dystrophy, 2: 68.
  See also chronic regional pain syndrome (CRPS)
Registry of Bone Sarcoma,
  3: 136–142
Rehabilitation Engineering and Assistive Technology Society of North America (RESNA), 2: 408, *408*
Rehabilitation Engineering Research Center, 2: 406
Reid, Bill, 1: 252–253, 255
Reidy, Alice Sherburne, 3: 334
Reidy, John A. (1910–1987)
  early life, 3: 331
  education and training, 3: 331
  effects of irradiation on epiphyseal growth, 3: 331
  Faulkner Hospital and, 3: 331
  fracture research and, 3: 334
  ganglionectomy in polio patient case, 3: 332
  as honorary orthopaedic surgeon,
    3: 398*b*
  marriage and family, 3: 334
  as MGH surgeon, 3: 74, 331
  Newton-Wellesley Hospital and,
    3: 331
  polio research, 3: 331–333

professional memberships and,
  3: 334
publications and research,
  3: 209, 331–334
RBBH and, 4: 35, 38, 89, 93
Slipped Capital Femoral Epiphysis,
  3: 294, 333
slipped capital femoral epiphysis research, 3: 331, 333–334;
  4: 237–238
on tendon transfers in lower extremities, 3: 332–333, *333*
Reilly, Donald, 4: 286
Reinertsen, James L., 4: 283
Reitman, Charles A., 4: 272*b*
Relton, J. E. S., 2: 334–335, *335*
Relton-Hall frame, 2: 334, *335*
Remarks on the Operation for the Cure of Club Feet with Cases (Brown), 1: 100
Remembrances (Coll Warren), 1: 83
Report of Cases in the Orthopedic Infirmary of the City of Boston (J.B. Brown), 1: *120*
Reports of Cases Treated at the Boston Orthopedic Institution (Brown and Brown), 1: *120*
Residency Review Committee (RRC), 1: 211
RESNA. *See* Rehabilitation Engineering and Assistive Technology Society of North America (RESNA)
Resurrectionists (Browne), 1: *21*
Reverdin, Jaques-Louis, 4: 216
Revere, Anne, 2: 272
Revere, John, 1: 293
Revere, Paul, 1: 8, 13–17, 19–20,
  22, 28, *28*; 2: 272
Reynolds, Edward, 3: 42
Reynolds, Fred, 4: 125
Reynolds, Fred C., 1: 162
rheumatic fever, 2: 171
Rheumatism Foundation Hospital,
  4: 96
rheumatoid arthritis
  body mechanics and, 4: 82–83
  boutonniere deformities of the hand, 4: 98
  children and, 2: 164, 171, 350
  foot surgery and, 4: 188, *188*
  gene therapy and, 2: 82
  genetics in, 4: 169
  of the hand, 4: 96–98, *98*
  hindfoot pain, 4: 188, *189*
  knee arthroplasty and,
    4: 70*b*–71*b*
  MacIntosh prothesis and, 4: 188
  McKeever prothesis and,
    4: 188–189

metacarpophalangeal arthroplasty,
  4: 97
mold arthroplasty and, 3: 239
nylon arthroplasty in, 4: *65*
opera-glass hand deformity, 4: 99
radiation synovectomy and,
  4: 136
release of contractures in arthroplasty, 4: 166
swan neck deformity, 4: 98
synovectomy of the knee in,
  4: 102
thumb deformities, 4: 97
total hip replacement and, 4: 134
total knee replacement and,
  4: 181
treatment for, 4: 97, 138
upper extremities and, 2: 137
wrist joint damage in, 4: 166–167, *168*
rheumatoid synovitis, 4: 166
rheumatology, 2: 321
Rhinelander, Frederic W., Jr. (1906–1990), 3: *335*
  Boston Children's Hospital and,
    3: 335
  burn care and, 3: 336
  Case Western Reserve University School of Medicine and,
    3: 337
  death of, 3: 337
  early life, 3: 335
  education and training, 3: 335
  HMS appointment, 3: 335
  honors and awards, 3: 337, 337*b*
  Letterman Army Hospital and,
    3: 336
  marriage and family, 3: 337
  as MGH surgeon, 3: 74, 335
  private medical practice, 3: 336
  publications and research,
    3: 335–336, *336*, 337
  Shriners Hospital for Children and, 3: 335
  University of Arkansas College of Medicine and, 3: 337
  University of California Hospital and, 3: 336–337
  US Army and, 3: 336
  US Army Legion of Merit,
    3: *337*
Rhinelander, Julie, 3: 337
Rhinelander, Philip Mercer, 3: 335
Rhode Island Hospital, 3: 401
Rhodes, Jonathan, 1: 90
Richard J. Smith Lecture, 3: 431
Richards, Thomas K. (1892–1965)
  Boston City Hospital and, 1: 258
  as football team physician,
    1: 258–262

as Harvard athletics surgeon, 1: 258, 262; 4: 303
Harvard Fifth Surgical Service and, 4: 303
on physician's role, 1: 259–262
scientific studies, 1: 262
as team physician for the Boston Red Sox, 1: 258
Richardson, Frank, 1: 255
Richardson, Lars C., 4: 287
Richardson, Mary R., 3: 75
Richardson, Maurice H., 3: 18, 94; 4: 274–275
Richardson, William, 4: 3
rickets, 1: 129; 2: 36, 114; 3: 83, 388
Riley, Donald, 1: 225; 4: 193
Riley, Maureen, 2: 414
Ring, David, 1: 167; 3: 410, 463
Riseborough, Bruce, 2: 400
Riseborough, Edward J. (1925–1985), 2: *395*
Boston Children's Hospital and, 2: 286, 399; 4: 127
Brigham and Women's Hospital and, 4: 163, 193
congenital kyphosis case, 2: 399–400
death of, 2: 400
distal femoral physeal fractures research, 2: 400
education and training, 2: 395
fat embolism syndrome research, 2: 397, *397*, 398
HMS appointment, 2: 395, 399
intercondylar fractures of the humerus research, 2: 397, *397*
marriage and family, 2: 400
MGH and, 2: 395; 4: 127
orthopaedics appointments, 2: 399
orthopaedics education and, 2: 398–399
PBBH and, 4: 163
professional memberships, 2: 400
publications and research, 2: 385, 396, *396*, 397, 399–400, *400*; 3: 322–323
rugby and, 2: 385, 400
Scoliosis and Other Deformities of the Axial Skeleton, 2: 398, *398*
scoliosis research, 2: 395–396, 399–400, *400*; 4: 127
trauma research, 2: 396, *396*, 397, 399
Riseborough, Jennifer, 2: 400
Risser, Joseph, 2: 335
Risser cast, 2: 178
RMS *Aurania*, 4: 431

Robbins, Anne Smith, 1: 123–125; 2: 114
Robbins, Chandler, 2: 5
Robert Breck Brigham Hospital Corporation, 4: 23–24, 25*b*
Robert Breck Brigham Hospital for Incurables, 4: 22, 23*b*, 30, 36
Robert Breck Brigham Hospital (RBBH), 4: *26, 28, 31, 35, 37, 40, 42*
affiliation with PBBH, 4: 34, 36, 39
annual reports, 4: *37*
arthritis clinic and, 3: 371; 4: 36
arthroplasties at, 4: 64
board of overseers, 4: 132
Chief of Orthopedic Service report, 4: 41*b*
chronic disease treatment at, 4: 23*b*, 25*b*, 27–28, 30, 30*b*, 32, 32*b*, 33, 36, 39*b*, 46
as Clinical Research Center, 4: 38, 40
clinical teaching at, 4: 32–33
Emergency Campaign speech, 4: 32, 32*b*
financial difficulties, 4: 25–26, 28–29, 31–32, 34, 35*b*, 37, 42
founding of, 4: 22–24
Goldthwait and, 3: 81, 84, 91–92; 4: 24–25, 25*b*, 26–28, 31, 36–38, 39*b*
Goldthwait Research Fund, 4: 27
grand rounds and, 4: 118
growth in patient volume, 4: 124*t*
history of, 4: 1
HMS students and, 4: 30, 69
laboratory at, 4: *35*
lawsuit on hospital mission, 4: 29–30, 30*b*
leadership of, 4: 31–33, 35–36, 38, 39*b*, 40, 41*b*, 42, 99, 127
Lloyd T. Brown and, 3: 257; 4: 25, 30–34, 36
military reconstruction hospital and, 4: 443–444
occupational therapy department, 4: 28, *29*
orthopaedic advancements at, 4: 40
orthopaedic research and, 4: 38, 41*b*
orthopaedic service chiefs at, 4: 43
orthopaedic surgery at, 1: 171; 4: 28, 31, 40, 41*b*, 115
orthopaedics and arthritis at, 4: 26–28, 43
orthopaedics as specialty at, 4: 1

orthopaedics instruction at, 1: 157; 4: 41*b*, 68
orthopaedics residencies, 1: 207–208; 4: 30, 40, 131
patient conditions and outcomes, 4: 29*t*
patient outcomes, 4: 31*t*
physical therapy and, 4: 28, 29
professorship in orthopedic surgery, 4: 114
Reconstruction Base Hospital No. 1 and, 4: 445, 447–448
rehabilitation service at, 4: 37, *38*
research at, 4: 33, 42, 117, 132
residencies at, 4: 34–35, 39–40, 42
rheumatic disease treatment, 4: 47, 136, 188
as specialty arthritis hospital, 4: 122–123
staffing of, 4: 25, 28, 32, *34*, 35–38, 45, 68, 131–132
statistics, 1945, 4: 34*t*
surgeon-scholars at, 4: 43, 79
surgery at, 4: *132*
surgical caseloads at, 4: 131, 131*t*, 132
total knee arthroplasty and, 4: 129–130, 131*t*
transition to Brigham and Women's Hospital, 4: 42, 69, 113–114, 116, 116*b*, 117–119, 121, 127, 132
World War I and, 4: 25–26, 79
World War II and, 4: 33
Robert Brigham Multipurpose Arthritis and Musculoskeletal Disease Center, 4: 184
Robert C. Hinckley and the Recreation of The First Operation Under Ether (Wolfe), 1: 59
Robert Jones and Agnes Hunt Orthopaedic Hospital, 3: 426
Robert Jones Orthopaedic Society, 2: 132
Robert Leffert Memorial Fund, 3: 415
Robert Salter Award, 2: 415
Robert W. Lovett Memorial Unit for the Study of Crippling Diseases, 2: 82
Robert W. Lovett Professorship, 2: 166; 4: 195*b*
Roberts, Ada Mead, 3: 338
Roberts, Elizabeth Converse, 3: 339
Roberts, Melita Josephine, 2: 143
Roberts, Odin, 3: 338
Roberts, Sumner N. (1898–1939), 3: *338*

cervical spine fracture research, 3: 340–341, *341*
Children's Hospital/MGH combined program and, 3: 338
congenital absence of the odontoid process case, 3: 340
death of, 3: 342
early life, 3: 338
education and training, 3: 338
fracture research and, 3: 339–341, *342*
HMS appointment, 2: 223; 3: 338–339; 4: 61
marriage and family, 3: 339
Massachusetts Eye and Ear Infirmary and, 3: 339
as MGH surgeon, 3: 187, 270, 339
private medical practice, 3: 338
professional memberships and, 3: 341–342
publications and research, 3: 339–341; 4: 63
RBBH and, 3: 339; 4: 31, 60
World War I and, 3: 338
Robinson, James, 1: 248
Robinson, Marie L., 2: 111–112
Robson, A. W. Mayo, 2: 91
Rockefeller Foundation, 1: 147
Rockefeller Institute, 2: 72
rocking beds, 2: *315*
Rocky Mountain Trauma Society, 3: 311
Rodriguez, Edward, 3: 410
Rodriquez, Ken, 4: 287
Roentgen Diagnosis of the Extremities and Spine (Ferguson), 4: 110
Roentgen Method in Pediatrics, The (Rotch), 2: 170
roentgenograms. *See also* x-rays
  arthritis and, 4: 64, *64*
  in curriculum, 1: 161
  diagnosis and, 2: 155; 3: 99
  discovery of, 2: 24, 54; 3: 57, 96
  MGH and, 3: 20–21
  Osgood and Dodd on, 2: 116
  slipped capital femoral epiphysis and, 4: 238
  total knee arthroplasty-scoring system, 4: 150
ROFEH International, 2: 363, *363*
Rogers, Carolyn, 1: 239
Rogers, Elizabeth Grace, 2: 258
Rogers, Emily, 3: 350
Rogers, Emily Ross, 4: 230
Rogers, Fred A., 1: 180
Rogers, Horatio, 4: 475
Rogers, Margaret, 4: 371

Rogers, Mark H. (1877–1941), 4: *224*
  American Journal of Orthopedic Surgery editor, 4: 226
  AOA resolution on orthopaedics, 4: 227
  as Beth Israel chief of orthopaedics, 4: 220, 223, 228–230, 289*b*
  Beth Israel Hospital and, 4: 208*b*
  as Boston and Maine Railroad orthopaedic surgeon, 4: 225
  Boston City Hospital and, 4: 229–230, 328
  Burrage Hospital and, 4: 226
  Clinics for Crippled Children and, 2: 230
  education and training, 4: 224
  Fort Riley base hospital and, 4: 452–453
  HMS appointment, 4: 226, 226*b*
  legacy of, 4: 230
  marriage and family, 4: 230
  Massachusetts Regional Fracture Committee, 3: 64
  MGH orthopaedics and, 1: 189; 3: 266, 268; 4: 224, 226, 226*b*
  as MGH orthopaedics chief, 3: 11*b*, 173, 227
  New England Deaconess Hospital and, 4: 225
  New England Regional Committee on Fractures, 4: 341
  orthopaedics education and, 4: 228–230
  professional memberships and roles, 4: 229*b*
  psoas abscess in the lumbar retroperitoneal lymph glands case, 4: 225
  publications and research, 4: 224–225, *225*, 226, 228–229, 242
  RBBH and, 4: 406
  rehabilitation of soldiers and, 4: 444
  Trumbull Hospital and, 4: 225
  tuberculosis research and, 4: 224–226
  Tufts appointment, 4: 226, 226*b*
  US Army Medical Corps and, 4: 226–227
Rogers, Orville F., Jr., 2: 119; 4: 389*b*
Rogers, Oscar H., 3: 343
Rogers, W. B., 3: 420
Rogers, William A. (1892–1975), 3: *343*

closed reduction of lumbar spine facture-dislocation case, 3: 347
death of, 3: 350
early life, 3: 343
education and training, 3: 343
fracture research and, 3: 343, 347–348
HMS appointment, 2: 223; 4: 60–61
honors and awards, 3: 350
Journal of Bone and Joint Surgery editor, 2: 165; 3: 161, 260, 344–347
legacy of, 3: 349
marriage and family, 3: 349–350
on mental attitude and spine fractures, 3: 349*b*
as MGH surgeon, 1: 158; 3: 187, 192, 270, 343–344, 348, 375
publications and research, 2: 297; 3: 184–185, 294, 347–349
RBBH and, 4: 31, 36, 93, 111
sacroiliac joint arthrodesis and, 3: 184–185
sling procedure for the foot and, 3: 294
spinal fusion and, 3: 321, 344
spinal research and, 3: 343–344, 347–349, *349*
Rogers, William Allen, 4: *200*
Roi Albert I Anglo-Belgian Hospital, 4: 401
Rokitanasky, Karl, 1: 82
Romney, Mitt, 3: 424
Roosevelt, Eleanor, 2: 72
Roosevelt, Franklin D.
  chair lift design, 2: 76, *76*
  Lovett and, 2: 72, *73*, *74*, 75–76, 271
  Lovett's diagram of muscle exam, 2: *75*
  nonstandard treatments and, 2: 77
  onset of poliomyelitis, 2: 71–72
  poliomyelitis treatment, 2: 72–78
  suggestions on treatment, 2: 76–77
  and Warm Springs Foundation, 2: 77–78
  World War II and, 4: 465–466, *466*
Roosevelt, James, 2: 72
Roosevelt, Theodore, 1: 248, 253; 4: 361
Roosevelt Hospital, 2: 248, 250–251
Root, Howard F., 4: 229
Roper, Jane, 4: 66
Ropes, Marian W., 3: 336

Rose, P., 3: 327
Rose, Robert M., 2: 407; 3: 327–328
Rosenau, Milton J., 4: 6, 210
Rosenberg, Benjamin, 2: 368
Rosenthal, Robert K. (1936–2021), 2: *401*
    Boston Children's Hospital and, 2: 401–402
    Brigham and Women's Hospital and, 4: 163, 193
    Cerebral Palsy Clinic and, 2: 402
    cerebral palsy research, 2: 401, *401*, 402
    education and training, 2: 401
    HMS appointment, 2: 401
    PBBH and, 4: 163
    professional memberships, 2: 402
    publications and research, 2: 401–402
Rossier, Alain B., 4: 152
Rotch, Thomas Morgan, 2: 13–14, 170
Roussimoff, André (Andre the Giant), 4: *251*, 252–253
Rowe, Carter R. (1906–2001), 3: *350, 359, 360, 361, 447, 461*; 4: *491*
    as AOA president, 3: 355, 355b, 360
    Bankart procedure and, 3: 351, *351*, 352–354, 357–359, *359*, 360
    Children's Hospital/MGH combined program and, 3: 237
    dead arm syndrome and, 3: 359–360
    death of, 3: 361
    early life, 3: 350
    education and training, 3: 350–351
    on Ernest Codman, 3: 143
    on Eugene Record, 3: 330
    Fracture course and, 3: *273*
    fracture research and, 3: 354
    on fractures in elderly patients, 3: *353*, 354, 354b
    Harvard Unit and, 1: 270, *270*
    HMS appointment, 3: 354, 360
    on Klein, 4: 236
    knee arthrotomy research, 3: 351
    legacy of, 3: 360–361
    Lest We Forget, 3: 61, 187, 257, 347, *357*, 360
    on Mankin, 3: 387
    marriage and family, 3: 361
    MGH Fracture Clinic and, 4: 464
    as MGH surgeon, 3: 354, 360, 398b
    MGH Ward 1 and, 3: 70b, 74
    105th General Hospital and, 3: 351; 4: 489, 490b–491b
    as orthopaedic surgeon for the Boston Bruins, 3: 356–357, 357b
    private medical practice, 3: 271, 448
    professional memberships and, 3: 354–355, 360
    publications and research, 3: 350–359, 448–449
    Shoulder, The, 3: 360
    shoulder dislocations and, 3: 352, *352*, 353, 355–356, *356*
    shoulder surgery and, 3: 352–354, 356
    on Smith-Petersen, 3: 187
    sports medicine and, 3: 356, 388t
    34th Infantry Division and, 4: 484
    on Thornton Brown, 3: 257
    US Army Medical Corps and, 3: 351
    voluntary shoulder dislocation case, 3: 355–356
    on William Kermond, 3: 299
    on William Rogers, 3: 347, 349
    World War II service, 4: 17
Rowe, George, 4: 3
Rowe, Mary, 3: 361, *361*
Roxbury Clinical Record Club (R.C.R.C.), 3: 161
Roxbury Ladies' Bikur Cholim Association, 4: 212
Roxbury Latin School, 1: 6, 20
Royal National Orthopaedic Hospital (London), 1: 106; 2: 333–334, *334*; 3: 412, 426
Royal Orthopaedic Hospital (Birmingham, England), 2: 181
Rozental, Tamara D., 3: 410; 4: 288
RRC. *See* Residency Review Committee (RRC)
Rubash, Harry E.
    Edith M. Ashley Professor, 3: 464b
    HCORP and, 1: 224–225
    Knee Biomechanics and Biomaterials Laboratory, 3: 464b
    as MGH clinical faculty, 3: 464b
    as MGH orthopaedics chief, 3: 11b, 228, 399, 462–463
Rubidge, J. W., 1: *34*
Rubin, S. H., 4: 199
Ruby, Leonard, 2: 250; 4: 99
Rudman, Warren, 2: 414
Rudo, Nathan, 2: 173, 175–176, 438
Ruggles, Timothy, 1: 13
Ruggles-Fayerweather House, 1: 22, *22*
Rugh, J. T., 3: 158
Rumford, Count Benjamin, 1: 292–293
Runyon, Lucia, 2: 291
Runyon, Robert C. (1928–2012), 2: *290–291*
    Boston Children's Hospital and, 2: 289–290
    death of, 2: 291
    education and training, 2: 289
    marriage and family, 2: 291
    MGH/Children's Hospital residency, 2: 289
    MIT Medical and, 2: 277, 290–291
    private medical practice, 2: 289
    publications of, 2: 291
    sports medicine and, 2: 290
Runyon, Scott, 2: 291
Rush, Benjamin, 1: 25, 293; 3: 23
Russell, Stuart, 3: 364
Ruth Jackson Orthopaedic Society, 2: 413, *414*
Ryerson, Edwin W., 1: 197; 2: 160; 4: 394
Ryerson, W. E., 2: 105

S

Sabatini, Coleen, 4: 190b
Sabin, Albert, 2: 191, 264, 315
sacrococcygeal chordoma, 3: 390
sacroiliac joint
    arthrodesis of, 3: 183–185
    fusion for arthritis, 3: 184–185
    fusion for tuberculosis, 3: 185
    ligamentous strain of, 3: 191
    low-back and leg pain, 3: 184
    orthopaedic surgeon opinions on fusion of, 3: 184–185
sacrospinalis, 2: 146–147
Saint Joseph Hospital, 4: 157
Salem Hospital, 1: 220, 224–225; 2: 270–272
Salib, Philip, 3: *238*, 239, 460b
Salk, Jonas, 2: 189
Salter, Robert B., 1: 167; 2: 209, 302, 334–335; 4: 351, 355–356
Salter innominate osteotomy, 2: 390–391
Salter–Harris classification system, 4: 351, 355–356
Saltonstall, Francis A. F. Sherwood, 3: 89
Salvati, Eduardo, 4: 134

Salve Regina College, 1: 216
Salzler, Matthew, 3: 463*b*
Salzman, Edwin W., 4: 251
Samilson, Robert, 3: *293*
San Diego Naval Center, 4: 246
Sancta Maria Hospital, 4: 342, 346
Sandell, L. J., 3: 445
Sanders, Charles, 3: 391
Sanders, James, 2: 378
Sanderson, Eric R., 4: 489
Sanderson, Marguerite, 4: 444
Sanhedrin, Mishnah, 4: 197
Santa Clara County Hospital, 3: 300
Santore, R. F., 4: 176, *176*, 177
Santurjian, D. N., 1: 179
sarcoidosis, 4: 98
Sarcoma Molecular Biology Laboratory, 3: 464*b*
Sargent, John Singer, 4: *424*
Sarmiento, Augusto, 3: 249
Sarni, James, 3: 463, 464*b*
Sarokhan, Alan, 2: 249
Sayre, Lewis A., 1: 119; 2: 26, 30, 48, 50–51, 63, *227*
Sayre, Reginald H., 2: 52
Scannell, David D., 4: 207, 439
scaphoid fracture, 3: 101–102; 4: 359–361, 368–369
Scardina, Robert J., 3: 396, 398*b*, 460*b*, 464*b*
scarlet fever, 1: 7; 2: 4, 52
Scarlet Key Society (McGill), 3: 253, *253*
Schaffer, Jonathan L., 4: 193, 195*b*
Schaffer, Newton M., 2: 47–48
Schaller, Bill, 4: 284
Scheuermann kyphosis, 2: 343, 359
Schiller, Arnold, 2: 369
Schlatter, Carl B., 2: 115
Schlens, Robert D., 2: 266
Schmitt, Francis O., 2: 321, 323; 3: 248, 455*b*
Schmorl, Georg, 3: 204; 4: 262
Schneider, Bryan, 2: 439*b*
School for Health Officers (HMS), 2: 42, 65–66
Schurko, Brian, 4: 190*b*
Schussele, Christian, 1: *57*
Schwab, Robert, 3: 286
Schwab, Sidney I., 3: 164
Schwamm, Lee, 3: 412–413
Schwartz, Felix, 4: 489
Schwartz, Forrest, 3: 463*b*
sciatica
    herniated disc as cause of, 3: 184
    laminectomy and, 3: 204, 206
    low-back pain research, 2: 396; 3: 184, 203–206
    nonoperative treatment of, 2: 373–374

ruptured intervertebral disc and, 3: 205–207, *207*
surgery for, 2: 373–374, 396
treatment of, 2: 152–153; 3: 203
use of chymopapain, 3: 254–255, 419, *421*
scoliosis
  Abbott Frame, 4: 232, *232*
  Adam's machine, 2: 86
  Boston brace, 2: 339–340, 358–359
  brace management of, 2: 339–340, 367
  Bradford and, 2: 35, *35*, *36*, 58
  Brewster and, 2: 223–228
  cadaver studies, 2: 56, 58, *58*
  celluloid jackets, 2: *85*
  collagen and, 2: 328
  congenital, 4: 62, 65
  devices for, 2: 35, *35*, *36*, 296–297, *297*
  diastematomyelia in, 2: 399–400
  Dwyer instrumentation, 2: 336
  Dwyer procedure, 2: 328
  early onset (EOS), 2: 360–361
  exercises for, 2: 59
  Forbes method of correction, 2: 87, *87*; 3: 229; 4: 232, *232*
  forward flexion test, 2: *367*
  Galeazzi method, 2: 227
  genetic background and, 2: 399, *400*
  growth-sparing surgery, 2: 360–361
  Hall and, 2: 334–335
  Harrington rods, 2: 316, 325, 335, 340
  Hibbs spinal fusion procedure, 2: 164
  idiopathic, 1: xxiii; 2: 334, 339, 341, 343, 358–359, 366–367, 399
  jackets for, 2: 59, *59*, 60, *60*, 61, 85–87
  kyphoscoliosis, 1: 97, 105
  latent psoas abscess case, 2: 365
  Lovett and, 2: 56–61, 79, 86, 223–225
  Lovett Board, 2: *59*, 86
  Lovett-Sever method, 2: 87
  measurement methods, 2: 366, *367*
  Milwaukee Brace, 2: 336
  pedicle screws, 2: 343
  pelvic machine design, 2: 86
  photography and, 2: 247
  posterior spinal fusion, 2: 341
  pressure correction apparatus (Hoffa-Schede), 3: *151*, 152

  Relton-Hall frame, 2: 334
  right dorsal, 3: *229*
  self-correction of, 2: *297*
  Sever and, 2: 84–86
  Soutter and, 2: 296
  spinal surgery and, 2: 334–335, 337–338, 340–343
  surgical procedures for, 2: *369*
  suspension and, 2: *336*
  tibial osteoperiosteal grafts, 2: 316
  treatment of, 1: xxi, xxii, 100, 106, 109, *116*; 2: 35, 84–88, 296, 316, 334, 366–367, 396; 3: 208–209, 229; 4: 232–233
  turnbuckle jacket, 2: 80, 223–226, 226*b*, 227, 227*b*, 316, *336*; 3: 209
  use of photographs, 2: 84
  vertebral transverse process case, 3: 229–230
  x-rays and, 2: 79
  Zander apparatus for, 3: *152*, *153*
Scoliosis and Other Deformities of the Axial Skeleton (Riseborough and Herndon), 2: 398, *398*
Scoliosis Research Society (SRS), 2: 338, 342, 347, 370, 400, 411, *411*
scoliosometer, 2: 36
Scollay, Mercy, 1: 19
Scott, Catherine, 4: 175
Scott, Dick, 1: 167
Scott, Richard D. (1943–), 4: *175*
  Brigham and Women's Hospital and, 4: 163, 181, 193
  CHMC and, 4: 176
  education and training, 4: 175
  HCORP and, 4: 175
  hip and knee reconstructions, 4: 175–178
  HMS appointment, 4: 176, 178
  honors and awards, 4: 180
  on importance of PCL preservation, 4: 181
  on metal tibial wedges, 4: 180, *180*
  metallic tibial tray fracture case, 4: 177
  MGH and, 4: 175
  New England Baptist Hospital and, 4: 181
  New England Deaconess Hospital and, 4: 280
  PBBH and, 4: 163
  PFC unicompartmental knee prothesis, 4: 177
  publications and research, 4: 176, *176*, 177–178, *178*, 180, *180*, 181, *181*, 189
  RBBH and, 4: 132, 175–176

Total Knee Arthroplasty, 4: 176
   on total knee replacement outcomes, 4: 178, 180–181
   unicompartmental prothesis and, 4: 176
Scott, S. M., 2: 212
Scudder, Abigail Taylor Seelye, 3: 55
Scudder, Charles L. (1860–1949), 3: *53, 57, 63, 65*
   ACS Committee on Fractures, 3: 64
   American College of Surgeons Board of Regents and, 3: 62–63
   Boston Children's Hospital and, 2: 438; 3: 54
   Boston Dispensary and, 2: 306
   clinical congress meeting, 3: 118
   club foot research and, 3: 54
   "Coll" Warren and, 3: 54–55
   death of, 3: 65
   early life, 3: 53
   education and training, 3: 53–54
   fracture treatment and, 3: 55–56, 56b, 58–65; 4: 340b
   HMS appointment, 3: 58, 61
   legacy of, 3: 64–65
   marriage and family, 3: 55, 64
   at MGH case presentation, 3: *54*
   MGH Fracture Clinic and, 2: 130; 3: 60, 60b, 371; 4: 464
   as MGH house officer, 1: 189; 3: 54
   as MGH surgeon, 3: 54, 58, 64, 266; 4: 472b
   New England Deaconess Hospital and, 4: 274
   professional memberships and, 3: 65
   publications and research, 1: 264; 3: 55–58, 64–65; 4: 335
   Treatment of Fractures, 1: 147; 3: 55–56, *57*, 58, 64, 99; 4: 312, 350
   Tumors of the Jaws, 3: 64
Scudder, Evarts, 3: 53
Scudder, Sarah Patch Lamson, 3: 53
Scudder Oration on Trauma, 3: 63
Scutter, Charles L., 2: 66
Seal of Chevalier du Tastevin, 2: 348, *348*
Sears, George, 4: 303
Seattle Children's Hospital, 4: 250
Section for Orthopedic Surgery (AMA), 2: 110–111, 176
Seddon, Herbert, 2: 135, 140; 3: 412
Sedgwick, Cornelius, 4: 276–277, 279

Seeing Patients (White and Chanoff), 4: *265*
Seelye, Abigail Taylor, 3: 55
Segond, Paul, 2: 91
Seider, Christopher, 1: 14
Sell, Kenneth, 3: 439
Selva, Julius, 2: 31
Semmelweis, Ignaz, 1: 81, 84, 193
sepsis. *See also* antisepsis
   amputations and, 3: 373
   ankle arthrodesis case, 3: 330
   following intramedullary fixation of femoral fractures, 2: 248; 3: 309–310
   hip fractures and, 3: 218
   infectious research and, 1: 91
   recurrence of, 3: 196, 301
septic arthritis, 2: 79
Sevenson, Orvar, 2: 302
Sever, Charles W., 2: 83
Sever, Elizabeth Bygrave, 2: 92, 97
Sever, James T., 2: 252
Sever, James W. (1878–1964), 2: *84, 98, 255*
   on astragalectomy, 2: 92–93
   on back disabilities, 2: 92
   birth palsies research, 2: 415, 417
   Boston Children's Hospital and, 1: 187; 2: 13, 40, 84, 90, 92, 274, 282, 296; 4: 338
   Boston City Hospital and, 4: 305b, 307–308, 308b, 328
   brachial plexus injury study, 2: 90, 96
   on Bradford, 2: 44, 92
   as Browne & Nichols School trustee, 2: 97
   calcaneal apophysitis study, 2: 88–90, 100
   clinical congress meeting, 3: 116
   death of, 2: 100
   early life, 2: 83
   foot research, 2: 107
   fracture research, 3: 340
   HMS appointment, 2: 92, 97; 4: 59
   HMS Laboratory of Surgical Pathology and, 2: 90
   on improvement of medicine, 2: 98
   marriage and family, 2: 92, 97
   Massachusetts Industrial Accident Board examiner, 2: 92
   Massachusetts Regional Fracture Committee, 3: 64
   medical appointments, 2: 84
   as medical director of the Industrial School, 2: 97
   medical education, 2: 83

   military surgeon training and, 4: 396
   New England Regional Committee on Fractures, 4: 341
   obstetrical paralysis study, 2: 89–90, *90*, 91, 94–96, 100
   on occupational therapy, 4: 359
   on orthopaedic surgery advances, 2: 99–100
   pelvic machine design, 2: 86
   Principles of Orthopedic Surgery, 2: 92, *93*
   Principles of Orthopedic Surgery for Nurses, The, 2: 92, *93*
   professional memberships, 2: 97–98
   publications of, 2: 84, 92, 223
   schools for disabled children, 2: 97
   scoliosis treatment, 2: 59, 61, 84–86
   Textbook of Orthopedic Surgery for Students of Medicine, 2: 92, *93*
   tibial tuberosity fracture treatment, 2: 91, 96–97
Sever, Josephine Abbott, 2: 97
Sever, Mary Caroline Webber, 2: 83
Sever procedure, 2: 90
Sever-L'Episcopo procedure, 2: 90, 100, 417
Sever's disease. *See* calcaneal apophysitis (Sever's Disease)
Seymour, N., 2: 211
Shaffer, Newton M., 2: 43, 48, *49*, 57, 99
Shanbhag, Arun, 3: 462, 464b
Shands, Alfred, 1: 99, 114, 180
Shands, Alfred R., Jr., 2: 165, 183; 3: 208, 290
Shands Hospital, 3: 432
Shapiro, Frederic (1942–), 2: *402*
   Boston Children's Hospital and, 2: 354, 403, 403b, 439b; 4: 280
   education and training, 2: 402–403
   HMS appointment, 2: 403, 403b
   honors and awards, 2: 403–404
   Pediatric Orthopedic Deformities, 2: 403, *404*
   professional memberships, 2: 403–405
   publications and research, 2: 400, 403–404, *404*
Sharpey, William, 1: 84
Sharpey-Schafer, Edward A., 2: 242
Shattuck, Frederick C., 2: 20, 39, 43; 3: 94
Shattuck, George Cheever, 4: 414–415

Shaw, A., 2: 115
Shaw, Amy, 1: 85
Shaw, Benjamin S., 2: 8
Shaw, Lemuel, 1: 302, 307, 310–311
Shaw, Robert Gould, 1: 303, 308
Shaw, Robert S., 3: 287
Shea, William D., 4: 163
Sheehan, Diane, 1: 239
Sheltering Arms (New York), 2: 5
Shephard, Margaret, 3: 219
Shepherd's Bush Military Hospital, 4: 398, *398*, 399, 402, 411, 444
Shepherd's Bush Orthopaedic Hospital, 3: 365
Sherman, Henry M., 3: 234
Sherman, William O'Neill, 3: 60–61; 4: 338, 339*b*, 340, 340*b*, *342*
Sherrill, Henry Knox, 3: 1
Shields, Lawrence R., 4: 116, 116*b*, 117, 128, 163
Shippen, William, 1: 25
shock, 4: 373
Shortell, Joseph H. (1891–1951), 4: *338*
    AAOS and, 4: 337
    American Expeditionary Forces and, 4: 338
    athletic injury treatment, 4: 342
    BCH Bone and Joint Service, 4: 307, 328, 333–334, 341, 380*b*
    BCH residencies and, 4: 377
    Boston Bruins and, 4: 342
    Boston Children's Hospital and, 2: 252, 274; 4: 338
    Boston City Hospital and, 1: 199; 3: 64; 4: 242, 338, 341
    death of, 4: 342
    education and training, 4: 338
    fracture treatment and, 4: 339*b*, 342
    hip fractures in elderly case, 4: 341
    HMS appointment, 4: 338, 341
    on industrial accidents, 4: 338, 341
    New England Regional Committee on Fractures, 4: 341
    professional memberships, 4: 341
    publications and research, 4: 338, 341
    Ted Williams and, 4: 342
Shortkroff, Sonya, 4: 136, 194
Shoulder, The (Codman), 2: 239; 3: 105, *105*, 115, 122, 140*b*
Shoulder, The (Rowe), 3: 360
shoulders
    acromioclavicular dislocation, 3: 449
    amputations, 1: 23
    anterior subluxation of, 3: 360
    arthrodesis outcomes, 2: 154
    Bankart procedure, 3: 351–354, 357–358, *359*, 450
    Bankart procedure rating sheet, 3: 358*t*
    brachial plexus injuries, 2: 90–91, 96; 3: 412, *412*, 413–414
    cleidocranial dysostosis, 2: 254
    Codman's Paradox, 3: 105
    dislocations and, 3: 352, *352*, 353, 355–356, *356*
    fracture treatment and, 3: 339
    frozen shoulder, 1: 277–278
    glenoid labrum composition, 3: 449
    instability and, 3: 352, 448–450, *450*
    posterior dislocations, 2: 417–418
    ruptures of the serratus anterior, 2: 253
    sports injuries and, 2: 288
    subacromial bursitis, 3: 104–105, 107–109
    subdeltoid bursa, 3: 95, 98, 103–105, 108
    supraspinatus tendon, 3: 108–109
    surgery, 1: 29
    transfers for, 2: 154
    transient subluxation of, 3: 359
    treatment of, 3: 107–110
Shriners Hospital for Crippled Children, 4: 378
Shriners Hospitals for Children, 2: 110, 212, 424; 3: 335
Sibley, John, 1: 307
sickle cell disease, 3: 403
SICOT. *See* International Society of Orthopaedic Surgery and Traumatology (SICOT)
Siffert, R. S., 1: 126
Silen, William, 1: 167; 4: 262, 283, 283*t*
silicone flexible implants, 4: 132, 166–167, *167*
Siliski, John M., 1: 217*b*; 3: 399, 460*b*, 464*b*
Silver, David, 2: 31, 64, 67, 87; 3: 87, 156, 158, 375; 4: 405, 412, 451
Simcock, Xavier C., 3: 463*b*; 4: 190*b*
Simmons, Barry P. (1939–), 4: *182*
    AO trauma fellowship, 4: 182
    Beth Israel Hospital and, 4: 182, 262
    Brigham and Women's Hospital and, 2: 375; 4: 163, 183, 193, 195*b*
    carpal tunnel syndrome research, 2: 375; 4: 183–184, *184*, 185, *185*, 186
    Children's Hospital/MGH combined program and, 4: 182
    CHMC and, 4: 182
    education and training, 4: 182
    focal scleroderma of the hand case, 4: 183
    hand surgery fellowship, 4: 116*b*, 182
    Hands, 4: 183
    Harvard University Athletics Department and, 4: 183
    HMS appointment, 4: 183
    honors and awards, 4: 186
    New England Baptist Hospital and, 4: 183
    Occupational Disorders of the Upper Extremity, 4: 168, 183
    orthopaedics education and, 4: 186
    outcomes movement and, 4: 186
    PBBH and, 4: 163, 182
    professional memberships, 4: 186
    publications and research, 4: 182–185, *185*, 186
    RBBH and, 4: 182, 184
    residency rotations, 4: 182, 182*b*
    Richard J. Smith Lecture, 3: 431
    US Navy and, 4: 182
    West Roxbury Veterans Administration Hospital and, 4: 182–183
Simmons, C. C., 4: 102
Simmons College, 2: 213, 413
Simon, Michael A., 3: 435–436, *436*
Simon, Sheldon R. (1941–), 2: *405*
    Albert Einstein College of Medicine and, 2: 408
    Boston Children's Hospital and, 2: 406–407
    Brigham and Women's Hospital, 4: 163
    Cave Traveling Fellowship and, 1: 217*b*
    cerebral palsy research, 2: 406–407
    computer-simulated planning and, 2: 389
    education and training, 2: 405–406
    foot and ankle treatment, 2: 407
    gait research, 2: 406–408, 439
    Glimcher and, 2: 406
    HMS appointment, 2: 406–407
    honors and awards, 2: 406–407, 407*b*
    MGH and, 2: 406

Ohio State University School of
Medicine and, 2: 407–408
orthopaedics appointments,
2: 408
PBBH and, 4: 163
*Practical Biomechanics for the
Orthopedic Surgeon*, 3: 328
professional memberships,
2: 407, 407*b*
publications and research,
2: 406, *406*, 407–408; 3: 326
RESNA and, 2: 408
study of Swiss method of treating
fractures, 2: 406
West Roxbury Veterans Administration Hospital and, 2: 406
Simon, William H., 3: 377
Simpson, Sir James, 1: 84
69th Field Ambulance, 4: 405*b*
Skaggs, David, 2: 379
skeletogenesis, 2: 439
skiagraphy, 2: 16
Skillman, John J., 4: 251
skin grafts, 1: 75, 77; 3: 310;
4: 204, 216–217
Skoff, Hillel, 4: 263, 286
Sledge, Clement (1930–), 4: *126*,
128, *133*
AAOS and, 4: 139–141
Affiliated Hospitals Center board
and, 4: 119
articular cartilage research,
4: 133, 136
on avascular necrosis, 4: 238
on Barr, 3: 213
BIH Board of Consultants,
4: 262–263
Boston Children's Hospital and,
2: 354–355
Brigham Orthopaedic Foundation (BOF) and, 4: 123, 191
Brigham Orthopedic Associates
(BOA) and, 4: 123, 191
BWH chair of orthopaedic
surgery, 1: 180, 284; 4: 132–
133, 143, 191–193, 195*b*–196*b*
Children's Hospital/MGH combined program and, 1: 210;
4: 126
chondrocyte metabolism in cell
culture research, 4: 133
on Codman, 4: 141
on diastematomyelia, 2: 236
education and training,
4: 125–127
embryonic cartilage research,
4: 127, *127*
Hip Society president, 4: 141
HMS appointment, 4: 127
honors and awards, 4: 142

John Ball and Buckminster
Brown Professorship, 3: 202;
4: 132, 195*b*
joint replacement research and
treatment, 4: 40, 133, *133*,
134–135, *135*
knee arthroplasty and, 4: 129–
130, 147, 149
mandate to unify orthopaedics
at Brigham Hospitals, 4: 116,
116*b*, 117–118
Marion B. Gebbie Research Fellowship, 4: 127
on merger of RBBH and PBBH,
4: 128
as MGH honorary orthopaedic
surgeon, 3: 398*b*
MGH orthopaedics department
and, 1: 210–211; 4: 127
on orthopaedic basic and clinical
research, 4: 141, *141*, 142
as PBBH chief of orthopaedic
surgery, 2: 269, 279; 4: 43,
115–117, 128–129, 132, 143,
191, 196*b*
as PBBH orthopaedic surgery
professor, 4: 43, 114–115
publications and research,
4: 127, 129–130, *130*, 131,
133–139, *139*
radiation synovectomy research,
4: 64, 136, *136*, 137
RBBH board of overseers, 4: 132
as RBBH chief of surgery,
2: 279; 4: 43, 115, 128–129,
131–132, 143, 191, 196*b*
as RBBH orthopaedic surgery
professor, 4: 43, 114–115
as research fellow in orthopaedic
surgery, 4: 126
rheumatoid arthritis treatment,
4: 138–139
Strangeways Research Laboratory
fellowship, 4: 126
US Navy and, 4: 125
Slipped Capital Femoral Epiphysis
(Joplin et al.), 3: 294, 333
Slipped Capital Femoral Epiphysis
(Klein et al.), 4: 238
slipped capital femoral epiphysis
(SCFE)
acetabular morphology in, 2: 392
Howorth procedure and, 4: 243
impingement treatment, 3: 189
internal fixation of, 2: 176
Klein's Line and, 4: 238–239, *239*
open reduction of, 2: 168; 4: 237
recommendations for, 2: 176
research in, 3: 294, 331, 333;
4: 237–238, 243

treatment of, 2: 137
treatment outcomes, 2: 380
use of roentgenology in, 3: 334
Slocum, Donald B., 1: 279
Slowick, Francis A., 2: 230
smallpox, 1: 8–9, 295; 2: 4
Smellie, William, 1: 6
Smith, Dale C., 4: 464
Smith, Ethan H., 3: 160*b*
Smith, Gleniss, 3: 427
Smith, H., 3: 210
Smith, H. W., 1: *31*
Smith, Homer B., 1: 253–254
Smith, Ida, 2: 431–432
Smith, J. V. C., 1: 97
Smith, Jacob, 3: 427
Smith, Job L., 2: 7
Smith, Lyman, 3: 254
Smith, Nellie, 3: 247
Smith, Richard J. (1930–1987),
3: *427*, *428*, *430*
ASSH and, 3: 428–429, *430*
death of, 3: 399, 429–430
early life, 3: 427
education and training, 3: 427
factitious lymphedema case,
3: 429
hand surgery and, 3: 385–386,
388*t*, 427–429, 460*b*
HMS appointment, 3: 428
Hospital for Joint Diseases and,
3: 413, 427
legacy of, 3: 430–431
Mankin on, 3: 427, 429–430
as MGH surgeon, 3: 395, 398*b*,
413, 428
professional memberships and,
3: 428, 430
publications and research,
3: 427–429
Smith Day lectures, 3: 431
*Tendon Transfers of the Hand and
Forearm*, 3: 428
Smith, Robert M., 2: 177, 234, 432
Smith, Rose, 3: 427
Smith, Theobold, 4: 6
Smith-Petersen, Evelyn Leeming,
3: 362
Smith-Petersen, Hilda Dickenson,
3: 198
Smith-Petersen, Kaia Ursin, 3: 179
Smith-Petersen, Marius N. (1886–
1953), 3: *174*, *179*, *197*, *198*
AAOS and, 4: 337
AAOS Fracture Committee and,
3: 191
adjustable reamer and, 3: 317
American Ambulance Hospital
and, 4: *388*, 389*b*, *390*

approach to wrist during arthrodesis, 3: 191
Brackett and, 3: 180–181
death of, 3: 198
early life, 3: 179
education and training, 3: 179–181
femoral neck fracture treatment, 3: 185–186, *186*, 189, *189b*, 190
femoral stem prothesis, 3: *293*
femoroacetabular impingement treatment, 3: 188–189
Harvard Surgical Unit and, 2: 119, 123–124; 3: 180, *180*, *370*
hip nailing and, 3: 237
hip surgery and, 3: 244
HMS appointment, 3: 183, 187, 192; 4: 59
innovation and, 3: 216–217
Knight's Cross, Royal Norwegian Order of St. Olav, 3: *198*
kyphosis treatment, 3: 239
legacy of, 3: 198–199
on Legg-Calve-Perthes disease, 2: 103
marriage and family, 3: 198
MGH Fracture Clinic and, 3: 60*b*, 315
MGH orthopaedics and, 1: 179, 189, 203–204; 2: 297; 3: 183, 269, 456*b*
as MGH orthopaedics chief, 3: 11*b*, 187–188, 191, 227, 375
MGH physical chemistry laboratory, 2: 322
military orthopaedics and, 4: 473
mold arthroplasty and, 3: 181, 183, 192, *192*, 193, 193*b*, 194, *194*, 195, *195*, 196, *196*, 198, 216, 238–239, 241, 292, 292*b*, 293
New England Rehabilitation Center and, 1: 272
orthopaedic surgery and, 1: 158
personality of, 3: 187–188
pillars of surgical care, 3: 187
private medical practice, 3: 183, 192
professional memberships and, 3: 197, 197*b*
publications and research, 2: 136; 3: 188, 192–193, 241–242, 302, 366
RBBH and, 4: 31, 36, 93, 111
sacroiliac joint treatment, 3: 183–185, 191

supra-articular subperiosteal approach to the hip, 3: 181, *181*, 182*b*
treatment of fractures, 3: 62
triflanged nail development, 3: 62, 185–186, *186*, 187, 189–190; 4: 237
World War II and, 3: 191
Smith-Petersen, Morten (1920–1999), 3: *361*
Children's Hospital/MGH combined program and, 3: 361
death of, 3: 362
early life, 3: 361
education and training, 3: 361
hip surgery and, 3: 362
HMS appointment, 3: 362
marriage and family, 3: 362
New England Baptist Hospital and, 3: 362
publications and research, 3: 362
Tufts appointment, 3: 362
US Naval Reserves and, 3: 361
Smith-Petersen, Morten, Sr., 3: 179
Smith-Petersen Foundation, 3: 198
Snedeker, Lendon, 2: 191
Snyder, Brian D. (1957–), 2: *409*
biomechanics research, 2: 410–411
Boston Children's Hospital and, 2: 409–411
Cerebral Palsy Clinic and, 2: 409
contrast-enhanced computed tomography and, 2: 411
education and training, 2: 409
fracture-risk research, 2: 411, *411*
HCORP and, 2: 409
HMS appointment, 2: 409
honors and awards, 2: 411
hospital appointments, 2: 409
modular spinal instrumentation device patents, 2: 412
orthopaedics appointments, 2: 409
professional memberships, 2: 412
publications and research, 2: 410, *410*, 411
Society for Medical Improvement, 3: 35
Society of Clinical Surgery, 3: 113*b*
Söderman, P., 3: 219
Sohier, Edward H., 1: 307, 310
Solomon, Dr., 4: 210
Soma Weiss Prize, 2: 319
somatosensory evoked potentials (SSEPs), 2: 342
Sons of Liberty, 1: 11, 13, 15–16
Soule, D., 2: 372

Southern Medical and Surgical Journal, 1: 63
Southmayd, William W., 1: 279; 4: 163, 193
Southwick, Wayne, 4: 258, 261
Soutter, Anne, 2: 292
Soutter, Charlotte Lamar, 2: 292
Soutter, D. R., 2: 34
Soutter, Helen E. Whiteside, 2: 292
Soutter, James, 2: 292
Soutter, Lamar, 2: 292, 293*b*
Soutter, Robert (1870–1933), 2: *292*, *293*
Boston Children's Hospital and, 2: 34, 292; 4: 338
Boston City Hospital and, 4: 305*b*
Bradford and, 2: 292, 297
cartilage transplantation, 2: 294
critique of shoes, 2: 293
death from blood poisoning, 2: 299, *299*
dislocated patella treatment, 2: 294–296
education and training, 2: 292
hip contracture treatment, 2: 294, 295*b*
hip disease treatment, 2: 293–294
HMS appointment, 2: 223, 298; 4: 59–60
hot pack treatment, 2: 264
letter to Catherine A. Codman, 1: *129*, 130
marriage and family, 2: 292, 293*b*
military surgeon training by, 2: 42, 66
New England Peabody Home for Crippled Children and, 2: 270, 292
orthopaedic device innovations, 2: 296–297
orthopaedic surgery and, 1: 171
orthopaedics appointments, 2: 292
professional memberships, 2: 292, 292*b*
"Progress in Orthopaedic Surgery" series, 2: 297
publications of, 2: 61, 293, 297
scoliosis treatment, 2: 296
surgical procedure innovations, 2: 294–296
Technique of Operations on the Bones, Joints, Muscles and Tendons, 2: 294, 297–298, *298*
Soutter, Robert, Jr., 2: 292
Soutter, Robert, Sr., 2: 292
Spalding, James Alfred, 1: 47, 49, 49*b*, 50
Spanier, Suzanne, 3: 390

Index

Spanish American War, 4: 310–311, *311*
Spanish Flu, 4: *11*
Sparks, Jared, 1: 310
Spaulding Rehabilitation Hospital, 1: 217, 225; 3: 387–388, 396, 426, 461
Spear, Louis M., 4: 23, 26–28, 31–32, 45, 79
"Special Orthopedic Hospital–Past and Present, The" (Platt), 1: 114
Spector, Myron, 4: 194, 195*b*
Speed, Kellogg, 4: *319*
Spencer, Herbert, 4: 466–467
Spencer, Hillard, 2: 367
Spencer, Upshur, 4: 190*b*
spina bifida
    Lovett on, 2: 51–52
    research in, 2: 370
    ruptures of sac, 2: 309–310
    treatment of, 2: 51–52
    University of Massachusetts clinic, 2: 364
Spinal Deformity Study Group, 2: 365
spinal dysgenesis, 2: 366
spinal fusion wake-up test, 2: 340–342
Spinal Surgery Service (Children's Hospital), 2: 359
spinal taps, 2: 72, 78
spinal tuberculosis, 1: *109*
    operative treatment for, 4: 343
    pediatric patients, 2: 11, 308–309; 3: 289
    research in, 3: 289
    treatment of, 1: 100, 106, 108–109; 2: 308–309; 4: 225
spine. *See also* scoliosis
    advances in, 2: 338
    anterior and posterior procedures, 2: 343–345, 360, 366; 3: 426
    apparatus for, 1: 107; 2: *35, 36*
    athletes and, 2: 385
    benefits of, 2: 373
    Boston Children's Hospital and, 2: 337–338, 338*t*
    Bradford Frame and, 2: 30
    cerebral palsy and, 2: 370
    children and, 1: 123; 2: 385
    closed reduction of lumbar facture-dislocation, 3: 347
    community-based physicians and, 2: 373
    computed tomography and, 3: 254
    congenital absence of the odontoid process, 3: 340
    degenerative stenosis, 4: 269–270
    Down syndrome and, 2: 370
    Dwyer instrumentation and, 2: 336
    for early-onset, 2: 360
    fractures and dislocations, 3: 349*b*, 349
    fusion in tubercular, 3: 148–149, 157–158, 158*b*; 4: 343
    halo-vest apparatus, 4: *152*, 153
    Harrington rods and, 2: 316, 325, 335–336, 338
    Hibbs spinal fusion procedure, 2: 164; 3: 155
    instability of lower cervical, 4: 261
    interpedicular segmental fixation (ISF) pedicle screw plate, 3: 420–421
    lumbar spinal stenosis, 2: 373–374
    measurement of, 2: *31*
    mental attitude and, 3: 349*b*
    MRI and, 3: 255
    myelodysplasia, 2: 359
    neurologic effects after surgery, 4: 269
    nutritional status and, 2: 361–362
    open anterior lumbosacral fracture dislocation, 3: 420, 425
    paraplegia and, 3: 319
    pedicle screws in, 2: 343; 3: 420
    posterior segment fixator (PSF), 3: 420
    Pott's Disease, 1: 97, 108–109; 3: 148–150
    pressure and pain, 2: 271
    prosthetic titanium rib and, 2: 360, *362*
    research in, 2: 343
    sacrococcygeal chordoma, 3: 390
    Scheuermann kyphosis, 2: 343, 359
    somatosensory evoked potentials (SSEPs), 2: 342
    spinal dysgenesis, 2: 366
    spinal fusion, 2: 271, 334–335, *335*, 343, 369; 3: 207–208
    spinal fusion wake-up test, 2: 340–342
    spinal height increases, 2: 367
    spondylolisthesis, 3: 421
    strengthening exercises for, 1: 100
    study of, 2: 57, *57*, 58, *58*, 59
    thoracic insufficiency syndrome, 2: 360
    tibial fracture, 4: 365
    treatment of, 1: 97–98, 100, 106; 2: 359; 4: 152
    vertebral column resections (VCRs), 2: 362–363
Spine Care Medical Group, 4: 263
Spine Patient Outcomes Research Trial (SPORT), 2: 371, 373
Spitzer, Hans, 2: 80
splints
    for drop-foot deformity, 4: *418*
    Eames molded plywood leg, 4: *470*
    first aid, 4: *418*
    Jones splints, 4: 389, 411
    manufacture of, 3: *167*, 168
    military orthopaedics and, 2: 120; 4: 389, 408–409, 416–417, *418*
    standardization of, 3: 167–168
    Thomas, 2: 20, *123*, *257*; 3: *168*; 4: 389, *391*, *408*, 409, 411, 417, *418*
    use during transportation, 3: 169, 169*b*; 4: 389
sports medicine. *See also* Harvard athletics
    acromioclavicular joint dislocation in, 1: 268, 277
    acute ligament injuries, 1: 277–278
    ankle injuries and, 1: 281
    assessment and treatment in, 1: 274
    athlete heart size, 1: 262, 267, 288
    athletic training and, 1: 248, 250–251, 258, 265–266
    BCH clinic for, 2: 287, 384
    caring for athletic injuries, 1: 268
    concussions in, 1: 247, 254, 275, 286–287; 2: 385
    dieticians and, 1: 258
    fatigue and, 1: 264–265
    foot and ankle treatment, 3: 348
    football injuries and, 1: 247–248, 252–255, 255*t*, 256, 258–262, 288
    frozen shoulder, 1: 277–278
    guidelines for team physicians, 1: 287
    Harvard athletics and, 2: 287
    ice hockey and, 1: 275, 286
    injury prevention and, 1: 265, 285–286
    knee joint injuries, 1: 267–268, 268*t*, 278–279, 285–287
    knee problems and, 2: 387
    MGH and, 3: 397
    Morton's neuroma, 2: 287
    musculoskeletal injuries, 1: 288
    myositis ossificans and, 1: 266–267
    neuromusculoskeletal genius and, 1: 279

orthopaedics curriculum and, 1: 165–166
pediatric, 2: 287, 385–387
physical therapy and, 3: 348
preventative strappings, 1: *269*, 274
professional teams and, 3: 348, 356–357, 397, 399, 448, 450
progress in, 1: 267
reconditioning and, 1: 271
rehabilitation and, 1: 275
scientific study of, 1: 250–251, 254–256, 262, 267–269, 277–278
spinal problems, 2: 385
sports teams and, 1: 248, 250–251
tenosynovitis of the flexor hallucis longus, 3: 348
torn meniscus, 1: 278
women basketball players and, 1: 285–286
Sports Medicine Bible for Young Adults, The (Micheli), 2: 385
Sports Medicine Bible, The (Micheli), 2: 385, *385*
Sports Medicine Fund, 2: 439*b*
Sports Medicine Service (MGH), 3: 356
Sprengel deformity, 2: 195, *196*
spring muscle test, 2: 70, *70*, 71
Springfield, Dempsey S. (1945–), 1: *242*; 3: *431*
  allograft research and, 3: 433, 435
  Association of Bone and Joint Surgeons and, 3: 436
  education and training, 3: 431–432
  Gaucher hemorrhagic bone cyst case, 3: 434
  HCORP and, 1: 242–243; 3: 435
  HMS appointment, 3: 432
  honors and awards, 3: 431, 436
  limb salvage surgery and, 3: 433
  as MGH surgeon, 3: 432
  Mount Sinai Medical School and, 3: 435
  Musculoskeletal Tumor Society and, 3: 436
  orthopaedic oncology and, 3: 399, 432, 435, 460*b*
  orthopaedics education and, 3: 435–436
  publications and research, 3: 432–433, 435–436
  on resident surgical case requirements, 3: 435–436, *436*
  Shands Hospital and, 3: 432
  surgical treatment of osteosarcoma, 3: 432–433
  University of Florida and, 3: 432
  US Army and, 3: 432
Spunkers, 1: 21, 32, 133
Spurling, Ina, 2: 144, 166
St. Anthony Hospital, 2: 111
St. Botolph Club (Boston), 2: *284*
St. George's Hospital, 1: 81, 83, 106
St. Louis Children's Hospital, 3: 165
St. Louis Shriners Hospital for Crippled Children, 3: 173
St. Luke's Home for Convalescents, 2: *307*
St. Luke's Hospital (New York), 2: 5, 20
St. Margaret's and Mary's Infant Asylum, 2: 256
St. Mary's Hospital (Nairobi, Kenya), 3: 379
St. Thomas's Hospital, 1: 37
Stack, Herbert, 2: 249
Stagnara, P., 2: 340
Staheli, Lynn, 2: 302; 4: 250
Stamp Act, 1: 11–13
Stamp Act Congress, 1: 13
Stanish, William, 2: 423
Stanton, Edwin, 3: 43
Staples, Mable Hughes, 3: 362
Staples, Nellie E. Barnes, 3: 362
Staples, O. Sherwin (1908–2002)
  Boston Children's Hospital and, 2: 438
  Children's Hospital/MGH combined program and, 3: 362
  Dartmouth Medical School appointment, 3: 363–364
  death of, 3: 364
  early life, 3: 362
  education and training, 3: 362
  on Edwin Cave, 3: 276
  as first orthopaedic surgeon in NH, 3: 363–364
  marriage and family, 3: 362
  Mary Hitchcock Memorial Hospital and, 3: 363–364
  as MGH surgeon, 3: 74, 362
  New England Peabody Home for Crippled Children and, 3: 362
  on osteochondritis in a finger, 3: 363
  private medical practice, 3: 271, 362
  publications and research, 3: 362
  6th General Hospital and, 4: 482
  White River Junction VA Hospital, 3: 364
  World War II service, 3: 362
Staples, Oscar S., Sr., 3: 362

Star and Garter Hospital, 4: 402
State Hospital School for Children (Canton), 2: 308
Statement by Four Physicians, 2: 6, *6*, 7
Steadman, Richard, 3: 446
Steadman Hawkins Clinic, 2: 378
Stearns, Peter N., 3: 83
Steele, Glenn, 4: 279
Steele, Mrs., 4: *128*
Steindler, Arthur, 2: 94; 3: 303; 4: 362
Steiner, Mark, 1: 217*b*, 289; 4: 194, 195*b*
Steinmann pin, 2: 237–238; 4: 166
Stelling, Frank H., 2: 351; 4: 19
Stephen J. Lipson, MD Orthopaedic and Spine lectureship, 4: 272, 272*b*
Stern, Peter, 3: 431
Stern, Walter, 1: xxiv
stethoscope, 1: 74
Stevens, James H., 2: 96, 415; 3: 109
Stevens, Samuel, 1: 6
Stevens, W. L., 3: 133
Stillman, Charles F., 2: 50–51
Stillman, J. Sidney, 4: 37, 40, 79
Stillman, James, 2: 253
Stillman Infirmary, 2: 253, *254*
Still's disease, 2: 171
Stimson, Lewis A., 1: 147
Stinchfield, Allan, 3: 332
Stinchfield, Frank, 3: 275
Stirrat, Craig, 4: 194, 195*b*
Stone, James S., 2: 146, 230, 307, 438; 4: 310
Stone, James W., 1: 308
Storer, D. Humphries, 3: 42
Storey, Elizabeth Moorfield, 2: 80
Strammer, Myron A, 4: 208*b*
Strangeways Research Laboratory, 4: 126
Stromeyer, Georg Friedrich Louis, 1: xxiii, 101, 105–106
Strong, Richard P., 4: 389*b*, 422*b*
Stryker, William, 3: 249; 4: 246
Stubbs, George, 1: *136*
Study in Hospital Efficiency, A (Codman), 3: 125, *125*, 127*b*, 128–131
Sturdevant, Charles L. (b. ca. 1913)
  Boston Children's Hospital and, 2: 299
  Crippled Children's Clinic and, 2: 299
  education and training, 2: 299
  HMS appointment, 2: 299
  Marlborough Medical Associates and, 2: 146, 269, 299

MGH orthopaedics residency, 3: 74
  PBBH and, 4: 18–20, 110
  publication contributions, 2: 300
Sturgis, Susan, 3: 30
Sturgis, William, 3: 30
subacromial bursitis, 3: 104–105, 108–109
subdeltoid bursa, 3: 95, 98, 103–105, 108
Subjective Knee Form (IKDC), 2: 381
Subjective Shoulder Scale, 2: 380
subscapularis tendon, 2: 95, *95*
subtrochanteric osteotomy, 2: 293
Such a Joy for a Yiddish Boy (Mankin), 3: 392, *392*
suction socket prosthesis, 1: 273
Suffolk District Medical Society, 3: 120–122
Sugar Act, 1: 11
Suk, Se Il, 2: 343
Sullivan, James T., 4: 233
Sullivan, Louis, 4: 266*b*
Sullivan, Patricia, 3: 460*b*
Sullivan, Robert, 1: 317
Sullivan, Russell F. (1893–1966), 4: *343*
  BCH Bone and Joint Service, 4: 343–344, 346, 380*b*
  Boston City Hospital and, 4: 307
  Boston Red Sox and, 4: 345
  Carney Hospital and, 4: 343
  death of, 4: 346
  education and training, 4: 343
  elbow joint fracture-dislocation case, 4: 345
  Lahey Clinic and, 4: 345
  marriage and family, 4: 346
  Melrose Hospital and, 4: 343
  private medical practice, 4: 344
  professional memberships, 4: 346
  publications and research, 4: 343, 344*b*
  spinal tuberculosis research, 4: 343, 344*b*
  Ted Williams and, 4: 345–346
  Tufts Medical School appointment, 4: 343
Sullivan, Thelma Cook, 4: 346
Sullivan, W. E., 3: 86
Sumner Koch Award, 2: 415
Sunnybrook Hospital, 2: 334
SUNY Downstate Medical Center, 3: 388
supraspinatus tendon, 3: 108–109
Surgeon's Journal, A (Cushing), 3: 369
surgery. *See also* orthopaedic surgery
  abdominal, 1: 81

antisepsis principles and, 1: 85, 141
Astley Cooper and, 1: 34, 36, 42, 44
Clavien-Dindo classification in, 2: 393
Coll Warren and, 1: 81–84
early training in, 1: 183–186
fracture care and, 4: 463–464
general anesthesia and, 1: 141
HMS curriculum for, 1: 140–141
infection from dirty, 3: 60
Jack Warren and, 1: 22–23, 25, 29, 40
John Collins Warren and, 1: 36–37, 53, 68
Joseph Warren and, 1: 6, 9, 15
long-bone fractures, 3: 60–61
pedagogy and, 1: 34, 137–138
plastic, 1: 71, 76–77
Richard Warren and, 1: 90
shoulder and, 1: 29
use of ether, 1: 55–65
Surgery (Keen), 3: 103
Surgery (Richard Warren), 1: 90
Surgery of Joints, The (Lovett and Nichols), 2: 52
Surgical After-Treatment (Crandon and Ehrenfried), 4: 217, *217*
surgical instruments, 3: 40–41
Surgical Observations with Cases and Operations (J. M. Warren), 1: 47, 75, 78
Surgical Treatment of the Motor-Skeletal System (Bancroft), 3: 316
Sutterlin, C. E., 3: 420
Sutton, Silvia Barry, 3: 259
Suzedell, Eugene, 2: 233
Swaim, Caroline Tiffany Dyer, 4: 51
Swaim, Joseph Skinner, 4: 51
Swaim, Loring T. (1882–1964), 4: *51*
  American Rheumatism Association and, 4: 57–58
  Arthritis, Medicine and the Spiritual Law, 4: 58, *58*
  back pain research and, 3: 203
  Body Mechanics in Health and Disease, 4: 53
  Buchmanism and, 4: 57
  chronic arthritis growth disturbances case, 4: 56
  chronic arthritis treatment and, 4: 54–58
  chronic disease treatment and, 4: 52–53
  Clifton Springs Sanatorium and, 3: 88; 4: 52–53
  death of, 4: 40, 59
  early life, 4: 51
  education and training, 4: 52

HMS appointment, 2: 223; 4: 57, 59–60
on importance of posture, 4: 52–54
marriage and family, 4: 59
MGH and, 3: 269; 4: 52, 54
Moral Re-Armament program and, 4: 57
on patient care, 4: 54, 55*b*, 58
private medical practice, 4: 53
professional memberships, 4: 58–59
publications and research, 2: 136, 297; 3: 91; 4: 52–55, 57–58, 60–61
RBBH and, 4: 93, 406
as RBBH chief of orthopaedics, 4: 48, 55–57, 79, 196*b*
RBBH orthopaedic surgeon, 4: 28, 31, 33, 35, 63
rehabilitation of soldiers and, 4: 444
World War I and, 4: 54
Swaim, Madeline K. Gill, 4: 59
Swartz, R. Plato, 2: 438
Sweet, Elliot, 3: 242, 243*b*
Sweetland, Ralph, 3: 396
Swinton, Neil, 2: 232
Swiontkowski, Marc, 2: 424–425
Syme, James, 1: 56, 84
synovectomy, 4: 64, 102, 371–372
synovial fluid, 3: 174, *174*, 175
syringes, 1: 80, *80*
System of Surgery (Holmes), 1: 81
systemic lupus erythematosus (SLE), 4: 98
systemic sclerosis, 4: 98

T

Tachdjian, Jason, 2: 305
Tachdjian, Mihran O. (1927–1996), 2: *300*
  birth palsies research, 2: 417
  Boston Children's Hospital and, 2: 301–302
  cerebral palsy treatment, 2: 300–301, *301*
  Children's Memorial Hospital (Chicago) and, 2: 302
  course on congenital hip dysplasia, 2: 302
  death of, 2: 305
  education and training, 2: 300
  Green and, 2: 301–304
  honors and awards, 2: 305*b*
  intraspinal tumors in children case, 2: 301–302
  marriage and family, 2: 305

Northwestern University and, 2: 302
PBBH and, 4: 20
Pediatric Orthopaedic International Seminars program, 2: 304
Pediatric Orthopaedic Society and, 2: 351
pediatric orthopaedics and, 2: 300–304
Pediatric Orthopedics, 2: 188, 303, *303*
professional memberships, 2: 304, 305*b*
publications and research, 2: 300–303, 303*b*, 304
Tachdjian, Vivian, 2: 305
Taft, Katherine, 4: 286
Taitsman, Lisa, 4: 190*b*
tarsectomy, 2: 23
Taylor, Charles Fayette, 1: 107; 2: 20, 22, 26, 47
Taylor back brace, 2: 247
Tea Act, 1: 15
Technique of Operations on the Bones, Joints, Muscles and Tendons (Souter), 2: 294, 297–298, *298*
Tegner Activity Scale, 2: 380
teleroentgenography, 2: 170, 170*t*
Temperance Society, 1: 40
tendon transfers
  ankles and, 2: 148
  flexor carpi ulnaris transfer procedure, 2: 172, 188, *199*
  hands and forearms, 3: 428
  iliotibial band and, 2: 109
  Ober on, 2: 147–149
  obstetrical paralysis and, 2: 96
  patella, 2: 294
  polio and, 2: 108–109
  polio patient lower extremities, 2: 265; 3: 332–333
  quadriplegic patient hands and, 2: 265
  Trendelenburg limp and, 2: 108, *108*
  for wrist flexion and pronation deformity, 2: 172
Tendon Transfers of the Hand and Forearm (Smith), 3: 428
tenosynovitis, 2: 89; 3: 315, 414, 438
tenotomy
  Achilles, 1: 100–101, 106; 2: 25
  club foot and, 1: 106, 118; 2: 25–26
  early study of, 1: xxiii, 100
  Guérin's, 1: 118
  physical therapy and, 1: 100

Stromeyer's subcutaneous, 1: 118, *118*
technique for, 1: 100–101
Terrono, A., 4: 167
Textbook of Disorders and Injuries of the Musculoskeletal System (Salter), 1: 167
Textbook of Orthopedic Surgery for Students of Medicine (Sever), 2: 92, *93*
thalidomide, 2: 334, *334*
Thane, George D., 2: 242
Thayer General Hospital, 4: 241, *241*
Theodore, George H. (1965–), 3: *437*
  education and training, 3: 437
  extracorporeal shockwave therapy (ESWT) research, 3: 437–438, *438*
  foot and ankle treatment, 3: 460*b*
  HCORP and, 3: 437
  HMS appointment, 3: 437
  as MGH clinical faculty, 3: 464*b*
  as MGH surgeon, 3: 348, 437
  plantar fasciitis treatment, 3: 437–438
  professional sports teams and, 3: 348
  publications and research, 3: 437–438
Theodore, Harry, 3: 437
Theodore, Marie, 3: 437
Therapeutic Exercise and Massage (Bucholz), 3: 269
Thibodeau, Arthur, 4: 91, 95, 333, 378
Thilly, William G., 4: 171
Thomas, Charles, 4: 187
Thomas, Claudia L., 4: 266*b*
Thomas, Hugh Owen, 1: xxiii; 2: 20, 22, 116
Thomas, John Jenks, 2: 90
Thomas, Leah C., 4: *235*, 236
Thomas, Margaret, 4: 189
Thomas, William H. (1930–2011), 4: *187*
  Brigham and Women's Hospital, 4: 163, 187
  Brigham Orthopedic Associates (BOA) and, 4: 123
  Children's Hospital/MGH combined program and, 4: 187
  death of, 4: 189
  education and training, 4: 187
  Florida Civil Air Patrol and, 4: 189
  on foot surgery and rheumatoid arthritis, 4: 188, *188*, *189*

HMS appointment, 4: 187–188
  honors and awards, 4: 189
  marriage and family, 4: 189
  on McKeever and MacIntosh prostheses, 4: 188–189
  MGH and, 4: 187
  PBBH and, 4: 116, 128–129, 161, 163, 187
  publications and research, 4: 69, 70*b*–71*b*, 134, 187–188, *189*
  RBBH and, 4: 40, 68, 116*b*, 129, 131, 187–188
  rheumatoid clinic and, 4: 188
  West Roxbury Veterans Administration Hospital and, 4: 187
Thomas B. Quigley Society, 1: *282*, 283
Thomas splint, 2: 20, *123*, 247; 3: *168*; 4: 389, *391*, *408*, 409, 411, 417, *418*
Thompson, Milton, 3: 192
Thompson, Sandra J. (1937–2003), 2: *412*, 413
  arthritis clinic and, 2: 413
  Boston Children's Hospital and, 2: 413
  death of, 2: 414
  education and training, 2: 412–413
  HMS appointment, 2: 413
  humanitarianism and, 2: 413
  Laboratory for Skeletal Disorders and Rehabilitation and, 2: 413
  pediatric orthopaedics and, 2: 414
  professional memberships, 2: 413–414
  prosthetic clinic and, 2: 413
  publications of, 2: 414
  Ruth Jackson Orthopaedic Society and, 2: 413
  Simmons College and, 2: 413
Thomson, Elihu, 2: 114; 3: 97–98
Thomson, Helen, 1: 317
thoracic insufficiency syndrome, 2: 360
thoracic outlet syndrome, 3: 415
thoracic spine, 4: 259–260
thoracostomy, 2: 360
Thorn, George W., 4: 79
Thorndike, Alice, 2: 312
Thorndike, Augustus (1863–1940), 2: *305*
  address to the American Orthopaedic Association, 2: 311
  Bar Harbor Medical and Surgical Hospital and, 2: 312
  Boston Children's Hospital and, 2: 34, 40, 307
  Boston Dispensary and, 2: 306

Index

Boston Lying-in-Hospital and, 2: 306
death of, 2: 312
disabled children and, 2: 307–308
education and training, 2: 305–306
hip infection treatment, 2: 108
HMS appointment, 2: 307
House of the Good Samaritan and, 2: 114, 115*b*, 306
Manual of Orthopedic Surgery, A, 2: 311, *312*
marriage and family, 2: 312
MGH and, 2: 306
on orthopaedic supervision in schools and sports, 2: 310
orthopaedic surgery and, 1: 171; 2: 311
poliomyelitis treatment, 2: 264
professional memberships, 2: 306–307, 312
publications and research, 2: 61, 308–309
rupture of the spina bifida sac case, 2: 309–310
schools for disabled children, 2: 36, 38, 308, 310–311; 3: 151
St. Luke's Home for Convalescents, 2: 307
tuberculosis treatment, 2: 308
Thorndike, Augustus, Jr. (1896–1986), 1: *263, 270*; 3: *450*; 4: *491*
on acromioclavicular joint dislocation in football, 1: 268
AMA Committee on the Medical Aspects of Sports, 1: 274, 280
Athlete's Bill of Rights and, 1: 279–281
Athletic Injuries. Prevention, Diagnosis and Treatment, 1: 265, *266*
Boston Children's Hospital and, 1: 264
clinical congress meeting, 3: 118
education and training, 1: 263–264
5th General Hospital and, 4: 484
first aid kit, 1: *270*
Harvard Department of Hygiene and, 2: 253
Harvard football team and, 1: 259, 263
Harvard University Health Service and, 1: 274, 277
legacy of, 1: 274–275
Manual of Bandaging, Strapping and Splinting, A, 1: 268
Massachusetts Regional Fracture Committee, 3: 64

military orthopaedics and, 1: 270–272
New England Regional Committee on Fractures, 4: 341
105th General Hospital and, 4: 489–491
preventative strappings, 1: *269,* 274
publications of, 1: 263–268, 271–274, 280–281
rehabilitation and, 1: 271–274
sports medicine and, 1: 264–269, 274–275
study of fracture treatment, 1: 264
suction socket prosthesis and, 1: 273
34th Infantry Division and, 4: 484
World War II active duty and, 1: 270–272; 2: 232; 4: 17
World War II civilian defense and, 1: 269–270
Thorndike, Charles, 3: 338
Thorndike, George, 4: 297
Thorndike, Olivia Lowell, 1: 263
Thorndike, William, 4: 297
Thornhill, Thomas S.
Brigham and Women's Hospital and, 4: 143, 163, 193–194, 195*b*
as BWH orthopaedics chief, 4: 172, 196*b*
John Ball and Buckminster Brown Professorship, 4: 195*b*
New England Deaconess Hospital and, 4: 280
PFC unicompartmental knee prothesis and, 4: 176–177
publications and research, 4: 180, *180*
Thrasher, Elliott, 2: 277, 290
Three Star Medal of Honour, 3: 451, *451*
thrombocytopenia, 3: 434
tibia
anterolateral bowing of, 2: 173
congenital pseudarthrosis of, 2: 173–176
pseudofracture of, 3: 341, *342*
tibial tubercle
lesions during adolescence, 2: 115, *116,* 117
nonunion of the humerus, 2: 96, *96,* 97, *97*
Osgood-Schlatter disease and, 2: 115, *116,* 117
Sever's study of, 2: 91, 96–97
treatment of, 2: 91, 96
Ticker, Jonathan B., 3: *145*

Tobin, William J., 3: 74
Toby, William, 4: 266*b*
Toldt, C., 2: 170
Tomaselli, Rosario, 4: 41*b*
Tomford, William W. (1945–), 3: *439, 461*
adult reconstruction and, 3: 460*b*
articular cartilage preservation research, 3: 442, *442*
on bone bank procedures, 3: 440–441, *442*
Children's Hospital/MGH combined program and, 3: 439
early life, 3: 439
education and training, 3: 439
HMS appointments, 3: 440, 440*b*
leadership of, 3: 443
MGH Bone Bank and, 3: 396, 439–441, 443
as MGH clinical faculty, 3: 464*b*
as MGH orthopaedics chief, 3: 11*b*, 228, 399, 443
as MGH surgeon, 3: 398*b*, 440, 440*b*
Musculoskeletal Tissue Banking, 3: 443
Naval Medical Research Institute and, 3: 439
orthopaedic oncology and, 3: 440
orthopaedic tumor fellowship program and, 3: 388
publications and research, 3: 440–443
rapid postoperative osteolysis in Paget Disease case, 3: 441
tissue banks and, 3: 386
transmission of disease through allografts research, 3: 442–443, *443*
US Navy and, 3: 439
Toom, Robert E., 2: 408
Toronto General Hospital, 2: 334
torticollis brace, 1: *99,* 100, *124*
Tosteson, Daniel, 4: 119
Total Care of Spinal Cord Injuries, The (Pierce and Nickel), 3: 321
total condylar prosthesis, 4: 130
total hip replacement
bladder fistula after, 4: 162
bone stock deficiency in, 3: 279
cemented/uncemented, 3: 223–224
Charnley and, 3: 218–219
Gibson posterior approach, 4: 170
Harris and hybrid, 3: 220
Hylamer acetabular liner complications, 4: *171,* 172
infections and, 4: 170
introduction to the U.S., 3: 218

osteoarthritis and, 3: 221, *222*
osteolysis after, 3: 220, *220*, 221–222, *222*, 223, 225
patient outcomes, 4: 134–135
pelvic osteolysis with acetabular replacement, 3: 279
radiographs of uncemented, 3: *223*
RBBH and, 4: 129
renal transplant infarction case, 4: 252–253
rheumatoid arthritis complications, 4: 134
sensitivity to heparin and, 3: 362
surgeon preferences in, 4: 170*b*
trochanteric osteotomy in, 4: 133–134
ultraviolet light and, 4: 162
use of bone ingrowth type prostheses, 3: 222–223
use of methylmethacrylate (bone cement), 3: 220, 222; 4: 129, 133, 171
total joint replacement
  BWH registry for, 4: 141, *172*, 173
  continuing medical education and, 3: 225
  implant design, 4: 137–138
  infection rates, 4: 164
  metals for use in, 2: 234
  patellofemoral joint, 4: 137
  patient outcomes and, 3: 277; 4: 134
  proximal femoral grafts and, 3: 435
  research in, 3: 326; 4: 133–134, 136
  tibial component fixation, 4: 137, 148
  ultraviolet light and, 4: 164
Total Knee Arthroplasty (Scott), 4: 176
total knee replacement
  Duocondylar prostheses and, 4: 178
  duopatellar prosthesis, 4: 180*t*
  gait and, 2: 408
  giant cell synovitis case, 4: 148
  inflammatory reactions, 3: 223
  kinematic, 4: 138–139
  Kinematic prosthesis, 4: 138–139, *139*, 147, 149–150
  Maine Medical Assessment Foundation, 2: 372
  McKeever prosthesis, 4: 40, 130
  metal and polyethylene prosthesis, 4: 147–148, *148*
  metallic tibial tray fracture, 4: 177

osteoarthritis and, 4: 177
preservation of PCL, 4: 130, 138–139, 147, 180–181
press-fit condylar knee (PFC), 4: 180, 180*t*
prosthesis development, 4: 137, 179*t*
at RBBH, 1950–1978, 4: 131*t*
research in, 4: 133, 135
roentgenographic arthroplasty-scoring system, 4: 150
soft tissue balancing and, 4: 139
tibial component fixation, 4: 148
tourniquet, 1: 55
Towle, Chris, 3: 386
Townsend, Nadine West, 3: 300
Townsend, Solomon Davis, 1: 59; 3: 14, 18, *31*
Townshend, Charles, 1: 13
Townshend Acts, 1: 13–15
tracheostomy, 2: 49, 51
traction
  Buck's, 1: 80
  continuous, 1: 108; 2: 32
  femoral neck fractures and, 3: 186, 189–190
  flexion injuries and, 3: 348–349
  for fractures and limb deformities, 2: 23, 25
  halo-femoral, 2: 342, 344, 399
  hip disease and, 2: 21–22, 32–33, 52–54; 3: 148
  lumbar fracture-dislocation and, 3: 347
  modification of, 2: 27
  reductions of dislocations and, 1: 10, *43*, 44, 52, 68
  scoliosis and, 2: 35, 296–297
  slipped capital femoral epiphysis (SCFE) and, 2: 176
  Sprengel deformity and, 2: 195–196
  Thomas splint, 3: *168*, 169
Tracy, Edward A., 4: 204
Trahan, Carol, 3: 386, 392
Training Administrators of Graduate Medical Education (TAGME), 1: 238
transmetatarsal amputation, 4: 276
trauma
  acute compartment syndrome of the thigh and, 3: 417
  amputations and, 3: 373
  bone cysts and, 2: 236
  cartilaginous labrum and, 3: 352
  in children, 2: 359, 365, 368, 378, 385
  coxa plana, 2: 104
  to the epiphysis, 2: 176, 193

fracture treatment and, 4: 339*b*–340*b*
fractures of the radial head and, 2: 396–397
hip dislocations, 2: 352–353
ischemia-edema cycle and, 2: 200
laparotomy and, 3: 55
lesions of the atlas and axis, 2: 117
military orthopaedics and, 3: 274, 301; 4: 393
olecranon fractures and, 3: 309
orthopaedic surgery and, 3: 220, 275, 376, 416; 4: 393
paralysis and, 2: 71
Sever's disease and, 2: 88–89
sports injuries and, 2: 279, 385
thoracic spine and, 4: 259
tibial tubercle and, 2: 115
treatment deficiencies, 4: 349
Trauma Management (Cave, et al.), 3: 62, 253, 273
Travis, Dorothy F., 2: 324
Travis Air Force Base, 3: 337
Treadwell, Ben, 3: 386
Treatise on Dislocations and Fractures of Joints, A (Cooper), 1: 35, 36, *42*, *43*
Treatise on Orthopaedic Surgery, A (Bradford and Lovett), 1: 108; 2: 29–30, *30*, 43, 50, *50*, 51
Treatise on the Disease of Infancy and Childhood (Smith), 2: 7
Treatment of Fractures, The (Scudder), 1: 147; 3: 55–56, *57*, *58*, 64, 99; 4: 312, 350
"Treatment of Infantile Paralysis, The" (Lovett), 2: 71
Tremont Street Medical School, 3: 26, 42
Trendelenburg limp, 2: 33, 108, *108*, 151
triceps
  brachioradialis transfer for weakness, 2: 148, 153–154, *154*
  tendon repair, 3: 309
  transfers for deltoid muscle paralysis, 2: 230
triflanged nail, 3: 62, 185–186, *186*, 187, 189, 189*b*, 190; 4: 237
triple arthrodesis
  foot deformities and, 2: 197, 228–229
  heel-cord lengthening and, 2: 172
  modification of, 2: 180–181
  Ober and, 2: 149
  stabilization of polio patients by, 2: 265

tendon transplantations and, 3: 333
weakness/paralysis of the foot and ankle, 2: 150–151
Trippel, Stephen B. (1948–), 3: *444*
    adult reconstruction and, 3: 460*b*
    articular cartilage research, 3: 445
    Cave Traveling Fellowship and, 1: 217*b*
    education and training, 3: 444
    Gordon Research Conference and, 3: 445
    growth-plate chondrocytes research, 3: *444*, 445
    HCORP and, 3: 444
    HMS appointment, 3: 444–445
    as MGH clinical faculty, 3: 464*b*
    as MGH surgeon, 3: 444–445
    professional memberships and, 3: 445
    publications and research, 3: 444–445
    University of Indiana School of Medicine and, 3: 445
trochanteric osteotomy, 4: 133, 145
Trott, Arthur W. (1920–2002), 2: *179*, 313–314
    AAOS and, 2: 314
    Boston Children's Hospital and, 2: 233, 301, 313–316
    Boston polio epidemic and, 2: 314–315
    Brigham and Women's Hospital and, 4: 163, 193
    on circulatory changes in poliomyelitis, 2: 264
    Crippled Children's Clinic and, 2: 314
    death of, 2: 318
    education and training, 2: 313
    Foot and Ankle, The, 2: 317
    foot and ankle treatment, 2: 316–317
    Green and, 2: 177, 286, 317–318
    on Grice, 2: 214
    Korean War and, 2: 313
    March of Dimes and, 2: 315
    marriage and family, 2: 313
    military service, 2: 313
    as naval hospital surgical consultant, 2: 313–314
    PBBH and, 2: 313; 4: 19–20, 22, 116, 128, 163
    poliomyelitis research and treatment, 2: 190, 314, *314*, 315–316
    private medical practice and, 2: 313

publications and research, 4: 243
    publications of, 2: 316–317
Trott, Dorothy Crawford, 2: 313, 318
Trout, S., 2: 417
Trowbridge, William, 2: 114
Truax, R., 1: 15
Trumble, Hugh C., 3: 367
Trumble, Thomas E., 3: 431
Trumbull, John, 1: *19*
Trumbull Hospital, 4: 225
Truslow, Walter, 2: 84; 3: 229
Tseng, Victor, 1: 217*b*
tuberculosis. *See also* spinal tuberculosis
    amputations and, 3: 374
    bone and joint, 2: 11, 16, 25, 308–309; 3: 148, 166
    decline due to milk pasteurization, 2: 16
    hip disease and, 2: 21–22
    of hips, 2: 52–53, *54*
    infected joints and, 1: 61, 73, 75, 81; 4: 225
    of the knee, 1: 73; 4: 225
    mortality due to, 2: 4
    open-air treatment of, 4: 363, 367
    pulmonary, 1: 56; 2: 16
    sacroiliac joint fusion for, 3: 185
    spinal, 1: 100, 106, 108–109, *109*; 2: 11; 3: 289; 4: 225
    synovial joints and, 4: 226
    treatment advances in, 2: 32
Tubiana, Raoul, 4: 182
Tucker, Sarah, 1: 4
Tufts Medical Center Hospital, 2: 306; 4: *311*
Tufts University School of Medicine
    affiliation with Beth Israel Hospital, 4: 213–214, 214*b*, 228
    affiliation with Boston City Hospital, 4: 228, 296–297
    Aufranc and, 3: 247
    Boston Pathology Course at, 1: 230
    Fitchet and, 2: 252
    hand fellowships and, 2: 250
    Karlin and, 2: 369–370
    Legg and, 2: 102
    Lovett and, 2: 64
    MacAusland and, 3: 308
    Ober and, 2: 165
    orthopaedics residencies, 4: 377–379
    Painter and, 3: 266
    Radin and, 3: 328
    Smith-Petersen and, 3: 362
    Webber and, 2: 9
Tukey, Marshall, 1: 304, 309

tumors
    Barr and Mixter on, 3: 204
    bone irradiation and, 2: 237
    Codman on, 3: 110
    femoral allograft transplantation, 3: 389–390
    giant-cell, 3: 390
    intraspinal in children, 2: 301–302
    knee fusion with allografts, 3: 435
    musculoskeletal, 3: 433, 435
    research in, 2: 236–237
    sacrococcygeal chordoma, 3: 390
Tumors of the Jaws (Scudder), 3: 64
turnbuckle jacket, 2: 80, 223–224, *224*, 225, *225*, 226, 226*b*, 227, 227*b*, 316, *336*; 3: 209
Turner, Henry G., 4: 434
Turner, Roderick H., 2: 397; 3: 246; 4: 187
Tyler, Charles H., 4: 303
typhoid fever, 2: 4

U

Ulin, Dorothy Lewenberg, 4: 244
Ulin, Kenneth, 4: 244
Ulin, Robert (1903–1978), 4: *242*
    BCH surgeon-in-chief, 4: 333
    as Beth Israel chief of orthopaedics, 4: 243–244, 289*b*
    Beth Israel Hospital and, 4: 242, 247
    Boston City Hospital and, 4: 242
    Boston VA Hospital and, 4: 242
    death of, 4: 244
    education and training, 4: 242
    Faulkner Hospital and, 4: 242
    fender fracture case, 4: 242
    HMS appointment, 4: 244
    Lowell General Hospital and, 4: 243
    marriage and family, 4: 244
    private medical practice, 4: 242–243
    professional memberships, 4: 244
    publications and research, 4: 229, 242–243
    silverwork by, 4: *242*, *243*, 244, *244*
    slipped capital femoral epiphysis research, 4: 243
    subdeltoid bursitis research, 4: 243
    Tufts Medical School appointment, 4: 242, 244
    US Army and, 4: 242–243
ultraviolet light, 4: 162–164, 164*t*
unicompartmental prosthesis, 4: 176, 178

Unit for Epidemic Aid in Infantile Paralysis (NFP), 2: 188–189
United Cerebral Palsy Association, 2: 401
United States General Hospital (Readville, Mass.), 2: 5
University of Arkansas College of Medicine, 3: 337
University of California Hospital, 3: 336–337
University of California in San Diego (UCSD), 3: 402
University of Chicago, 3: 382
University of Edinburgh, 1: 7
University of Florida, 3: 432
University of Indiana School of Medicine, 3: 445
University of Iowa, 3: 303
University of Maryland Health Center, 4: 263–264
University of Maryland Medical Center, 4: 157
University of Massachusetts, 2: 286–288, 364
University of Massachusetts Medical School, 2: 293, 371
University of Miami Tissue Bank, 3: 442
University of Michigan Medical Center, 4: 254–255
University of Missouri, 4: 372
University of Pennsylvania Medical School, 1: 7; 2: 424
University of Pittsburgh School of Medicine, 3: 382–383, 385; 4: 111
University of Southern California, 2: 266
Upper Extremity Injuries in the Athlete (Pappas and Walzer), 2: 288
Upton, Joseph, III, 3: 431
Urist, Marshall R., 3: 433
US Air Force Hospital, 3: 323
US Army
 Boston-derived base hospitals, 4: 420t
 curative workshops and, 4: 403
 Division of Orthopedic Surgery, 2: 65; 4: 411–412
 Harvard Unit and, 1: 270
 hospital reconditioning program, 1: 271–272
 Hospital Train, 4: *414*
 levels of medical care by distance, 4: 475t
 Medical Officer instructions for, 4: 410b
 recruiting poster, 4: *397*
 staffing of ambulances with medics, 4: 387

US Army 3rd General Hospital (Mt. Sinai), 4: 88
US Army 3rd Southern General Hospital (Oxford), 3: 365
US Army 7th General Hospital (St. Alban's, England), 4: 90
US Army 11th General Hospital, 4: 420, 422b, *424–425*
US Army 13th General Hospital (Boulogne, France), 4: 422b
US Army 22nd General Hospital, 4: 415
US Army 42nd General Hospital, 4: 488, 490
US Army 105th General Hospital, 4: *490*
 Biak Island deployment, 4: 491, 491b, 492, *492*
 camaraderie at, 4: 492
 Cave and, 3: 271; 4: 489
 closing of, 4: 493
 construction of, 4: 489
 in Gatton, Australia, 1: 270; 4: 488–489, *489*
 Harvard Unit and, 1: 270–271; 2: 231–232; 4: 484, 487–489
 hospital beds at, 4: 490
 malaria treatment and, 4: 491
 MGH and, 4: 493
 orthopaedic staff at, 4: 489–490
 patient rehabilitation and, 1: 271; 4: 490–491
 plaque commemorating, 4: *492*
 Rowe and, 3: 351; 4: 489, 490b–491b
 Sheldon Hall Surgical Building, 4: *490*
 tent ward, 4: *491*
 Thorndike and, 4: 489–491
US Army 118th General Hospital, 4: 488
US Army 153rd Station Hospital (Queensland), 4: 488
US Army Base Hospital No. 5 (Boulogne, France), 4: *424, 426*
 commemoration of Harvard Unit, 4: *428*
 Cushing and, 4: 420, 420t, 422–423
 demobilization of, 4: 426
 first two years at, 4: 422b
 Harvard Unit and, 1: 270; 4: 420, 423–424, *428*
 hazards and mortality rate at, 4: 424–425
 map of, 4: *427*
 Ober and, 2: 145
 officers of, 4: *422*
 operating room at, 4: *427*

 Osgood and, 2: 125; 4: 405, 421b, 422
 patient ward in, 4: *428*
 PBBH and, 4: 420t
 training in, 4: 420–421
 US and British medical staff in, 4: 422–423, 425
US Army Base Hospital No. 6 (Talence, France)
 Adams and, 3: 232; 4: 433–434
 buildings at, 4: *432*
 demobilization of, 4: 437
 expansion of, 4: 433–434
 map of, 4: *429*
 MGH orthopaedists and, 3: 313; 4: 420t, 429–432
 operating room at, 4: *431*
 patient census at, 4: 436, 436t, 437
 patient flow process at, 4: 435–436
 patients treated at, 4: *434*
 reconstruction and occupational aides, 4: 436b
 release of equipment to Base Hospital No. 208, 4: 437
 surgical & orthopaedic wards, 4: *431*
 surgical ward at, 4: *433*
 use of the Petit Lycée de Talence, 4: *429*, 432
 Ward in Lycée building, 4: *430*
 WWII reactivation of, 4: 474
US Army Base Hospital No. 7 (Tours, France), 4: *438*
 Boston City Hospital and, 1: 256; 4: 420t, 438–439
 Harvard Unit and, 4: 437–439
 Nichols and, 4: 438–439
 Ward 6, 4: *437*
US Army Base Hospital No. 8 (Savenay, France), 3: 365
US Army Base Hospital No. 9 (Chateauroux, France), 4: 409
US Army Base Hospital No. 10 (Roxbury, Mass.), 2: 258
US Army Base Hospital No. 18 (Bazoilles-sur-Meuse, France), 2: 221–222
US Army Base Hospital No. 114 (Beau-Desert, France), 3: 232
US Army Base Hospital No. 208, 4: 437
US Army Evacuation Hospital No. 110 (Argonne), 4: 439
US Army Hospital (Landstuhl, Germany), 3: 418
US Army 34th Infantry Division, 4: 484

US Army Medical Board, 2: 124; 3: 168
US Army Medical Corps, 2: 124, 130, 220, 222; 3: 282, 288, 291, 313, 351, 365, 370; 4: 387, 420
US Army Medical Reserve Corps, 2: 66, 268; 3: 61, 89, 232
US Army Mobile Unit No. 6 (Argonne), 4: 426
US Army Nurse Corps, 4: 492
US Army ROTC, 3: 300
US Food and Drug Administration (FDA), 3: 249
US General Hospital No. 2 (Fort McHenry, Maryland), 4: 452
US General Hospital No. 3 (Camp Shanks, Orangeburg, New York), 4: 88
US General Hospital No. 3 (Colonia, N.J.), 4: 452
US General Hospital No. 5, 4: *487*
   in Belfast, Ireland, 4: 484–485
   closing of, 4: 487
   construction of, 4: *486*
   facilities at, 4: 485–486
   Fort Bragg and, 4: 484
   Harvard Unit and, 1: 270, 277; 3: 271; 4: 484
   in Normandy, France, 4: 486, *486*, 487
   nursing at, 4: *487*
   in Odstock, England, 4: 486
   operating room at, 4: *487*
   personnel and training, 4: 484
   ward tent, 4: *486*
US General Hospital No. 6
   Aufranc and, 3: 239, 240*b*
   bivouac and staging area in Maddaloni, Italy, 4: *479*
   in Bologna, Italy, 4: *481*, 482
   Camp Blanding and, 4: 474–475
   Camp Kilmer and, 4: 475
   in Casablanca, 4: 476–477, *477*, 480*b*
   closing of, 4: 482, 484
   commendation for, 4: 485*b*
   experiences at, 4: 483*b*
   hospital ward in Naples, 4: *479*
   Instituto Buon Pastore and, 4: *480*, 481
   leadership of, 4: 482*b*
   main entrance, 4: *481*
   medical staff, 4: *476*
   MGH and, 3: 239, 362; 4: 474, 485*b*
   mobilization of, 4: 475–476
   operating room at, 4: *481*
   organization of, 4: 477
   orthopaedics section of, 4: 482, 483*b*
   Peninsular Base Station and, 4: 481–482
   personnel and training, 4: 474–475
   prisoners of war and, 4: 484
   relocation of, 4: 479, 481
   in Rome, Italy, 4: 481–482
   surgical services at, 4: 478, *478*
   temporary camp in Italy, 4: *480*
   wards at, 4: *478*
US General Hospital No. 10, 4: *328*, *445*, 446
   Cotton and, 4: 452
   Elks' Reconstruction Hospital and, 4: 447–448
   Massachusetts Women's Hospital and, 4: 447–448
   as a model for civilian hospitals, 4: 450–451
   RBBH and, 4: 447–448
   West Roxbury plant (Boston City Hospital), 4: 447–448
US Medical Department, 4: 439
US Naval Hospital, 3: 201, 207
US Naval Medical Corps, 3: 248
US Navy Tissue Bank, 3: 439–440, 442
US Public Health Service, 4: 165
US War Department, 4: 474
USS *Arizona*, 4: *465*
USS *Okinawa*, 3: 446, *447*
USS *West Point*, 4: 488

V

Vail Valley Medical Center, 3: 446
Vainio, Kauko, 4: 96
Valley Forge Army Hospital, 2: 279
Van Dessel, Arthur, 1: 193
Van Gorder, George W. (1888–1969), 3: *364*
   arthrodesis procedures, 3: 368, *368*
   Brackett and, 3: 365
   Cave on, 3: 368
   chronic posterior elbow dislocation case, 3: 366
   Clinics for Crippled Children and, 2: 230; 3: 365
   death of, 3: 368
   early life, 3: 364
   education and training, 3: 364–365
   femoral neck fracture research and treatment, 3: 185–186, *186*, 367, *367*
   fracture research and, 3: 334, 366–367
   hip nailing and, 3: 237
   HMS appointment, 3: 365
   hospital appointments, 3: 365
   marriage and family, 3: 365
   MGH Fracture Clinic and, 3: 60*b*, 314, 366
   as MGH house officer, 1: 189
   as MGH orthopaedics chief, 1: 199; 3: 11*b*
   as MGH surgeon, 3: 187, 192, 365, 367–368
   Peking Union Medical College and, 3: 365
   private medical practice, 3: 365
   professional memberships and, 3: 368
   publications and research, 3: 365–368
   Trumble technique for hip fusion and, 3: 367, *367*
   US Army Medical Corps and, 3: 365
   World War I volunteer orthopaedics, 4: 407
Van Gorder, Helen R. Gorforth, 3: 365
Vanguard, The, 4: *421*
Vanishing Bone (Harris), 3: 225, *225*
vascular anastomosis, 4: 216
vastus slide, 3: 278
Vauzelle, C., 2: 340
Venel, Jean-Andrew, 1: xxii
VEPTR (Vertical Expandable Prosthetic Titanium Rib), 2: 360, *362*
Verdan, Claude, 4: 96
Vermont Department of Health, 2: 221
Vermont Medical Association, 2: 221
Vermont State Medical Society, 2: 147
vertebral column resections (VCRs), 2: 362–363
Veterans Administration Hospital (La Jolla, Calif.), 3: 402
Veterans Administration Medical Center (Richmond, Virginia), 4: 153
Veterans Administration Prosthetic and Sensory Aids Service, 1: 273
Veterans Administration Rehabilitation Research and Development Programs, 4: 152
Vincent, Beth, 2: 119; 4: 389*b*
Virchow, Rudolf, 1: 82
visceroptosis, 3: 83–84, 84*b*, 86–88
Vogt, E. C., 3: 341, *342*
Vogt, Paul, 2: 115
volar plate arthroplasty, 2: 248
Volkmann ischemic contracture, 2: 200–201, *201*, 249–250

Volunteer Aid Association,
    3: 152–153
Von Kessler, Kirby, 2: 325
Vose, Robert H., 4: 389*b*
Vrahas, Mark, 1: 167, 235; 3: 462,
    464*b*; 4: 194
Vresilovic, Edward J., Jr., 4: 288

W

Wacker, Warren E .C., 4: 132
Wagner, Katiri, 3: 410
Wagner spherical osteotomy,
    2: 390–392
Waite, Frederick C., 4: 50
Waldenström, Johann H., 2: 104
Waldo County General Hospital,
    2: 371
Walford, Edward, 1: *34*
Walker, C. B., 4: 10
Walker, Irving, 4: 305
Walker, Peter, 4: 130, 137–138,
    147, 152, 176, 178
Walker, Thomas, 3: 132–133
Wallis, Oscar, 3: 25
Walsh, Francis Norma, 2: 333
Walter, Alice, 4: 109
Walter, Carl, 4: 109
Walter, Carl Frederick, 4: 104
Walter, Carl W. (1905–1992),
    4: *104, 106, 108*
  aseptic technique interest,
      4: 105–106
  Aseptic Treatment of Wounds,
      4: 106, *106*, 107*b*
  blood storage bag, 4: 107, *107*,
      108
  canine surgical scenarios and,
      4: 105
  death of, 4: 109
  education and training, 4: 104
  fracture treatment and, 1: 204;
      4: 16, 18
  HMS appointment, 4: 105, 107*b*
  HMS Surgical Research Laboratory, 4: 105, *106*, 107–108
  marriage and family, 4: 109
  medical device development,
      4: 107–108
  PBBH and, 4: 16, 18–20, 79,
      104–105
  PBBH blood bank and,
      4: 107–108
  PBBH fracture service,
      4: 108–109
  professional memberships, 4: 109
  publications and research, 4: 106
  renal dialysis machine modification, 4: 108
  on ultraviolet light use, 4: 164

Walter, David, 4: 109
Walter, Leda Agatha, 4: 104
Walter, Linda, 4: 109
Walter, Margaret, 4: 109
Walter, Margaret Davis, 4: 109
Walter, Martha, 4: 109
Walter Reed General Hospital,
    3: 168; 4: 327, *450*, 451, 488, *488*
Walzer, Janet, 2: 288
War of 1812, 1: 40–41
Ware, John, 1: 296, 299, 302
Warman, Matthew, 2: 439, 439*b*
Warner, Jon J. P., 3: *145*, 462, 464*b*;
    4: 194, 195*b*
Warren, Abigail Collins, 1: 24, 28,
    31
Warren, Amy Shaw, 1: 85, 87
Warren, Anne Winthrop, 1: 55
Warren, Annie Crowninshield,
    1: 76–78
Warren, Edward (author), 1: 46, 68
Warren, Edward (son of Jack), 1: 24,
    28, 31
Warren, Elizabeth, 1: 4
Warren, Elizabeth Hooton, 1: 9, 15,
    21
Warren, Gideon, 1: 4
Warren, Howland (1910–2003),
    1: 90–91
Warren, Howland Shaw, Jr. (1951–),
    1: 71, 91
Warren, John (1874–1928), 1: *88*
  anatomical atlas and, 1: 88–89
  anatomy instruction at Harvard
      Medical School, 1: 71, 88;
      2: 296; 4: 82
  enlistment in WWI, 1: 88
  injury and death of, 1: 89
  medical education, 1: 87–88
  *Outline of Practical Anatomy,
      An*, 1: 88
Warren, John (ca. 1630), 1: 4
Warren, John Collins (1778–1856),
    1: 31, 33, *67, 68*
  American mastodon skeleton and,
      1: 51, *51*, 52
  amputations and, 1: 52–53, 61
  apprenticeship with father, 1: 33
  birth of, 1: 24, 31
  on chloroform, 3: 31
  community organizations and,
      1: 69
  daily routine of, 1: 39
  death of, 1: 66–67, 77
  diagnostic skills, 1: 52–53
  dislocated hip treatment, 3: 13,
      13*b*
  donation of anatomical museum,
      1: 66
  early life, 1: 31

  educational organizations and,
      1: 38–39
  Etherization, 1: 62, *62*; 3: 33
  European medical studies,
      1: 33–37, 54
  on father's death, 1: 29–30
  first use of ether at MGH,
      1: 56–59, *59*, 60–62, *63*,
      64–65, 77; 3: 27–28, 28*b*, 29,
      29*b*, 30, 32–34
  founding of Boston Medical
      Association, 1: 38
  founding of MGH, 1: 31, 41–42,
      71; 3: 5, *5*, 6*b*–7*b*, 12–13
  fundraising for hospital in Boston,
      1: 41
  Genealogy of Warren, 1: 4
  at Harvard College, 1: 31–32
  Harvard Medical School and,
      1: 38–40, 66, 68–69, 299;
      3: 30, 94
  as Hersey Professor of Anatomy
      and Surgery, 1: 29, 66, 68
  hip dislocation case, 1: 42,
      44–46, *46*, 47–50, 68; 3: 36
  home of, 1: *38, 51*
  influence of Astley Cooper on,
      1: 36–37
  influence on Mason, 1: 72, 75
  interest in exercise, 1: 54
  John Ball Brown and, 1: 97–99
  legacy of, 1: 68–69
  "Letter to the Honorable Isaac
      Parker," 1: 45, *45*
  marriage to Anne Winthrop, 1: 55
  marriage to Susan Powell Mason,
      1: 37–38
  medical and surgical practice,
      1: 37–39, 51–55, 66
  medical studies at Harvard,
      1: 32–33
  orthopaedics curriculum and,
      1: 136–137
  orthopaedics specialty and,
      1: 99–100, 119
  Parkman on, 1: 296
  postsurgical treatment and,
      1: 52–53
  publications of, 1: 46, 52, *52*,
      53, 62, *62*, 69*b*
  reputation of, 1: 51–53
  retirement and, 1: 65–66
  Spunkers and bodysnatching,
      1: 32–33
  surgical apprenticeship, 1: 33–37
  surgical practice at MGH,
      1: 52–55, 57–58, 65
  Temperance Society and, 1: 40
  thumping skills, 1: 37

Index

Warren, John Collins "Coll" (1842–1927), 1: *79*, *80*, *82*; 3: *19*
  antisepsis principles and, 1: 85–86; 3: 45
  Charles L. Scudder and, 3: 54–55
  as Civil War hospital surgeon, 1: 79–80
  death of, 1: 87
  European medical studies, 1: 81–84
  fundraising for cancer research, 1: 87
  fundraising for Harvard Medical School, 1: 85, 87; 4: 3
  Harvard Medical School campus and, 1: 87
  Henry Bowditch and, 1: 82
  honorary degrees, 1: 87
  as house pupil at MGH, 1: 80–81
  influence of father on, 1: 80
  influence of Lister on, 1: 84
  Lowell hip dislocation and, 1: 49
  medical and surgical practice, 1: 84–85, *85*, 86; 2: 3
  medical education, 1: 79–81
  professorship at Harvard Medical School, 1: 87; 2: 32
  publications of, 1: 87
  Remembrances, 1: 83
  research laboratory at MGH, 1: 71
  study of tumors, 1: 85
  as supervisor at MGH, 2: 20
  surgical training, 1: 81–84
  treatment of tumors and, 1: 82
Warren, John "Jack" (1753–1815), 1: *23*
  admission tickets to lectures, 1: *27*
  anatomical studies, 1: 22–25
  anatomy lectures, 1: 24, 26–29
  anti-slavery sentiment, 1: 24
  apprenticeships by, 1: 15, 21, 25, 33
  attendance certificates, 1: *28*
  community affairs and, 1: 29
  death of, 1: 29–30, 41
  early life, 1: 21
  establishment of medical board, 1: 29
  father's death and, 1: 3–4
  founding of Boston Medical Association, 1: 25
  founding of Harvard Medical School, 1: 21, 25–29, 40, 71
  at Harvard College, 1: 21
  institutionalization of Boston medicine and, 1: 30
  marriage and family, 1: 24, 28, 31
  Masons and, 1: 29
  medical studies at Harvard, 1: 6
  military service, 1: 22
  orthopaedics curriculum and, 1: 134
  as pioneer of shoulder surgery, 1: 29
  private medical practice, 1: 22, 24, 28
  publications of, 1: 29
  as senior surgeon for Continental Army, 1: 22–24
  smallpox inoculations and, 1: 9, 29
  Spunkers and bodysnatching, 1: 21
Warren, Jonathan Mason (1811–1867), 1: *71*, *76*
  birth of, 1: 38
  chronic illness, 1: 72, 76–78
  European medical studies, 1: 53, 73–76
  fracture care and, 1: 76
  influence of father on, 1: 72, 75
  influence on Coll, 1: 80
  instrument case, 1: *77*
  introduction of plastic surgery to the U.S., 1: 71–72, 77
  legacy of, 1: 78–79
  on Lowell's autopsy, 1: 47–50
  medical practice with father, 1: 76–77
  medical studies at Harvard, 1: 72
  MGH and, 1: 53; 3: 15, *31*
  Norwalk train accident and, 1: 77
  orthopaedic surgery and, 1: 81
  plastic surgery techniques, 1: 76–77
  publications of, 1: 78
  scientific method and, 1: 71, 74
  support for House of the Good Samaritan, 1: 124
  Surgical Observations with Cases and Operations, 1: 47, 75, 78
  use of ether, 1: 57, 63
  as visiting surgeon at MGH, 1: 77
  Warren Triennial Prize and, 1: 78
Warren, Joseph (1663–1729), 1: 4
Warren, Joseph (1696–1755), 1: 3–4
Warren, Joseph (1741–1775), 1: *3*, *11*, 18
  apprenticeships by, 1: 15
  Boston Massacre oration, 1: 15–16
  Boston Massacre report, 1: 14
  Bunker Hill battle, 1: 18–19
  command of militia, 1: 18
  death at Bunker Hill, 1: 3, 19, *19*, 20, 22
  early career, 1: 6
  father's death and, 1: 3–4
  as founder of medical education in Boston, 1: 15
  marriage to Elizabeth Hooten, 1: 9
  Masons and, 1: 10–12
  medical studies at Harvard, 1: 6
  Mercy Scollay and, 1: 19
  obstetrics and, 1: 9
  orthopaedic practice and, 1: 10
  physician apprenticeship, 1: 6, 8
  as physician to the Almshouse, 1: 15
  as president of the Third Provincial Congress, 1: 18
  private medical practice, 1: 8–10, 15
  publications and, 1: 12
  as Revolutionary War leader, 1: 10–20
  smallpox inoculations and, 1: 8–9
  Suffolk Resolves and, 1: 16
  tea party protest and, 1: 16
Warren, Joseph (1876–1942), 1: 87, 90
Warren, Margaret, 1: 4
Warren, Martha Constance Williams, 1: 90
Warren, Mary, 1: 19
Warren, Mary Stevens (1713–1803), 1: 3–4, 10
Warren, Peter, 1: 4
Warren, Rebecca, 1: 96
Warren, Richard (1907–1999), 1: 71, 90–91, 270; 3: 330; 4: 20
Warren, Richard (d. 1628), 1: 4
Warren, Shields, 4: *277b*
Warren, Susan Powell Mason, 1: 37–38, 72
Warren Anatomical Museum, 1: 28, 49–50, 52, 66; 3: 38
Warren family
  early years in Boston, 1: 4
  Harvard Medical School (HMS) and, 1: 71
  history of, 1: 4*b*
  lineage of physicians in, 1: 3, 5, 6, 71
  Massachusetts General Hospital (MGH) and, 1: 71
Warren Russet (Roxbury) apples, 1: 3, *4*
Warren Triennial Prize, 1: 78
Warren's Atlas, 1: 89
Warshaw, Andrew, 3: 146

Washburn, Frederick A., 1: 188;
3: 1, 70b, 174; 4: 420t, 429–430,
432, 433
Washington, George, 1: 19, 22–23
Washington University, 3: 163–165
Washington University Base Hospital
No. 21, 3: 166
Washington University School of
Medicine, 3: 165, 170, 404–405
Watanabi, Masaki, 2: 279
Waterhouse, Benjamin, 1: 25, 40
Waters, Peter (1955–), 2: 414
 birth palsies research, 2: 415,
 417, 417, 418–419, 419, 420
 Boston Children's Hospital and,
 2: 415, 415b, 420, 439b
 education and training, 2: 414
 hand surgery and, 2: 414–415
 hand trauma research, 2: 415
 HMS appointment, 2: 415, 415b
 honors and awards, 2: 415
 John E. Hall Professorship in
 Orthopaedic Surgery, 2: 439b
 as orthopaedic chair, 2: 15b
 orthopaedics curriculum and,
 1: 216, 225
 orthopaedics education and,
 2: 416b
 posterior shoulder dislocation
 case, 2: 417–418
 professional memberships,
 2: 416b
 publications and research,
 2: 415, 417, 417, 418–420
 radiographic classification of glenohumeral deformity, 2: 419t
 on Simmons, 4: 186
 visiting professorships and lectures, 2: 415, 416b
Watkins, Arthur L., 1: 273; 3: 269,
285–286, 286, 454b
Watts, Hugh G. (1934–), 2: 420
 Boston brace and, 2: 423–424,
 424
 Boston Children's Hospital and,
 2: 422–423
 Brigham and Women's Hospital
 and, 4: 193
 Children's Hospital of Philadelphia and, 2: 424
 education and training, 2: 420
 on gait laboratories, 2: 424
 global public health and, 2: 421,
 424–425
 HMS appointment, 2: 422
 humanitarianism and, 2: 421
 on the Krukenberg procedure,
 2: 425
 limb-salvage procedure by,
 2: 422, 423b

McIndoe Memorial Research
 Unit and, 2: 422
 PBBH and, 4: 163
 on pediatric orthopaedics,
 2: 303–304
 professional memberships, 2: 425
 publications and research,
 2: 421–422, 422, 423–424,
 424, 425
 scoliosis research, 2: 423
 University of California and,
 2: 425
 University of Pennsylvania and,
 2: 424
Wayne County Medical Society,
 2: 135
Weaver, Michael J., 3: 463b
Webber, S. G., 2: 5, 9
Webster, Daniel, 1: 54, 307
Webster, Hannah White, 1: 298
Webster, Harriet Fredrica Hickling,
 1: 299
Webster, John W., 1: 299
 confession of, 1: 312–313
 debt and, 1: 302–303
 detection of arsenic poisoning,
 1: 301–302
 education and training, 1: 299
 Ephraim Littlefield and,
 1: 303–304
 execution of, 1: 313, 314
 on guilt of, 1: 314–318
 HMS chemistry professorship,
 1: 296, 298–301
 home of, 1: 302
 letters on behalf of, 1: 309, 309,
 310–311
 Manual of Chemistry, 1: 299,
 301
 murder of George Parkman,
 1: 305–312, 315, 315, 318
 publications of, 1: 299–301
 trial of, 1: 307, 307, 308–311,
 314–316; 3: 40
Webster, Redford, 1: 298
Weed, Frank E., 4: 409
Weigel, Louis A., 2: 56
weight training, 3: 281–282
Weiland, Andrew J., 3: 431
Weiner, David, 2: 436
Weiner, Norbert, 2: 326
Weinfeld, Beverly D. Bunnin,
 4: 101, 103
Weinfeld, Marvin S. (1930–1986),
 4: 101
 Beth Israel Hospital and, 4: 247
 Brigham and Women's Hospital,
 4: 163
 death of, 4: 103
 education and training, 4: 101

HMS appointment, 4: 102–103
 hospital appointments, 4: 102
 knee arthroplasty evaluation,
 4: 103
 marriage and family, 4: 101, 103
 on McKeever and MacIntosh
 prostheses, 4: 189
 MGH and, 4: 101
 osteogenic sarcoma research,
 4: 102
 PBBH and, 4: 163
 private medical practice, 4: 102
 professional memberships, 4: 103
 publications and research,
 4: 102–103
 RBBH and, 4: 41b, 68, 80,
 102–103, 116b, 131
 synovectomy of the knee research,
 4: 40, 102–103
 total elbow replacement and,
 4: 129
 US Army Medical Corps and,
 4: 101
Weinstein, James N., 2: 371;
4: 266b
Weiss, Charles, 3: 385–386, 395,
413, 460b
Weiss, Soma, 3: 350; 4: 79
Weissbach, Lawrence, 3: 460b
Weld, William, 3: 424
Weller, Thomas, 2: 234
Wellesley Convalescent Home, 2: 9,
189, 191
Wellington, William Williamson,
1: 59
Wells, Horace, 1: 56–57, 60
Welsh, William H., 1: 185
Wenger, Dennis, 2: 403
Wennberg, Jack, 2: 372, 374, 374
Wennberg, John, 4: 185
Wesselhoeft, Walter, 3: 120
West Roxbury Veterans Administra-
tion Hospital
 DeLorme and, 3: 285
 Ewald and, 4: 144
 HCORP residencies and,
 1: 199–200, 206–208, 218,
 220, 224–225
 MacAusland and, 3: 312
 McGinty and, 2: 279; 4: 22
 orthopaedic biomechanics labora-
 tory, 4: 137
 orthopaedics residencies, 4: 378
 RBBH and, 4: 36
 Simon and, 2: 406
 spinal cord injury research and
 treatment, 4: 152
 Spinal Cord Injury Service,
 4: 152–153
 training program at, 4: 117

Index

West Virginia University School of Medicine, 3: 328
Weston, Craig, 1: 217*b*
Weston, G. Wilbur, 2: 438
Weston, Nathan, 1: 44–45, 50
Weston Forest and Trail Association, 4: 91, *91*
Whipple, John Adams, 1: *31*
Whipple, Martha Ellen, 2: 113
White, Anita Ottemo, 4: 266
White, Arthur H., 4: 263
White, Augustus A., III (1936–), 4: *257, 263*
    "Analysis of the Mechanics of the Thoracic Spine in Man," 4: 259, *259*
    AOA Alfred R. Shands Jr. lecture, 4: 264
    back pain research and, 4: 258
    as Beth Israel chief of orthopaedics, 4: 262–264, 289*b*
    as Beth Israel chief of surgery, 4: 223, 255
    BIDMC teaching program and, 4: 286
    BIH annual reports, 4: 262–263
    biomechanics research, 4: 260–261
    Brigham and Women's Hospital and, 4: 163, 193
    Cervical Spine Research Society president, 4: 265
    Clinical Biomechanics of the Spine, 4: 262
    clinical research protocols at BIH and, 4: 262
    Delta Upsilon fraternity and, 4: 258
    diversity initiatives in orthopaedics, 4: 264–265
    education and training, 4: 257–258
    Ellen and Melvin Gordon Professor of Medical Education, 4: 264, 266
    Federation of Spine Associations president, 4: 265
    Fort Ord US Army Hospital and, 4: 259
    HMS appointment, 4: 262, 264, 266
    honors and awards, 4: 264–265
    legacy of, 4: 265–266
    marriage and family, 4: 266
    MGH and, 3: 398*b*
    nonunion of a hangman's fracture case, 4: 261
    Oliver Wendell Holmes Society and, 4: 264
    orthopaedic biomechanics doctorate, 4: 259
    professional memberships and activities, 4: 265
    publications and research, 4: 259–262, 264
    Seeing Patients, 4: 265
    spine fellowship program and, 4: 263
    spine research, 4: 259–261, *261*, 262, 264
    University of Maryland Health Center presidency offer, 4: 263–264
    US Army Medical Corps and, 4: 258–259
    Yale University School of Medicine and, 4: 259–260, 262
White, D., 1: 258
White, George Robert, 3: 75
White, Hannah, 1: 298
White, J. Warren, 2: 197
White, John, 3: 191
White, Kevin, 4: 379
White, Paul Dudley, 4: 431
Whitehill, W. M., 2: 11
White's Apothecary Shop, 1: 39–40
Whiteside, Helen E., 2: 292
Whitman, Armitage, 4: 233
Whitman, Royal, 2: 31, 93
Whitman's foot plate, 2: 244–245
Whitman's operation (astragalectomy), 2: 92–94
Whittemore, Wyman, 4: 211, 283*t*
whooping cough, 2: 4
Wickham, Thomas W., 4: 371
Wiggin, Sidney C., 4: 330
Wigglesworth, George, 3: 124
Wigglesworth, Marian Epes, 4: 83
Wilcox, C. A., 3: 34
Wilcox, Oliver D., 3: 34
Wild, Charles, 1: 96
Wilensky, Charles F., 1: 158
Wilkins, Early, 3: 448
Willard, DeForest P., 1: 197; 2: 78, 160
Willard, Joseph, 1: 25
Willard Parker Hospital, 1: 276
Willert, H. G., 3: 220
William H. and Johanna A. Harris Professorship, 3: 464*b*
William H. Thomas Award, 4: 189, 190*b*
William T. Green Fund, 2: 436
William Wood and Company, 2: 50–51
Williams, Harold, 1: 250
Williams, Henry W., 1: 138
Williams, Ted, 1: 258; 4: 342, 345–346
Wilson, Edward, 3: 369
Wilson, George, 1: 56
Wilson, Germaine Parfouru-Porel, 3: 370
Wilson, H. Augustus, 3: 234
Wilson, James L., 2: 78, 191
Wilson, John C., Sr., 1: 189
Wilson, Louis T., 4: 313
Wilson, Marion, 4: 389*b*
Wilson, Michael G., 3: 248; 4: 193–194, 195*b*
Wilson, Philip D., Sr. (1886–1969), 3: *369*, 375
    American Ambulance Hospital and, 4: 389*b*, *390*
    American Appreciation, An, 3: 369
    amputation expertise, 3: 371, 373–374; 4: 472*b*
    arthroplasty of the elbow, 4: 63
    back pain research and, 3: 204
    on Cobb, 2: 225–226
    death of, 3: 376
    displacement of proximal femoral epiphysis case, 3: 372
    early life, 3: 369
    education and training, 3: 369
    Experience in the Management of Fractures and Dislocations, 3: 376
    fracture research and, 3: 371–373
    Fractures, 3: 315
    Fractures and Dislocations, 3: 371, *371*
    Harvard Unit and, 2: 119, 123; 3: *180*, 369
    HMS appointment, 3: 371
    Hospital for the Ruptured and Crippled, 3: 376
    Human Limbs and Their Substitutes, 3: 376
    knee flexion contracture approach, 3: 374–375, *375*
    Management of Fractures and Dislocations, 3: 62, 273
    marriage and family, 3: 370
    MGH Fracture Clinic and, 3: 60*b*, 61, 314, 371, 373, 376
    as MGH house officer, 1: 189
    as MGH surgeon, 3: 187, 269, 370
    military orthopaedics and, 4: 473
    New York Hospital for the Ruptured and Crippled and, 1: 89
    on Osgood, 2: 138
    private medical practice, 3: 338
    professional memberships and, 3: 376

publications and research,
2: 136, 297; 3: 371–373, *373*,
374–376; 4: 60, 363
RBBH and, 4: 28, 31, 55
Robert Breck Brigham Hospital
and, 3: 370
Scudder Oration on Trauma,
3: 63
slipped capital femoral epiphysis
treatment, 4: 237
US Army Medical Corps, 3: 370
World War II volunteers and,
4: 363
Wilson, Philip, Jr., 4: 134
Wiltse, Leon, 3: 249
Wimberly, David, 1: 233
Winchester Hospital, 2: 218–219;
3: 299, 417; 4: 169, 214
Winter, R. B., 2: 343
Winthrop, Anne, 1: 55
Winthrop Group, 2: 317
Wirth, Michael, 2: 288
Wislocki, George B., 1: 179
Wistar, Casper, 1: 39
Wittenborg, Dick, 2: 234
Wojtys, Edward, 1: 286
Wolbach, S. Burt, 2: 234; 4: *6*
Wolcott, J. Huntington, 2: 5
Wolfe, Richard J., 1: 59
Wolff, Julius, 1: xxiii
women
    ACL injuries, 1: 285–286
    admission to HMS, 1: 138,
138*b*, 239
    chronic illness treatment,
1: 123–124, 129
    as MGH house officers, 1: 239
    nursing training, 1: 41; 2: 7–8;
4: 208
    opposition to medical studies by,
3: 44
women orthopaedic surgeons
    first HCORP resident, 1: 239
    limited teaching residencies for,
1: 200
    Ruth Jackson Orthopaedic Society and, 2: 413
Wong, David A., 4: 272*b*
Wood, Bruce T., 4: 117, 129, 163,
193
Wood, Edward Stickney, 3: 94
Wood, G. W., 3: 420
Wood, Leonard, 4: 337
Woodhouse, Charles, 4: 378
Woods, Archie S., 2: 82
Worcester, Alfred, 1: 259, 262–263
workers' compensation
    Aitken and, 4: 353–354
    carpal tunnel syndrome and,
2: 375; 4: 186

Cotton and, 4: 325, 444
major medical problems and,
3: *379*
rehabilitation goals and, 4: 354
surgical interventions and,
2: 373; 4: 352
treatment protocols and,
4: 353–354
Yett and, 4: 253
World Health Organization, 1: 168
World War I. *See also* American Expeditionary Forces (AEF); British
Expeditionary Forces (BEF)
    American Ambulance Hospital
(Neuilly, France), 2: 117–119,
119, 120; 3: 166, 180, *180*;
4: 9, 386, *386*, 387, *387*
    American base hospitals,
4: 419–420
    American Expeditionary Forces,
2: 126, 128, 221
    American experience in, 4: 405*b*
    American Field Service Ambulance, 4: 386, *386*, 387, *387*,
388
    American medical volunteers,
1: 256; 2: 117–119; 4: 387–
396, 398–399, *399*, 402, 404,
406–409, 412*b*–413*b*, 425
    AOA and orthopaedic hospitals,
2: 64
    British Expeditionary Forces,
4: 10
    curative workshops, 4: 399–403,
403
    end of, 4: *453*
    facilities for wounded soldiers,
4: 414–416
    femur fracture treatment, 4: 408
    field ambulances, 4: 414–415,
415
    field hospital equipment, 4: 393*b*
    field hospitals, 4: *414*
    First Goldthwait Unit, 4: *399*
    Harvard Medical School and,
2: 41, 64, 117–120, 125, 145
    hospital trains, 4: *414*, 416
    impact of posture-related conditions, 4: 233
    impact on medical education,
4: 397
    impact on orthopaedics, 4: 453–
454, 463–464
    impact on US economy, 4: 465
    military hospitals and, 1: 270
    military reconstruction hospitals
and, 4: 439–441
    military surgeon training and,
1: 148; 2: 65–69

    New England Dressings Committee (Red Cross Auxiliary), 4: *10*
    orthopaedic contributions before,
2: 50–63
    orthopaedic surgery, 2: 119–126
    postural treatments and, 3: 83
    recruiting poster, 4: *397*
    rehabilitation of soldiers and,
2: 67–68; 4: *396*
    scheme of British hospitals, 4: *414*
    splints and, 3: 167–169, 169*b*;
4: 389, *391*, *408*, 409, 411,
416–417
    standardization of equipment,
2: 124; 3: 167–168
    transport of injured, 3: 169,
169*b*, *170*
    trench warfare in, 4: 385, 389,
390
    US Army Hospital Train, 4: *414*
    US declaration of war on Germany, 4: *396*
    US entry into, 4: 409
    wound treatment during, 4: 385,
389, *390*, 391, 395–396, 407,
471
World War II
    American medical volunteers,
4: 363
    bombing of Pearl Harbor,
4: *465*, 466
    civilian defense and, 1: 269–270
    civilian surgery specialists,
4: 471–472
    field hospitals and, 4: 468
    Fifth Portable Surgical Hospital,
4: 489
    Fourth Portable Surgical Hospital
(4PSH), 2: 232–233; 4: 489
    Harvard Unit (5th General Hospital), 1: 270, 277; 3: 271;
4: 17, 484
    Harvard Unit (105th General Hospital), 1: 270–271;
2: 231–232; 4: 488–489
    HMS surgeons and, 1: 270;
2: 232
    Hospital Trains, 4: *478*
    impact on training programs,
4: 467
    impact on US economy, 4: 465
    impact on US hospitals,
4: 467–468
    military hospitals in Australia,
4: 488–489
    military surgery and, 4: 469–470
    mobile army surgical hospitals
(MASHs), 2: 231–232, *232*,
233; 4: 468–469, *470*
    mobile warfare in, 4: 468–469

orthopaedic surgery and, 4: 463, 473, 493
physician preparation for war injury treatment, 3: 367
US Army 5th General Hospital, 4: 484–487
US Army 6th General Hospital, 4: 474–478, *478*, 479, 480*b*, 481–482, 483*b*, 484, 484*b*
US Army 105th General Hospital, 1: 270; 2: 232; 3: 351; 4: 487–493
US Army levels of medical care, 4: 475*t*
US entry into, 4: *466*, 467
wound management and, 3: 274; 4: 469, 469*b*, 470–473
wound management
amputations, 4: *469*
aseptic treatment of, 4: 107*b*, 469
changes from WWI to WWII, 4: 471, 473
evidence-based practices and, 2: 379
gunshot injuries, 2: 66, 119, 161, 233; 3: 43; 4: 437, 441
impact of World War II on, 3: 274; 4: 469, 469*b*, 470–472
military orthopaedics and, 2: 121, 128, 233; 3: 43
in osteomyelitis, 3: 301
standardization of, 4: 470
wounded soldiers and, 4: 385, 391, 398–399, 432, 434–435, 437, 451
WWI Medical Officer instructions for, 4: 410*b*
Wright, John, 1: 216, 224–225; 2: 378
Wright, R. John, 4: 193, 195*b*
Wright, Wilhelmine, 2: 70
Wrist and Radius Injury Surgical Trial (WRIST), 3: 409–410
wrists. *See also* hands
arthrodesis procedures, 3: 191, 239; 4: 166–167
avascular necrosis case, 3: 403
carpal injuries, 3: 101–102
distal radius fractures, 3: 408–409
flexor carpi ulnaris transfer procedure, 2: 172, 188, 198–199, *199*, 200
fusion and, 2: 198, 200; 4: 167
lunate dislocation, 3: 101–102
reconstruction of, 2: 248
rheumatoid arthritis and, 4: 166–167, *167–168*
scaphoid fracture, 4: 361

tendon transfers and, 2: 172
ulnar nerve compression and, 3: 405–406
vascularity and, 3: 403
Wry neck, 2: 256
Wulfsberg, Karen M., 1: 231
Wyman, Edwin T., Jr. (1930–2005), 3: *377, 378, 380, 461*
Children's Hospital/MGH combined program and, 3: 376
death of, 3: 380
education and training, 3: 376
fracture research and, 3: 376–378
fracture service and, 3: 388*t*
HMS appointment, 3: 380
medical cost research, 3: 379, 379*t*
metastatic pathological fracture case, 3: *376*, 377–378
as MGH clinical faculty, 3: 464*b*
MGH Fracture Clinic and, 3: 378
MGH operations improvement and, 3: 378–379
as MGH surgeon, 3: 376, 398*b*
MGH trauma unit and, 3: 396, 399, 460*b*
Omni Med and, 3: 379
orthopaedics education and, 3: 378
private medical practice, 3: 310
publications and research, 3: *376*, 377–379, *379*
Wyman, James, 1: 308
Wyman, Jeffries, 1: 306, *306*; 3: 25
Wyman, Stanley, 3: 241
Wynne-Davies, Ruth, 2: 399, *400*

X

x-rays. *See also* roentgenograms
accidental burns, 3: 100
American Surgical Association on, 3: 58
bone disease diagnosis and, 3: 101–103
bone lesions and, 4: 110
of bullet fragments, 3: *98*
calcaneal apophysitis (Sever's Disease) and, 2: *88*
clinical use of, 3: 97, 99–100
discovery of, 3: 58
Dodd and, 3: *20*, 20, 21, 96, 99
experiments with, 3: 96
fluoroscope and, 3: 96–97
MGH and, 3: 20
orthopaedic surgeons and, 2: 56
publication of, 3: 97, *97*, 98, *99*
safety of, 3: 99–100
scoliosis and, 2: 79

skin injury and, 3: 97–98

Y

Yale University School of Medicine, 4: 259–260
Yanch, Jacquelyn C., 4: 136
Yee, Lester B. K., 3: 351; 4: 489
Yett, Harris S. (ca. 1934–), 4: *250*
Andre the Giant and, 4: 252–253
as Beth Israel chief of orthopaedics, 4: 251, 289*b*
Beth Israel Hospital and, 4: 248, 251, 253, 262–263
BIDMC and, 4: 253
BIDMC teaching program and, 4: 286–287
Boston Orthopaedic Group, 4: 251
Children's Hospital/MGH combined program and, 4: 250–251
deep vein thrombosis research, 4: 251–252
education and training, 4: 250
HMS appointment, 4: 251
honors and awards, 4: 251
hospital appointments, 4: 251
MGH and, 4: 251
professional memberships, 4: 253
publications and research, 4: 251–253
renal transplant infarction case, 4: 252–253
Y-ligament, 3: 35–36, 38
Yoo, Won Joon, 2: 379
Yorra, Alvin, 3: 258
Yosifon, David, 3: 83
Young, E. B., 2: 115
Young, Thomas, 1: 14
Yount, Carl, 2: 153, 294
youth sports, 2: 384–385, *385*, 386
Yovicsin, John, 1: 275
Yun, Andrew, 1: 217*b*

Z

Zaleske, David J., 3: 401, 460*b*, 464*b*
Zander, Gustav, 3: *69, 71, 152*, 264–265
Zarins, Antra, 3: 383, 386
Zarins, Bertram (1942–), 3: *359*, 388*t*, *446–447, 461*
anterior interosseous nerve palsy case, 3: 449
arthroscopic surgery and, 3: 422, 446, 448
as Augustus Thorndike Professor, 3: 464*b*

Cave Traveling Fellowship and, 1: 217b
Children's Hospital/MGH combined program and, 3: 446
early life, 3: 446
education and training, 3: 446
glenoid labrum composition research, 3: 449
Harvard University Health Services and, 3: 450
HMS appointment, 3: 448, 450
honors and awards, 3: 450–451
Latvian Medical Foundation and, 3: 451
leadership roles, 3: 451b
as MGH clinical faculty, 3: 464b
as MGH surgeon, 3: 398b, 450
posterior cruciate ligament (PCL) research, 3: 450
private medical practice, 3: 448
professional sports teams and, 3: 448, 450
publications and research, 3: 359, 448–450, *450*
shoulder surgery and research, 3: 448–450
sports medicine and, 3: 396, 399, 422, 446, 448, 450, 460b
sports medicine fellowship program director, 3: 448
Three Star Medal of Honour and, 3: 451
US Navy and, 3: 446
Vail Valley Medical Center and, 3: 446
as Winter Olympics head physician, 3: 448

Zausmer, Elizabeth, 2: 260, *260*
Zechino, Vincent, 2: 299
Zeiss, Fred Ralph, 2: 438
Zeleski, David, 1: 225
Zevas, Nicholas T., 3: 420
Zilberfarb, Jeffrey, 4: 286–287
Zimbler, Seymour "Zeke" (ca. 1932–2021), 4: *245, 247*
 as Beth Israel chief of orthopaedics, 4: 247–249, 251, 289b
 Beth Israel Hospital and, 4: 246–247
 Boston Children's Hospital and, 2: 279, 439b; 4: 245–250
 breast carcinoma and chondrosarcoma case, 4: 247–249
 Charleston Naval Hospital and, 4: 246
 Children's Hospital/MGH combined program and, 4: 245
 education and training, 4: 245
 on Green, 2: 182
 HCORP and, 4: 247–248
 HMS appointment, 4: 247
 Legg-Perthes Study Group and, 2: 425; 4: 250
 MGH and, 3: 401; 4: 250
 New England Medical Center and, 4: 249
 pediatric orthopaedics and, 4: 248–250
 private medical practice, 4: 247, 249
 publications and research, 4: 246–247, 250
 on shoes with correctives, 4: 250
 Simmons College physical therapy lectures, 4: 246
 Tufts Medical School appointment, 4: 248–249
 US Navy and, 4: 246
Zimmerman, C., 4: 253
Zurakowski, D., 2: 380

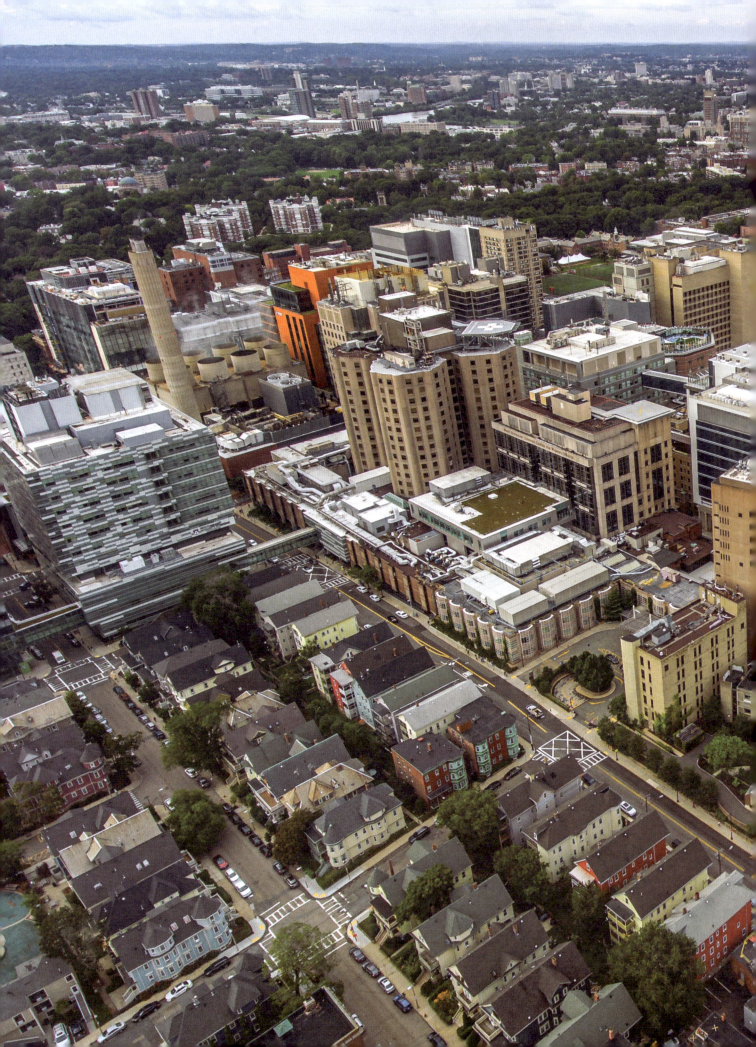